Value in Pediatric Orthopaedics

William L. Hennrikus • Richard M. Schwend
Editors

Value in Pediatric Orthopaedics

A Case-Based Guide

Springer

Editors
William L. Hennrikus
Professor Emeritus and Distinguished Educator
Pennsylvania State College of Medicine
Hershey, PA, USA

Richard M. Schwend
Professor, Children's Mercy Hospital
Kansas City, MO, USA

ISBN 978-3-032-19569-2 ISBN 978-3-032-19570-8 (eBook)
https://doi.org/10.1007/978-3-032-19570-8

This Springer imprint is published by the registered company Springer Nature Switzerland AG
The registered company address is: Gewerbestrasse 11, 6330 Cham, Switzerland

"We dedicate this book to our wives and families, for whose support and love we are forever grateful"

together make decisions that are supported by literature and efficacious. I congratulate Drs. Hennrikus, Schwend, and each of the authors for creating such a valuable must-read resource for all healthcare professionals who care for children including orthopaedic surgeons, primary care physicians, residents, nurse practitioners, and physician assistants.

Vice Dean for Educational Affairs
Penn State College of Medicine
Hershey, PA, USA

Kevin B. Black, MD

Preface

Value in health care is often defined by Michael E Porter's equation: *Value = Outcomes / Costs*. While efforts to improve value appropriately focus on reducing unnecessary tests and procedures, this equation underscores that value can also be enhanced by improving outcomes. Ultimately, a key measure of value lies in the outcomes experienced by patients.

In April 2012, the ABIM Foundation and Consumer Reports launched the *Choosing Wisely* campaign, initially identifying the top five unnecessary tests and treatments from nine specialty societies. Over time, the campaign expanded to include 80 specialty societies. Using a semi-structured Delphi process, the Pediatric Orthopaedic Society of North America (POSNA) and the American Academy of Pediatrics Section on Orthopaedics (AAP SOOr) collaborated to develop a list of 30 unwarranted practices in pediatric orthopaedics. This list was ultimately refined to five key recommendations, published in *CWOrthopaedics.pdf* (aap.org) in 2018. These recommendations include:

1. Not ordering a screening hip ultrasound for newborns with a normal exam and no risk factors
2. Choosing conservative management for young children with in-toeing
3. Avoiding shoe inserts for children with flexible flat feet
4. Not ordering advanced imaging without first obtaining an appropriate history, physical exam, and plain radiographs
5. Not ordering follow-up radiographs for buckle fractures

Although many unnecessary tests and procedures were identified, the *Choosing Wisely* list was ultimately limited to these five items.

A survey conducted by the ABIM revealed that nearly three-quarters of physicians view unnecessary tests and procedures as a significant problem within the healthcare system. The three most frequently cited reasons for ordering these interventions were concerns about malpractice (52%), a desire to practice cautiously (36%), and the need for additional information to reassure patients (30%). These motivations often reflect a shift toward emotional-based decision-making rather than evidence-based medicine. It is our hope that this book offers insights to support a more evidence-driven, value-focused approach to care.

We are deeply grateful to the 38-chapter authors, leading experts on their topic, who generously contributed their knowledge and experience to this book. Through the examination of various conditions, our goal is to advance value within the specialty by highlighting clinical practices that improve outcomes, reduce unnecessary tests and procedures, limit costs, and optimize care. We also extend our sincere thanks to our Content Editor at Springer, Miranda Finch, and our Project Coordinator and Production Editor, Sinchu Mohan, for their guidance and support. Most importantly, we thank our patients, whose experiences continue to teach us lessons and inspire our work.

We hope this book stimulates new perspectives on delivering value in the care of children with musculoskeletal conditions. Your feedback is important to us as we strive to improve future editions. Please share your comments and suggestions by contacting us at Whennrikus@pennstatehealth.psu.edu and rmschwend@cmh.edu.

Hershey, PA, USA William L. Hennrikus
Kansas City, MO, USA Richard M. Schwend

Contents

Part I

Trauma

Buckle Fractures of the Distal Radius: Stability Adds Value

1

Andrew J. M. Gregory

Introduction

Fractures of the forearm are among the most common injuries in children. The distal radius is the most frequent site of forearm fracture occurrence. A buckle fracture typically involves a compression injury to one side of the cortex with an intact cortex on the other side of the bone [1]. Due to the one-sided cortical compression injury, buckle fractures are inherently stable. These injuries are common. About 10–15% of all pediatric fractures are distal radius buckle fractures. The incidence of buckle fractures of the distal radius in the United States is estimated at 17.3 per 100,000 people per year [2]. Distal radius buckle fractures occur in about 1 in 25 children and account for 50% of pediatric wrist fractures [3]. There is considerable variation in the management of distal radius buckle fractures, including the type of immobilization, time off from activities, the need for follow-up visits, and the need for repeat radiographs. This variation presents opportunities for standardizing care, reducing costs, and enhancing value.

Value-Based Themes

1. *No Routine Radiographs Beyond the Initial Injury Films*

If a fracture is suspected, initial anterior posterior (AP) and lateral radiograph of the wrist should be obtained (Fig. 1.1). A buckle fracture is characterized by bulging of the cortex at the metaphyseal-diaphyseal junction due to the axial compression forces on the bone [1]. The buckle is often best appreciated on the lateral view.

A. J. M. Gregory (✉)
Orthopedics and Pediatrics, Vanderbilt University Medical Center, Nashville, TN, USA
e-mail: Andrew.gregory@vumc.org

W. L. Hennrikus, R. M. Schwend (eds.), *Value in Pediatric Orthopaedics*,
https://doi.org/10.1007/978-3-032-19570-8_1

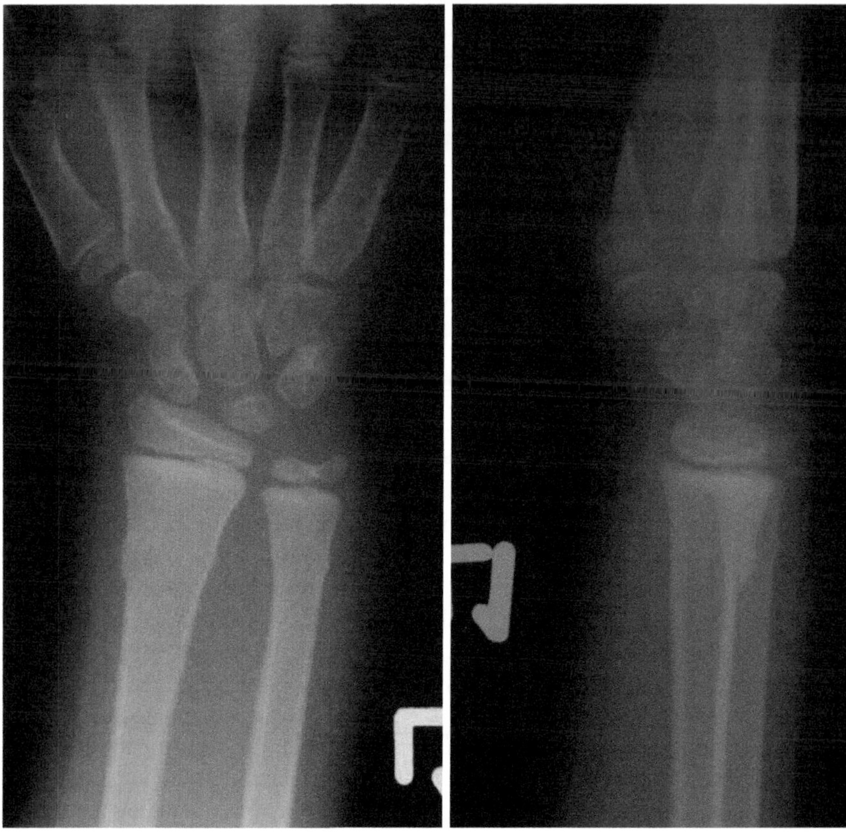

Fig. 1.1 AP and lateral X-rays demonstrating buckle fractures of the distal radius/ulna

Follow-up radiographs are unnecessary for distal radius buckle fractures because buckle fractures do not displace. Eliminating unnecessary follow-up radiographs reduces costs and minimizes radiation exposure without compromising outcomes.

2. *Treat with Removable Splints Instead of Casts*

Evidence supports the use of removable (Velcro ® Brand) splints or braces over traditional circumferential casts to treat distal radius buckle fractures [4–6]. This approach enhances comfort, hygiene, and convenience, while also reducing costs and minimizing potential complications associated with casting. Immobilizing the wrist in a splint reduces pain and prevents further injury. The wrist splint consists of a soft canvas brace with metal stays on the volar and dorsal aspects to hold the wrist in a neutral position, secured with Velcro. A wrist splint is as effective as a short arm cast for treating buckle fractures of the distal radius [4, 6]. The wrist splint offers additional benefits, including ease of bathing, improved function, and greater parental preference [5]. One study has even shown that use of a soft bandage may be equivalent to rigid immobilization, with no difference in pain at 3 days or 6 weeks post injury [7].

3. *Distinguish Buckle Fractures from Other Fractures About the Distal Radius*

It is important to differentiate a buckle fracture from other fractures, such as physeal and greenstick fractures. AP and lateral radiographs of the distal radius can distinguish buckle fractures from physeal fractures and greenstick fractures. Physeal fractures involve the growth plate and are often displaced (Fig. 1.2), while greenstick fractures consist of an traction fracture on one side of the bone, often with angulation (Fig. 1.3). In addition, a scaphoid fracture should be considered if there is tenderness over the anatomic snuff box. If radiographs are normal, and the examination suggests a scaphoid fracture, then obtain an additional scaphoid radiographic view (Fig. 1.4) to diagnose an occult scaphoid fracture. For radiologists, accuracy for distinguishing between a stable buckle fracture and a potentially unstable

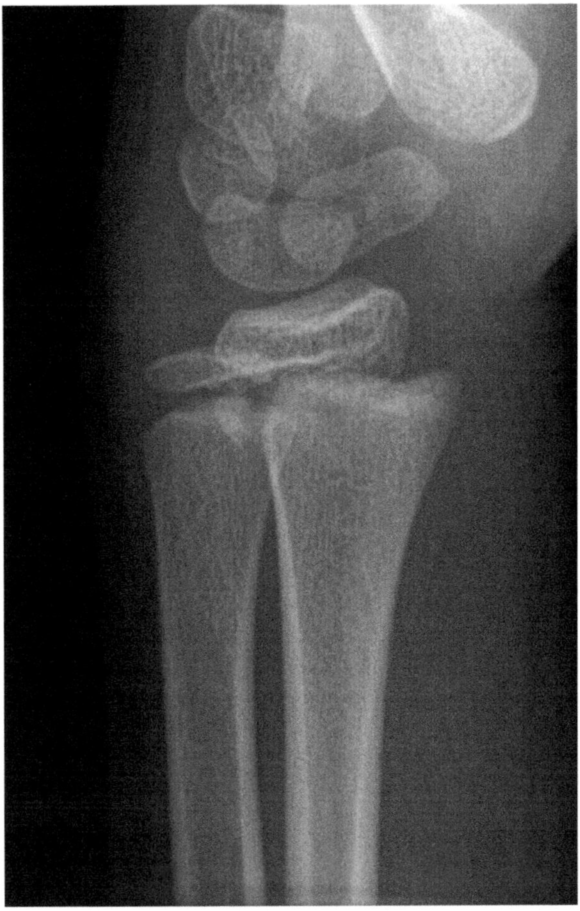

Fig. 1.2 A Salter Harris II fracture of the distal radius with 5 mm of displacement through the distal radius physis

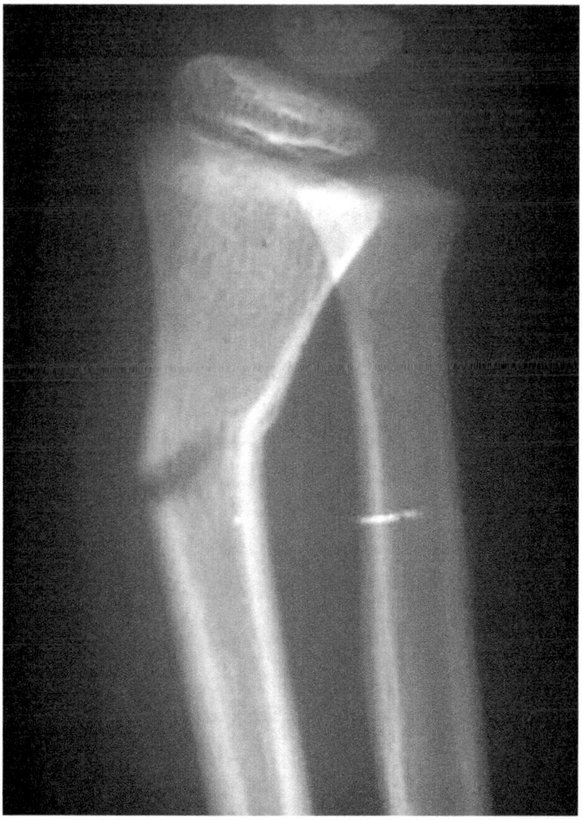

Fig. 1.3 A greenstick fracture of the distal radius with angulation

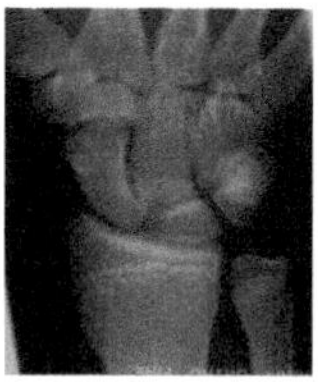

Fig. 1.4 A nondisplaced scaphoid fracture in a patient with open distal radius and ulna physes

"slipper" distal radius fracture in children [8] is improved through education, standardized reporting, and measurement tools [9]. A slipper fracture can initially present as a nondisplaced fracture of both sides of the bone and then "slip" or displace during immobilization. A Velcro splint is not indicated for these fractures. Instead, treatment for distal radius physeal fractures, greenstick fractures, and slipper fractures includes a cast and radiographic follow-up. A thumb spica cast and follow-up films, or even surgery if displaced, may be indicated for a scaphoid fracture.

4. *Early Return to Function and Activities*

Buckle fractures are stable, so immobilization for 3–4 weeks is sufficient. Parents should be informed that their child can return to activities, including sports, once pain has resolved [10]. No prolonged absences from school or sports are indicated. In addition, return to playing while in a splint for certain noncontact sports is permitted, although a note from the doctor may be required.

5. *No Routine Orthopedic Clinic Follow-Up or Follow-Up Radiographs*

Traditionally, distal radius buckle fractures have been overtreated with casting, multiple clinic visits, and repeat follow-up radiographs. However, today, children with distal radius buckle fractures can be treated with a Velcro splint, discharged from care after the initial diagnosis, and managed at home with appropriate parental education [4, 5]. Follow-up can be limited to a nurse phone call to check patient progress at 1–2 weeks. In-person follow-up visits can be reserved for atypical cases. A standardized protocol that uses a splint, avoids follow-up imaging, and minimizes follow-up clinic visits improves efficiency, minimizes parents' time off from work, saves costs, and enhances value. A study from England found that adherence to the National Institute for Health and Care Excellence (NICE) guidelines for distal radius buckle fractures led to better patient management [11]. The NICE guidelines recommend *not using a cast for buckle fractures of the distal radius and discharge children after the first assessment, advising parents that further review is generally unnecessary* [12]. *There is significant cost savings if at-home management is used instead of physician follow-up and repeat X-rays (on the order of $100–300)* [13, 14].

6. *Ultrasound May Be a Reasonable Alternative to Radiographs for Diagnostic Imaging*

Ultrasound, rather than radiographs, performed by a variety of clinicians, can be used for diagnosing clinically nondeformed distal forearm fractures in children and adolescents [15, 16]. As musculoskeletal (MSK) ultrasound becomes more widely available and accepted, MSK ultrasound may serve as an alternative to radiographs. Not all primary care offices or urgent care clinics have access to radiographic imaging; however, portable MSK ultrasound may be more readily accessible.

7. *Primary Care Management of Distal Radius Buckle Fractures*

There is increasing evidence in the literature supporting the management of distal radius buckle fractures by primary care physicians [17, 18]. When primary care physicians manage these injuries with a Velcro wrist splint, a doctor's note, and parental education, the outcomes are equally excellent. By omitting an orthopedic referral, the costs of specialty consultation, additional imaging, and potentially unnecessary treatments are avoided, thereby enhancing value. An orthopedic consultation should be obtained for other distal radius fractures (i.e., greenstick and physeal fractures).

Case Example

Julia is a 7-year-old female who presented with a right wrist injury sustained the previous day. She was riding her Heelys in the street when she hit a rock and fell onto her right forearm. Since the fall, she has experienced right wrist pain and swelling. The pain worsened with motion but improved with rest. Her mom has been managing the injury with ice and ibuprofen. She has had no history of previous fractures.

On examination, there was mild swelling of the right wrist. Limited wrist supination and extension were noted, accompanied by pain. Tenderness of the distal radius and ulna was present. She was neurovascularly intact. Radiographs revealed a buckle fracture of the dorsal cortex of both the distal radius and ulna.

Julia was fitted with a Velcro wrist splint to be worn during activities for the next month. She was provided with instructions on the proper use of the splint and guidance on when to discontinue its use. She was given a doctor's note for no contact sports for 4 weeks. A follow-up phone call by the clinic nurse was arranged for 2 weeks. No return to clinic follow-up was necessary or scheduled.

Author Pearls

1. Maintain a high index of suspicion for a distal radius buckle fracture in children who present with a fall, no deformity, and wrist pain.
2. The physical examination may often be subtle or unremarkable.
3. X-ray findings can also be quite subtle.
4. It's important to distinguish between buckle fractures and other types of fractures (e.g., physeal, greenstick, "slipper," and scaphoid fractures).
5. Buckle fractures heal very well with a splint.
6. Casting is unnecessary.
7. Follow-up visits and repeat radiographs are unnecessary.

Summary

Buckle fractures of the distal radius are common injuries in children and can be diagnosed with AP and lateral radiographs. Rule out other fractures that may present similarly, such as greenstick, physeal, or scaphoid fractures. Distal radius buckle fractures can be treated with a Velcro wrist splint, a doctor's note for temporary modified activities, and parental education. Children can resume physical activity and sports when pain subsides. This chapter presents practical recommendations that reduce costs, maintain excellent outcomes, and enhance value.

Editor Comments

WLH

The current chapter demonstrates that value is enhanced when distal radius buckle fractures are treated with home management using a removable splint after a single clinic evaluation. Buckle fractures are stable, heal quickly, and do not require surgery, repeat X-rays, or follow-up visits. In fact, as Dr. Gregory has indicated, distal radius buckle fractures can be managed by the primary care doctor without an orthopedic referral.

RMS

In the case of a simple buckle fracture of the distal radius, definitive management is achieved when the pediatrician applies a removable splint, provides clear instructions to the family, and takes responsibility for follow-up (e.g., a nurse's phone call at 2 weeks). Since current procedural terminology (CPT) code 25600 describes closed treatment without manipulation and includes all necessary follow-up within the global period, it is appropriate to bill under this code even if no cast is applied and no in-person follow-up visits are required. This example highlights how value in care can be defined not only by avoiding unnecessary casting and visits but also by properly recognizing the work involved by the physician in managing the fracture.

References

1. Light TR, Ogden DA, Ogden JA. The anatomy of metaphyseal buckle fractures. Clin Orthop Relat Res. 1984;188:103–11.
2. Sandefur, et al. Estimated incidence of pediatric distal radius buckle fractures in the United States. J Pediatr Soc North Am. 2024;8:100075.
3. Naranje SM, Erali RA, Warner WC Jr, et al. Epidemiology of pediatric fractures presenting to emergency departments in the United States. J Pediatr Orthop. 2016;36(4):e45–8.
4. Boutis K, Willan A, Babyn P, Goeree R, Howard A. Cast vs splint in children with minimally angulated fractures of the distal radius: a randomized, controlled trial. CMAJ. 2010;182:1507–12.
5. Kuba M, Izuka B. One brace: one visit: treatment of distal radius buckle fractures. J Pediatr Orthop. 2018;38:e338–3442.
6. Plint AC, Perry JJ, Correll R, et al. A randomized, controlled trial of removable splinting versus casting for wrist buckle fractures in children. Pediatrics. 2006;117:691–7.
7. Perry DC, et al. Immobilization of torus fractures of the wrist in children (FORCE): a randomised equivalence trial. Lancet. 2022;400(10357):39–47.
8. Alvarez C, Chen J, Pilla N, Hennrikus W. The slipper fracture: re-visited. Cureus. 2023;15:e38607.
9. Ruess L, Chmil M, Singh S, Samora J. Improving diagnostic accuracy for distinguishing buckle fractures from other distal radius fractures in children. Pediatr Qual Saf. 2022;7(2):e547.
10. Bhanushali A, Bright R, xu L, Cundy P, Williams N. Return to sport after forearm fractures in children: a scoping review and survey. J Child Orthop. 2023;17(2):164–72.

11. Zaib J, Ahamad J, Kumar K. Enhancing patient management and financial efficiency: adherence to National Institute for Health and Care Excellence (NICE) guidelines for pediatric distal radius buckle fractures. Cureus. 2023;15(8):e44198.
12. NICE. Fractures (non-complex): assessment and management. Nice.org.uk. 2016.
13. Colaco K, et al. Home management versus primary care physician follow up of patients with distal radius buckle fractures: a randomized controlled trial. Ann Emerg Med. 2021;77(2):163–73.
14. Woo CY, Wong PLK, Mahadev A. The single visit treatment of pediatric distal radius buckle fractures—a center's experience with the treatment algorithm. Injury. 2020;51(10):2186–91.
15. Morello PR, Mariani F, Snelling P, Buonsenso D. Point-of-care ultrasound for the diagnosis of distal forearm fractures in children and adolescents: a scoping review. Eur J Pediatr. 2024;184(1):19.
16. Snelling PJ, et al. Ultrasonography or radiography for suspected pediatric distal forearm fractures. N Engl J Med. 2023;389(1):12–22.
17. Koelink E, Schuh S, Howard A, Stimec J, Barra L, Boutis K. Primary care physician follow up of distal radius buckle fractures. Pediatrics. 2016;137:1542–5.
18. Koelink E, Boutis K. Pediatric office follow up of common fractures. Paediatr Child Health. 2014;19:407–12.

2 Value-Based Care for Pediatric Salter-Harris I Distal Fibula Ankle Fractures

Sara Buckley and Melissa Bent

Introduction

Lateral ankle injuries are among the most common musculoskeletal injuries in children, typically including Salter-Harris Type I distal fibula fractures and ankle sprains. These injuries often result from sports participation, recreational play, or accidents and are generally associated with excellent long-term outcomes when appropriately managed. Despite their high prevalence and favorable prognosis, treatment approaches vary, leading to inconsistencies in care and unnecessary healthcare costs [2]. For pediatric and adolescent athletes, these injuries may lead to time lost from competition, diminished performance upon return to play, and a burden on the healthcare system [2].

Value-based care offers a framework to address these challenges by emphasizing outcomes while minimizing costs [2–5]. There has been a shift from volume-based to value-based care, with a focus on maximizing quality relative to cost [3]. Regulatory structures have been introduced that have maintained patient outcomes while reducing the cost of care [6]. For Salter-Harris Type I distal fibula and ankle

S. Buckley
Charles R. Drew University of Medicine and Science, Physical Medicine and Rehabilitation, Los Angeles, CA, USA

M. Bent (✉)
Charles R. Drew University of Medicine and Science, Physical Medicine and Rehabilitation, Los Angeles, CA, USA

Jackie and Gene Autry Orthopedic Center, Children's Hospital Los Angeles, Los Angeles, CA, USA

KeckSchool of Medicine, University of Southern California, Los Angeles, CA, USA
e-mail: mbent@chla.usc.edu

W. L. Hennrikus, R. M. Schwend (eds.), *Value in Pediatric Orthopaedics*,
https://doi.org/10.1007/978-3-032-19570-8_2

sprains, this approach involves standardizing treatment protocols, minimizing non-essential interventions, and prioritizing high-value practices.

Value-Based Themes (Fig. 2.1)

When Less Is More: Selective Imaging for Salter-Harris I Distal Fibula Fractures

Lateral ankle sprains account for over two million emergency department (ED) visits annually in the United States and Canada [1, 8, 9]. In Salter-Harris Type I injuries, patients typically present with tenderness over the distal fibula without radiographic evidence of a fracture. These injuries are often first evaluated in the ED and traditionally managed with immobilization, orthopedic follow-up, and repeat imaging [10]. The Ottawa Ankle Rules (OAR) can guide the decision-making process for obtaining radiographs of ankle and midfoot injuries, which have been validated for children >5 years of age [11]. Many clinicians rely on a combination of physical examination and serial X-ray films to differentiate between a Salter-Harris Type I distal fibula fracture and a ligamentous ankle sprain [2]. However, it is important to consider the radiation associated with imaging. For example, a single plain film radiograph exposes the patient to 0.005–0.02 millisieverts (mSv) of radiation, which is roughly equivalent to 1–2 days of natural background radiation at sea level and less than a chest radiograph. With the advent of improved imaging techniques, as low as reasonably achievable (ALARA) guidelines, and pediatric dosing, the

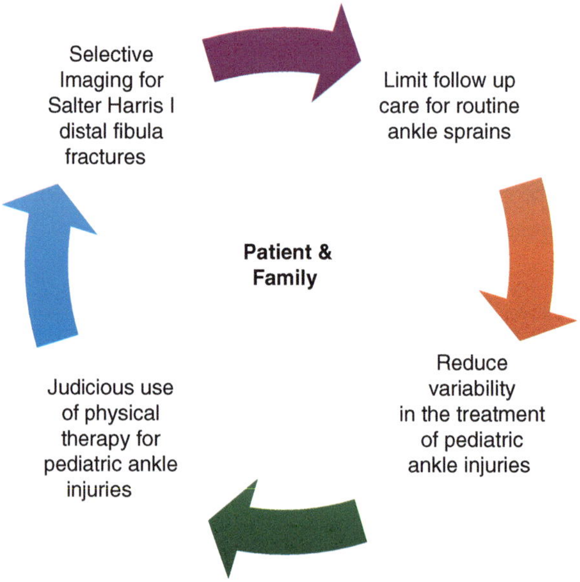

Fig. 2.1 Patient and family-value-centered themes [7]

cumulative exposure to unnecessary radiation falls well below thresholds associated with lifetime cancer risk [12].

The cost of radiographs should also be considered. The initial evaluation of an ankle injury may involve charges for ED services, facility fees, medications, and technical and professional imaging fees. X-ray imaging costs vary depending on the health system and patient insurance. A study analyzing the Nationwide Emergency Department Sample reported a median charge of $1029 USD per event for all ankle sprains [13]. The cost of X-ray imaging alone can be several hundred dollars [14, 15, 16].

Radiation-sparing imaging is an alternative to standard radiographs. For example, a 2022 study reported point-of-care ankle ultrasound to have a sensitivity of 78%, specificity of 71%, and a positive likelihood ratio of 2.7. Use of the OAR alone reduced radiograph use by 18% with one missed fracture, while combining ultrasound with OAR yielded a 17% reduction with no missed fractures. Due to its high safety profile, ultrasound imaging may be particularly valuable in detecting radiographically occult ankle fractures [17, 18]. However, the effectiveness of ultrasound imaging remains operator-dependent [19]. Magnetic Resonance Imaging (MRI) is an option, but it is more expensive and carries anesthesia-related risks for the younger pediatric patient [1].

Reduce Variability in the Treatment of Pediatric Ankle Injuries

Variability exists in the treatment of pediatric ankle injuries among pediatric orthopedic surgeons. Compared to emergency medicine physicians, orthopedic surgeons more frequently utilize cast immobilization over the use of controlled ankle motion (CAM) boots [2, 10]. Casting has the risks of pressure sores and thermal cast saw burns, which can result in medicolegal claims and increased healthcare costs [20, 21]. Total payments related to cast saw burns ranged from $2995 to $25,000 per claim at one institution. Notably, the emergency department was identified as the setting with the highest risk of cast saw burns [20, 21].

A 2022 survey demonstrated that the CAM boot has surpassed casting as the most used immobilization method for Salter-Harris Type I distal fibula fractures among orthopedic surgeons, especially among younger physicians [2]. Boutis et al. reported no difference in functional outcomes between fractures and ligamentous injuries when both were treated with a removable boot [1]. Immobilization remains the primary treatment approach for Salter-Harris Type I distal fibula fractures, with weight-bearing as tolerated recommended in the boot [2].

Limit Follow-Up Care for Routine Ankle Sprains

In pediatric patients, less severe acute lateral ankle sprains are often managed with functional rehabilitation, which has been shown to be more effective than immobilization. For more severe sprains, a brief period of immobilization followed by rehabilitation is recommended [22]. Most children recover fully and return to preinjury activity levels [23]. Studies have demonstrated no difference in functional outcomes between intermediate-to-high-grade ankle sprains and Salter-Harris Type I distal fibula fractures when treated with immobilization [1]. Given the evidence demonstrating favorable outcomes and the advantages of less restrictive immobilization, management of pediatric ankle injuries has shifted toward targeted and minimal casting [1, 24, 25]. Primary care physicians can rely on patient symptoms to guide return-to-play decisions and reserve orthopedic referral for cases with displaced fractures or delayed recovery [1, 25].

Judicious Use of Physical Therapy for Pediatric Ankle Injuries

Physical therapy is more commonly recommended for lateral ankle sprains than for Salter-Harris Type I fractures [2]. Exercise initiated after acute lateral ankle sprains has been shown to reduce the risk of recurrent injuries and improve functional stability [26]. For isolated Salter-Harris Type I distal fibula fractures, studies support early removal of immobilization and a return to weight-bearing, which promotes functional loading and facilitates fracture healing [10, 24, 25]. From a value-based care perspective, limited physical therapy, combined with a home exercise program, supports strength and range-of-motion gains and potentially reduces the risk of future injury.

Outcomes

A 2022 survey of the Pediatric Orthopaedic Society of North America (POSNA) members found that most patients experienced no complications following lateral ankle injuries [2]. Complication rates were low: 8.7% among Salter-Harris Type I fractures and 6.6% among ankle sprains. Reported complications included persistent pain, growth disturbances, prolonged healing, recurrent injury, and infection. Salter-Harris Type I injuries also carry small risks of fracture displacement, growth disturbance, and nonunion [2].

Unlike bone, ligamentous injuries heal with altered collagen architecture and reduced tensile strength, which may contribute to a small risk of chronic ankle instability. In contrast, bone healing restores original structural integrity. Overall, the diagnosis of a Salter-Harris Type I fracture does not necessitate a treatment approach different from that of an ankle sprain [1].

Case Examples: The Story of Two Ankles

Case 1 A 13-year-old boy sustained an inversion injury to his right ankle while playing basketball. On physical examination, he had pain with weight-bearing and tenderness over the lateral malleolus and proximally along the distal fibula. Since he

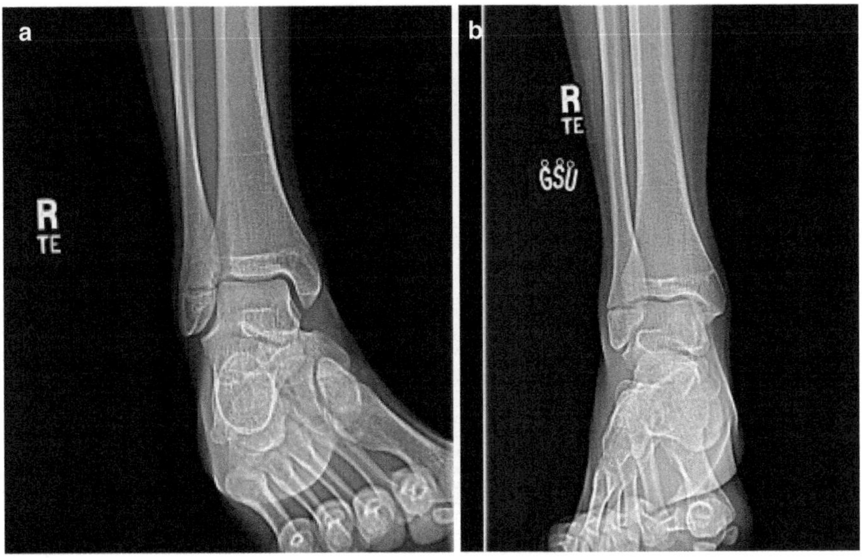

Fig. 2.2 (**a**, **b**) Anterior-Posterior (AP) and lateral radiograph of a 13-year-old boy with Salter-Harris type I of the distal fibula. Note that there is no displacement of the talus in its articulation with the tibia plafond. The distal tibia physis is almost completely closed

had tenderness over the fibula (OAR), radiographs were obtained (Figs. 2.2a,b), and he was diagnosed with a Salter-Harris Type I fracture of the distal fibula. He was treated with a controlled ankle motion (CAM) boot and weight-bearing as tolerated. Although he still experienced pain with weight-bearing after 10 days, his symptoms gradually improved. Formal physical therapy was not prescribed, and he progressed well with a home exercise program

Case 2 A 9-year-old boy also sustained an inversion injury during basketball. He had pain distal to the lateral malleolus (Fig. 2.3a). He was placed in a CAM boot initially, and his symptoms resolved within 2 weeks. He had no pain at the time of follow-up and was thus treated as an ankle sprain. Both cases illustrate the importance of physical examination and judicious follow-up based on the patient's symptoms

Summary

The current chapter outlines four practical recommendations aimed at improving value by reducing diagnostic and follow-up costs, minimizing variability, reducing radiation exposure, and maintaining excellent clinical outcomes in the management of Salter-Harris Type I distal fibula fractures and ankle sprains. Table 2.1 summarizes this care pathway.

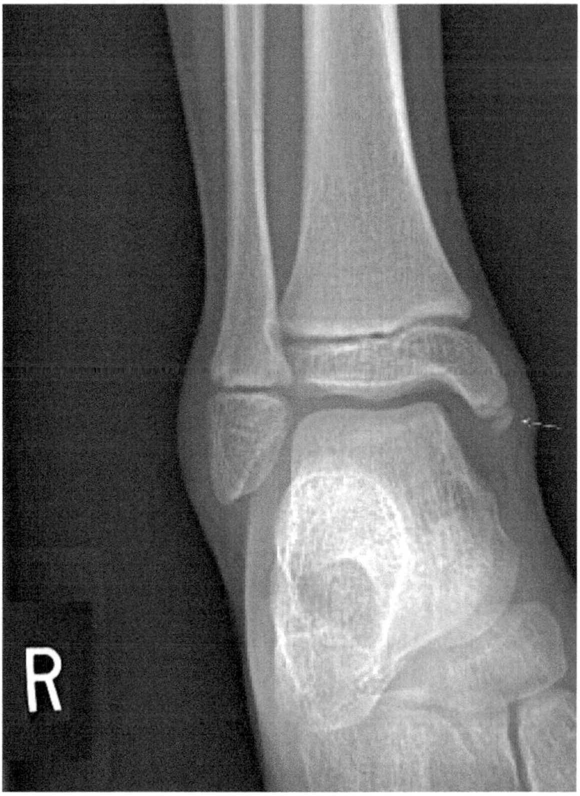

Fig. 2.3 AP radiograph of a 9-year-old boy. Note that there is no Salter-Harris fracture of the distal fibula or any displacement of the talus in its articulation with the tibia plafond. The distal tibia and fibula physes are both open

Table 2.1 High-value care pathway for lateral ankle injuries

Clinical step	Recommended high-value practice
Initial evaluation	Apply Ottawa Ankle Rules (OAR) to determine the need for radiographs (bone tenderness/can't weight bear); avoid imaging in low-risk cases.
Imaging	Limit imaging to cases meeting OAR criteria; consider ultrasound in select cases as a radiation-free alternative.
Immobilization	Prefer removable CAM boot over casting; avoid unnecessary rigid immobilization.
Specialist referral	Refer to orthopedics only for displaced fractures or delayed recovery.
Follow-up	Minimize follow-up visits; base return-to-play decisions on symptom resolution and functional status.
Physical therapy	Recommend home exercise program; reserve formal physical therapy (PT) for instability, recurrent sprain, or slow recovery.
Patient/family education	Provide reassurance and clear guidance on natural course, recovery expectations, and return to activity.

Author Pearls

- Lateral ankle injuries are common in children
- Treatment with a brief period of immobilization followed by return to play results in good outcomes
- Complications are rare
- A value-based care model should be applied, including cost, time to appointments, and radiation exposure
- The Ottawa Ankle Rules can help reduce unnecessary imaging

Editors Comments

WLH

Low-risk lateral ankle injuries not requiring radiographs, as defined by the OARs, as well as x-ray negative lateral ankle injuries, can be treated symptomatically by the primary care physician in a removable CAM boot. Return to activity is typically 3–4 weeks and can be determined by the patient as their symptoms improve. Patients with an X-ray-identified displaced fracture or with a delayed recovery should be referred to orthopedics.

RMS

This chapter offers a clear, evidence-based framework for managing low-risk pediatric lateral ankle injuries through a value-based lens. As with many common injuries, the challenge lies not in the treatment but in avoiding over-treatment. The authors outline practical strategies to reduce unnecessary imaging, limit immobilization, and minimize follow-up, while maintaining excellent clinical outcomes. Value in pediatric care also extends beyond direct medical costs to include time lost from school or sports and time off work for the parents. Consideration of access to care, particularly the availability of removable boots or imaging in resource-limited settings, is another important component of delivering equitable value.

References

1. Boutis K, et al. Radiograph-negative lateral ankle injuries in children: occult growth plate fracture or sprain? JAMA Pediatr. 2016;170(1):e154114.
2. Beck JJ, et al. Treatment variability and complications associated with pediatric lateral ankle injuries: a POSNA quality, safety, and value initiative survey. Orthop J Sports Med. 2022;10(6):23259671221100223.
3. Orman S, et al. Health economics in pediatric orthopaedic surgery. J Pediatr Orthop Soc N Am. 2020;2(2):103.

4. Kocher MS. Value of pediatric orthopaedic surgery. J Pediatr Orthop. 2015;35(5 Suppl 1):S9–13.
5. Waters PM. Value in pediatric orthopaedic surgery health care: the role of time-driven activity-based cost accounting (TDABC) and standardized clinical assessment and management plans (SCAMPs). J Pediatr Orthop. 2015;35(5 Suppl 1):S45–7.
6. Teisberg E, Wallace S, O'Hara S. Defining and implementing value-based health care: a strategic framework. Acad Med. 2020;95(5):682–5.
7. Buckley S, Patient and family value centered themes. in Biorender.com. 2025.
8. Herzog MM, et al. Epidemiology of ankle sprains and chronic ankle instability. J Athl Train. 2019;54(6):603–10.
9. Steiger C, et al. A retrospective epidemiological cohort study of ankle fractures in children and teenagers. J Child Orthop. 2023;17(4):348–53.
10. Zomorrodi A, et al. Consistency between emergency department and orthopedic physicians in the diagnosis and treatment of distal fibular Salter Harris I fractures. Pediatr Emerg Care. 2011;27(4):301–3.
11. Stiell IG, et al. Implementation of the Ottawa ankle rules. JAMA. 1994;271(11):827–32.
12. Wheeler JA, et al. Radiation exposure in patients with isolated limb trauma: acceptable or are we imaging too much? J Clin Med. 2020;9(11):3609.
13. Shah S, et al. Incidence and cost of ankle sprains in United States emergency departments. Sports Health. 2016;8(6):547–52.
14. Moore BJ, Liang L. Costs of emergency department visits in the United States, 2017. In: Healthcare Cost and Utilization Project (HCUP) statistical briefs. Rockville; 2020.
15. Cost, N.H. Cost estimates: X-ray of Ankle, 2-views. Health costs [Webpage] [cited 2025 05/05/2025]; Available from: https://nhhealthcost.nh.gov/costs/medical/result/x-ray-of-ankle-2-views.
16. Children's, N. Nationwide Children's Hospital Price Information. Price information 05/05/2025; Available from: https://www.nationwidechildrens.org/your-visit/billing-and-insurance/pay-my-bill/price-information-list.
17. Simanovsky N, et al. Sonographic detection of radiographically occult fractures in paediatric ankle injuries. Pediatr Radiol. 2005;35(11):1062–5.
18. Nadler A, Tsung JW, Rabiner JE. Point-of-care ultrasonography for ankle injuries in children. Pediatr Emerg Care. 2022;38(1):e17–22.
19. Song JH, et al. Use of a comprehensive systemic ultrasound evaluation in the diagnosis and analysis of acute lateral region ankle sprain. BMC Musculoskelet Disord. 2023;24(1):517.
20. Shore BJ, et al. Epidemiology and prevention of cast saw injuries: results of a quality improvement program at a single institution. J Bone Joint Surg Am. 2014;96(4):e31.
21. Drake DF, Ritzman TF. Cast-related complications. Orthop Clin North Am. 2021;52(3):231–40.
22. Gill LE, Klingele KE. Management of foot and ankle injuries in pediatric and adolescent athletes: a narrative review. Orthop Res Rev. 2018;10:19–30.
23. Michels F, et al. The evolution of patient-reported outcome measures after a first lateral ankle sprain: a prospective study. Foot Ankle Surg. 2024;30(7):568–75.
24. Tay JY, et al. Non-surgical interventions for isolated Salter-Harris type I distal fibula fractures: a systematic review. J Orthop Rep. 2024;3(3):100319.
25. Macneille R, Hennrikus W. Value based treatment of common pediatric fractures by primary care. Clin Pediatr. 2018;15:1378–84.
26. Beck JJ, et al. Low energy, lateral ankle injuries in pediatric and adolescent patients: a systematic review of ankle sprains and nondisplaced distal fibula fractures. J Pediatr Orthop. 2020;40(6):283–7.

Methods to Improve Value When Treating Pediatric/Adolescent Diaphyseal Clavicle Fractures

3

Katherine Eigo, Brian Li, Stephanie Stuerzel, and Wojciech Czoch

Introduction

Direct impact to the shoulder during sports activities is the most common mechanism of clavicle fractures, which comprise 8–15% of all skeletal injuries in children [7]. Other causes include rough play, biking accidents, falls, and motor vehicle collisions [7]. Clavicle fractures show a strong demographic trend, with adolescents aged 13–20 years experiencing twice the incidence seen in other age groups [7]. In addition, male predominance (79%), sports-related trauma (88%), and nondominant side fracture (56%) are common [7].

The diaphyseal region is fractured in 85% of cases, followed by the lateral third (10%) and medial third (5%) [1–4]. This susceptibility of the diaphyseal region to fracture is attributed to the anatomical transition in the midshaft, where the clavicle changes from concave to convex in the frontal plane and from round to flat in cross-section [10, 11]. Additionally, the junction between the middle and outer third is the thinnest part of the clavicle and the only segment lacking muscular or ligamentous attachments, further increasing its vulnerability to fracture [8, 12].

The first classification system for clavicle fractures was introduced by Allman in 1967, categorizing fractures based on anatomical location: Type I for the middle third, Type II for the lateral third, and Type III for the medial third [13]. Later, the modified Neer classification expanded upon this by providing a more detailed system for distal (lateral third) clavicle fractures [2, 14–16]. The AO Foundation/

K. Eigo · S. Stuerzel · W. Czoch (✉)
Department of Pediatric Orthopaedics, Northwell Health, Cohen Children's Medical Center, New Hyde Park, NY, USA
e-mail: keigo@northwell.edu; sstuerzel@northwell.edu; wczoch@northwell.edu

B. Li
Donald and Barbara Zucker School of Medicine, Hempstead, NY, USA
e-mail: bli5@northwell.edu

W. L. Hennrikus, R. M. Schwend (eds.), *Value in Pediatric Orthopaedics*,
https://doi.org/10.1007/978-3-032-19570-8_3

Orthopaedic Trauma Association (AO/OTA) classification added more detail, categorizing fractures by segment and articular involvement for medial fractures, fracture pattern for diaphyseal fractures, and displacement and ligament disruption for lateral fractures [12]. The AO/OTA system is valuable in complex trauma settings, while the modified Neer system is useful for lateral third fractures. However, the Allman classification remains the most widely used in clinical practice due to its simplicity and clear anatomical divisions [2].

Management of pediatric diaphyseal clavicle fractures differs from that in adults. Children possess exceptional healing potential due to active physes and a thick periosteum with a robust vascular supply [8, 17]. The medial clavicular physis is the last to close, typically between 22 and 25 years of age. The clavicle periosteum not only enhances healing but also helps maintain fracture alignment, making severely displaced fractures less common in the pediatric and adolescent populations [7, 8, 12].

Value-Based Themes

Nonoperative Treatment and Primary Care–Directed Treatment Adds Value

Non-operative treatment remains the standard of care for most pediatric and adolescent diaphyseal clavicle fractures due to high union rates and excellent remodeling potential. In skeletally immature patients, the thick periosteal sleeve often results in incomplete fracture patterns. Up to two-thirds of pediatric clavicle fractures present with some degree of displacement [8, 18]. Despite displacement, reliable remodeling over time typically corrects angulation and displacement.

Some complex displaced clavicle fractures may require surgical intervention. The decision to proceed with surgery is influenced by patient age > 15 years old, open injury, fracture shortening greater than 2 cm, nonmidshaft location, or associated vascular, neurological, or soft tissue injury [2, 8, 19]. The most common surgical indications include older patient age, severe displacement, and soft tissue interposition [20, 21]. The rate of surgical fixation has increased in recent years; however, the surgical rate is relatively low—currently around 12% of all pediatric cases, up from 5% in the early 2000s [20, 21].

Except for a few specific operative indications, simple sling immobilization remains the preferred treatment for most pediatric clavicle fractures due to the outstanding clinical outcomes and low cost. In fact, operative management of diaphyseal clavicle fractures in adolescents incurs costs nearly 19 times higher than nonoperative treatment [22]. In addition, long-term studies have shown lower rates of nonunion with immobilization alone compared to surgical intervention in pediatric patients [15, 23]. Conservative treatment also avoids surgical scarring, reduces postoperative pain, and minimizes cosmetic concerns [24].

Non-operative treatment typically involves sling or figure-of-eight brace immobilization. Immobilization continues for about 4 weeks, followed by gradual shoulder range-of-motion home exercises. Return to sports usually occurs at about

8–12 weeks [9]. Figure-of-eight bracing is associated with higher pain scores and greater patient dissatisfaction compared to arm slings [25]. In one prospective, randomized study, 26% of patients treated with figure-of-eight bracing reported dissatisfaction, versus only 7% of those treated with a sling [25]. Additionally, figure-of-eight braces are more expensive [25]. Therefore, we recommend sling immobilization due to superior comfort, lower cost, higher patient and parent satisfaction rates, and improved value.

Minimizing Emergency Room Visits and Optimizing Clinic Follow-Up and Imaging Adds Value

Many children with clavicle fractures initially present to the emergency department (ED). Orthopaedic surgical consultation is recommended for fractures when operative indications are present [20, 21]. However, nondisplaced diaphyseal clavicle fractures can be treated with added value by a primary care doctor. Management of a nondisplaced fracture is straightforward, focusing on pain control with ibuprofen or acetaminophen, application of a simple arm sling, and a note for gym or sports [26, 27]. In addition, patients who present initially to an outpatient setting such as pediatric primary care clinics or urgent care centers with a nondisplaced fracture do not typically require referral to the emergency department. Such referrals may lead to unnecessary delays, increased financial burden, and added stress for both the child and their parents. Instead, the primary care physician in the outpatient clinic can apply a simple arm sling and arrange follow-up. Adequate follow-up for nondisplaced diaphyseal clavicle fractures that minimizes radiation can include a 4-week follow-up visit with an AP clavicle radiograph to confirm healing and alignment, begin shoulder range of motion, and then a second follow-up at 8 weeks to assess healing and return the patient to sports. If any signs of delayed healing are present at the 4-week or 8-week visit, the patient can be referred to an orthopedic surgeon [26, 27].

Surgery for Select Cases Adds Value

Operative treatment for diaphyseal clavicle fractures is indicated in cases of open fractures, skin compromise, significant displacement >2 cm overlap, vascular injury, neurological injury, select refractures, and nonunions [9]. The Canadian Orthopaedic Trauma Society conducted a multicenter randomized clinical trial comparing nonoperative and operative treatment of displaced midshaft clavicle fractures in patients aged 16 years and older [28]. For fractures with >2 cm overlap, operative management demonstrated improved self-reported shoulder function, fewer complications, and greater cosmetic satisfaction [28]. Accordingly, when indications for surgery are present, operative treatment may offer meaningful benefits and add value.

Type of Instrumentation

We recommend standardizing instrumentation to reduce variability and improve cost efficiency. Open reduction and internal fixation using plate and screw constructs for diaphyseal clavicle fractures is recommended [5]. Both reconstruction plates and precontoured plates are effective, though precontoured plates facilitate easier placement [12]. Locked plates have also been used but offer minimal advantage in young patients with good bone quality, making the higher cost of locked plates unjustified [9, 14].

Placement of the Plate

Plates can be placed either in the anterosuperior or anteroinferior position. Anterosuperior plating offers improved biomechanical stability. However, anteroinferior plating is often preferred due to the advantages in surgical safety and patient comfort. For example, drilling for an anteroinferior plate directs the drill away from the subclavian vessels and lungs. Placing the plate anteroinferior avoids the incision site and minimizes soft tissue irritation, discomfort, and the later need for implant removal [14]. In contrast, anterosuperior plating risks injury to the subclavian vessels and lung and results in higher rates of painful implants and more frequent need for later removal [19]. Plate removal increases healthcare costs and reduces value. Plate removal also exposes the patient to additional radiation, surgical risks, and potential complications.

Outcome

The open physis and thick periosteum contribute to favorable healing outcomes [5]. Pediatric patients experience low rates of nonunion (< 1%) and symptomatic malunion (< 2%) [5, 6]. In addition, even in cases of malunion, children rarely exhibit deficits in shoulder motion, strength, or comfort [29]. While both operative and nonoperative treatments carry a small risk of malunion or nonunion, surgical intervention introduces additional risks, including infection and implant failure or need for later removal. For nonoperative treatment, immobilization with a simple sling for about 4 weeks is recommended, and nondisplaced fractures can be managed by a primary care doctor. Outcomes are typically excellent.

Case Report

A 14-year-old male ice hockey player presented to the emergency department (ED) with acute right shoulder pain following a collision during a game. He reported immediate pain and reduced ability to move his right arm after sustaining a direct impact during play. He had no significant past medical history or prior fractures. On examination, there was moderate tenderness over the midshaft of the right clavicle, with crepitus and pathologic motion noted on gentle palpation. There was no evidence of skin tenting or compromise. Active shoulder abduction was limited to 20°,

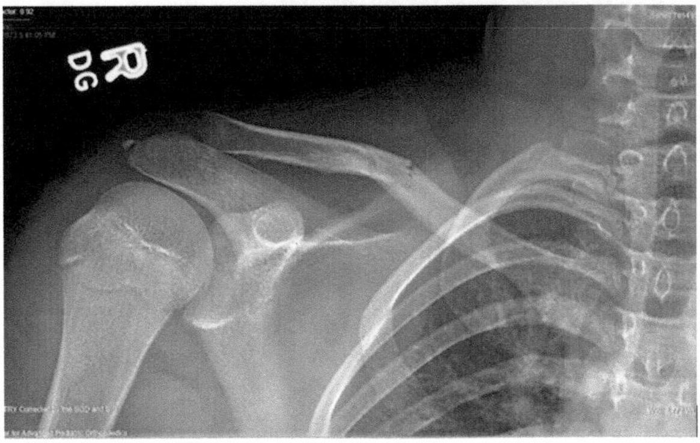

Fig. 3.1 Injury radiograph

and forward flexion to 30° due to pain. Neurovascular examination was normal. Radiographs revealed a minimally angulated fracture of the right midshaft clavicle (Fig. 3.1). There was no displacement or shortening. Conservative management was initiated using a simple arm sling. Over-the-counter ibuprofen was recommended for pain control, and the family was provided with detailed instructions on proper sling use and a note for activity restriction.

At follow-up 4 weeks post-injury in the primary care sports medicine clinic, he demonstrated improvement, with active forward flexion to 90°, abduction to 80°, and external rotation to 30°. Radiographs showed early signs of healing with maintained alignment (Fig. 3.2). The sling was discontinued, and home exercises were initiated, including pendulum exercises and gentle active-assisted range of motion.

Eight weeks after the injury, he had marked improvement, with forward flexion and abduction both reaching 160°, and external rotation to 70°. Radiographs confirmed appropriate healing with evidence of bridging callus formation. A gradual return to sports was initiated (Fig. 3.3).

Summary

Pediatric and adolescent diaphyseal clavicle fractures are common. Due to a thick periosteum and active growth plates, children have excellent healing potential. Most of these fractures can be effectively managed nonoperatively with simple sling immobilization.

The current chapter challenges practices that contribute to reduced value, such as unnecessary ED visits, excessive imaging, formal physical therapy, and follow-up exclusively by an orthopedic surgeon. A standardized follow-up protocol can ensure fracture monitoring, minimize radiation exposure, and reduce the burden on parents. Formal physical therapy is rarely indicated, and most children recover well after sling immobilization with home exercises. Surgical intervention is reserved for select cases, such as open fractures, fractures in patients >15 years of age with

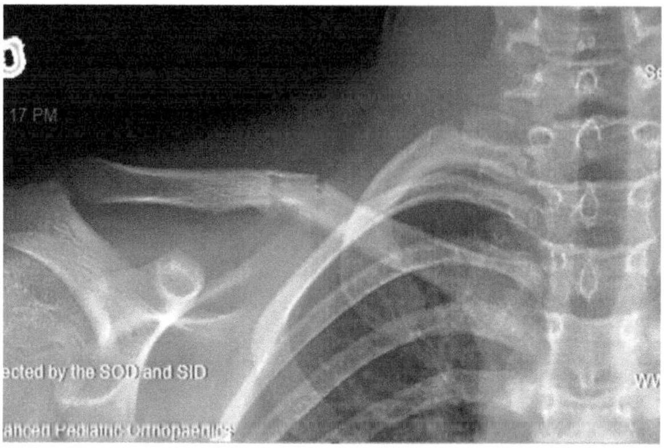

Fig. 3.2 Radiograph 4 weeks post injury

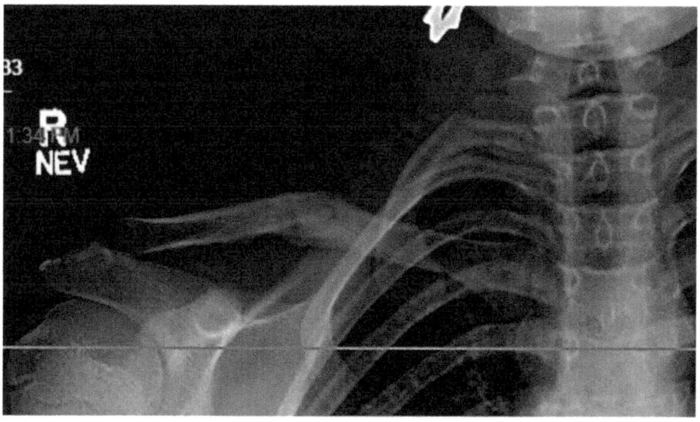

Fig. 3.3 Radiograph 8 weeks post injury

overlap >2 cm, or fractures with associated neurovascular injuries. When surgery is indicated, standardized instrumentation and meticulous surgical planning are essential to optimize outcomes.

Author Pearls

- Most pediatric diaphyseal clavicle fractures heal reliably with a simple sling immobilization.
- An arm sling is preferred over a figure-of-eight brace because a sling provides superior comfort, compliance, cost, and overall satisfaction.
- Primary care doctors can manage uncomplicated diaphyseal clavicle fractures. Uncomplicated clavicle fractures can be managed in an outpatient setting. Reserve emergency department visits for complex clavicle fractures such as open fractures and fractures with neurovascular compromise or significant displacement.

- Minimize radiation exposure by standardizing imaging to include an injury radiograph, a 4-week follow-up radiograph, and, in select cases, an 8-week film.
- Prioritize home exercise programs over formal physical therapy.
- When surgery is indicated, consider anteroinferior plate placement for greater safety, to minimize implant irritation and reduce the likelihood of needing later removal.

Comments by the Editors

WLH

The clavicle is one of the most fractured bones in children. The current chapter highlights multiple common-sense methods that enhance value when treating pediatric clavicle fractures, including treatment with a simple sling, management of nondisplaced fractures by primary care doctors, minimizing follow-up x-rays, minimizing the use of physical therapy, reserving surgery for specific fracture indications, and using anteroinferior plates when surgery is performed.

RMS

Shared decision-making (SDM) is important when deciding on surgical management of pediatric midshaft clavicle fractures, where most children heal well without surgery, but select cases may benefit from operative treatment. Unlike adults, where displaced fractures often require fixation, children, especially those under 15 years, typically achieve excellent outcomes nonoperatively. However, older adolescents, high-demand athletes, or those with markedly displaced fractures may warrant surgical consideration. In these cases, SDM helps families weigh the modest potential benefits of surgery against its risks, recovery, and the child's natural healing potential, ensuring that care is individualized, transparent, and aligned with patient and family goals. What is of value to the child and family may be different than what is of value to the medical system and insurer.

References

1. Nordqvist A, Petersson C. The incidence of fractures of the clavicle. Clin Orthop Relat Res. 1994;300:127–32. https://doi.org/10.1097/00003086-199403000-00016.
2. van der Meijden OA, Gaskill TR, Millett PJ. Treatment of clavicle fractures: current concepts review. J Shoulder Elb Surg. 2012;21(3):423–9. https://doi.org/10.1016/j.jse.2011.08.053.
3. Landin LA. Fracture patterns in children: analysis of 8,682 fractures with special reference to incidence, etiology and secular changes in a Swedish urban population 1950–1979. Acta Orthop. 1983;54(S202):1–109. https://doi.org/10.3109/17453678309155630.

4. Mukhtar IA, Yaghmour KM, Ahmed AF, Ibrahim T. Flexible intramedullary nailing versus nonoperative treatment for paediatric displaced Midshaft clavicle fractures. J Child Orthop. 2018;12(2):104–10. https://doi.org/10.1302/1863-2548.12.170185.
5. Jasty NM, Heyworth BE. Evaluation and management of Midshaft clavicle fractures in adolescents. J Pediatr Orthop Soc North Am. 2020;2(3) https://doi.org/10.55275/jposna-2020-172.
6. Heyworth BE, Pennock AT, Li Y, et al. Two-year functional outcomes of operative vs nonoperative treatment of completely displaced Midshaft clavicle fractures in adolescents: results from the prospective multicenter FACTS study group. Am J Sports Med. 2022;50(11):3045–55. https://doi.org/10.1177/03635465221114420.
7. Ellis HB, Li Y, Bae DS, et al. Descriptive epidemiology of adolescent clavicle fractures: results from the FACTS (function after adolescent clavicle trauma and surgery) prospective, multicenter cohort study. Orthop J Sports Med. 2020;8(5):2325967120921344. https://doi.org/10.1177/2325967120921344.
8. Shannon EG, Hart ES, Grottkau BE. Clavicle fractures in children: the essentials. Orthop Nurs. 2009;28(5):210–4. https://doi.org/10.1097/NOR.0b013e3181b57a27.
9. Pandya NK, Namdari S, Hosalkar HS. Displaced clavicle fractures in adolescents. J Am Acad Orthop Surg. 2012;20(8):498–505. https://doi.org/10.5435/JAAOS-20-08-498.
10. Finnegan M. Skeletal trauma in children, vol. 3. J Bone Joint Surg. 1994;76(5):796. https://doi.org/10.2106/00004623-199405000-00027.
11. Nawar K, Eliya Y, Burrow S, Peterson D, Ayeni O, Darren d SA. Operative versus non-operative management of mid-diaphyseal clavicle fractures in the skeletally immature population: a systematic review and meta-analysis. Curr Rev Musculoskelet Med. 2020;13(1):38–49. https://doi.org/10.1007/s12178-020-09604-4.
12. Markes AR, Garcia-Lopez E, Halvorson RT, Swarup I. Management of displaced Midshaft Clavicle fractures in pediatrics and adolescents: operative vs nonoperative treatment. Orthop Res Rev. 2022;14:373–81. https://doi.org/10.2147/ORR.S340538.
13. Allman FL. Fractures and ligamentous injuries of the clavicle and its articulation. J Bone Joint Surg Am. 1967;49(4):774–84. https://doi.org/10.2106/00004623-196749040-00024.
14. Moverley R, Little N, Gulihar A, Singh B. Current concepts in the management of clavicle fractures. J Clin Orthop Trauma. 2020;11:S25–30. https://doi.org/10.1016/j.jcot.2019.07.016.
15. Neer CS. Fractures of the distal third of the clavicle. Clin Orthop Relat Res. 1968;58:43–50. https://doi.org/10.1097/00003086-196805000-00007.
16. Stenson J, Baker W. Classifications in brief: the modified Neer classification for distal-third clavicle fractures. Clin Orthop Relat Res. 2021;479(1):205–9. https://doi.org/10.1097/CORR.0000000000001456.
17. Jeray KJ. Acute midshaft clavicular fracture. J Am Acad Orthop Surg. 2007;15(4):239–48. https://doi.org/10.5435/00124635-200704000-00007.
18. van der Water L, Macken AA, Eygendaal D, van Bergen CJA. Pediatric clavicle fractures and congenital pseudarthrosis unraveled. Children (Basel). 2022;9(1):49. https://doi.org/10.3390/children9010049.
19. Curtis RJ. Operative management of children's fractures of the shoulder region. Orthop Clin North Am. 1990;21(2):315–24. https://doi.org/10.1016/s0030-5898(20)31547-9.
20. Patel M, Heyworth BE, Dehghan N, Mehlman CT, McKee MD. Clavicular fractures in the adolescent. J Bone Joint Surg. 2023;105(9):713–23. https://doi.org/10.2106/JBJS.22.01036.
21. Fanter NJ, Kenny RM, Baker CL, Baker CL. Surgical treatment of clavicle fractures in the adolescent athlete. Sports Health. 2015;7(2):137–41. https://doi.org/10.1177/1941738114566381.
22. Feldman L. Volume and costs of operative vs. nonoperative Tx of Diaphyseal clavicle fractures in adolescents treated at U.S. children's hospitals from 2009 to 2013. In: POSNA; 2015.
23. Rowe CR. An atlas of anatomy and treatment of midclavicular fractures. Clin Orthop Relat Res. 1968;58:29–42. https://doi.org/10.1097/00003086-196805000-00006.
24. Luo TD, Ashraf A, Larson AN, Stans AA, Shaughnessy WJ, McIntosh AL. Complications in the treatment of adolescent clavicle fractures. Orthopedics. 2015;38(4):e287–91. https://doi.org/10.3928/01477447-20150402-56.

25. Lenza M, Faloppa F. Conservative interventions for treating middle third clavicle fractures in adolescents and adults. Cochrane Database Syst Rev. 2016;2016(12):CD007121. https://doi.org/10.1002/14651858.CD007121.pub4.
26. MacNeille R, Hennrikus WL. Value-based treatment of common pediatric fractures by primary care. Clin Pediatr. 2018;57(12):1378–84. https://doi.org/10.1177/0009922818775743.
27. Stepanyan H, Gendelberg D, Hennrikus W. Management of simple clavicle fractures by primary care physicians. Clin Pediatr. 2017;56:467–71.
28. McKee MD, Kreder HJ, Mandel S, et al. Nonoperative treatment compared with plate fixation of displaced midshaft clavicular fractures: a multicenter, randomized clinical trial. J Bone Joint Surg. 2007;89(1):1–10. https://doi.org/10.2106/JBJS.F.00020.
29. Bae DS, Shah AS, Kalish LA, Kwon JY, Waters PM. Shoulder motion, strength, and functional outcomes in children with established malunion of the clavicle. J Pediatr Orthop. 2013;33(5):544–50. https://doi.org/10.1097/BPO.0b013e3182857d9e.

Casting and Splinting Pearls: Methods to Improve Value

4

Elia Newman and James E. Toledano

Introduction

Mastering casting techniques enhances value by improving patient outcomes and reducing healthcare costs. Casting is becoming a lost art. For example, elbow extension casting, cast wedging, pressure injury prevention, and wet cast prevention and treatment are casting topics sometimes forgotten but reemphasized in the current chapter. By refining these casting practices, clinicians can reduce reintervention rates, optimize resource utilization, and deliver safe and superior care.

Value-Based Themes

Elbow Extension Casting in Pediatric Fractures

Elbow extension casting is a less commonly utilized yet highly effective alternative to traditional 90° flexed-elbow casting for specific pediatric upper extremity fractures (Fig. 4.1). Extension casting offers substantial value by improving fracture stability and minimizing the need for repeat reductions.

One study examining children with closed, displaced forearm fractures found no cases of secondary displacement in the 60 children treated with an extension cast. In

E. Newman
Pediatric Orthopaedics, Center for Orthopaedics, Arnold Palmer Hospital for Children, Orlando, FL, USA
e-mail: Elia.newman@orlandohealth.com

J. E. Toledano (✉)
Director of Pediatric Orthopaedics, Center for Orthopaedics, Arnold Palmer Hospital for Children, Orlando, FL, USA
e-mail: james.toledano@orlandohealth.com

W. L. Hennrikus, R. M. Schwend (eds.), *Value in Pediatric Orthopaedics*,
https://doi.org/10.1007/978-3-032-19570-8_4

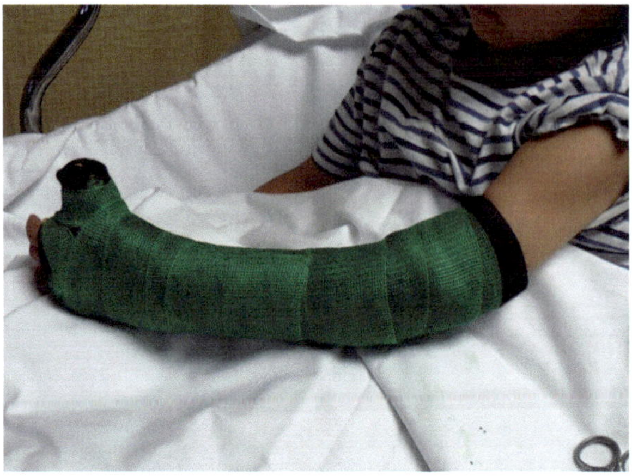

Fig. 4.1 Application of a well-padded long arm cast with the elbow in 20° of flexion. A firm interosseous mold maintains fracture reduction, while a supracondylar mold and thumb spica extension help prevent cast slippage

contrast, 18% of the 51 children treated with a flexed-elbow cast experienced loss of alignment [1]. Another series reported a 5% repeat reduction rate (4 out of 86 cases) for extension casting of displaced diaphyseal both-bone forearm fractures, which was significantly lower than the pooled average from the literature of 15% repeat reduction rate for flexed-elbow casts [2].

Concerns about elbow stiffness with extension casting are largely unfounded. Most children regain full range of motion within a few weeks to 3 months after cast removal, usually without physical therapy [1, 3, 4]. While the extended position may initially seem awkward, children adapt quickly, and basic activities such as dressing and eating are similarly limited in both flexed and extended positions [1, 5].

Extension casting may be easier for trainees to apply effectively. For example, one study reported lower loss of reduction rates when trainees applied extension casting for both-bone forearm fractures (2 of 54 cases, or 4%) compared to flexion casting (7 of 71 cases, or 10%) [6].

Consider using a long arm cast with the elbow in extension for the following pediatric fractures:

- *Proximal both-bone forearm fractures*: Especially useful in the short, stout forearms of young children, where flexed casts fail to control ulnar alignment [7].
- *Olecranon fractures*: For minimally displaced olecranon fractures, extension casting neutralizes the displacing pull of the triceps muscle, promoting fracture stability and union [7].
- *Flexion-type supracondylar humerus fractures*: Immobilization in extension is biomechanically advantageous for flexion-type fractures [7, 8], both after closed reduction with casting and pinning. One series of 14 cases reported good to excellent results in ten children treated with extension casting postmanipulation [8].

- *Type II Monteggia fractures*: For ulna fractures with posterior dislocation of the radial head, applying traction with the elbow in full extension helps reduce the radial head. Immobilizing the arm in this extended position afterward supports ulnar alignment and stability [7].

Cast Wedging: Techniques and Tips

Cast wedging is a valuable, minimally invasive technique for correcting unacceptable angulation following initial closed treatment of pediatric long-bone fractures, particularly in the tibia and forearm [9–11].

When performed correctly, cast wedging can improve fracture alignment, potentially eliminating the need for repeat reduction under anesthesia or surgical intervention. Cast wedging improves outcomes, saves time and resources, and reduces healthcare costs [9, 11–13]. Below are the key tips for effective cast wedging:

Timing

Perform cast wedging typically 5–10 days after the initial injury or casting [9, 10, 13]. This timeframe allows initial swelling to subside, making the procedure more comfortable for the child [13]. On the other hand, cast wedging is not effective 3 weeks post injury because callus formation limits mobility at the fracture site.

Analgesia

Consider administering ibuprofen or acetaminophen 30–40 min prior to wedging to alleviate pain and reassure parents that their child's comfort is a priority.

Wedging Technique

- *Localize the fracture site:*
  - Start by taping a paper clip to the cast where you *think* the fracture is, then get an X-ray. On the image, measure how far proximal or distal the paper clip sits in relation to the fracture. Now, go back to the cast, measure that same distance from the paper clip, and mark the location of the fracture apex.
  - Alternatively, check the X-ray to see how far the fracture is from a fixed landmark, such as the distal edge of the cast. Then just measure that same distance on the cast itself and mark the spot (Fig. 4.2).
  - For distal-third radius or tibia shaft fractures, place the wedge about 5 cm *proximal* to the fracture apex. This creates a longer lever arm, enhancing the effectiveness of the correction [10].

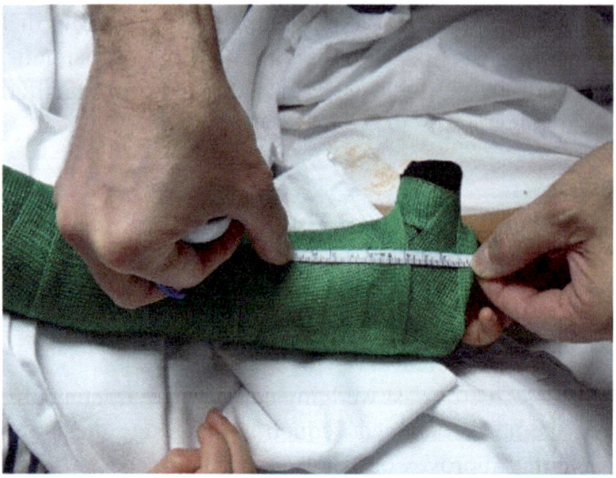

Fig. 4.2 Measure the distance from the fracture site to the cast edge on the X-ray, then replicate that measurement on the patient's limb using a ruler, starting from the distal edge of the cast

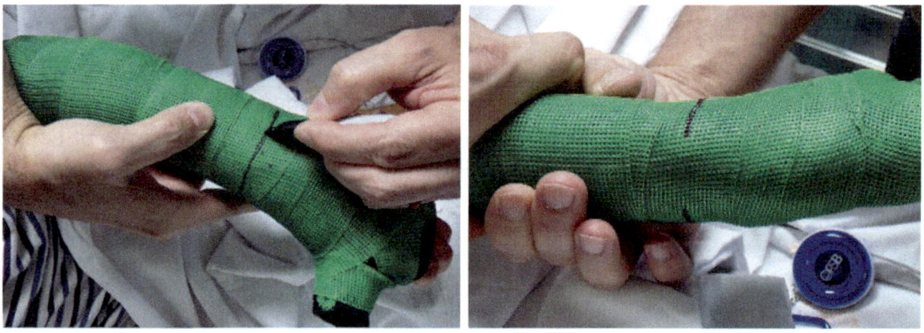

Fig. 4.3 Outline the cast cut by marking two-thirds of the cast's diameter, leaving a small hinge on the convex side of the fracture apex

- *The cut:* On the concave side of the deformity, make a circumferential cut at the level of the fracture, cutting through approximately two-thirds of the cast's diameter and perpendicular to the bone's long axis [13]. Leave a hinge of intact cast material on the convex side of the deformity (Fig. 4.3).
- *The wedge*: On the concave side, gently open the cast cut using a cast spreader until the desired correction is achieved. Then insert a firm, radiolucent spacer (e.g., plastic, cork, or wood) to maintain the correction [10]. Obtain radiographs to confirm alignment, adjusting the wedge size as needed. Once satisfied with the correction, fill the gap with soft cast padding to reduce skin irritation and prevent window edema [14]. Finally, overwrap the area with 2–3 layers of casting material to secure the construct (Fig. 4.4).
- *Limitations:* Cast wedging is a reliable technique, with success rates of up to 96% for tibial shaft fractures and 94% for radial shaft fractures [10]. However, wedging has its limitations. Typically, you can correct up to 5° in the coronal

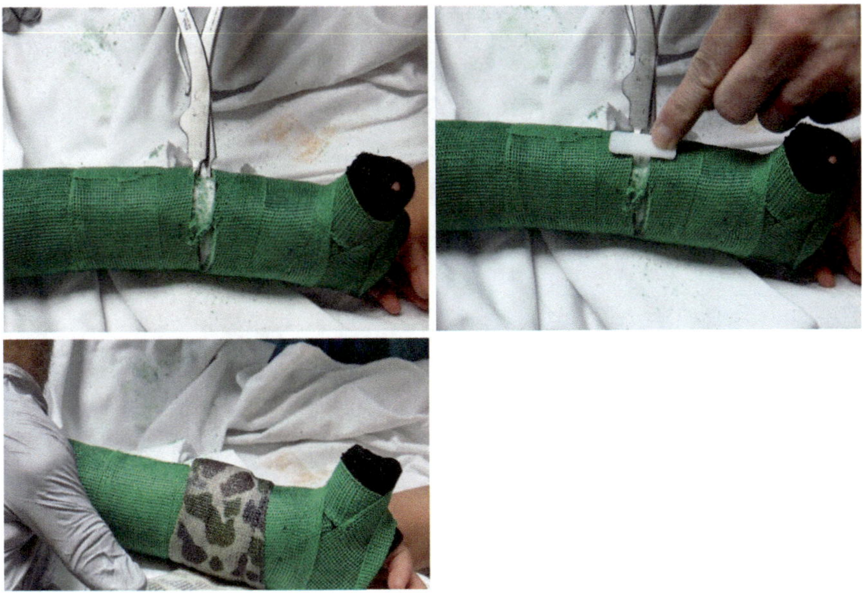

Fig. 4.4 Open the cut with a cast spreader; insert wedge. Repeat x-rays to confirm satisfactory deformity correction, apply additional cast padding and overwrap to secure the wedge in place

plane [10] and 15° in the sagittal plane [9, 11]. If the initial angulation is too severe or postwedging radiographs still show unacceptable alignment, discontinue wedging. In such cases, proceed with closed reduction and recasting under sedation, or consider surgical fixation.

- *Post-wedge care:* Obtain postwedging X-rays to confirm satisfactory correction. Follow up with X-rays about 10 days later to ensure the alignment is maintained. Instruct families to call the office if the child develops new or worsening pain or swelling that doesn't resolve with elevation. This could indicate pressure injury from a cast crease or sharp edge, or in rare instances, compartment syndrome [12].

How to Pad and Cast to Prevent Pressure Injury

Patients especially vulnerable to pressure injuries include nonverbal children, those with impaired sensation or mobility, including spina bifida patients, children requiring prolonged immobilization, and intubated or neurologically impaired trauma patients. Preventing cast-related pressure injuries reduces patient discomfort, minimizing unplanned cast changes and avoiding the burden of wound care or prolonged treatment [15]. Fortunately, most pressure injuries can be prevented with thoughtful padding and early detection.

The heel is the most common site for pressure injury in short leg, long leg, and clubfoot casts [16, 17]. Difazio et al. [18] showed that adding extra padding to the heel reduced skin complications by 56% in both short and long leg casts. Heel ulcers

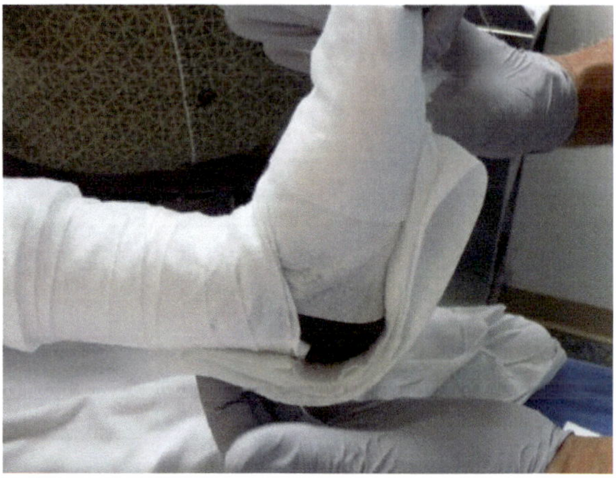

Fig. 4.5 Application of additional layers of cast padding over the heel to reduce the risk of pressure ulcers

were most frequent in short leg casts, likely due to the smaller surface area available for pressure distribution compared to long leg casts. We recommend adding about four extra layers of cast padding directly over the heel, as shown below (Fig. 4.5), followed by an overwrap of cast padding to secure the additional layers in place.

The prominent metatarsal heads are another high-risk area for cast-related pressure injury. A common issue with leg casts is insufficient space around the toes. To prevent this, place a small roll of cast padding under the stockinette next to the small toe before casting (Fig. 4.6). Once the cast sets, remove the padding to create a larger toe box. This method ensures adequate space around the first and fifth metatarsal heads, minimizing compression of the toes.

In upper extremity casts, the first webspace is a common site of pressure irritation. The following image series demonstrates a reliable technique to prevent cast-related rubbing in this area, improving comfort and reducing the risk of skin breakdown (Figs. 4.7, 4.8 and 4.9).

Parent Involvement in Pressure Injury Prevention

Parents play a key role in identifying early signs of cast-related pressure issues. Teach the parents to watch for symptoms such as burning discomfort under the cast, foul odors, drainage, or persistent soreness. Increased fussiness or difficulty settling can also be a sign. Addressing these issues early and adjusting the cast as needed can prevent minor irritations from progressing into serious skin pressure injuries.

Pain Away from the Fracture: A Red Flag

Subtle or vague reports of discomfort, particularly if located away from the fracture site, should raise concern for early skin compromise. Children may not always be able to clearly articulate the problem [17]. Do not dismiss these concerns; instead,

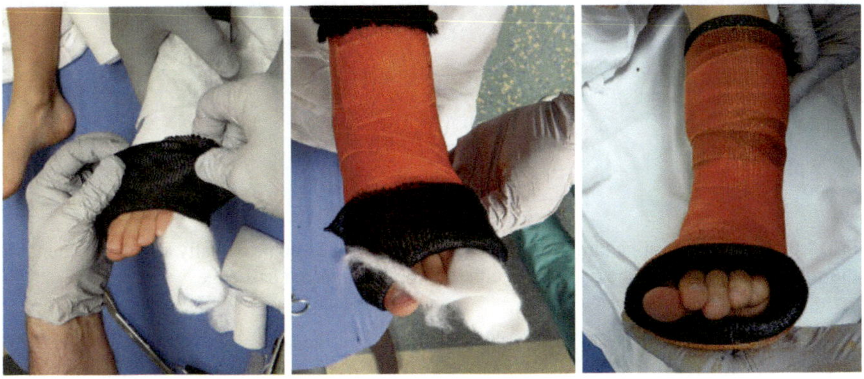

Fig. 4.6 Placement of a temporary cast padding roll under the stockinette to create a larger toe box, reducing pressure on the metatarsal heads

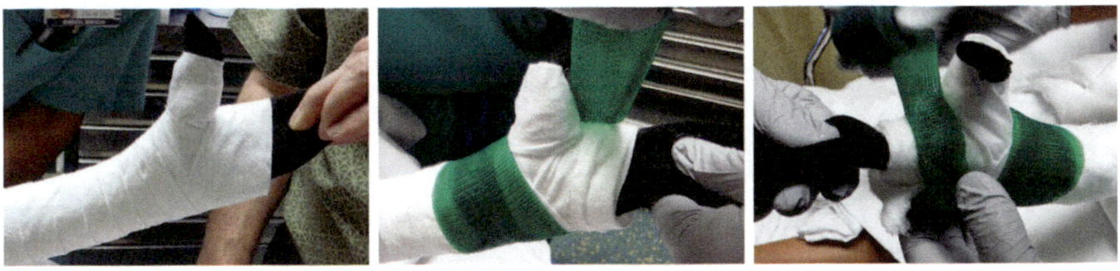

Fig. 4.7 Apply stockinette and padding to the thumb and hand, even if you're applying a standard arm cast without a thumb spica extension, as shown here. Apply the first cast layer. When passing the webspace, pinch and fold it in half

check the cast immediately. If a pressure issue is suspected, cut a window over the area of concern or remove the cast to evaluate the underlying skin [19]. Early intervention can make the difference between a minor skin mark versus a full-thickness pressure injury requiring wound care or surgical treatment.

Cast Slippage Mitigation

Preventing cast slippage is crucial in pediatric fractures and clubfoot management. Cast slippage can result in loss of fracture reduction, malunion, skin pressure injury, additional clinic or emergency department visits, and increased patient discomfort and healthcare costs [20]. Utilizing meticulous casting techniques can reduce these risks.

Here are our top pearls for preventing cast slippage::

General Pearls

- *Avoid excessive padding:* Too much padding can lead to limb motion within the cast, causing slippage and loss of reduction and pressure injury.

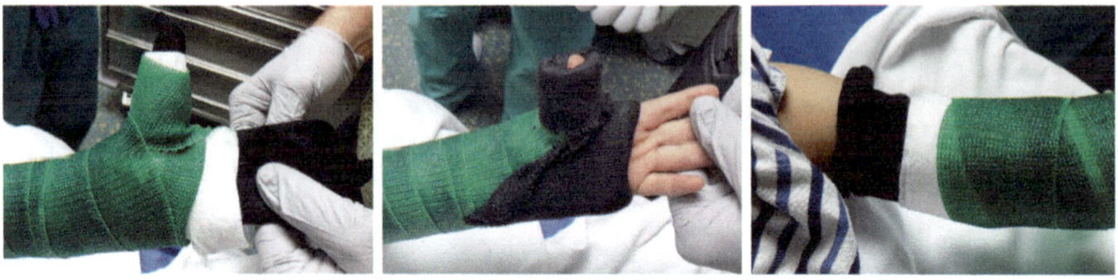

Fig. 4.8 Leave a cuff of padding exposed distally at the hand and proximally at the arm, then fold the stockinette back over the padding to create smooth, protected cast edge

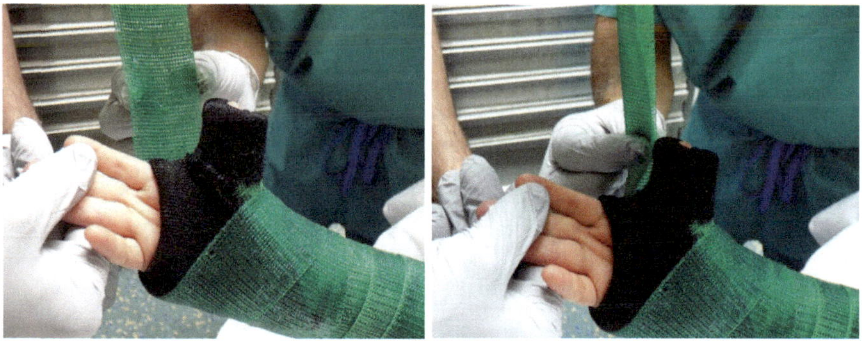

Fig. 4.9 Apply another cast layer to secure the stockinette. Pinch and fold the cast in half when passing through the webspace

- *Optimal cast shape:* Mold casts to fit snugly around the limb's anatomical curves, avoiding cylindrical or banana-shaped loose casts (Fig. 4.10) [20]. For distal radius fractures, aim for a cast index (the ratio of sagittal to coronal cast width at the fracture site) of ≤ 0.8, as this cast index has been shown to reduce the risk of loss of fracture reduction [21].

Upper Extremity Casts

- For children under 5 years of age with a forearm or wrist fracture requiring a cast, use a long arm cast well molded above the medial and lateral epicondyles (Fig. 4.11).
- For the pediatric "escape artists," consider adding a thumb spica extension.

Lower Extremity Casts

- Mold around the malleoli and heel to prevent cast pistoning.

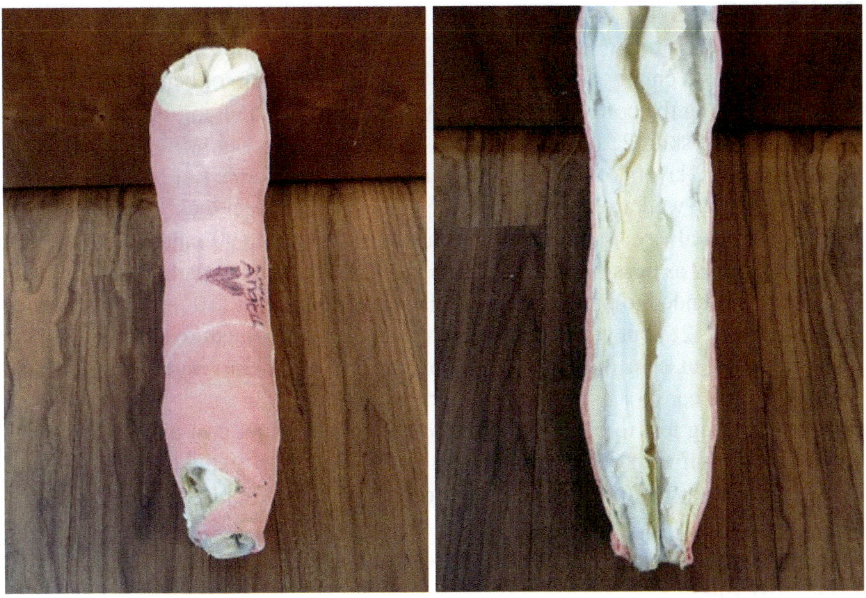

Fig. 4.10 Long arm cast without any molding and excess padding. It was Sir John Charnley who said, "a curved plaster is necessary to make a straight limb."

Fig. 4.11 Supracondylar mold

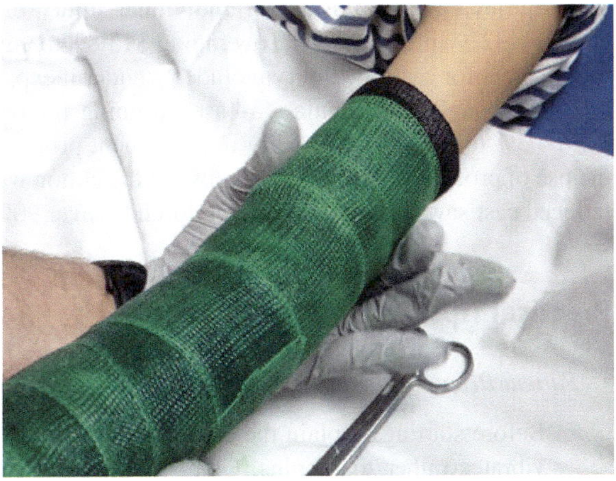

- For long leg casts, add a mold just above the femoral condyles with the knee flexed at 20°–30°.
- For children under 5 years of age, consider using long leg casts instead of short leg casts, as the malleoli are not prominent enough to effectively prevent slippage.

Clubfoot Casts

- In infants with chubby legs and stubby feet, apply tincture of benzoin to the skin before placing the cotton roll. This acts as an adhesive, helping the cast padding adhere to the skin [22, 23].
- Use thin, 1–2 layers of padding to ensure a close and stable fit [24].
- Mold the cast well around the heel to create a secure "heel lock" [25, 26].
- For clubfeet, always apply a long leg cast, flex the knee to 90° and extend the cast as proximally as possible (to the groin) [27]. Three layers of padding at the groin are recommended to prevent rubbing. Flexing the knee to 110°–120° can reduce slippage [27, 28] but can cause skin irritation in the popliteal fossa [23]. Placing petroleum gauze in the fossa or anterior ankle can help reduce irritation and demonstrate care for the delicate skin of newborns.
- Perform a tug test to check the snugness of the clubfoot cast after application. Hold the thigh with one hand and gently pull the cast with the other. If slippage occurs, such as the toes slipping inward into the cast, reapply the cast [26].

Cast Saw Safety

Cast saw safety is very important. Complications such as abrasions, burns, and lacerations occur in up to 4% of cast removals [29–31]. The financial impact of cast saw injuries can be substantial. Individual injury claims range from $2995 to $25,000 [32], with one hospital averaging $15,898 per injured patient annually [31]. Risk factors for cast saw injury include provider inexperience and equipment issues [29, 30]. Thankfully, simulation-based training for residents reduces injury rates from 4.3% to 0.7% [32]. Quality improvement programs, including education and the use of protective strips placed between the cotton webril and the fiberglass, have reduced cast saw complications in children by over 90% [33].

Practical Tips, Tricks, and Pearls

- *Patient Preparation and Communication*
  - Before starting, explain the cast saw in simple terms and demonstrate that it vibrates rather than spins. Gently touching the moving blade to your own palm can ease fears and build trust.
  - Noise: The saw is loud. Offer ear protection, especially for younger or anxious children.
  - Encourage the child to speak up if they feel any heat, tingling, or pain, so immediate adjustments can be made to prevent injury.

- *Cutting Technique*
  - Perform an “in-and-out” cutting motion instead of dragging the saw along the cast. Dragging increases friction, heat, and the risk of catching skin [29, 30]. Think of the cast saw as perforating the cast rather than sawing wood.
  - Keep your thumb on the cast while sawing to maintain control and prevent the blade from going too deep (Fig. 4.12).
  - Periodically touch the side of the blade. If it’s too hot for your finger, it’s too hot for the patient’s skin. To prevent thermal injury, frequently lift the blade, pause, and cool it with a damp cloth, as temperatures above 50°C can cause burns [31, 32].
  - Avoid cutting directly over bony prominences, such as the malleoli, ulnar styloid, or olecranon, as these areas have less protective subcutaneous tissue [30].
  - Avoid flexion creases: Do not cut directly over flexion creases (e.g., antecubital fossa, popliteal fossa), as the cast material bunches and padding thins, increasing the risk of injury [19].

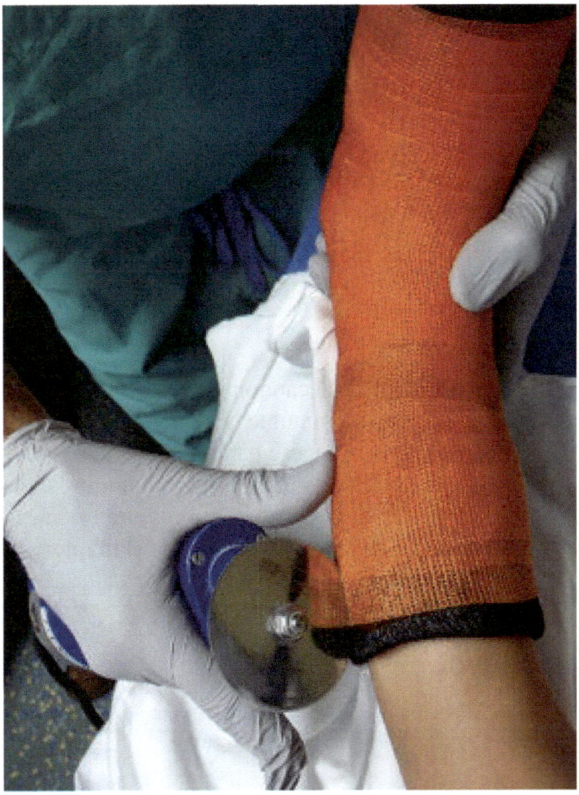

Fig. 4.12 Rest your thumb on cast for better control when cutting

- *Protective Barriers*
  - If you did not apply the cast, exercise caution, as the padding depth and quality are unknown. Waterproof undercast materials provide less thermal protection than cotton. When in doubt, insert a thin plastic "zip stick" between the cast and padding to guide the saw and protect the skin [19].
  - Use commercially made protective strips, placed on top of the cast padding (Fig. 4.13). These strips provide a reliable physical barrier, significantly reducing the risk of blade-to-skin contact injuries [33]. The strips also help mitigate heat transfer during cast removal [31, 33].

- *Equipment*
  - Vacuum attachment: Use a cast saw with a vacuum attachment to cool the blade and reduce dust [30, 34, 35].
  - Always inspect the saw blade before use. A dull blade generates more heat and requires increased pressure, raising the risk of thermal injury and loss of control [31, 35]. Studies show that without a vacuum, blades may need replacement after just 30–60 bivalved plaster casts, whereas with a vacuum, they can last up to 100 casts before exceeding safe temperature thresholds [34]. Establish a regular blade inspection and replacement protocol at your office, emergency department, and operative suite.

- *Train Your Staff*
  - Implement a standardized training program for all personnel involved in cast removal, focusing on proper cast saw handling and injury prevention techniques [19, 32]. Simulation-based training for residents and in-experienced staff reduces injury rates and is cost-effective [32].

- *Special Considerations*
  - Exercise additional caution with sedated, anesthetized, or nonverbal children, as they cannot communicate pain or burning sensations. The risk of cast saw injury is higher in these patients [29, 30, 33].
  - Freshly applied or wet casts: Avoid cutting casts that are still curing or wet. Softer material requires more pressure to cut, reducing tactile feedback and control, which increases the risk of skin injury beneath the cast [30].

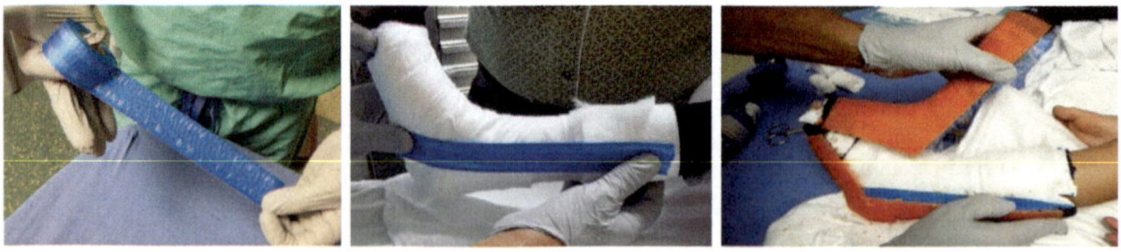

Fig. 4.13 Application of protective strips. These strips help prevent blade-to-skin contact and reduce heat transfer during cast cutting

- Thick casts: Thick casts require more time and generate more heat during removal [35]. Take frequent pauses to cool the cast saw blade.
- Safely removing a cast depends, in part, on how the cast is applied. Just as aircraft are designed for safety, a well-made cast should incorporate both longitudinal splints and circular material. The cast should be thin, with material applied in both directions. For example, spine, spica, and limb casts should include longitudinal splints over areas that won't be cut with the cast saw, typically the anterior and posterior aspects of the cast. This ensures that the saw cuts over thinner lateral areas of the cast, generating less heat and reducing the risk of cast saw burns to the child.
- Avoid using warm or hot water in the operative suite. Burns have occurred in the operative suite due to the use of hot water when applying a cast. Cold water is safer. Warm or hot water can increase the heat generated during material curing in a patient under anesthesia. In addition, do not place the new cast on a plastic pillow. Placing the fresh cast on a plastic pillow can further increase the cast heat.
- When a child is under general anesthesia, the protective reflexes of the middle ear, mediated by the stapedius and tensor tympani muscles, are inactive. These muscles usually contract in response to loud sounds, reducing sound transmission to the inner ear. Without this reflex, loud noises, such as a cast saw near the ear, can transmit unchecked sound energy to the cochlea, increasing the risk of inner ear damage. To minimize this risk, avoid using loud cast saw equipment near the patient's head while the child is under anesthesia.

Wet Casts: Prevention and Solutions

Wet casts are a leading cause of cast-related emergency room visits in children, accounting for nearly 29% of returns [36]. Moisture-related complications, such as maceration, odor, ulcers, and infection, can lead to unplanned cast changes, treatment delays, and worse outcomes [18, 37]. With effective prevention strategies such as waterproof casting options, unplanned recasting rates can drop from 24% to 7% [38], improving patient outcomes, reducing the emergency department burden, and improve patient and parent satisfaction [39].

Traditional Casts: Keeping Them Dry and Managing Mishaps

While the adage "keep your cast dry"is a standard recommendation, reinforcing how and addressing accidental wetting is key.

- Prevention pearls:
  - Provide clear, practical guidance on keeping the cast dry during bathing. We recommend using commercially available reusable cast protectors or the DIY method with plastic bags, as outlined below.

  - Use two sturdy plastic bags (e.g., kitchen trash bags) large enough to fully cover the cast and extend several inches above the cast.
  - Secure the top edges of both bags to the skin above the cast using duct tape. First, seal the inner bag directly to the skin, then place the second bag over it and tape it securely. Ensure the tape does not touch the cast, as moisture can wick under the tape and soak into the cast [40].
  - This double-bag method prevents about 99.6% of external water absorption and costs about 30 cents per use [40].
  - It is important to explain that this DIY method serves as a secondary barrier and is not intended for full immersion, such as bathing or swimming. For children or individuals who cannot manage cast care independently with this method, sponge baths or other localized hygiene methods are safer and suitable alternatives [40].
  - Avoid using single bags with rubber bands or wrapping the cast in cling plastic film [41].

- If a traditional cast gets wet, instruct parents to act quickly. They should use a hairdryer on a cool setting to dry the cast (hot air can cause thermal injury). A damp cast, especially postop, may need to be replaced. Serious infections, including osteomyelitis, have been seen in children with pin fixation after supracondylar fractures when wet casts were not addressed. Prompt action can prevent complications. Be vigilant for signs of maceration, erythema, blistering, or secondary infection.

  - Every August, we see a familiar scenario in our office: A boy with a supracondylar humerus fracture, pinned and casted, decides to swim in a pond. At this time of year, just before school starts, the pond is teeming with bacteria. We've seen serious infections, including osteomyelitis, in these cases if treatment is delayed. A quick visit to the clinic for action can prevent complications. Reinforce that prevention and early intervention can turn a major problem into a minor issue.

Waterproof Casts

Waterproof cast liners/padding offer a valuable alternative to traditional cotton padding in nonsurgical fracture care. Waterproof padding is combined with a fiberglass cast outer shell [37–39]. The benefits are clear. Patients can shower, bathe, and swim without compromising cast integrity or risking skin maceration. This leads to improved hygiene, enhanced comfort, and reduced odor. From a cost-effectiveness standpoint, unplanned recasting rates drop from 24% with standard cotton padded casts to 7% with waterproof cast padding [42]. While waterproof padding adds about $17 in material costs per cast, the overall cost-effectiveness remains favorable, with around $81 saved per recast avoided [42]. Waterproof casts consistently outperform traditional casts in patient and parent satisfaction [38, 39]. From the child's perspective, these casts allow continued participation in water-related activities and improve quality of life during recovery.

- Pearls for waterproof casts:
  - Ensure the waterproof liner/padding is applied smoothly and wrinkle-free to prevent skin irritation [37]. Apply two layers, with a third layer over bony prominences for added protection.
  - Remind patients and parents that while waterproof casts can get wet, drying the cast thoroughly is still important. While the liner/padding allows water to drain and evaporate, the skin underneath may remain damp. Encourage air drying or gently patting the cast with a towel. Most liners dry within 30–90 min [37, 38]. Advise against swimming right before bedtime to prevent causing damp sheets and potential skin irritation.
  - After swimming in chlorinated or saltwater, advise rinsing the cast and limb with fresh water to remove any chlorine or salt residue to protect the skin.
  - Have a clear conversation with the parents about costs. Waterproof liners are often not covered by insurance, so families should be aware that they will have to pay for the waterproof materials [43].
  - Be mindful that waterproof cast liners and padding do not mold as effectively as a traditional cast. One study found waterproof casts had a higher cast index compared to traditional cotton padding casts, although the clinical significance of fracture stability remains unclear [44].
  - Although waterproof liners are generally well-tolerated, minor skin irritation or contact dermatitis can occur [37]. Instruct families to report any persistent itching, redness, or discomfort so that issues can be addressed early.
  - Do not use a waterproof cast when there are incisions or percutaneous pins under the cast.

Summary

The current chapter provides practical, evidence-based strategies to help clinicians improve outcomes and reduce costs when applying and removing casts in children.

Editor Comments

WLH

The authors have written a practical and helpful chapter that every physician, NP, PA, MA, resident, and cast tech should keep in their library. Casting is a lost art, and complications from casting are becoming more commonplace. Value-based topics emphasized in the current chapter include casting in extension, cast wedging, cast padding tips, cast saw pearls, wet cast wisdom, waterproof casting techniques, and more.

RMS

The term “pressure injury“offers a more comprehensive and accurate description of the range of tissue damage that can occur due to pressure. In the current chapter, this pressure comes from a cast. The term pressure injury reflects both early and advanced stages of injury, which is essential terminology for early detection and intervention for best practices in wound care. This shift in terminology potentially contributes to better patient outcomes by improving communication, fostering quicker recognition of issues, and encouraging timely interventions.

References

1. Bochang C, Jie Y, Zhigang W, Wiegl D, Bar-On E, Katz K. Immobilisation of forearm fractures in children. Extended versus flexed elbow. J Bone Joint Surg Series B [Internet]. 2005;87(7):994–6. [cited 2025 May 18]; Available from: https://pubmed.ncbi.nlm.nih.gov/15972919/
2. Neal KM, Osterbur TA, Kiebzak GM. Improving quality in the treatment of pediatric forearm fractures: minimizing the need for repeat intervention with long-arm extension casting. J Pediatr Orthop [Internet]. 2020;40(7):329–33. [cited 2025 May 18]; Available from: https://pubmed.ncbi.nlm.nih.gov/32032216/
3. Yadav P, Phalak MO, Patel S, Chaudhari T, Nair A, Gurnani S. Functional outcome of closed reduction and extension casting in forearm fractures in children. Cureus [Internet]. 2022;14(2) [cited 2025 May 18]; Available from: https://pubmed.ncbi.nlm.nih.gov/35371711/
4. Walker JL, Rang M. Forearm fractures in children. Cast treatment with the elbow extended. J Bone Joint Surg B [Internet]. 1991;73(2):299–301. [cited 2025 May 18]; Available from: https://pubmed.ncbi.nlm.nih.gov/2005160/
5. Shaer JA, Smith B, Turco VJ. Mid-third forearm fractures in children: an unorthodox treatment. Am J Orthop (Belle Mead NJ). 1999;28(1):60–3.
6. Babazadeh S, Mason TG, Petterwood J, Taylor SW, Chapman N, Fettke GR. Extension casting for both-bone forearm fractures in children. Acta Orthop Belg. 2017;83(3):445–8.
7. Reynolds AW, Hennrikus WL, Adebayo T, Winthrop Z, Gendelberg D. Utility of a long arm extension cast in management of pediatric fractures: a technique revisited. Trauma Case Rep [Internet]. 2018;17:14. [cited 2025 May 18]; Available from: https://pmc.ncbi.nlm.nih.gov/articles/PMC6178488/
8. Williamson DM, Cole WG. Flexion supracondylar fractures of the humerus in children: treatment by manipulation and extension cast. Injury [Internet]. 1991;22(6):451–5. [cited 2025 May 18]; Available from: https://pubmed.ncbi.nlm.nih.gov/1757135/
9. Samora JB, Klingele KE, Beebe AC, Kean JR, Klamar J, Beran MC, et al. Is there still a place for cast wedging in pediatric forearm fractures? J Pediatr Orthop [Internet]. 2014;34(3):246–52. [cited 2025 May 4]; Available from: https://pubmed.ncbi.nlm.nih.gov/24045589/
10. Kattan JM, Leathers MP, Barad JH, Silva M. The effectiveness of cast wedging for the treatment of pediatric fractures. J Pediatr Orthop B [Internet]. 2014;23(6):566–71. [cited 2025 May 4]; Available from: https://gemini.google.com
11. Gaukel S, Leu S, Fink L, Skovgaard SR, Ramseier LE, Vuille-Dit-bille RN. Cast wedging: a systematic review of the present evidence. J Child Orthop [Internet]. 2017;11(5):398–403. [cited 2025 May 4]; Available from: https://gemini.google.com
12. Ho CA. Tibia shaft fractures in adolescents: how and when can they be managed successfully with cast treatment? J Pediatr Orthop [Internet]. 2016;36(4):S15–8. [cited 2025 May 4]; Available from: https://pubmed.ncbi.nlm.nih.gov/27078230/

13. Freislederer F, Berberich T, Erb TO, Mayr J. Pain during cast wedging of forearm shaft and distal forearm fractures in children aged 3 to 12 years—a prospective, observational study. Children [Internet]. 2020;7(11):229. [cited 2025 May 4]; Available from: https://pmc.ncbi.nlm.nih.gov/articles/PMC7697833/
14. Mencio GA, Frick SL, Green NE. Green's skeletal trauma in children. Elsevier; 2020.
15. Singh CD, Anderson C, White E, Shoqirat N. The impact of pediatric pressure injury prevention bundle on pediatric pressure injury rates. J Wound Ostomy Continence Nurs [Internet]. 2018;45(3):209–12. [cited 2025 May 3]; Available from: https://pubmed.ncbi.nlm.nih.gov/29722749/
16. Vrankovic MI, Annaheim S, Willibald J, Lieber J, van Hedel HJA, Schlüer AB, et al. Assessment of compression forces in a digitally modified short leg cast for pressure injury risk monitoring in healthy children. Front Pediatr [Internet]. 2023;11. [cited 2025 May 2]; Available from: https://pubmed.ncbi.nlm.nih.gov/38304440/
17. Nie AM. Pressure injury prevention and treatment in critically Ill children. Crit Care Nurs Clin North Am [Internet]. 2020;32(4):521–31. [cited 2025 May 2]; Available from: https://pubmed.ncbi.nlm.nih.gov/33129411/
18. Difazio RL, Harris M, Feldman L, Mahan ST. Reducing the incidence of cast-related skin complications in children treated with cast immobilization. J Pediatr Orthop [Internet]. 2017;37(8):526–31. [cited 2025 May 2]; Available from: https://journals.lww.com/pedorthopaedics/fulltext/2017/12000/reducing_the_incidence_of_cast_related_skin.3.aspx
19. Ellsworth BK, Bram JT, Haeberle HS, DeFrancesco CJ, Scher DM. Back to basics: pediatric casting techniques, pearls, and pitfalls. Iowa Orthop J [Internet]. 2023;43(2):79. [cited 2025 May 3]; Available from: https://pmc.ncbi.nlm.nih.gov/articles/PMC10777705/
20. Dipaola MJ, Abzug JM, Pizzutillo PD, Herman MJ. Incidence and etiology of unplanned cast changes for fractures in the pediatric population. J Pediatr Orthop [Internet]. 2014;34(6):643–6. [cited 2025 May 2]; Available from: https://pubmed.ncbi.nlm.nih.gov/24787307/
21. Kamat AS, Pierse N, Devane P, Mutimer J, Horne G. Redefining the cast index: the optimum technique to reduce redisplacement in pediatric distal forearm fractures. J Pediatr Orthop [Internet]. 2012;32(8):787–91. [cited 2025 May 2]; Available from: https://pubmed.ncbi.nlm.nih.gov/23147621/
22. Ibrahim S. Tincture of Benzoin to prevent cast slippage in clubfoot. Malays Orthop J [Internet]. 2016;10(3):62. [cited 2025 May 1]; Available from: https://pmc.ncbi.nlm.nih.gov/articles/PMC5333691/
23. Mosca VS, Ignacio V, Ponseti. Clubfoot: biomechanics and practical principles-based application of the Ponseti method. Global HELP Organization. [cited 2025 May 2]; Available from: www.orthobooks.org
24. Youn SB, Ranade AS, Agarwal A, Belthur MV. Common errors in the management of idiopathic clubfeet using the Ponseti method: a review of the literature. Children [Internet]. 2023;10(1) [cited 2025 May 2]; Available from: https://pubmed.ncbi.nlm.nih.gov/36670703/
25. Barrie A, Varacallo MA. Clubfoot. StatPearls [Internet]. 2023. [cited 2025 May 2]; Available from: https://www.ncbi.nlm.nih.gov/books/NBK551574/
26. Sinha SK, Garg V, Singh V. The tug test and modified Ponseti casting: a simple and reliable method to improve the efficacy of casting in complex clubfoot. Indian J Orthop [Internet]. 2023;57(7):1147. [cited 2025 May 1]; Available from: https://pmc.ncbi.nlm.nih.gov/articles/PMC10293533/
27. Radler C. The Ponseti method for the treatment of congenital club foot: review of the current literature and treatment recommendations. Int Orthop [Internet]. 2013;37(9):1747. [cited 2025 May 2]; Available from: https://pmc.ncbi.nlm.nih.gov/articles/PMC3764299/
28. Lohan I. Iris Lohan treatment of congenital clubfoot using the Ponseti method workshop manual. 2nd ed. [cited 2025 May 1]; Available from: www.ponseti.info
29. Shore BJ, Hutchinson S, Harris M, Bae DS, Kalish LA, Maxwell W, et al. Epidemiology and prevention of cast saw injuries: results of a quality improvement program at a single institution. J Bone Joint Surg [Internet]. 2014;96(4) [cited 2025 May 10]; Available from: https://pubmed.ncbi.nlm.nih.gov/24553900/

30. Halanski MA. How to avoid cast saw complications. J Pediatr Orthop [Internet]. 2016;36(4):S1–5. [cited 2025 May 10]; Available from: https://pubmed.ncbi.nlm.nih.gov/27152901/
31. Stork NC, Lenhart RL, Nemeth BA, Noonan KJ, Halanski MA. To cast, to saw, and not to injure: can safety strips decrease cast saw injuries? Clin Orthop Relat Res [Internet]. 2016;474(7):1543–52. [cited 2025 May 10]; Available from: https://pubmed.ncbi.nlm.nih.gov/26847455/
32. Bae DS, Lynch H, Jamieson K, Yu-Moe CW, Roussin C. Improved safety and cost savings from reductions in cast-saw burns after simulation-based education for orthopaedic surgery residents. J Bone Joint Surg Am Vol [Internet]. 2017;99(17) [cited 2025 May 10]; Available from: https://pubmed.ncbi.nlm.nih.gov/28872536/
33. Balch Samora J, Samora WP, Dolan K, Klingele KE. A quality improvement initiative reduces cast complications in a pediatric hospital. J Pediatr Orthop [Internet]. 2018;38(2):e43–9. [cited 2025 May 10]; Available from: https://pubmed.ncbi.nlm.nih.gov/29227371/
34. McNeil DS, Trenholm JAI. Establishing safety parameters for orthopaedic cast saw blade usage. J Pediatr Orthop [Internet]. 2021;41(10):E884–8. [cited 2025 May 10]; Available from: https://pubmed.ncbi.nlm.nih.gov/34516468/
35. Monroe KC, Sund SA, Nemeth BA, Noonan KJ, Halanski MA. Cast-saw injuries: assessing blade-to-skin contact during cast removal: does experience or education matter? Physician Sportsmed [Internet]. 2014;42(1):36–42. [cited 2025 May 10]; Available from: https://pubmed.ncbi.nlm.nih.gov/24565820/
36. Nguyen S, Schlechter J, McDowell M. Casting: pearls and pitfalls learned while caring for children's fractures. World J Orthop [Internet]. 2016;7(9):539. [cited 2025 May 13]; Available from: https://pmc.ncbi.nlm.nih.gov/articles/PMC5027008/
37. Shannon EG, DiFazio R, Kasser J, Karlin L, Gerbino P. Waterproof casts for immobilization of children's fractures and sprains. J Pediatr Orthop [Internet]. 2005;25(1):56–9. [cited 2025 May 13]; Available from: https://pubmed.ncbi.nlm.nih.gov/15614060/
38. Derksen RJ, Commandeur JP, Deij R, Breederveld RS. Swim cast versus traditional cast in pediatric distal radius fractures: a prospective randomized controlled trial. J Child Orthop [Internet]. 2013;7(2):117–21. [cited 2025 May 13]; Available from: https://pubmed.ncbi.nlm.nih.gov/24432069/
39. Stevenson AW, Gahukamble AD, Antoniou G, Pool B, Sutherland LM, Cundy P. Waterproof cast liners in paediatric forearm fractures: a randomized trial. J Child Orthop [Internet]. 2013;7(2):123. [cited 2025 May 13]; Available from: https://pmc.ncbi.nlm.nih.gov/articles/PMC3593019/
40. Udall D, Zimmerman R, Bast N, Schlechter J. Efficacy of DIY cast covers: an in vivo study. J Pediatr Orthop. 2024;44(3):164–7.
41. McDowell M, Nguyen S, Schlechter J. A comparison of various contemporary methods to prevent a wet cast. J Bone Joint Surg [Internet]. 2014;96(12):e99(1). [cited 2025 May 13]; Available from: https://pubmed.ncbi.nlm.nih.gov/24951750/
42. Clifford AL, Jennings A, Baez C, Boschert E, Ihnow S, Mcquerry J. Financial implications associated with the use of waterproof casting material in pediatric patients. J Pediatr Orthop [Internet]. 2025; [cited 2025 May 13]; Available from: https://pubmed.ncbi.nlm.nih.gov/40214133/
43. VanInwegen A. The incidence and determinants of waterproof casting in pediatric patients. Biomed J Sci Tech Res. 2018;2(4). https://doi.org/10.26717/BJSTR.2018.02.000787.
44. Nolte MT, Luchetti TJ, Bohl DD, Kogan M. Comparison of waterproof versus cotton cast liners on cast index in pediatric forearm fractures. Acta Orthop Belg [Internet]. 2022;88(4):733–7. [cited 2025 May 13]; Available from: https://pubmed.ncbi.nlm.nih.gov/36800657/

Value-Based Care for Pediatric Supracondylar Humerus Fractures

5

Richard M. Schwend and William L. Hennrikus

Introduction

Supracondylar humerus fractures are the most common operative fracture in children. About 80,000 children in the United States sustain a supracondylar fracture each year, with 24% receiving operative treatment [2]. The estimated annual cost of this treatment is about $480 million [3, 4]. Improving value for pediatric health care has a potentially greater impact due to children's longer lifespan and potential for productivity [1]. Although the modified Gartland fracture classification (Fig. 5.1) is used to guide treatment decisions [5], variation in factors such as surgical time, anesthesia time, postoperative immobilization, number of postoperative visits, and number of radiographs offers opportunities for standardization and cost reduction [7].

R. M. Schwend
Children's Mercy Hospital, Kansas City, MO, USA
e-mail: rmschwend@cmh.edu

W. L. Hennrikus (✉)
Pennsylvania State College of Medicine, Hershey, PA, USA
e-mail: whennrikus@pennstatehealth.psu.edu

W. L. Hennrikus, R. M. Schwend (eds.), *Value in Pediatric Orthopaedics*,
https://doi.org/10.1007/978-3-032-19570-8_5

Fracture Type	Modified Gartland Classification
Type I	Nondisplaced, minimally displaced
Type II	Displaced in extension. Posterior cortical contact with posterior hinge IIA - no displacement on coronal or axial plane IIB - Rotational displacement or angulation in the axial or coronal plane
Type III	Complete displacement. No useful cortical contact
Type IV	Multidirectional instability. Incompetent periosteal hinge with instability in flexion and extension during the reduction attempt. This type is diagnosed at the time of surgery.

Fig. 5.1 Modified Gartland classification for supracondylar humerus fractures

Value-Based Themes

Nonoperative Care Is Appropriate for Type I and IIA Fractures

The decision for surgical management is based on the child's age and severity of the injury [6]. Type I fractures are nondisplaced with minimal risk for complications or poor outcomes. Three weeks of immobilization is usually sufficient. The traditional 1-week check-up visit can be omitted if the splint or cast is applied well. In select cases, such as a child who lives far away, the parents can remove the splint or soft cast at home. More typically, the immobilization is removed in the clinic at 3 weeks. A radiograph at this visit is not required and rarely has value [9].

The decision to do surgery has a great influence on the cost of care [7]. This decision can be controversial for Gartland type IIA fractures, which are stable with angulation purely in the sagittal plane. Especially for a child less than 5 years old with a type IIA fracture, a splint or cast for 3 weeks is appropriate, and remodeling can correct the hyperextension deformity. Multiple recent systematic reviews and prospective studies confirm that many Type IIA fractures can be managed nonoperatively, with similar functional outcomes and patient satisfaction, but a higher rate of residual sagittal deformity and treatment failures requiring surgery [8–11]. Predictors of failure include rotational/coronal deformity and a shaft-condylar angle of <30 [10, 11]. For the patient older than 5 years with a type IIA fracture, closed reduction under sedation with immobilization can be performed [2, 12]. The elbow is immobilized at less than 90° of flexion to avoid the risk of vascular compromise and compartment syndrome [13].

If surgical management is chosen, a community hospital setting has been shown to deliver this care at 44% less than a teaching hospital due to lower operating room and anesthesia costs [6]. Ambulating surgery centers are as safe as hospitals and more cost-effective [14]. Although the AAOS recommends reduction and pin fixation of all displaced type II fractures, this recommendation can result in unnecessary surgery in 72% of patients with this fracture type [15] [12]. For example, Liebs reported that 141 of 143 type II fractures were treated successfully with closed reduction and simple immobilization [16]. Treatment should be individualized by the child's age, degree of angulation, and surgeon's experience. At 3 weeks, if a splint or soft cast was used, the parents can remove at home.

Delayed Care and Surgery Center for IIB Fractures

Remodeling does not reliably occur for displaced Gartland IIB fractures due to the added rotational and coronal plane deformity [17]. Type IIB fractures can fail simple reduction or be unstable in a cast. Therefore, adding pin fixation is recommended [18]. However, closed reduction percutaneous pinning (CRPP) for type IIB fractures is not an emergency. For type IIB fractures, the elbow can be splinted, and the child discharged from the emergency room or urgent care with surgery scheduled for the same day surgical unit within several days [9, 17]. Since 2009, there has been an increased use of outpatient surgical management for Type II fractures with no change in outcomes, but at 60% of the cost of inpatient care [19]. Local fracture site injections of bupivacaine can reduce the need for postoperative opioids [20]. In addition, after secure fixation and immobilization, there is no need for a 1-week postoperative visit. Only one postop visit is needed at 3 weeks to remove the splint/cast and pins [21]. In most cases, no additional radiographs or routine use of physical therapy is necessary [22].

Minimizing Unnecessary Transfers from Emergency Rooms

Community hospitals typically have lower costs than academic centers, and it is sometimes not cost-effective to transfer a patient with a supracondylar fracture to an academic center if the local orthopedic surgeon is experienced, willing, and available [23]. All orthopedic surgeons have passed the American College of Graduate Medical Education (ACGME) milestone during residency for treating supracondylar fractures [24]. However, as practicing orthopedic surgeons, some prefer not to come to the emergency room to evaluate a child with a supracondylar fracture when on call. This can lead to type I and type II supracondylar fractures being unnecessarily transferred in the middle of the night [23]. In addition, the cost and inconvenience to families having to travel longer distances for this care should be considered in the decision to transfer to another hospital [21, 23, 25].

Less night-time surgery, less fluoroscopy, shorter surgical times, and less open reductions have been reported when pediatric orthopedic surgeons perform the surgery for supracondylar fractures [9, 20, 21]. However, outcomes and complications of treatment of supracondylar fractures are similar for pediatric orthopedic surgeons compared to general orthopedic surgeons [6, 26–28] and orthopedic trauma surgeons [29, 30]. In some academic settings, with a shared call schedule, general orthopedic surgeons have similar training, skill, and experience to treat these fractures as pediatric orthopedic surgeons [31]. The individual surgeon, the fracture type, and the surgical time are the main factors contributing to the $6345 average surgical charge when treating a supracondylar fracture [32]. The high cost of operating room time is one area of focus that surgeons and hospital leadership can improve, regardless of hospital type or location [32].

Next Morning Surgery Is Generally Appropriate for Most Type III Fractures

After-hours surgical treatment of displaced Gartland type III fractures can have higher rates of mal-reduction and poor fixation. The latest literature shows that time-to-surgery (e.g., 18 h) does not affect outcomes, challenging current quality metrics [33]. These uncommon events can increase costs due to revision surgery [29, 34]. In cases with intact vascularity, the surgery can be safely performed the next day during working hours without an increased risk of open reduction, iatrogenic nerve injury, pin site infection, or reoperation [35, 36].

Most supracondylar fractures can be treated with closed reduction and percutaneous pinning, estimated to have a cost savings of US $2312 compared to open reduction [37]. The rate of open reduction, mostly performed for irreducible fractures rather than for vascular concerns, ranges from 0% to 15% among surgeons, representing another opportunity for standardization and cost reduction [38]. Some fractures present with a "pucker sign," representing a more severe soft tissue injury, but can often be "milked" for successful closed reduction [39]. Open type III supracondylar fractures are rare, but can be treated with timely antibiotics, wound management, and fracture reduction with fixation, and have similar outcomes to closed fractures [13, 40].

When Is It Safer to Do Surgery at Night?

Displaced supracondylar fractures presenting with an abnormal vascular exam should have emergency surgery, including surgery in the middle of the night [41]. In addition, while in the operating room, after reduction and pinning, the surgeon should perform an examination for hand perfusion and document the exam in the operative report. If the hand is pale (> 3-s capillary refill time) and the pulse is absent (pink/pulseless), the AAOS Appropriate Use Criteria (AUC) for pediatric supracondylar humerus fracture recommends additional immediate emergency surgery by the orthopedic surgeon, often in collaboration with a plastic or vascular surgeon, to restore the pulse [42]. The brachial artery may be caught in the fracture site and can be freed, or if damaged, then vascular repair is done. If after closed reduction and pinning, the hand is pink, perfused (capillary refill time < 3 s), but no palpable/Dopplerable pulse (pink/pulseless), the patient is admitted for 24–48 h of observation. Lastly, if after reduction and pinning, there is a palpable pulse, and the hand is well perfused (< 3 s capillary refill), the patient can be discharged home after a few hours of observation.

Splash and Dash: Minimal Draping

A seldom-used method to improve value when treating displaced supracondylar fractures is the semisterile surgical technique, in which the limb is prepped, but with minimal draping and no surgical gown (Fig. 5.2). This technique has been shown to be safe and cost-effective [43, 44] and can decrease surgical time by 10 min [45]. Draping time was decreased by 75%, anesthesia time by 17%, and medical waste by

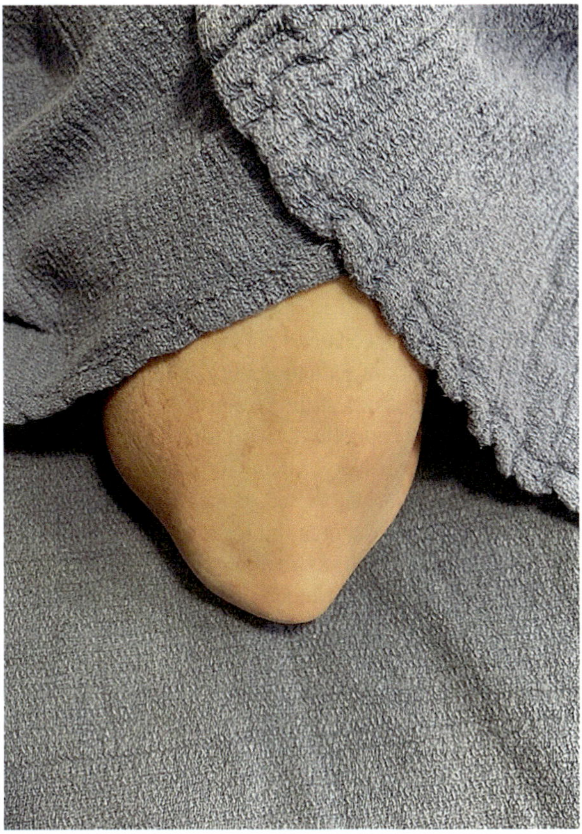

Fig. 5.2 Semisterile technique. Prep and minimal draping after closed reduction with C-arm control. The surgeon wears sterile gloves, but no gown. Mask is optional

88% [44]. In one study of 1270 patients, semisterile draping with no gown or mask was compared to full sterile draping [43]. Three deep infections occurred—all in the full sterile draping group. Potential national cost savings in gown, masks, draping, and 10 min less surgical time were estimated at about $four million/year [43, 46].

No Antibiotics Please

Antibiotics add drug costs and may lead to adverse effects or resistance, so a simple and effective method to improve value when treating supracondylar fractures with closed reduction and percutaneous pinning is to omit giving perioperative antibiotics [47]. This practice change has been demonstrated to be safe and effective [48, 49]. In a placebo-controlled trial of preoperative antibiotics of 160 patients, there was no difference in infection rates between the antibiotic group (1.2%) versus the placebo group (1.3%) [50]. Use of antibiotics in the post-operative period is also commonly performed; however, there is no benefit to this expensive practice [51].

The negligible infection difference underscores that prophylactic antibiotics provide no value and may even cause harm.

Standardize the Pin Configuration

The quality of the intraoperative reduction utilizing the periosteal hinge and having stout pins engage bone securely with bicolumnar fixation are the keys to regain fracture stability [52, 53] . The advantage of using three pins rather than only two is that if one of the pins is not secure, there are still two pins holding the reduction. Common pin configurations are 2–3 lateral pins or two lateral pins with one medial pin. Cross-pinning is more stable with less risk of loss of reduction but has higher risk of ulna nerve injury [54–58]. Gottschalk recommended a stronger construct that resists rotational forces, with the lateral pin started in the capitellum, larger pin size, and maximum spread of the pins [59]. We also recommend pins larger than 0.062″, such as 5/64″ for children over 5 years of age, since larger pins are more secure and are less likely to fail. We recommend lateral pinning for type IIB fractures and for many type III fractures.

However, for type III and IV fractures, in about 20% of cases, lateral pin fixation is not stable enough, and a medial pin is needed. For example, oblique fracture patterns, medial comminution, highly unstable fractures, an unstable reduction, open fractures, and an unreliable child are relative indications for medial pin fixation [13, 60, 61]. Methods of safe medial pin insertion have been reported [62, 63] including a mini-open exposure of the ulnar nerve when placing the medial pin [57, 58, 64]. In addition, Edmonds reported a simple technique of first stabilizing the reduced fracture with 1–2 lateral pins, then extending the elbow to relax the ulnar nerve, palpating the medial epicondyle to assure that the ulnar nerve is not overlying, then placing the medial pin percutaneously [65]. Figure 5.3 illustrates our technique of palpation of the medial

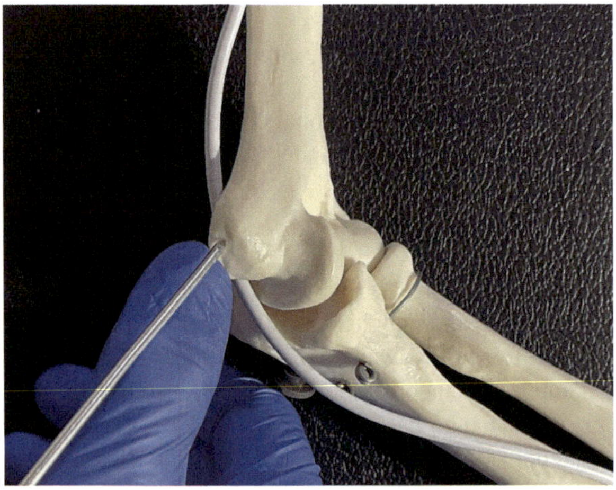

Fig. 5.3 After fixation of the lateral column with two pins, the elbow is extended to less than 90 deg. and the medial epicondyle is palpated. This ensures that the ulnar nerve remains posterior to the medial epicondyle and the medial pin can safely be inserted

epicondyle to ensure that the ulnar nerve is not at risk. We have used a similar technique and stimulated the medial pin after insertion with a disposable nerve stimulator (Fig. 5.4c). The decision to use a medial pin is made on a case-by-case basis based on the fracture severity, pattern, stability, and surgeon experience.

Minimize Aftercare

Another method to improve value when treating supracondylar fractures with surgery is to minimize the aftercare. For example, 5 cc of 0.25% bupivacaine injection with epinephrine into the fracture site or olecranon fossa after pinning for pain relief, use of postoperative non-steroidal anti-inflammatory drug (NSAIDs), avoidance of opioids, and earlier discharge to home have high value [20, 66–68]. Local

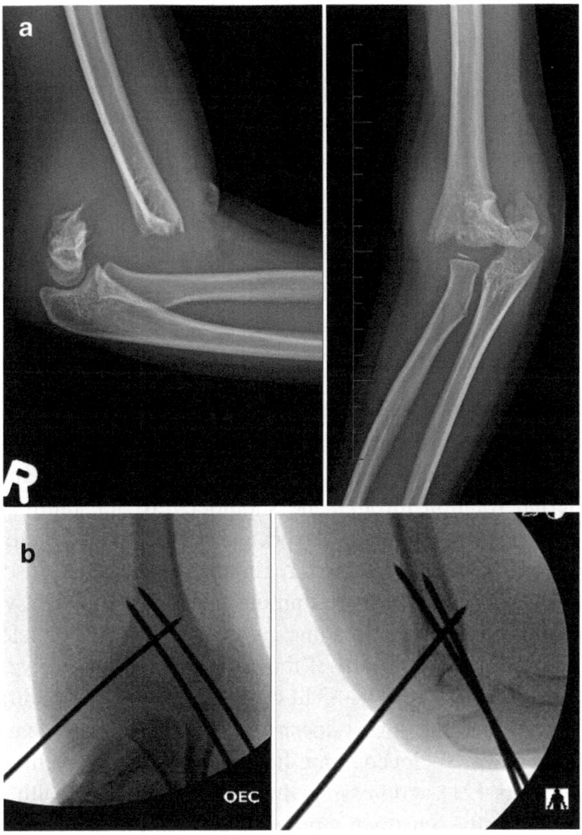

Fig. 5.4 (**a**) Anteroposterior and lateral radiographs of a right elbow demonstrating a type III supracondylar fracture with complete posterior-medial displacement of the distal humerus. (**b**). Intraoperative fluoroscopic images showing fixation using 5/16″ crossed Steinman pins. There is proper placement of the pins using a "cross-pinned" technique. (**c**) Intraoperative application of the VARI-STIM® III Nerve Locator (Medtronic, Minneapolis, MN, USA) to the pins with a grounding wire in the distal triceps brachii muscle

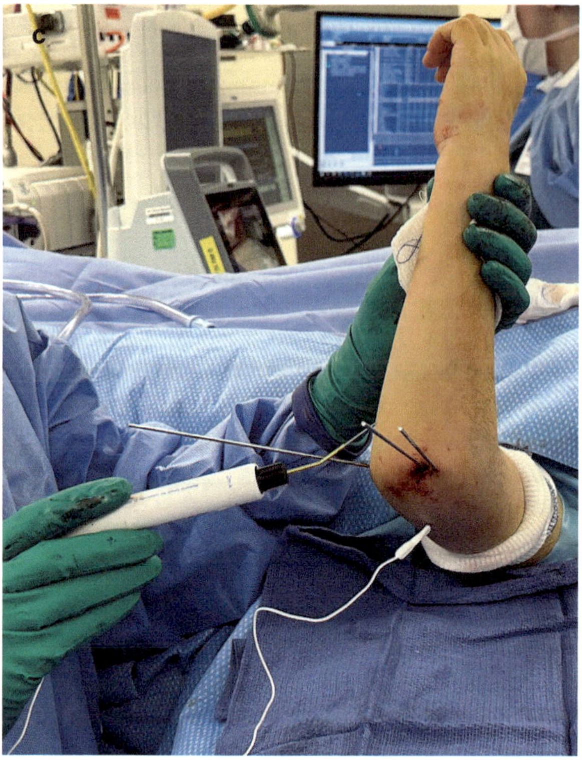

Fig. 5.4 (continued)

infiltration and nonopioid regimens achieve adequate pain control at lower costs than routine nerve blocks, which should be avoided. If a cast is used, we recommend placing the cast at <90° of elbow flexion, completely bi-valving, and using a sling to prevent external rotation through the shoulder. Provide families with written instructions on pain management and expectations. Educating families can reduce anxiety, improve adherence to nonopioid regimens, and decrease unscheduled visits.

With solid pin fixation and secure immobilization, the 1-week visit and radiographs can be omitted [21, 69]. In some cases, a phone call or telehealth visit at 1 week may be preferred, especially if the patient has a long drive to clinic [70]. This can provide an estimated $48–$344 cost savings [71]. In addition, waiting in the clinic is omitted, and the parent doesn't miss work [70]. Recent data highlight that patients from lower socioeconomic backgrounds are more likely to miss follow-up appointments [21]. Addressing this by offering telehealth, transportation assistance and culturally sensitive communication improves value by preventing complications and readmissions. At the 3-week postoperative visit, the cast and pins are removed [72]. Radiographs are only needed at that visit if there is obvious deformity, unexplained pain, or a severe fracture pattern [21, 73]. By avoiding the radiograph at 3 weeks, clinic flow is improved and the child's anxiety is decreased [74]. In cases in which a radiograph is performed, additional value occurs by having the orthopedic surgeon read and document interpretation of the radiograph rather than the radiologist [75]. Physical therapy is rarely needed after the cast and pins are removed, since function and motion gradually improve spontaneously [22]. An occasional 6-week postop visit may be used for unresolved neuropraxia, concern for cubitus varus, or for persistent stiffness.

Outcome

Regardless of fracture severity, direction of displacement, classification, or the child's age, children typically recover well [76, 77]. Return of motion may take up to 1 year in older children and those with more severe displaced fractures, so parents should be informed upfront [78]. Even after good treatment, cubitus varus occasionally occurs, and if the extension component of the fracture is not reduced, limited elbow flexion can persist [79]. Late osteotomy for these deformities may be needed.

Case Example

A 6-year-old boy fell from a 6′ monkey bar, sustaining a right Gartland type III supracondylar humerus fracture (Fig. 5.4a). He was seen at a small rural hospital emergency room that did not have an orthopedic surgeon. The elbow was splinted in 70° flexion, and he was transferred to the children's hospital 3 h away. Examination in the pediatric emergency room at 0100 by the orthopedic resident showed that there was an anterior lateral bruise, no puckering of the skin, inability to extend the thumb, pink and perfused fingers, 2-s capillary refill time, and a palpable pulse.

He was scheduled for surgery at 0730 am the next day in the trauma room. No perioperative antibiotics were used. Reduction was performed using the posterior-medial periosteal hinge, and bicolumnar fixation was done with three 5/64" Steinman pins, two lateral and one medial (Fig. 5.4b). The pins were stimulated at 2 MA with a disposable nerve stimulator, with no finger twitches noted (Fig. 5.4c). Total 5 cc of 0.25% bupivacaine with epinephrine was injected posteriorly into the fracture through the distal triceps. Soft cast padding and a single roll of 3-inch fiberglass (lighter, less material = less cost) was applied with 80° of elbow flexion. The cast was bivalved. Pulse and perfusion were normal before leaving the operating room. He was discharged that morning after a few hours of observation with only NSAIDs for pain relief and a sling to keep the shoulder from externally rotating. His father reported via a follow-up phone call at 1 week that he was doing well. During the 3-week visit, the radial nerve was fully functioning. There was no deformity. Radiographs were not done. The pins were removed, and no follow-up examination was scheduled. The parents were instructed to call if there was concern of deformity or stiffness after 6 weeks.

Summary

In summary, the latest literature strongly supports outpatient, community-based, and resource-conserving approaches for common pediatric orthopedic procedures, with robust cost-effectiveness and safety data. Multiple value-added methods can be used to improve the routine care of supracondylar fractures in children. Value = outcomes/costs [1]. This chapter highlights nine practical recommendations that improve value by reducing costs and maintaining excellent outcomes.

Author Pearls

- Type I—are splinted or casted.
- Type II—many can be treated with sedation, reduction, and immobilization. IIB fractures with axial or coronal plane deformity generally need reduction and lateral pin fixation.
- Type III and IV—surgery can be done the next morning during daylight hours unless vascular concern.
- Adopting semisterile techniques and reducing unnecessary disposables has less healthcare waste and supports sustainable orthopedic practice.
- Use of the mini C-arm can reduce radiation and cost.
- Three large lateral well-spread pins are appropriate for most fractures.
- For about 20% of fractures, one medial and 2 lateral pins are better for stability. In these cases, there are several techniques to place the medial pin safely.
- Opioids can be avoided by using local injection of 5 cc of 1/4% bupivacaine into the fracture site.
- Physical therapy is rarely needed to regain motion.
- Regardless of fracture type, 3–4 weeks of immobilization is sufficient.
- Surgery by general orthopedic surgeons at community hospitals is appropriate.

Comments by the Editors

WLH

Value = outcomes/costs. This chapter focuses on multiple value-based care changes that the orthopedic surgeon can add to their practice. Costs are reduced and outcomes are typically excellent.

RMS

Much of what has been considered "standard of care," such as treating these fractures in the middle of the night, sterile prep and draping, and perioperative antibiotics, is not evidence-based medicine (EBM) and continues to be practiced as "emotional-based medicine." This is slowly changing as surgeons report their experience and perform quality studies.

References

1. Porter ME. What is value in health care? New Engl J Med. 2010;363(26):2477–81.
2. Holt JB, Glass NA, Bedard NA, Weinstein SL, Shah AS. Emerging U.S. National Trends in the treatment of pediatric supracondylar humeral fractures. J Bone Joint Surg Am. 2017;99(8):681–7.
3. Bae DS, Kadiyala RK, Waters PM. Acute compartment syndrome in children: contemporary diagnosis, treatment, and outcome. J Pediatr Orthop. 2001;21(5):680–8.
4. Mulpuri K, Wilkins K. The treatment of displaced supracondylar humerus fractures: evidence-based guideline. J Pediatr Orthop. 2012;32(Suppl 2):S143–52.
5. Omid R, Choi PD, Skaggs DL. Supracondylar humeral fractures in children. J Bone Joint Surg Am. 2008;90(5):1121–32.
6. Chaudhry S. Value-driven pediatric supracondylar humerus fracture care: implementing evidence-based practices. J Am Acad Orthop Surg Glob Res Rev. 2024;8(4):e24.00058.
7. Holt JB, Glass NA, Shah AS. Understanding the epidemiology of pediatric supracondylar humeral fractures in the United States: identifying opportunities for intervention. J Pediatr Orthop. 2018;38(5):e245–e51.
8. Sanders JS, Ouillette RJ, Howard R, Boutelle K, Carroll AN, Bastrom TP, et al. Nonoperative versus operative treatment of type IIA supracondylar humerus fractures: a prospective evaluation of 99 patients. J Pediatr Orthop. 2023;43(1):e9–e16.
9. Gunes Z, Beydemir A, Mergen EK, Demirkiran HG, Yilmaz G, Aksoy MC, et al. Comparison of surgical and conservative treatments for Gartland type II supracondylar humerus fractures: evaluation of the need for surgical treatment. J Pediatr Orthop. 2025;45(1):7–15.
10. Baumann AN, Anaspure O, Patel S, Shams K, Yoder RG, Mistovich RJ. Examining outcomes and complications for operative versus nonoperative treatment of pediatric type II supracondylar humerus fractures: a systematic review of comparative studies. J Pediatr Orthop. 2025;45(1):e1–9.
11. Silva M, Delfosse EM, Park H, Panchal H, Ebramzadeh E. Is the "appropriate use criteria" for type II supracondylar humerus fractures really appropriate? J Pediatr Orthop. 2019;39(1):1–7.
12. Silva M, Ebramzadeh E. Is the "appropriate use criteria" for type II supracondylar humerus fractures really appropriate? J Pediatr Orthop. 2019;39(7):e563–e4.
13. Pan T, Widner MR, Chau MM, Hennrikus WL. Open supracondylar humerus fractures in children. Cureus. 2021;13(3):e13903.
14. Eguia FA, Gottlich CP, Vora M, Klyce W, Hassan S, Sponseller PD, et al. Radiographic assessments of pediatric supracondylar fractures and mid-term patient-reported outcomes. Medicine (Baltimore). 2020;99(41):e22543.
15. Quinn RH, Brown GA, Shea KG, Chen AF, Cummins DS, Sevarino KS. Is the "appropriate use criteria" for type II supracondylar humerus fractures really appropriate? J Pediatr Orthop. 2018;38(6):343.
16. Liebs TR, Burgard M, Kaiser N, Slongo T, Berger S, Ryser B, et al. Health-related quality of life after paediatric supracondylar humeral fractures. Bone Joint J. 2020;102-b(6):755–65.
17. Sinikumpu JJ, Victorzon S, Pokka T, Lindholm EL, Peljo T, Serlo W. The long-term outcome of childhood supracondylar humeral fractures: a population-based follow up study with a minimum follow up of ten years and normal matched comparisons. Bone Joint J. 2016;98-b(10):1410–7.
18. Spencer HT, Dorey FJ, Zionts LE, Dichter DH, Wong MA, Moazzaz P, et al. Type II supracondylar humerus fractures: can some be treated nonoperatively? J Pediatr Orthop. 2012;32(7):675–81.

19. Modest JM, Brodeur PG, Lemme NJ, Testa EJ, Gil JA, Cruz AI Jr. Outpatient operative management of pediatric supracondylar humerus fractures: an analysis of frequency, complications, and cost from 2009 to 2018. J Pediatr Orthop. 2022;42(1):4–9.
20. Gunda B, Tamburini LM, Hamilton-Hall MN, Block AM, Weaver A, Chaudhry S. Improving postoperative pain management in pediatric supracondylar humerus fractures with local anesthesia. J Pediatr Orthop. 2025;46:e8.
21. Zhao G, Trottier ER, Ng K, Murphy A, Moll S, Morrison SA, et al. Eliminating rote postoperative radiographs for surgically managed pediatric supracondylar humerus fractures. Can J Surg. 2024;67(3):E236–E42.
22. Schmale GA, Mazor S, Mercer LD, Bompadre V. Lack of benefit of physical therapy on function following supracondylar humeral fracture: a randomized controlled trial. J Bone Joint Surg Am. 2014;96(11):944–50.
23. Mowrer GS, Pilla NI, Sorenson SM, Armstrong DG, Hennrikus WL. Emergency pediatric orthopaedic transfer criteria: a pilot study. J Surg Orthop Adv. 2023;32(3):182–6.
24. Albanese s. Orthopaedic surgery milestones: The Accreditation Council for Graduate Medical Education. 2021. Available from: http://www.acgme.org/portals/0/pdfs/milestones/orthopaedicsurgerymilestones.pdf.
25. Macnab AJ. Paediatric inter-facility transport: the parents' perspective. Soc Work Health Care. 1992;17(3):21–9.
26. Osateerakun P, Thara I, Limpaphayom N. Surgical treatment of pediatric supracondylar humerus fracture could be safely performed by general orthopedists. Musculoskelet Surg. 2019;103(2):199–206.
27. Mets EJ, Grauer JN, McLynn RP, Frumberg DB. Pediatric supracondylar Humerus fracture outcomes by pediatric and nonpediatric orthopedists. Orthopedics. 2021;44(2):e203–e10.
28. Chen J, Yang A, Patterson M, Kwok E, Updegrove G, Hennrikus W. Pediatric supracondylar humerus fractures: treatment by a pediatric orthopedic surgeon versus a non-pediatric orthopedic surgeon. Cureus. 2024;16(6):e63476.
29. Albrahim IA, AlOmran AK, Bubshait DA, Tawfeeq Y, Alumran A, Alsayigh J, et al. Time of surgery and surgeon level in supracondylar humerus fractures in pediatric patients: a retrospective study. World J Orthop. 2023;14(11):791–9.
30. Sullivan MH, Stillwagon MR, Nash AB, Jiang H, Lin FC, Chen AT, et al. Complications with surgical treatment of pediatric supracondylar humerus fractures: does surgeon training matter? J Pediatr Orthop. 2022;42(1):e8–e14.
31. Farley FA, Patel P, Craig CL, Blakemore LC, Hensinger RN, Zhang L, et al. Pediatric supracondylar humerus fractures: treatment by type of orthopedic surgeon. J Child Orthop. 2008;2(2):91–5.
32. Su AW, Lee MC. The cost and educational experience of treating supracondylar humerus fractures: a pilot analysis on standardizing surgical care. J Am Acad Orthop Surg Glob Res Rev. 2020;4(6):e20.00063.
33. Gupta N, Kay RM, Leitch K, Femino JD, Tolo VT, Skaggs DL. Effect of surgical delay on perioperative complications and need for open reduction in supracondylar humerus fractures in children. J Pediatr Orthop. 2004;24(3):245–8.
34. Aydoğmuş S, Duymuş TM, Keçeci T, Adiyeke L, Kafadar AB. Comparison of daytime and after-hours surgical treatment of supracondylar humeral fractures in children. J Pediatr Orthop B. 2017;26(5):400–4.
35. Farrow L, Ablett AD, Mills L, Barker S. Early versus delayed surgery for paediatric supracondylar humeral fractures in the absence of vascular compromise: a systematic review and meta-analysis. Bone Joint J. 2018;100-b(12):1535–41.
36. Familiari F, Zappia A, Gasparini G, Mercurio M, Tedesco G, Riccelli DA, et al. Pediatric supracondylar humerus fracture: when should we surgically treat? A case-series. J Clin Med. 2025;14(1):237.
37. Striano BM, Talwar D, Flynn JM, Williams BA, Mitchell SL, Shah AS. High-volume hospitals have lower open reduction rates and lower cost of care for pediatric supracondylar humerus fractures. J Pediatr Soc North Am. 2023;5(1):422.

38. DeFrancesco CJ, Shah AS, Brusalis CM, Flynn K, Leddy K, Flynn JM. Rate of open reduction for supracondylar humerus fractures varies across pediatric orthopaedic surgeons: a single-institution analysis. J Orthop Trauma. 2018;32(10):e400–e7.
39. Smuin DM, Hennrikus WL. The effect of the pucker sign on outcomes of type III extension supracondylar fractures in children. J Pediatr Orthop. 2017;37(4):e229–e32.
40. Lewine E, Kim JM, Miller PE, Waters PM, Mahan ST, Snyder B, et al. Closed versus open supracondylar fractures of the humerus in children: a comparison of clinical and radiographic presentation and results. J Pediatr Orthop. 2018;38(2):77–81.
41. Goh WCK, Ong EJY, Lee NKL, Mahadev A, Wong KPL. Systematic review of paediatric pulseless pink humerus supracondylar fractures. J Pediatr Orthop B. 2024;33(5):468–76.
42. Brandt AM, Wally MK, Casey VF, Clark CC, Paloski MD, Scannell BP, et al. Appropriate use criteria for treatment of pediatric supracondylar humerus fractures with vascular injury: do our hospital practice patterns agree with current recommendations? J Pediatr Orthop. 2020;40(10):549–55.
43. Wilson JM, Schwartz AM, Farley KX, Devito DP, Fletcher ND. Doing our part to conserve resources: determining whether all personal protective equipment is mandatory for closed reduction and percutaneous pinning of supracondylar humeral fractures. J Bone Joint Surg Am. 2020;102(13):e66.
44. Wang GQ, Wang QF, Wang XD. A comprehensive comparison between the semi-sterile and sterile technique for closed reduction and percutaneous pinning of pediatric supracondylar humerus fractures. Front Surg. 2020;7:594027.
45. Dua K, Blevins CJ, O'Hara NN, Abzug JM. The safety and benefits of the Semisterile technique for closed reduction and percutaneous pinning of pediatric upper extremity fractures. Hand (N Y). 2019;14(6):808–13.
46. Rider CM, Hong VY, Westbrooks TJ, Wang J, Sheffer BW, Kelly DM, et al. Surgical treatment of supracondylar humeral fractures in a freestanding ambulatory surgery center is as safe as and faster and more cost-effective than in a children's hospital. J Pediatr Orthop. 2018;38(6):e343–e8.
47. Rupp M, Schafer C, Heiss C, Alt V. Pinning of supracondylar fractures in children – strategies to avoid complications. Injury. 2019;50(Suppl 1):S2–9.
48. Iobst CA, Spurdle C, King WF, Lopez M. Percutaneous pinning of pediatric supracondylar humerus fractures with the semisterile technique: the Miami experience. J Pediatr Orthop. 2007;27(1):17–22.
49. Bloomer AK, Coe KM, Brandt AM, Roomian T, Brighton B, Scannell BP. Hold the antibiotics: are preoperative antibiotics unnecessary in the treatment of pediatric supracondylar humerus fractures? J Pediatr Orthop. 2022;42(5):e474–e9.
50. Gupta SK, Esposito ER, Phillips R, Schwab PE, Leary EV, Hoernschemeyer DG. Effect of antibiotic prophylaxis on infection rates in pediatric supracondylar humerus fractures treated with closed reduction and percutaneous pinning: a prospective double-blinded randomized controlled trial. J Am Acad Orthop Surg. 2024;32(9):410–6.
51. Schroeder NO, Seeley MA, Hariharan A, Farley FA, Caird MS, Li Y. Utility of postoperative antibiotics after percutaneous pinning of pediatric supracondylar humerus fractures. J Pediatr Orthop. 2017;37(6):363–7.
52. Smuin D, Hatch M, Winthrop Z, Gidvani S, Hennrikus W. The reduction maneuver for pediatric extension type 3 supracondylar humerus fractures. Cureus. 2020;12(7):e9213.
53. Leitch KK, Kay RM, Femino JD, Tolo VT, Storer SK, Skaggs DL. Treatment of multidirectionally unstable supracondylar humeral fractures in children. A modified Gartland type-IV fracture. J Bone Joint Surg Am. 2006;88(5):980–5.
54. Carrazzone OL, Barbachan Mansur NS, Matsunaga FT, Matsumoto MH, Faloppa F, Belloti JC, et al. Crossed versus lateral K-wire fixation of supracondylar fractures of the humerus in children: a meta-analysis of randomized controlled trials. J Shoulder Elb Surg. 2021;30(2):439–48.
55. Kwok SM, Clayworth C, Nara N. Lateral versus cross pinning in paediatric supracondylar humerus fractures: a meta-analysis of randomized control trials. ANZ J Surg. 2021;91(5):980–5.

56. Dekker AE, Krijnen P, Schipper IB. Results of crossed versus lateral entry K-wire fixation of displaced pediatric supracondylar humeral fractures: a systematic review and meta-analysis. Injury. 2016;47(11):2391–8.
57. Xing B, Dong B, Che X. Medial-lateral versus lateral-only pinning fixation in children with displaced supracondylar humeral fractures: a meta-analysis of randomized controlled trials. J Orthop Surg Res. 2023;18(1):43.
58. Zhao H, Xu S, Liu G, Zhao J, Wu S, Peng L. Comparison of lateral entry and crossed entry pinning for pediatric supracondylar humeral fractures: a meta-analysis of randomized controlled trials. J Orthop Surg Res. 2021;16(1):366.
59. Gottschalk HP, Sagoo D, Glaser D, Doan J, Edmonds EW, Schlechter J. Biomechanical analysis of pin placement for pediatric supracondylar humerus fractures: does starting point, pin size, and number matter? J Pediatr Orthop. 2012;32(5):445–51.
60. Silva M, Knutsen AR, Kalma JJ, Borkowski SL, Bernthal NM, Spencer HT, et al. Biomechanical testing of pin configurations in supracondylar humeral fractures: the effect of medial column comminution. J Orthop Trauma. 2013;27(5):275–80.
61. Bloom T, Robertson C, Mahar AT, Newton P. Biomechanical analysis of supracondylar humerus fracture pinning for slightly malreduced fractures. J Pediatr Orthop. 2008;28(7):766–72.
62. Garg S, Weller A, Larson AN, Fletcher ND, Kwon M, Schiller J, et al. Clinical characteristics of severe supracondylar humerus fractures in children. J Pediatr Orthop. 2014;34(1):34–9.
63. Kwak-Lee J, Kim R, Ebramzadeh E, Silva M. Is medial pin use safe for treating pediatric supracondylar humerus fractures? J Orthop Trauma. 2014;28(4):216–21.
64. Rees AB, Schultz JD, Wollenman LC, Moore-Lotridge SN, Martus JE, Schoenecker JG, et al. A mini-open approach to medial pinning in pediatric supracondylar humeral fractures may be safer than previously thought. J Bone Joint Surg Am. 2022;104(1):33–40.
65. Edmonds EW, Roocroft JH, Mubarak SJ. Treatment of displaced pediatric supracondylar humerus fracture patterns requiring medial fixation: a reliable and safer cross-pinning technique. J Pediatr Orthop. 2012;32(4):346–51.
66. Kim K, Armstrong D, Hennrikus W. Methods to reduce opioid use during surgical treatment of pediatric supracondylar fractures – a pilot study. Injury. 2021;52(6):1331–5.
67. Marshall BJ, Koschmeder KT, Glass NA, Demers AJ, Kowalski HR. Opioid versus non-opioid postoperative pain management for pediatric supracondylar humerus fractures. Iowa Orthop J. 2025;45(1):137–43.
68. Rupp GE, Langner JL, Manhard CE, Bryl A, Upasani VV. A quality improvement initiative to reduce opioid prescriptions following surgical treatment of supracondylar humerus fractures in children. J Pediatr Soc North Am. 2023;5(3):696.
69. Acosta AM, Li YJ, Bompadre V, Mortimer A, Trask M, Steinman SE. The utility of the early postoperative follow-up and radiographs after operative treatment of supracondylar humerus fractures in children. J Pediatr Orthop. 2020;40(5):218–22.
70. Makarewich CA, Cheminant JR, Biddle NC, Brennan JN, San JA. Telehealth follow-up in the postoperative care of surgically treated pediatric supracondylar humerus fractures. J Pediatr Orthop B. 2024;33(2):192–7.
71. Jungbauer WN Jr, Gudipudi R, Brennan E, Melvin CL, Pecha PP. The cost impact of telehealth interventions in pediatric surgical specialties: a systematic review. J Pediatr Surg. 2023;58(8):1527–33.
72. Sorenson SM, Hennrikus W. Pain during office removal of K-wires from the elbow in children. J Pediatr Orthop. 2015;35(4):341–4.
73. Karalius VP, Stanfield J, Ashley P, Lewallen LW, DeDeugd CM, Walker J, et al. The utility of routine postoperative radiographs after pinning of pediatric supracondylar humerus fractures. J Pediatr Orthop. 2017;37(5):e309–e12.
74. Schlechter JA, Dempewolf M. The utility of radiographs prior to pin removal after operative treatment of supracondylar humerus fractures in children. J Child Orthop. 2015;9(4):303–6.
75. Du JY, Tamer P, Wang JH, Liu RW. Is there value in radiology reads for pediatric supracondylar fractures in the outpatient clinic? J Pediatr Orthop. 2019;39(6):e452–e5.

76. Ernat J, Ho C, Wimberly RL, Jo C, Riccio AI. Fracture classification does not predict functional outcomes in supracondylar humerus fractures: a prospective study. J Pediatr Orthop. 2017;37(4):e233–e7.
77. Ippolito E, Caterini R, Scola E. Supracondylar fractures of the humerus in children. Analysis at maturity of fifty-three patients treated conservatively. J Bone Joint Surg Am. 1986;68(3):333–44.
78. Spencer HT, Wong M, Fong YJ, Penman A, Silva M. Prospective longitudinal evaluation of elbow motion following pediatric supracondylar humeral fractures. J Bone Joint Surg Am. 2010;92(4):904–10.
79. Simanovsky N, Lamdan R, Mosheiff R, Simanovsky N. Underreduced supracondylar fracture of the humerus in children: clinical significance at skeletal maturity. J Pediatr Orthop. 2007;27(7):733–8.

Value-Based Care for Patients with a Pediatric Tibia Toddler Fracture: Less Is More

6

Caleb Grote and William L. Hennrikus

Introduction

Value is defined as health outcomes achieved per dollar spent (value = outcomes/cost) [1]. The purpose of the current chapter is to present strategies to improve value when treating tibial toddler fractures in children. Toddler fractures are nondisplaced, stable injuries that occur in children between 1 and 4 years of age. The injury was first described by Dunbar in 1964 as a stable, oblique, nondisplaced fracture of the distal tibia in toddlers [2] (Fig. 6.1). These injuries are inherently stable due to the thick periosteum present in young children, the presence of an intact fibula, and the lack of displacement. Patients often present with limping or limited weight-bearing following a low-energy simple fall while running or sliding. In some cases, parents may not recall a specific traumatic event, as the initial injury is often minor and easily overlooked.

Clinical evaluation begins with a careful history, physical examination, and X-rays of the affected tibia. The physical exam is often unremarkable but may reveal point tenderness over the tibia. One finding sometimes present is the child assuming a one-legged "flamingo" stance when attempting to bear weight. Anterior-Posterior (AP) and lateral x-rays of the tibia/fibula are usually sufficient for the diagnosis. Occasionally, when clinical suspicion remains high despite normal standard X-ray views, an additional oblique view may be obtained [3]. Traditional

C. Grote (✉)
University of Missouri School of Medicine, Children's Mercy Hospital, Kansas City, MO, USA
e-mail: cwgrote@cmh.edu

W. L. Hennrikus
Pennsylvania State College of Medicine, Hershey, PA, USA
e-mail: whennrikus@pennstatehealth.psue.edu

W. L. Hennrikus, R. M. Schwend (eds.), *Value in Pediatric Orthopaedics*,
https://doi.org/10.1007/978-3-032-19570-8_6

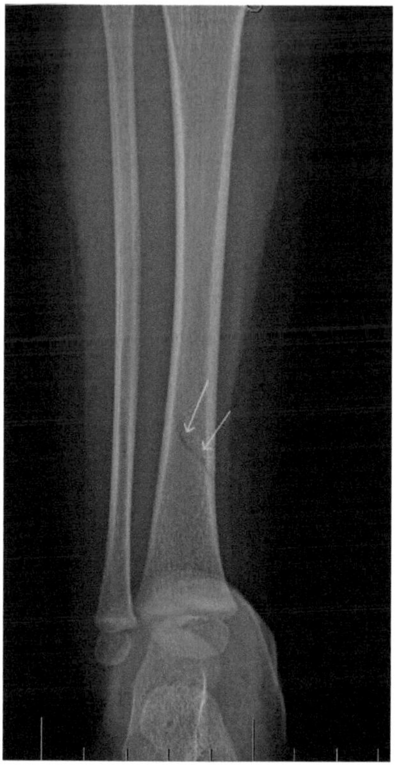

Fig. 6.1 Toddler fracture: Oblique nondisplaced distal tibia fracture and intact fibula

treatment has consisted of immobilization in a long leg cast for about 4 weeks, followed by repeat radiographs, to assess fracture healing [1, 4–6].

Toddler fractures are a common pediatric injury, accounting for up to 2.5 per 1000 pediatric emergency department visits [7–9]. Toddler fractures heal very well, with 0% rates of nonunion, refracture, and malunion [10, 11]. However, iatrogenic complications stemming from treatment with a cast, brace, or boot are common. Immobilizing a squirming young child's tibia is not easy. Padding may slip, boney prominences may remain at risk, and the foot may be mistakenly placed into plantar flexion. In addition, young children in a cast or brace often have limited ability to follow cast instructions/limitations and decreased communication skills to report pain or discomfort under the cast [12]. As a result, immobilization of a 3-year-old child's tibia can result in skin pressure injury in 40% [11] and skin breakdown in up to 17% of cases [13, 14]. Skin pressure injuries add increased costs due to additional clinic visits, lost time from work for parents, and potential plastic surgery (Fig. 6.2).

Modifying treatment strategies to simple observation, education, and monitoring can help mitigate risks to the skin and prevent pressure injuries. Limiting unnecessary clinical visits also offers direct and indirect cost savings. For instance, reducing the number of visits for cast removal and eliminating redundant radiographs can decrease imaging costs and reduce radiologists' fees. These changes in toddler fracture management require collaboration among the orthopedic doctors and buy-in

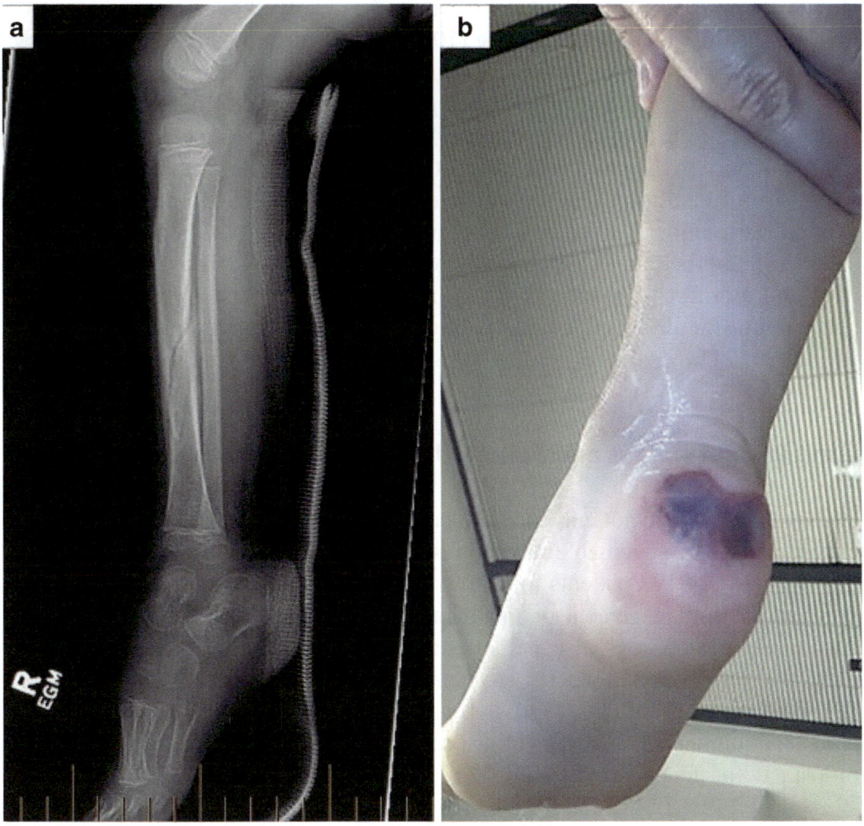

Fig. 6.2 Toddler fracture with a pressure injury to the heel from a poorly padded splint placed in equinus. (Reproduced with permission from: Noe MC et al. Toddler's fractures. J of Pediatr Orthop B 2025;34:193–197)

from the emergency department, urgent care centers, and referring facilities. Additionally, parent education and reassurance are key. Parents often experience anxiety when their child is diagnosed with a fracture but not placed in a cast or scheduled for repeat radiographs. Clear discussions with parents at the first visit to set expectations will help avoid overtreatment, minimize complications, and lower costs.

Value-Based Themes

Treatment

Traditional treatment for toddler fractures involved applying a long leg cast for 4 weeks, followed by repeat radiographs and clinical examination [2, 4–6].

However, the treatment of toddler fractures has evolved over recent years from long leg casting to short leg casting [10, 15], to controlled ankle motion (CAM) boots [14, 16, 17], and to observation and monitoring with no immobilization at all [18–21]. Long leg casting, short leg casting, and CAM boots all can cause skin pressure injuries [10, 14, 16–19]. In addition, removing a cast in the clinic risks skin burn to the child with the cast saw. Although some have suggested that a CAM boot results in less skin injuries than a cast [17], Boutin reported that skin pressure injuries were more common when using CAM boots compared to casts [16]. On the other hand, treating toddler fractures with observation, education, and monitoring results in no skin complications, faster return to weight-bearing, no fracture displacement, no refractures, and equal pain control [4, 11, 14, 18, 20, 21].

Limit Repeat X-Rays and Follow-Up Visits

Follow-up X-rays do not influence clinical outcomes. Instead, the additional X-rays expose children to avoidable radiation without clinical benefit [10]. For example, Bauer's study of 192 patients found 0% displacement on repeat radiographs, with no changes in management or treatment based on those follow-up images [10]. Avoiding repeat X-rays also helps reduce unnecessary clinic follow-ups, saves costs, and results in a broader socioeconomic impact on indirect costs of care [22, 23]. For example, in 2006, Morris et al. reported that each 100 pediatric fracture clinic appointments resulted in 54 lost school days, 25 lost workdays, and 18 days of lost pay for the parent [23].

Education

A key challenge when implementing any management change in medicine is securing buy-in from all stakeholders. For toddler fractures, the key stakeholders include parents, urgent care staff, emergency department staff, orthopedic schedulers, and the orthopedic staff. Reducing skin complications, lowering costs, limiting unnecessary visits, minimizing radiation, and improving value are the goals. The path to achieving these goals can be complex. We recommend starting with education sessions for all stakeholders. Develop an evidence-based care guideline and distribute the guideline to all stakeholders. The hospital's leadership team and safety council can be included. Develop a toddler fracture educational handout for parents and families. Suggested themes to mention in the parent handout include: Toddler fractures are common and heal well without a cast or brace. Healing takes about 3–4 weeks. Most patients with toddler fractures start bearing weight in about 2 weeks but often have a limp and walk with an externally rotated foot. This altered gait may last for 8 weeks or longer. No long-term complications have been reported.

Primary Care Management of Toddler Fractures

There is increasing evidence in the literature supporting the management of toddler fractures by primary care physicians [6, 10, 11]. When primary care physicians manage these injuries with observation, education, and reassurance, the outcomes are equally excellent. By bypassing an orthopedic referral, the costs of specialty consultation, additional imaging, and potentially unnecessary treatments are avoided, thereby enhancing value. An orthopedic consultation should be initiated for any nontoddler tibia fractures [6].

Case Example

You are the pediatric orthopedic surgeon on call at your children's hospital, a pediatric trauma center. At midnight, the transfer operator calls to connect you with a physician assistant (PA) from a community hospital located 2 h away. The PA has a 3-year-old child in the emergency department (ED) with a toddler fracture. The child fell at home in the kitchen. The child has no other injuries or medical problems. The PA initially consulted with the on-call orthopedic surgeon at the community hospital; however, that surgeon stated, "I don't take care of children," and recommended transferring the patient.

You ask the PA to send a copy of the X-ray image to your cell phone, and you confirm the injury is a toddler fracture. You explain to the PA that the current treatment for a toddler fracture involves observation, education, and reassurance. You suggest that the child can follow up in the morning with the on-call orthopedic surgeon locally or with another orthopedic surgeon in the community. You also send the PA links to two recent PubMed articles on the management of toddler fractures. The PA responds that she doesn't have time to review the articles and that her supervising physician in the ED, an adult oncologist by day, told her to transfer the child. You then advise her not to apply a splint to the child's leg.

The child is placed in a posterior splint by a tech at the community hospital and transferred to your trauma center children's hospital via ambulance. The mother follows the ambulance in her car. At 3:30 AM, the child arrives at your ED. The orthopedic resident on call removes the splint and notices a small red spot on the heel. The resident offers to treat the injury with a CAM boot, but the mother insists on a cast. The orthopedic resident, along with a medical student, applies a short leg cast, provides the mother with an educational/instructional handout about toddler fractures, and discharges the child with instructions for follow-up in your clinic in 3 weeks. The child leaves the ED at 5:00 AM.

Three weeks later, the child returns to your clinic with his mother and two siblings: a 1-year-old and a 5-year-old. The cast tech removes the cast as per instructions from the ED visit. The tech informs you that the child was a bit rambunctious during the cast removal process, the siblings were anxious when the cast saw was turned on, and that the child now has a one-inch cast burn on the side of the leg.

You enter the examination room, greet the mother warmly, and apologize for the cast burn. The child is otherwise doing well. The mother demands another X-ray and informs you that her husband is a trial attorney. The X-ray shows no changes compared to the injury film. Mom is satisfied when you confirm that the fracture has "healed properly." You offer a follow-up appointment in 2 weeks to check the child's progress. After the family leaves the clinic, you contact the risk management office at your hospital and go to see your next patient.

Summary

Toddler fractures are stable, low-energy injuries. Traditional treatment with a cast, splint, or boot, often results in a high rate of skin complications. Traditional treatment is often worse than the injury itself. Instead, a treatment approach focused on observation, education, and reassurance is recommended. For toddler fractures, less is truly more. Minimalist treatment reduces complications and costs, preserves excellent outcomes, and enhances value. Education and buy-in from all stakeholders are key for successfully implementation of this treatment approach.

Author Pearls

1. Toddler fractures are stable injuries that heal reliably without long-term sequelae.
2. Traditional treatment of 4 weeks in a long leg cast with repeat imaging leads to unnecessary cost, excess radiation, and potential skin pressure injuries.
3. Patients with a toddler fracture can be effectively managed with observation, education, and reassurance without the need for immobilization or repeat imaging and with minimal clinic follow-up.
4. Educating all stakeholders is key.

Editor Comments

WLH

Traditional treatment for toddler fractures often does more harm than good. The evolving management of these injuries challenges the practice of defensive medicine and the well-intentioned desire to meet parental expectations. This chapter aligns nicely with the goals of the 2012 Choosing Wisely Campaign, which seeks to identify and question unnecessary treatments and tests, encouraging open discussions with patients. The focus of the current chapter is not only on cost reduction but also on minimizing harm, improving outcomes, and enhancing value.

RMS

If a child presents from an outside facility in a posterior splint, be sure to remove it to check that the skin over the heel pad is intact and unharmed. I recommend removing any cast or splint applied by another provider if the child experiences discomfort, as you assume responsibility for the cast once the child is under your care. Any child in a cast or splint who complains of pain or appears uncomfortable should have the device removed immediately and the skin inspected. While the bone will heal without issue in a toddler fracture, the soft tissues may not. Lastly, current procedural terminology (CPT) coding for toddler fracture is simple: 22750 closes treatment, no manipulation. This code works for treatment with observation, cast, brace, or boot.

References

1. Porter ME. What is value in health care. N Engl J Med. 2010;363:2488–1.
2. Dunbar JS, et al. Obscure tibial fracture of infants—the toddler's fracture. J Can Assoc Radiol. 1964;15:136–44.
3. Tenenbein M, Reed MH, Black GB. The toddler's fracture revisited. Am J Emerg Med. 1990;8:208–11.
4. Halsey MF, et al. Toddler's fracture: presumptive diagnosis and treatment. J Pediatr Orthop. 2001;21:152–6.
5. John SD, Moorthy CS, Swischuk LE. Expanding the concept of the toddler's fracture. Radiographics. 1997;17:367–76.
6. MacNeille R, Hennrikus W. Value-based treatment of common pediatric fractures by primary care. Clin Ped. 2018;57:1378–84.
7. Clancy J, et al. Toddler's fracture. J Accid Emerg Med. 1996;13:366–7.
8. Shravat BP, Harrop SN, Kane TP. Toddler's fracture. J Accid Emerg Med. 1996;13:59–61.
9. Sapru K, Cooper JG. Management of the Toddler's fracture with and without initial radiological evidence. Eur J Emerg Med. 2014;21:451–4.
10. Bauer JM, Lovejoy SA. Toddler's fractures: time to weight-bear with regard to immobilization type and radiographic monitoring. J Pediatr Orthop. 2019;39:314–7.
11. Adamich JS, Camp MW. Do toddler's fractures of the tibia require evaluation and management by an orthopaedic surgeon routinely? Eur J Emerg Med. 2018;25:423–8.
12. Abzug JM, Schwartz BS, Johnson AJ. Assessment of splints applied for pediatric fractures in an emergency department/urgent care environment. J Pediatr Orthop. 2019;39:76–84.
13. Schuh AM, Whitlock KB, Klein EJ. Management of toddler's fractures in the pediatric emergency department. Pediatr Emerg Care. 2016;32:452–4.
14. Bradman K, et al. Randomised controlled trial comparing immobilisation in above-knee plaster of Paris to controlled ankle motion boots in undisplaced paediatric spiral tibial fractures. Emerg Med J. 2021;38:600–6.
15. MacNeille R, Gockley A, Hennrikus W. Outcomes of short versus long leg casts for childhood accidental spiral tibial cast fractures. Pediatr Emer Care. 2021;37:e252–4.
16. Boutin A, Colaco K, Stimec J, et al. Removable boot vs casting of toddler's fractures: a randomized clinical trial. JAMA Pediatr. 2025;179:713–21.
17. Noe MC, Jarka DE, Sinclair MK, Grote CW. Toddler's fracture: an updated guide on evaluation and management. J Pediatr Orthop B. 2025;34:193–7.
18. Fox J, et al. Observation versus cast treatment of toddler's fractures. J Pediatr Orthop. 2022;42:e480–5.
19. Leffler LC, Tanner SL, Beckish ML. Immobilization versus observation in children with toddler's fractures: a retrospective review. J Surg Orthop Adv. 2018;27:142–7.

20. Seguin J, Brody D, Li P. Nationwide survey on current management strategies of toddler's fractures. CJEM. 2018;20:739–45.
21. Townley S, et al. Is immobilisation required for toddler's fracture of the tibia? BMJ. 2022;379:e071764.
22. Holm AG, Luras PH, Randsborg PH. The economic burden of outpatient appointments following paediatric fractures. Injury. 2016;47:1410–3.
23. Morris MW, Bell MJ. The socio-economical impact of paediatric fracture clinic appointments. Injury. 2006;37:395–7.

Methods to Enhance Value When Treating Pediatric Lateral Condyle Fractures of the Elbow

7

N. M. Campbell and M. J. Herman

Introduction

Lateral humeral condyle fractures are the second most common pediatric elbow fracture [1], typically occurring in children between 4 and 10 years of age, with a peak incidence around 6 years [2]. The most common mechanisms of injury include falls onto an outstretched hand, direct trauma, and valgus impaction [1, 3]. These fractures present unique challenges for orthopedic surgeons due to their intraarticular nature, significant cartilaginous involvement, and proximity to the physis. They are associated with higher rates of nonunion, malunion, and avascular necrosis compared to other pediatric elbow fractures [4].

Value-based care focuses on reducing costs while improving care quality, patient outcomes, and physician performance. Key aspects of managing lateral humeral condyle fractures—such as advanced imaging, follow-up protocols, duration of immobilization, fixation methods, and the potential need for physical therapy—offer opportunities for standardization. By optimizing these factors, surgeons can enhance both efficiency and cost-effectiveness in treating these fractures.

Value-Based Themes

Imaging (Radiographs, Ultrasound, MRI, and Arthrogram)

The disruption of the articular surface is a key factor in determining the treatment method for lateral humeral condyle fractures. The joint surface can be evaluated using various imaging modalities, including radiographs, ultrasound imaging,

N. M. Campbell · M. J. Herman (✉)
St. Christopher's Hospital for Children, Philadelphia, PA, USA
e-mail: nancy.campbell@towerhealth.org; martin.herman@towerhealth.org

W. L. Hennrikus, R. M. Schwend (eds.), *Value in Pediatric Orthopaedics*,
https://doi.org/10.1007/978-3-032-19570-8_7

magnetic resonance imaging (MRI), and arthrography. The choice of imaging studies plays a significant role in the overall cost of care. Plain radiographs remain the primary tool for evaluating lateral humeral condyle fractures, typically including anterior posterior (AP), lateral, and internal oblique views. Among these, the internal oblique view provides the most accurate measurement of fracture displacement, as the fracture line typically runs in a posterolateral direction, making the internal oblique image crucial for guiding treatment decisions [5].

For clearly displaced injuries, radiographs are sufficient to determine the appropriate treatment. However, treatment decisions become less straightforward in cases of minimally displaced fractures or fractures in young children, where the cartilaginous articular surface may not be visible on radiographs. In these situations, additional imaging modalities—such as ultrasound, MRI, computerized tomography (CT), and arthrography—can help guide treatment. High-resolution ultrasound can assess whether a fracture line extends through the cartilaginous joint surface and whether there is displacement, but its utility is limited by the skill of the technologist [6–8] and the surgeon's experience with this imaging modality. As a result, ultrasound has primarily been described in small case series. MRI is effective in reliably detecting the integrity of the cartilaginous hinge [9, 10], but its routine use is hindered by limited access, high cost, and the need for sedation in younger children. CT scans can provide detailed information about the articular surface and fracture displacement; however, the inability to clearly visualize osseocartilaginous fragments, greater radiation exposure, and high costs limit its use [11].

When treating minimally displaced fractures operatively, arthrography is a crucial intraoperative tool for assessing the articular surface of the distal humerus. An arthrogram may be performed prior to reduction to better define the fracture characteristics and guide the decision between open versus closed reduction. In addition, an arthrogram may be performed after reduction to confirm the anatomic alignment of the joint surfaces [4]. Intraoperative arthrography can alter the surgical plan in 8–21% of cases [12, 13]. Although useful, arthrography has its limitations and requires anesthesia, and interpreting an elbow arthrogram can be challenging, even for experienced surgeons.

We recommend standard radiographs, including AP, lateral, and internal oblique views, for all lateral humeral condyle fractures. If there are concerns regarding articular displacement or fracture stability, we recommend arthrography in the operating room as the preferred advanced imaging modality, with immediate fixation based on the findings of the arthrogram.

Minimally and Nondisplaced Fractures

Lateral humeral condyle fractures that are nondisplaced or displaced by less than 2 mm are typically treated with cast immobilization and close follow-up [2, 4]. A long arm cast is applied with the elbow in 90 degrees of flexion and the forearm in neutral rotation. A sling is recommended. Close follow-up with radiographs is essential, as research indicates that 8–15% of nondisplaced or minimally displaced fractures may later displace [14, 15]. The definition of "close follow-up" varies across studies, with different recommendations for radiographs at various intervals, both in and out of the cast. However, recent studies suggest that a single follow-up 10–15 days after injury, followed by another at 4–6 weeks, with radiographs out of the cast including AP, lateral, and internal oblique views, is sufficient to safely manage nondisplaced and minimally displaced lateral humeral condyle fractures [16]. If fracture displacement is detected during the 2-week visit, surgical intervention can be performed without adversely affecting outcomes. This strategy is more cost-effective, reducing the number of visits and radiographs.

Open Versus Closed Reduction

Surgical indications for lateral humeral condyle fractures include displacement greater than 2 mm, malrotation, progressive displacement on follow-up radiographs, and failure of conservative treatment with delayed healing beyond 8 weeks [4]. Surgical options involve either closed or open reduction and fixation, using pins or screws.

Closed reduction and fixation are typically used for minimally displaced fractures, fractures without rotation, and those showing progressive displacement on follow-up imaging [5, 17]. Minimally displaced fractures are defined as those with a displacement of 2 mm (up to 4 mm), accompanied by an intact articular hinge. After closed reduction, it is crucial that the fracture is reduced to less than 2 mm of displacement and that the articular surface is congruent. Congruency can be confirmed with postreduction arthrography [2, 4]. Closed reduction for minimally displaced fractures generally results in shorter surgical times—over 20 min less than open reduction—without negatively impacting outcomes [18–20]. Given that the average operating room costs range from $21 to $133 per minute, with an average of $62 per minute, reducing surgical time presents an important opportunity for more cost-effective care [21].

Fractures with greater than 4 mm of initial displacement or malrotation, as well as fractures that cannot be reduced by closed means, are indications for open reduction [5, 17]. Attempting to treat these more displaced fractures with closed reduction can result in longer surgical times compared to open reduction and fixation [22].

For these reasons, we recommend an initial attempt at closed reduction for minimally displaced fractures. On the other hand, fractures with greater than 4 mm displacement or malrotation should be treated with open reduction. The most important factor in treating lateral condyle fractures is achieving an anatomic reduction of the joint surface. Therefore, any method employed by the treating surgeon can be acceptable, provided that anatomic reduction is successfully achieved.

Screw Versus Pins

There is currently no consensus on whether K-wires or screws provide optimal fixation for lateral condylar fractures, as both options have their respective pros and cons. When using K-wires, they are typically inserted percutaneously, with one wire placed parallel to the joint, and others aimed obliquely toward the proximal medial metaphysis of the humerus [2]. The pin construct can impact fracture stability. Using two divergent bicortical pins at a 60-degree angle is superior to other two-pin constructs, and three divergent pins offer increased stability compared to two [23].

The debate between exposed and buried K-wires has also been explored. Buried K-wires require a second trip to the operating room for removal, while exposed K-wires can be removed in the office, without increasing the risk of infection or other complications. As a result, exposed K-wires are preferred, as they provide more cost-effective care [24].

When comparing infection risk between K-wires and screws, the data remains inconclusive. Some studies have found an increased risk of superficial infections with K-wires [28, 30], while others have found no significant difference in infections between the two fixation methods [25, 26].

Screw fixation is typically performed with cannulated screws ranging from 3.5 mm to 4.5 mm in diameter. Fixation with a single 4.0 mm lag screw provides a biomechanically stronger construct than pin fixation using two divergent 0.062" K-wires [27]. Screw fixation also offers compression across the fracture site, enabling earlier mobilization compared to K-wire fixation [28, 29]. This may explain why postoperative stiffness is more common after K-wire fixation [29, 30], although not all studies support this finding [25, 26].

A major drawback of screw fixation is the increased cost. Screws are more expensive than K-wires and require a second procedure for removal. The cost of pediatric implant removal has been reported to exceed $11,000 per case [33].

For the most cost-effective care, we recommend smooth, exposed K-wire fixation for most lateral humeral condyle fractures, typically using two or three pins. After fixation, fluoroscopic or direct visual stress tests should be performed. If there is any concern about stability—especially with larger fracture fragments in older patients or rotated fragments—alternative fixation with a screw may be considered.

Standardized Postop Protocol

The evidence-based literature regarding postoperative protocols for lateral condyle fractures is limited. For fractures treated with K-wire fixation, the wires are typically left in place for a minimum of 3–4 weeks [2]. The wires are then removed in the office, and a cast is reapplied for an additional 2–4 weeks, depending on radiographic healing [2]. For fractures treated with screw fixation, postoperative immobilization may be shorter—based on radiographic healing. At our institution, we remove the pins at 4 weeks after surgery and recast for an additional 2 weeks, totaling 6 weeks of casting. Patients are scheduled for a follow-up visit 4–6 weeks after cast removal to assess range of motion.

When to Do Physical Therapy

While temporary elbow stiffness is common after lateral condyle fractures, most children treated for these injuries do not require physical therapy. A rapid recovery of motion is typically seen immediately after cast removal, with continued improvements up to a year following the injury [31]. Risk factors for postoperative stiffness include older age, concomitant elbow dislocation, and treatment with open reduction [32]. Patients who undergo surgical treatment should return to the clinic 4 to 6 weeks after cast removal for a range of motion assessment. Approximately 10% of these patients, regardless of whether they are treated with open or closed reduction, will require physical therapy [19]. We recommend waiting until this follow-up visit to determine the need for physical therapy, as this helps avoid over-treating patients who will regain motion without intervention.

Case Example

A 4-year-old male sustained a right lateral humeral condyle fracture after falling off his bike (Fig. 7.1a). He was initially evaluated in the outpatient clinic, where radiographs confirmed the injury. On examination, his upper extremity was swollen, but his neurovascular status was intact. He was placed in a long arm cast and scheduled for outpatient surgery 2 days later.

Given the degree of displacement, an arthrogram of the elbow was performed in the operating room to further assess the fracture and articular surface. Two cc of dilute contrast dye were injected into the posterior elbow via the olecranon fossa. Radiographic views showed that the joint surface was congruent, and the lateral condylar cortex was reducible with gentle pressure, forearm supination, wrist extension, and elbow valgus (Fig. 7.1b). Three lateral pins were then introduced from lateral to medial. Another arthrogram was performed after pinning to confirm the reduction of the articular surface (Fig. 7.1c). The patient was placed in a well-padded and molded long arm cast at 90 degrees elbow flexion and neutral rotation and discharged the same day with nonnarcotic over-the-counter pain medication as needed.

He was seen for follow-up at postoperative weeks 1, 4, and 6, with radiographs taken at each visit. At 4 weeks, the pins were removed, and a new long arm cast was applied for an additional 2 weeks. At 6 weeks postop, the cast was removed, and at the 1-month follow-up after cast removal, the patient had regained nearly full range of motion.

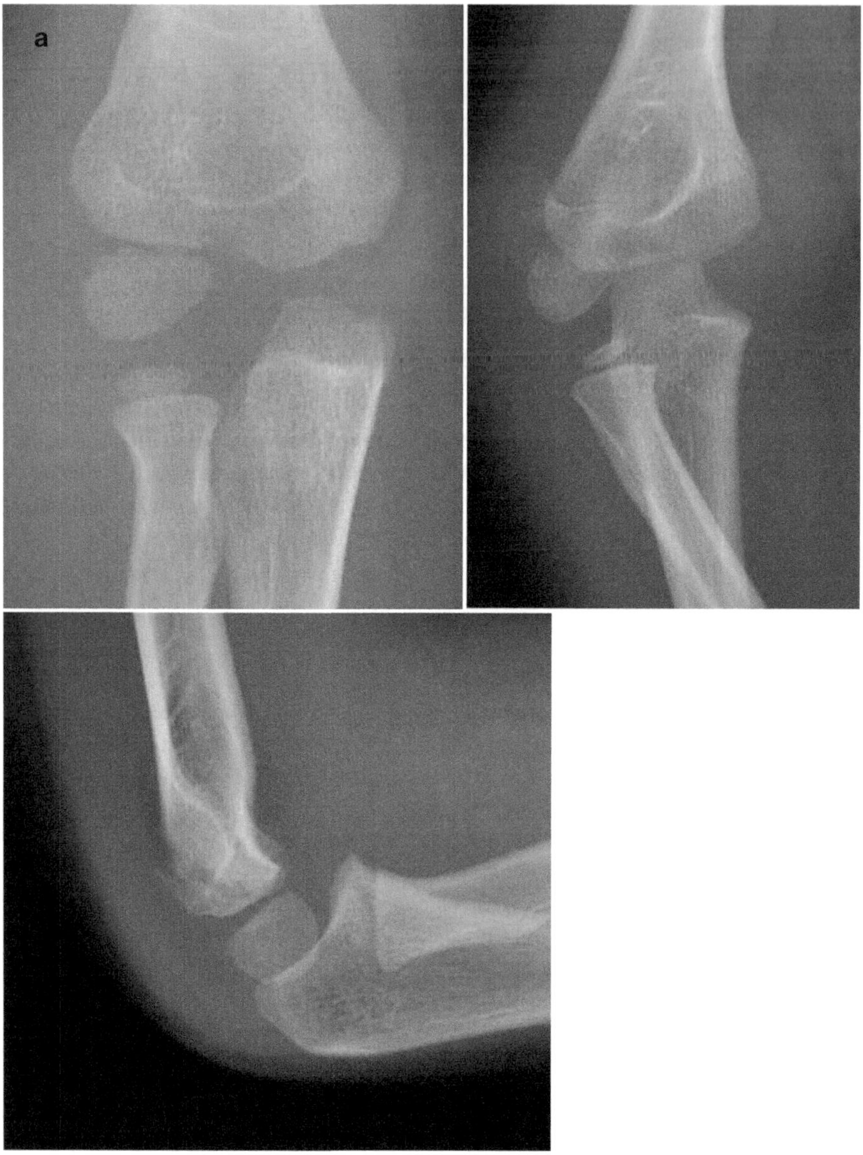

Fig. 7.1 (**a**): AP, internal oblique, and lateral radiographs of a right elbow demonstrating a displaced lateral humeral condyle fracture. (**b**): Intraoperative arthrogram demonstrating alignment of the articular surface with closed reduction. (**c**): Postreduction and pinning arthrogram confirming reduction of the articular surface.

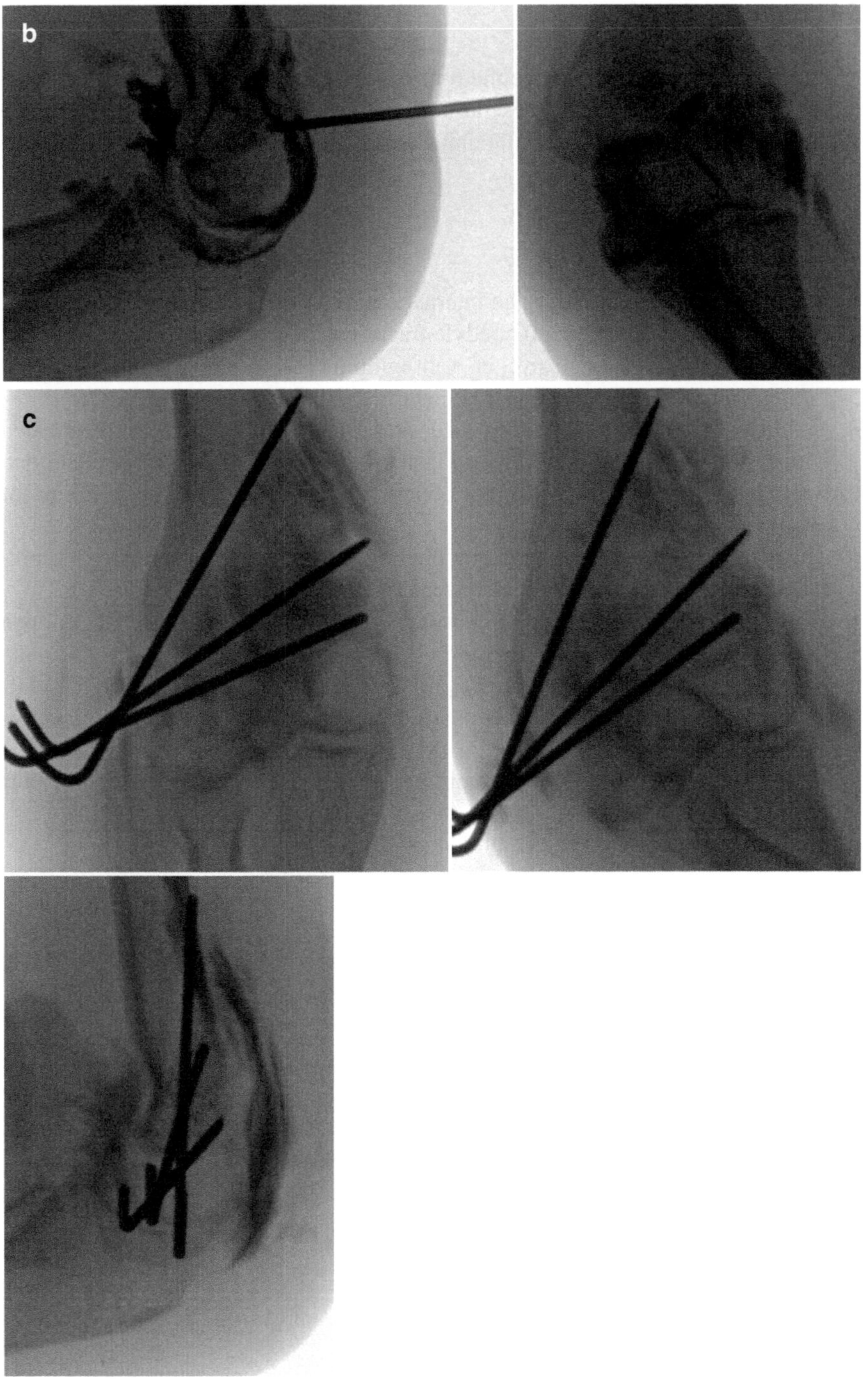

Fig. 7.1 (continued)

Summary

Multiple approaches can enhance the routine care of lateral humeral condyle fractures in children. This chapter presents six practical recommendations that improve value by reducing costs while maintaining excellent outcomes.

Author Pearls

- Elbow radiographs, including an internal oblique view, are the best initial imaging choice for lateral humeral condyle fractures.
- If radiographs are inconclusive, an arthrogram in the operating room is the next best imaging modality to guide treatment.
- Nondisplaced or minimally displaced lateral condyle fractures can be treated with casting, with the first follow-up visit scheduled 10–15 days after the injury. Radiographs (including an internal oblique view) should be taken to check for displacement.
- Closed reduction and percutaneous pinning with exposed K-wires is the preferred treatment for minimally displaced fractures.
- Fractures with >4 mm displacement or if rotated should be treated with open reduction and percutaneous pinning.
- Exposed percutaneous pins are the preferred choice for fixation. In older children, with mal-rotated fragments, or if instability persists after pinning, screws may be considered.
- Most operatively treated fractures are immobilized for a total of 6 weeks. Pins are removed at 4 weeks.
- Physical therapy should be prescribed only on an as-needed basis.

Comments by the Editors

WLH

An awesome value-packed chapter on a common peds ortho fracture! The authors have presented 6 practical recommendations to improve value when treating pediatric lateral humeral condyle fractures: The internal oblique X-ray view is key, indications for an intraop arthrogram, when to do a closed reduction vs an open reduction, exposed K-wires are the go-to fixation method, standardize the postop protocol, and utilize physical therapy only if stiff 4 weeks after final cast removal.

RMS

Percutaneous pins are readily available in all operating rooms and are cost-effective for fractures treated by closed or open reduction. Three well-spread pins are preferred, since if one of the pins is not ideally placed or needs to be removed for superficial infection, then there are still two pins in place to maintain the fracture reduction. Percutaneous pins are easy to remove in the clinic at 4 weeks, since by then they are starting to loosen and are no longer needed.

References

1. Milch H. Fractures and fracture dislocations of the humeral condyles. J Trauma. 1964;4(5):592–607.
2. Abzug JM, Dua K, Kozin SH, Herman MJ. Current concepts in the treatment of lateral condyle fractures in children. J Am Acad Orthop Surg [Internet]. 2020;28(1):e9–19. [cited 2025 Mar 12]; Available from: https://journals.lww.com/jaaos/abstract/2020/01010/current_concepts_in_the_treatment_of_lateral.4.aspx
3. Pirker ME, Weinberg AM, Höllwarth ME, Haberlik A. Subsequent displacement of initially nondisplaced and minimally displaced fractures of the lateral humeral condyle in children. J Trauma Inj Infect Crit Care. 2005;58(6):1202–7.
4. Schroeder K, Gilbert S, Ellington M, Souder C, Yang S. Pediatric lateral humeral condyle fractures. J Pediatr Orthop Soc North Am. 2020;2(1):82.
5. Song KS, Kang CH, Min BW, Bae KC, Cho CH, Lee JH. Closed reduction and internal fixation of displaced unstable lateral condylar fractures of the humerus in children. J Bone Joint Surg Am Vol. 2008;90(12):2673–81.
6. Vocke-Hell AK, Schmid A. Sonographic differentiation of stable and unstable lateral condyle fractures of the humerus in children. J Pediatr Orthop B. 2001;10(2):138–41.
7. Zhang J, Chen H. Ultrasonography for non-displaced and mini-displaced humeral lateral condyle fractures in children. Chin J Traumatol (English Edition). 2008;11(5):297–300.
8. Li XT, Shen XT, Wu X, Chen XL. A novel transverse ultrasonography technique for minimally displaced lateral humeral condyle fractures in children. Orthop Traumatol Surg Res. 2019;105(3):557–62.
9. Thévenin-Lemoine C, Salanne S, Pham T, Accadbled F, Baunin C, Sales De Gauzy J. Relevance of MRI for management of non-displaced lateral humeral condyle fractures in children. Orthop Traumatol Surg Res [Internet]. 2017;103(5):777–81. Available from: https://www.sciencedirect.com/science/article/pii/S1877056817301524
10. Qi Y, Guo L, Sun M, Wang Z. Clinical value of MRI in evaluating and diagnosing of humeral lateral condyle fracture in children. J Orthop Surg Res. 2021;16(1):617.
11. Chapman VM, Grottkau BE, Albright M, Salamipour H, Jaramillo D. Multidetector computed tomography of pediatric lateral condylar fractures. J Comput Assist Tomogr. 2005;29(6):842–6.
12. Vorhies JS, Funk S, Elliott M, Riccio A, Ramo B. The utility of intraoperative arthrogram in the management of pediatric lateral condyle fractures of the humerus. Orthopedics. 2020;43(1):30–5.
13. Lari A, Alenezi A, Abughaith J, AlShehawy H, Hammady W, AlSaifi S. Intraoperative arthrography favorably impacts the early outcome of operatively managed fractures of the lateral humeral condyle displaced 1–5 mm in children. J Orthop Surg Res. 2022;17(1):569.
14. Knapik DM, Gilmore A, Liu RW. Conservative management of minimally displaced ($\leq$2 mm) fractures of the lateral humeral condyle in pediatric patients. J Pediatr Orthop. 2017;37(2):e83–7.
15. Zale C, Winthrop Z, Hennrikus W. Rate of displacement of Jakob type 1 lateral condyle fractures treated with a cast. J Child Orthop. 2018;12:117–22.
16. Kraft DB, Moore TJ, Pargas C, Rogers K, Thacker MM. Minimally displaced lateral humeral condyle fractures: optimizing follow-up and minimizing cost. J Pediatr Orthop. 2022;43(1):1–6.
17. Weiss JM, Graves S, Yang S, Mendelsohn E, Kay RM, Skaggs DL. A new classification system predictive of complications in surgically treated pediatric humeral lateral condyle fractures. J

Pediatr Orthop [Internet]. 2009;29(6):602–5. [cited 2020 Mar 7]; Available from: https://www.ncbi.nlm.nih.gov/pubmed/19700990
18. Silva M, Cooper SD. Closed reduction and percutaneous pinning of displaced pediatric lateral condyle fractures of the humerus. J Pediatr Orthop. 2015;35(7):661–5.
19. Pennock AT, Salgueiro L, Upasani VV, Bastrom TP, Newton PO, Yaszay B. Closed reduction and percutaneous pinning versus open reduction and internal fixation for type II lateral condyle humerus fractures in children displaced >2 mm. J Pediatr Orthop. 2016 Dec;36(8):780–6.
20. Zhu S, Zheng Y, Jiang Y, Yin H, Zhu D. Open versus closed reduction internal fixation for lateral condyle humeral fractures in children: a systematic review and meta-analysis. J Orthop Surg Res. 2023;18(1):322.
21. Saul B, Ketelaar E, Yaish A, Wagner M, Comrie R, Brannan GD, et al. Assessing root causes of First Case On-time Start (FCOTS) delay in the orthopedic department at a busy level II community teaching hospital. Spartan Med Res J. 2022;7(2):36719.
22. Weng L, Cao Y, Zhang G, Zhou H, Liu X, Zhang Y. A comparative study on closed reduction vs. open reduction techniques in the surgical treatment of rotated lateral condyle fractures of the distal humerus in children. Front Pediatr [Internet]. 2022;10. [cited 2024 Apr 16]; Available from: https://www.ncbi.nlm.nih.gov/pmc/articles/PMC9201398/
23. Bloom T, Chen LY, Sabharwal S. Biomechanical analysis of lateral humeral condyle fracture pinning. J Pediatr Orthop. 2011;31(2):130–7.
24. Qin YF, Li ZJ, Li CK, Bai SC, Li H. Unburied versus buried wires for fixation of pediatric lateral condyle distal humeral fractures. Medicine (Baltimore). 2017 Aug;96(34):e7736.
25. Li WC, Xu RJ. Comparison of Kirschner wires and AO cannulated screw internal fixation for displaced lateral humeral condyle fracture in children. Int Orthop. 2011;36(6):1261–6.
26. Ganeshalingam R, Donnan A, Evans O, Hoq M, Camp M, Donnan L. Lateral condylar fractures of the humerus in children. Bone Joint J. 2018;100-B(3):387–95.
27. Schlitz RS, Schwertz JM, Eberhardt AW, Gilbert SR. Biomechanical analysis of screws versus K-wires for lateral humeral condyle fractures. J Pediatr Orthop. 2015;35(8):e93–7.
28. Stein BE, Ramji AF, Hassanzadeh H, Wohlgemut JM, Ain MC, Sponseller PD. Cannulated lag screw fixation of displaced lateral humeral condyle fractures is associated with lower rates of open reduction and infection than pin fixation. J Pediatr Orthop. 2017 Jan;37(1):7–13.
29. Gilbert SR, MacLennan PA, Schlitz RS, Estes AR. Screw versus pin fixation with open reduction of pediatric lateral condyle fractures. J Pediatr Orthop B [Internet]. 2016;25(2):148–52. [cited 2025 Feb 28]; Available from: https://journals.lww.com/jpo-b/pages/articleviewer.aspx?year=2016&issue=03000&article=00012&type=Fulltext
30. Cummings JE, Schwabe MT, Rivera AE, Sanders J, Denning JR, Neal K, et al. K-wire versus screw fixation in displaced lateral condyle fractures of the humerus in children: a multicenter study of 762 fractures. J Pediatr Orthop. 2023;43(4):e284–9.
31. Bernthal NM, Hoshino CM, Dichter D, Wong M, Silva M. Recovery of elbow motion following pediatric lateral condylar fractures of the humerus. J Bone Joint Surg. 2011;93(9):871–7.
32. Tippabhatla A, Torres-Izquierdo B, Pereira DE, Goldstein R, Sanders J, Neal K, et al. Risk factors for stiffness after surgical treatment of pediatric humeral lateral condyle fractures: results of a multicenter study. J Pediatr Orthop. 2024;44(4):208–12.
33. Boulos A, DeFroda SF, Kleiner JE, Thomas N, Gil JA, Cruz AI. Inpatient orthopaedic hardware removal in children: a cross-sectional study. J Clin Orthop Trauma. 2017;8(3):270–5.

Methods to Improve Value for Femoral Shaft Fractures in Children

8

Jimmy Daher, Benjamin D. Martin, and Matthew E. Oetgen

Introduction

Femoral shaft fractures account for 2% of all pediatric fractures [1, 2] and are among the most common lower extremity injuries in children, with an annual incidence of approximately 20 per 100,000 in the United States [3]. Among patients under 18 years of age, diaphyseal femur fractures make up nearly 68% of all femur fractures [3], with the majority occurring in males between 6 and 12 years [4–6]. This sex discrepancy is attributed to the higher participation of males in high-energy and sports activities [4].

The etiology of femoral shaft fractures varies by age. In younger children, low-energy mechanisms, such as simple falls, are the cause. However, in nonambulatory infants, nonaccidental trauma (NAT) is a common etiology of femoral shaft fractures [7]. High-energy trauma, such as motor vehicle accidents and sports-related injuries, accounts for many cases in the older child and adolescent [3, 4, 7]. Less common causes include pathologic fractures associated with conditions such as osteogenesis imperfecta, cerebral palsy, fibrous dysplasia, and low bone density or osteoporosis [3, 4, 8].

Age-Based Algorithm for Treatment

Multiple treatment options exist for pediatric femoral shaft fractures. Nonoperative methods include traction, Pavlik harness, and spica casting, while operative treatments consist of elastic intramedullary nails, rigid intramedullary nails,

J. Daher · B. D. Martin · M. E. Oetgen (✉)
Children's National Hospital, Washington, DC, USA
e-mail: Jdaher@childrensnational.org; bmartin@childrensnational.org; moetgen@childrensnational.org

W. L. Hennrikus, R. M. Schwend (eds.), *Value in Pediatric Orthopaedics*,
https://doi.org/10.1007/978-3-032-19570-8_8

submuscular plating, open plating, and external fixation [3, 9]. A flexible algorithm based on age and weight is suggested.

Neonates and Infants (<6 Months)

Young infants with diaphyseal femoral fractures are usually treated with a Pavlik harness [10, 11]. Children in this age group show rapid healing and exceptional remodeling potential, making the Pavlik harness an effective treatment option [10, 11]. This intervention is cost-effective, adjustable, easy to use, shortens hospitalization, and supports diapering and nursing care [10].

Children (6 Months–5 Years)

Immediate or early hip spica casting is standard treatment for femoral shaft fractures in this age group. Although early traction followed by delayed spica casting was once common, current evidence shows that immediate spica casting is safe and effective, resulting in excellent radiographic and functional outcomes. Typically, spica casting is required for 4–6 weeks to allow for fracture healing. Serial radiographic follow-up is essential for comminuted or unstable fractures because maintaining proper angulation and length in these fractures may be challenging with spica casting alone [12, 13]. Fractures that shorten >2.5 cm may need a change in treatment to prevent excessive shortening [13].

Children (6–12 Years)

In this age group, surgery is common. Surgery allows for easier mobilization and weight-bearing, reduces the social burden on parents, shortens hospitalization, and reduces immediate costs [13]. Several surgical options are available, including, but not limited to, elastic intramedullary nailing (EIN), submuscular plating, and external fixation. Additional costs are incurred at the time of implant removal.

Elastic Intramedullary Nailing

Elastic intramedullary nailing (EIN) is most suitable for length-stable, short-oblique, or transverse femoral shaft fractures [14]. EIN is performed frequently in patients over 5 years of age due to its advantages over spica casting [15, 16], plating [17], and external fixation [3]. EIN requires minimal surgical exposure, allows for rapid rehabilitation, shortens hospital stays, and is associated with few complications [18, 19]. EIN provides relative stability, promoting callus formation [18] while not injuring the physis [20]. Both titanium and stainless steel nails are available, with the choice depending on patient age and weight (suggested cutoff:

11 years or 49 kg). Titanium nails are more flexible than stainless steel nails and reduce stress shielding but are more prone to angular deformity in heavier or older patients [22, 23]. In these cases, more rigid stainless steel nails can be utilized [21].

Submuscular Plate Fixation

Submuscular plating is usually reserved for fractures that are not suitable for EIN. Submuscular plating provides rigid stability for length-unstable, comminuted, proximal or distal fractures, as well as fractures in obese patients [24, 25]. Theoretically, EIN involves minimal exposure, which helps preserve the periosteal blood supply and reduces soft-tissue damage [26]. However, higher rates of non-union, malunion, and leg-length discrepancy have been reported compared to EIN, partly because plating is often used for more complex fractures.

External Fixation

External fixation is an option when neither EIN nor plating is suitable. It is mostly used for open fractures, cases with severe soft tissue, neurovascular compromise, or in polytrauma. External fixation is relatively fast to perform, spares the physis, and can provide reliable temporary stabilization in complex cases [12, 27].

Adolescents (12 Years to Skeletal Maturity)

Rigid intramedullary nailing is accepted for this age group, offering satisfactory outcomes in terms of alignment, length, healing time, and complications. The minimum reported age for rigid nailing is 8 years [28] as longitudinal growth of the greater trochanteric apophysis is typically complete by this age [29]. However, some experts recommend delaying the procedure until age 13 to further minimize the risk to the trochanteric growth plate [30].

The recommended entry point for rigid nails in adolescents is along the lateral aspect of the greater trochanter, which reduces the risk of avascular necrosis compared to the traditional piriformis fossa entry [31, 32]. The piriformis entry carries a higher risk of disrupting the proximal femoral blood supply and is not recommended [32].

Value-Based Care in Pediatric Femur Fractures

Age-based treatment algorithms for pediatric femoral shaft fractures are well accepted; however, ongoing advancements in implant design and availability have shifted operative management to younger ages. For example, Niknam and colleagues analyzed the Pediatric Health Information System (PHIS) database to assess national trends between 2015 and 2020 [33]. They reported a decline in spica casting among 4- to 6-year-olds, accompanied by increases in intramedullary nailing

(+34%) and plating (+25%). While the study did not report outcomes, these trends are likely to increase costs and reduce value.

Prior comparative studies on pediatric femur fracture treatment have focused on surgical and radiographic outcomes [15, 16, 34–36]. A 2020 meta-analysis by Chen et al. included 1627 patients across 23 studies, comparing casting, EIN, plating, and external fixation [9]. The analysis found that EIN demonstrated superior clinical outcomes. Casting was associated with the lowest infection rates. EIN had the lowest malunion rates, reduced joint stiffness, faster healing, and better outcomes compared to other surgical methods. Malunion did not differ significantly between EIN and plating; however, casting resulted in more malunions. Union times were comparable with casting, EIN, and external fixation. Plating demonstrated slower union time.

Other studies support the superiority of EIN [15, 16, 37]. Fractures treated with EIN demonstrated faster healing, earlier ambulation, quicker return to school, higher parental satisfaction, and less limb length discrepancy compared to spica casting [15, 16, 37]. Spica casting offered the advantage of shorter procedure times.

Most studies have focused on traditional surgical outcomes such as alignment, union rates, complications, and reoperation. Other outcomes such as school absenteeism, parental work loss, caregiver burden, quality of life, and opioid use remain underreported, although they likely play a role in value. A recent study on shared decision-making highlighted this variability: Families prioritizing the avoidance of complications often chose spica casting, while those concerned with parent burden and time away from school preferred flexible nailing [38]. These findings underscore that the concept of value varies across families. Further research is needed to fully define the complex theme of value in pediatric femur fracture care.

Value-Based Themes

Accepting Imperfect Radiographic Alignment

Due to the remodeling potential in children, anatomic reduction is not the primary goal in treating femoral shaft fractures [38, 39]. Stabilization should be tailored to the patient's age and size, while minimizing complications and unnecessary reoperations. Accepting residual angulation and shortening within established parameters can improve value by reducing procedures, repeat anesthesia, and parental anxiety.

Age	Varus/valgus (degrees)	Anterior/posterior (degrees)	Shortening (mm)
Birth to 2 year	30	30	15
2–5 year	15	20	20
6–10 year	10	15	15
11 year to maturity	5	10	10

Acceptable angulation and shortening: Adapted from Beaty JH and Kasser JR, Rockwood and Wilkins Fractures in Children, seventh Ed. (Beaty JH, 2010 #133)

Early Spica Casting: No Traction Required

Traditional treatment with traction, which often lasted for up to 2 weeks, followed by delayed spica casting, has been replaced by immediate spica casting. Immediate spica casting results in equivalent outcomes for union, alignment, and limb length, compared to traction with delayed casting, but with shorter hospitalizations and less cost [40–42].

Standardized Clinical Pathways

A pathway that spans from the time of evaluation to discharge is key to maximizing value. Components include:

- *Nonaccidental trauma screening*: Pediatric femur fractures in young children who are not yet ambulating are associated with nonaccidental trauma (NAT). The AAOS clinical practice guideline recommends that all young children be evaluated for abuse [7]. While some pediatric hospitals have dedicated child protection teams, most hospitals do not. Protocols should be tailored to institutional resources to ensure consistent screening and reduce the risk of missing a case of NAT [43].
- *Site of care:* Children treated with spica casts do not always need hospital admission or operating room care. Spica application can be safely performed in the emergency department (ED), reducing hospital charges and length of stay without increasing complication rates [44].
- *Discharge readiness*: Regardless of whether casting is performed in the emergency department or operating room, care pathways should specify who provides immediate cast-care education and car seat fitting or safe transport alternatives. At many hospitals, this is done in the recovery area, allowing patients to be discharged directly after casting, avoiding the need for inpatient admission and reducing costs.
- *Single-leg spica reduces family burden*: Spica casting can disrupt family function, for school-aged children with working parents. Single-leg spica casts allow for greater mobility and may enable ambulation by the child, reducing parental burden. Cast wedging may be needed more often when using a single-leg spica to maintain alignment [45–48].
- *Functional bracing:* Functional bracing is an alternative to spica casting in young children and aims to reduce the limitations and costs associated with a spica. In a randomized prospective study, Andras and colleagues compared prefabricated functional braces applied at the bedside with spica casts placed in the operating room under anesthesia [49]. They reported equivalent radiographic outcomes at 6 weeks and 1 year, with no malunions in either group. Functional bracing avoided the need for anesthesia and casting, without increasing complications. In a second similar study, Casey et al. reported that in children aged 1–5 years, bracing had significantly lower admission rates, shorter lengths of stay, no exposure to general anesthesia, equal fracture union rates, similar time to weight-bearing, and no malunions [50]. Functional bracing adds value.

- *Limit follow-up radiographs once healed:* Practice variation exists in the follow-up of pediatric femur fractures [51]. Since nonunion is exceedingly rare [52], routine serial radiographs after healing are unnecessary and do not change management. Clinical examination and functional evaluation can then guide care, reducing costs and radiation exposure.
- *The age guidelines are flexible:* Some children fall near the transition point in age/weight treatment algorithms. For example, while immediate spica casting is recommended for children up to age 5 years, a spica is not indicated for a large 5-year-old hit by a car with a comminuted femur fracture and 4 cm of shortening. In a case like this, surgery should be performed. Similarly, a thin 7-year-old weighing 40 kg may be best treated with a 1-leg spica.

Case Example

A 5-year-old boy sustained a closed left diaphyseal femur fracture after a classmate ran into him on the playground, falling onto his leg (Fig. 8.1a, b). He was initially evaluated at a community hospital and was subsequently transferred to our children's hospital after splint immobilization. On examination at 3 am, the limb was painful; however, the child had normal motor strength in all muscle groups of the limb, intact light touch sensation throughout, and 2+ dorsalis pedis pulses. His single mother, with no other support and limited time off from work, was involved in the decision-making. After discussing the options, we decided to stabilize the femur with elastic flexible titanium nails, enabling the child to get about with crutches.

At 7 am, the patient was taken from the emergency department to the urgent fracture operating room. The fracture was stabilized with two 3.5 mm titanium flexible nails. Two small distal femoral incisions were used to place the nails in a retrograde manner (Fig. 8.2a, b). In the postoperative care unit (PACU), the patient was evaluated by nursing and physical therapy staff. Our protocol for crutch fitting, instructions, and mobility was implemented. The PACU case manager assisted the family in arranging a rental wheelchair for school and long-distance mobility. He was discharged from the PACU a few hours later, without formal hospital admission.

Six weeks postoperatively, he was seen for a follow-up, and radiographs showed excellent alignment with good early fracture site callus formation (Fig. 8.3a, b). He was comfortable, walking well with crutches and without crutches at home. He was off all pain medications. Activity restrictions were

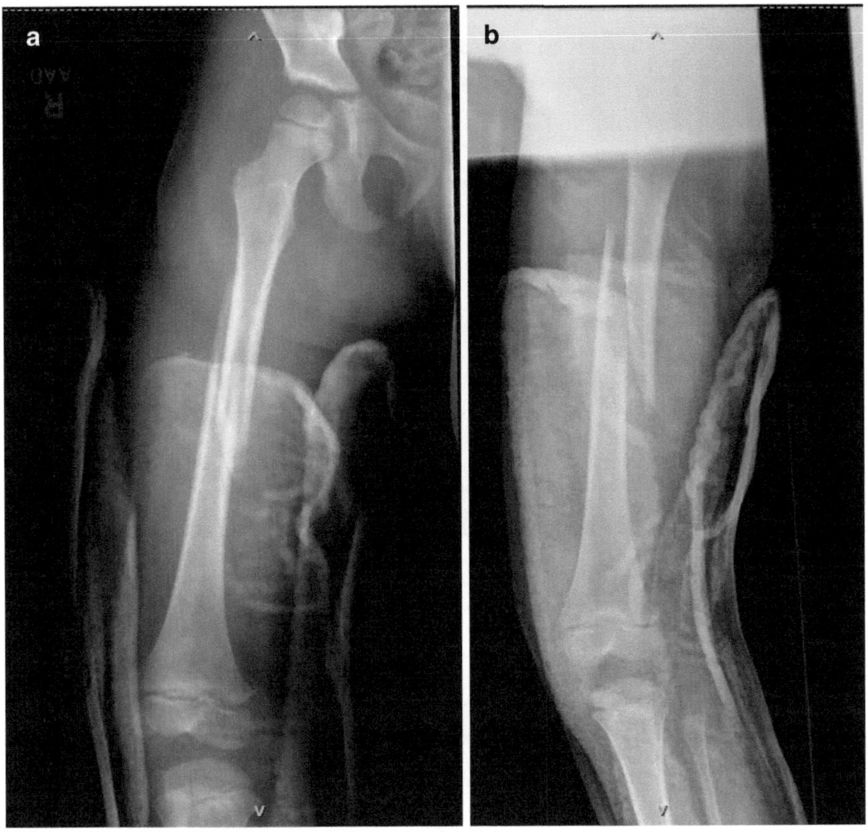

Fig. 8.1 (**a**, **b**): Anteroposterior (AP) and lateral radiographs of the left femur demonstrating a midshaft left oblique diaphyseal femur fracture

liberalized, allowing for an increase in activity as tolerated. A final follow-up visit was scheduled for 12 weeks postop, without the need for additional radiographs. During this visit, he had a stable gait and was running. Limb lengths were equal, with full, painless range of motion in both the left hip and knee. He was cleared for full activities and was advised to follow up 1 year later to discuss and plan implant removal.

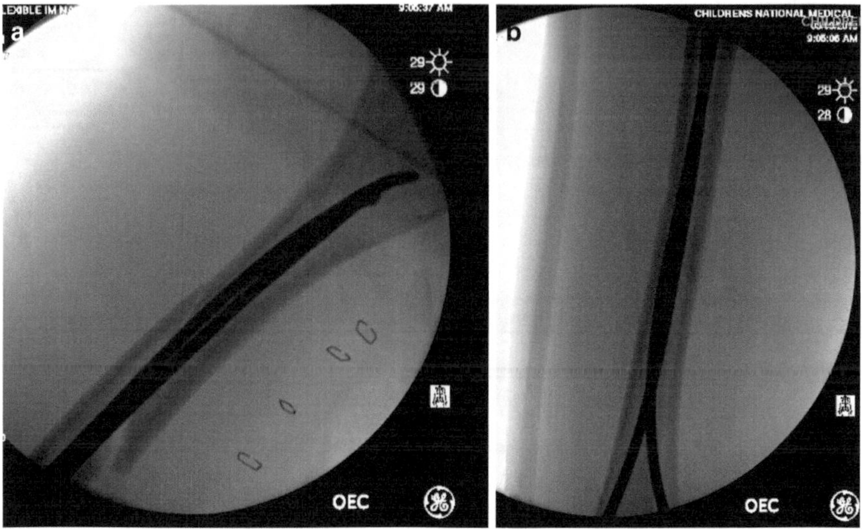

Fig. 8.2 (**a**, **b**): Intraoperative fluoroscopic images demonstrating excellent fracture reduction and stabilization with two retrograde titanium elastic femoral nails

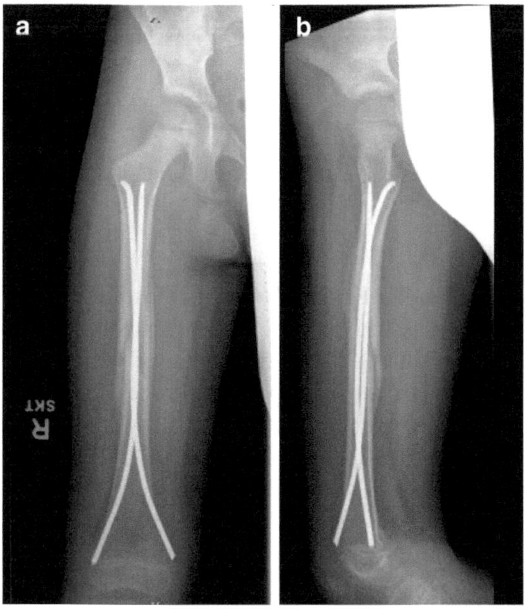

Fig. 8.3 (**a**, **b**): AP and lateral radiographs of the left femur fracture at 6 weeks postoperative demonstrating excellent fracture alignment and robust early bridging callus at the fracture site

Summary

Diaphyseal femur fractures are among the most common pediatric injuries. An established, age-based treatment algorithm guides care. By minimizing repeat surgeries and complications, while promoting early patient mobilization and reducing clinician workload, this approach ensures optimal value-based care for femur fractures in children.

Author Pearls

- *Patient age* is the primary factor in determining treatment: a Pavlik harness for patients <6 months, immediate spica casting for those 6 months to 5 years, elastic flexible nails for ages 5–11, and rigid intramedullary nails for those >11 years.
- *Pediatric femur fractures* heal well, so conservative use of postoperative radiographs is reasonable.
- *Anatomic reduction* is not necessary, particularly in younger children, as pediatric diaphyseal femur fractures have excellent remodeling potential.
- *Shared decision-making* with parents to select the most appropriate treatment, balancing surgical risk with family impact, adds value.
- Daycare restrictions may influence families who must get back to work to prefer flexible elastic nailing over spica casting.

Editor Comments

WLH

A splendid chapter that nicely summarizes methods to improve value in the treatment of pediatric femur fractures: Use a brace instead of a spica cast when possible; apply the spica in the ED rather than the OR; opt for a single-leg spica when casting; consider the possibility of child abuse in nonambulatory children; position metal implants to avoid the need for later removal; and minimize follow-up X-rays.

RMS

Value-based decisions in pediatric femur fracture care often consider family and social circumstances as much as fracture patterns or age. For instance, some daycare centers may not accept a young child in a spica cast but will accommodate a child mobilizing after flexible elastic nailing (FEN), which can influence both parents' and surgeons' decision-making. In adolescents with a femur fracture who require a rigid nail, antegrade FEN placed through the greater trochanter and left long proximally allows for simplified removal later. In older infants, a molded J-splint can serve as definitive treatment, avoiding the need for a trip to the operating room for spica application. These examples highlight how individualized choices, balancing medical outcomes with family needs and available resources, can enhance value.

References

1. McCartney D, Hinton A, Heinrich SD. Operative stabilization of pediatric femur fractures. Orthop Clin North Am. 1994;25:635–50.
2. Sahlin Y. Occurrence of fractures in a defined population: a 1-year study. Injury. 1990;21:158–60.
3. Liau GZQ, Lin HY, Wang Y, Nistala KRY, Cheong CK, Hui JHP. Pediatric femoral shaft fracture: an age-based treatment algorithm. Indian J Orthop. 2021;55:55–67.
4. Loder RT, O'Donnell PW, Feinberg JR. Epidemiology and mechanisms of femur fractures in children. J Pediatr Orthop. 2006;26:561–6.
5. Macha AP, Temu R, Olotu F, Seth NP, Massawe HL. Epidemiology and associated injuries in paediatric diaphyseal femur fractures treated at a limited resource zonal referral hospital in northern Tanzania. BMC Musculoskelet Disord. 2022;23:360.
6. Rewers A, Hedegaard H, Lezotte D, Meng K, Battan FK, Emery K, Hamman RF. Childhood femur fractures, associated injuries, and sociodemographic risk factors: a population-based study. Pediatrics. 2005;115:e543–52.
7. American Academy of Orthopaedic Surgeons: Treatment of pediatric diaphyseal femur fractures evidence-based clinical practice guideline. 2020; At <https://www.aaos.org/globalassets/quality-and-practice-resources/pdff/pdffcpg.pdf>.
8. Ortiz EJ, Isler MH, Navia JE, Canosa R. Pathologic fractures in children. Clin Orthop Relat Res. 2005:116–26. https://doi.org/10.1097/01.blo.0000155375.88317.6c.
9. Chen Z, Han D, Wang Q, Li L. Four interventions for pediatric femoral shaft fractures: network meta-analysis of randomized trials. Int J Surg. 2020;80:53–60.
10. Rush JK, Kelly DM, Sawyer JR, Beaty JH, Warner WCJ. Treatment of pediatric femur fractures with the Pavlik harness: multiyear clinical and radiographic outcomes. J Pediatr Orthop. 2013;33:614–7.
11. Mahajan J, Hennrikus W, Piazza B. Overgrowth after femoral shaft fractures in infants treated with a Pavlik harness. J Pediatr Orthop B. 2016;25:7–10.
12. Sanzarello I, Calamoneri E, D'Andrea L, Rosa MA. Algorithm for the management of femoral shaft fractures in children. Musculoskelet Surg. 2014;98:53–60.
13. Khoriati A-A, Jones C, Gelfer Y, Trompeter A. The management of paediatric diaphyseal femoral fractures: a modern approach. Strat Trau Limb Recon. 2016;11:87–97.
14. Nascimento FP, Santili C, Akkari M, Waisberg G, Dos Reis Braga S, De Barros Fucs PMM. Short hospitalization period with elastic stable intramedullary nails in the treatment of femoral shaft fractures in school children. J Child Orthop. 2010;4:53–60.
15. Shemshaki HR, Mousavi H, Salehi G, Eshaghi MA. Titanium elastic nailing versus hip spica cast in treatment of femoral-shaft fractures in children. J Orthop Traumatol. 2011;12:45–8.
16. Buechsenschuetz KE, Mehlman CT, Shaw KJ, Crawford AH, Immerman EB. Femoral shaft fractures in children: traction and casting versus elastic stable intramedullary nailing. J Trauma. 2002;53:914–21.
17. Park KC, Oh CW, Byun YS, et al. Intramedullary nailing versus submuscular plating in adolescent femoral fracture. Injury. 2012;43:870–5.
18. Lohiya R, Bachhal V, Khan U, et al. Flexible intramedullary nailing in paediatric femoral fractures. A report of 73 cases. J Orthop Surg Res. 2011;6:64.
19. Furlan D, Pogorelić Z, Biočić M, et al. Elastic stable intramedullary nailing for pediatric long bone fractures: experience with 175 fractures. Scand J Surg. 2011;100:208–15.
20. Fricka KB, Mahar AT, Lee SS, Newton PO. Biomechanical analysis of antegrade and retrograde flexible intramedullary nail fixation of pediatric femoral fractures using a synthetic bone model. J Pediatr Orthop. 2004;24:167–71.

21. Shaha J, Cage JM, Black S, Wimberly RL, Shaha SH, Riccio AI. Flexible intramedullary nails for femur fractures in pediatric patients heavier than 100 pounds. J Pediatr Orthop. 2018;38:88–93.
22. Li Y, Stabile KJ, Shilt JS. Biomechanical analysis of titanium elastic nail fixation in a pediatric femur fracture model. J Pediatr Orthop. 2008;28:874–8.
23. Flynn JM, Hresko T, Reynolds RA, Blasier RD, Davidson R, Kasser J. Titanium elastic nails for pediatric femur fractures: a multicenter study of early results with analysis of complications. J Pediatr Orthop. 2001;21:4–8.
24. May C, Yen YM, Nasreddine AY, Hedequist D, Hresko MT, Heyworth BE. Complications of plate fixation of femoral shaft fractures in children and adolescents. J Children's Orthop. 2013;7:235–43.
25. Abdelgawad AA, Sieg RN, Laughlin MD, Shunia J, Kanlic EM. Submuscular bridge plating for complex pediatric femur fractures is reliable. Clin Orthop Relat Res. 2013;471:2797–807.
26. Claes L, Heitemeyer U, Krischak G, Braun H, Hierholzer G. Fixation technique influences osteogenesis of comminuted fractures. Clin Orthop Relat Res. 1999;365:221–9. https://doi.org/10.1097/00003086-199908000-00027.
27. Kong H, Sabharwal S. External fixation for closed pediatric femoral shaft fractures: where are we now? Clin Orthop Relat Res. 2014;472:3814–22.
28. Keeler KA, Dart B, Luhmann SJ, Schoenecker PL, Ortman MR, Dobbs MB, Gordon JE. Antegrade intramedullary nailing of pediatric femoral fractures using an interlocking pediatric femoral nail and a lateral trochanteric entry point. J Pediatr Orthop. 2009;29:345–51.
29. Knapik DM, McCarthy C, Liu RW. Developmental patterns of the greater trochanter in skeletally immature patients. J Pediatr Orthop. 2019;39:e412–6.
30. González-Herranz P, Burgos-Flores J, Rapariz JM, Lopez-Mondejar JA, Ocete JG, Amaya S. Intramedullary nailing of the femur in children. Effects on its proximal end. J Bone Joint Surg Br. 1995;77:262–6.
31. Garner M, Bhat S, Khujanazarov I, Flynn J, Spiegel D. Fixation of length-stable femoral shaft fractures in heavier children: flexible nails vs rigid locked nails. J Pediatr Orthop. 2011;31:11–6.
32. Townsend D, Hoffinger S. Intramedullary nailing of femoral shaft fractures in children via the trochanter tip. Clin Orthop Relat Res. 2000;376:113–8.
33. Niknam K, Gatto A, Swarup I. Trends in the management of femur fractures in young children. J Pediatr Soc North Am. 2023;5:766.
34. Coyte PC, Bronskill SE, Hirji ZZ, Daigle-Takacs G, Trerise BS, Wright JG. Economic evaluation of 2 treatments for pediatric femoral shaft fractures. Clin Orthop Relat Res. 1997;336:205–15. https://doi.org/10.1097/00003086-199703000-00029.
35. Madhuri V, Dutt V, Gahukamble AD, Tharyan P. Interventions for treating femoral shaft fractures in children and adolescents. Cochrane Database Syst Rev. 2014;2014:CD009076.
36. Reeves RB, Ballard RI, Hughes JL. Internal fixation versus traction and casting of adolescent femoral shaft fractures. J Pediatr Orthop. 1990;10:592–5.
37. Hwaizi L, Saeed a, Mahmood M. Diaphyseal femoral fractures in children: comparison between elastic stable intramedullary nailing and conservative management. TOORTHJ. 2018;12:435–44.
38. Kumar CA, Reddy J, Jose MP, Gahukamble A, Palocaren T, Madhuri V. Remodeling of rotational Malunion of femoral shaft in children. Indian J Orthop. 2024;58:89–97.
39. Naik P. Remodelling in children's fractures and limits of acceptability. Indian J Orthop. 2021;55:549–59.
40. Younis MH, Mahmoud K, Kawas A, Ibrahim T. Early versus late hip spica casting for paediatric femoral shaft fractures. J Pediatr Orthop B. 2019;28:122–6.
41. Tisherman RT, Hoellwarth JS, Mendelson SA. Systematic review of spica casting for the treatment of paediatric diaphyseal femur fractures. J Child Orthop. 2018;12:136–44.
42. Wright JG. The treatment of femoral shaft fractures in children: a systematic overview and critical appraisal of the literature. Can J Surg. 2000;43:180–9.

43. Escobar MAJ, Pflugeisen BM, Duralde Y, Morris CJ, Haferbecker D, Amoroso PJ, Lemley H, Pohlson EC. Development of a systematic protocol to identify victims of non-accidental trauma. Pediatr Surg Int. 2016;32:377–86.
44. Mansour AA 3rd, Wilmoth JC, Mansour AS, Lovejoy SA, Mencio GA, Martus JE. Immediate spica casting of pediatric femoral fractures in the operating room versus the emergency department: comparison of reduction, complications, and hospital charges. J Pediatr Orthop. 2010;30:813–7.
45. Flynn JM, Garner MR, Jones KJ, D'Italia J, Davidson RS, Ganley TJ, Horn BD, Spiegel D, Wells L. The treatment of low-energy femoral shaft fractures: a prospective study comparing the "walking spica" with the traditional spica cast. J Bone Joint Surg Am. 2011;93:2196–202.
46. Hughes BF, Sponseller PD, Thompson JD. Pediatric femur fractures: effects of spica cast treatment on family and community. J Pediatr Orthop. 1995;15:457–60.
47. Leu D, Sargent MC, Ain MC, Leet AI, Tis JE, Sponseller PD. Spica casting for pediatric femoral fractures: a prospective, randomized controlled study of single-leg versus double-leg spica casts. J Bone Joint Surg Am. 2012;94:1259–64.
48. Kocher M, Ciarlo M, Feroe A, Dichtel L, Traver J. Impact on family functioning of immediate Spica casting for pediatric femur fractures: an ecological study: original research. JPOSNA. 2022;4:389.
49. Andras LM, Sanders JS, Phan TN, Purtell SR, Gasca J, Wren TAL, Sim AT, Skaggs D, Kramer A, Chavez M, et al. A prospective, randomized comparison of functional bracing and Spica casting for femoral fractures showed equivalent early outcomes. J Bone Joint Surg Am. 2025;107:1769–76.
50. Casey VF, Chandler CC, Graham GD, Frick SL. Dynamic femur fracture brace vs hip spica cast for pediatric femoral shaft fractures: a retrospective comparative cohort study. J Pediatr Soc North Am. 2025;12:100203.
51. Sanatani GE, Habib E, Bone JN, Sandhu A, Schaeffer EK, Mulpuri K. Variability in the follow-up Management of Pediatric Femoral Fractures. J Am Acad Orthop Surg Glob Res Rev. 2022;6:e20.00084.
52. Zura R, Kaste SC, Heffernan MJ, Accousti WK, Gargiulo D, Wang Z, Steen RG. Risk factors for nonunion of bone fracture in pediatric patients: an inception cohort study of 237,033 fractures. Medicine (Baltimore). 2018;97:e11691.

Part II

General Pediatric Orthopaedics

Rethinking Flat Feet Value in Children

9

Blaise Nemeth

Introduction

When children first begin standing and walking, most will show flattening of their arches. Regardless of how the shape of the arch or "flat feet" is defined, the majority of children will develop a "normal" arch before reaching the prepubertal growth spurt [1–3]. Approximately 4–14% will still have a flexible flat foot into later childhood [1–5]. Around 6% of adults with flat foot will develop a tight Achilles tendon, with approximately 10% of this group experiencing more significant deformities. Rigid flat feet are seen in about 2% of military recruits [4]. There is a disappointing lack of substantial studies on interventions and their benefits.

A flexible flat foot is characterized by a normal arch when nonweight-bearing but shows arch flattening under body weight. Key components of the deformity include hindfoot valgus/eversion, lateral shift of the navicular on the talus, and often pronation of the forefoot. This condition can also resolve when the great toe is extended (Jack test) or when the child rises onto tiptoes, causing the hindfoot to roll into varus (Fig. 9.1). Common examination findings among children who develop functional problems are a tight Achilles tendon and forefoot supination [6].

Since the majority of children with persistent flexible flat feet experience no issues, the most practical approach is to avoid unnecessary treatment. Early identification of children who may develop problems could allow for cost savings through conservative management, potentially preventing the need for surgery. Surgery should be reserved for those with clear functional issues, and only if there are safe interventions with proven positive outcomes.

B. Nemeth (✉)
Department of Orthopedics and Rehabilitation, University of Wisconsin School of Medicine and Public Health, American Family Children's Hospital, Madison, WI, USA
e-mail: nemeth@ortho.wisc.edu

W. L. Hennrikus, R. M. Schwend (eds.), *Value in Pediatric Orthopaedics*,
https://doi.org/10.1007/978-3-032-19570-8_9

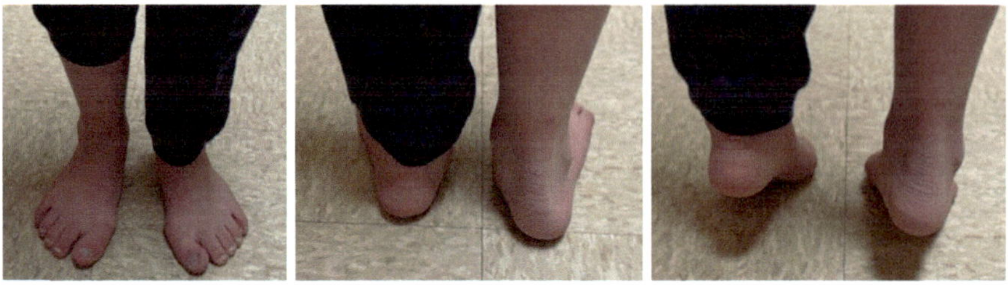

Fig. 9.1 Demonstration of the clinical appearance of a flexible flat right foot in a patient with Trisomy 21 who has collapse of the arch, forefoot pronation and hindfoot valgus (left and middle), with an arch that reconstitutes when on tiptoes and hindfoot moves into varus (right)

Value-Based Themes

Barefoot Is Okay

Arches develop best with less restrictive or no footwear. There are no high-quality studies on the best methods for encouraging normal foot development, nor is it clear whether "normal" arches prevent future foot problems. Therefore, attempting to prevent symptomatic flexible flat foot remains an unachievable goal. However, insight comes from an observational cohort study conducted in India, which found that among children who wore shoes, the rate of flat feet was 13.6% [4], a figure consistent with findings in Western cultures [1, 2, 5]. Similarly, in the Congo, flat feet occurred in 6% of children who wore sandals [3], but in only 2.8% of children who grew up barefoot. These findings suggest that allowing children to be barefoot or wear minimal, unsupportive footwear may promote better foot development, with little to no additional cost compared to traditional western footwear.

No Radiographs

Radiographs offer no additional value over physical examination when evaluating asymptomatic flat feet in children. Since flexible flat feet deform under weight-bearing and appear normal when nonweight-bearing, radiographs do not help differentiate a symptomatic flat foot from an asymptomatic one, despite the ability to measure various parameters with radiographs [7, 8]. For symptomatic feet, no studies have evaluated the cost-benefit of radiographs beyond the physical exam. However, clinically indicated imaging may be necessary to confirm suspected pathologies in cases with atypical presentations, such as rigid flat feet, pain, unilateral flat foot, or other deformities. Radiographs can help identify specific surgical conditions such as tarsal coalition, congenital vertical talus, excessive tibio-talar valgus, pronounced lateral talo-1st metatarsal (Meary) angle, and/or lateral displacement of the navicular on the talus.

No Corrective Footwear

Corrective footwear does not induce arch development. Wenger's classic study demonstrated that corrective shoes and inserts do not alter the natural course of foot development [9], findings that have been recently reaffirmed [10]. To give the foot the best chance to develop naturally, it is recommended that children be barefoot as much as possible, and wear thin, flexible footwear when going barefoot is not possible [4]. There is no evidence to suggest that additional interventions or more expensive footwear options provide any benefit.

No Orthotics

Orthoses do not induce arch development or improve pain. Numerous studies have evaluated the effect of orthoses in children with flexible flat feet. While some studies report improved alignment and gait mechanics, there is no evidence to suggest that orthoses influence the natural progression of arch development [9, 11]. In fact, one study comparing orthoses with physical therapy suggested that orthoses may inhibit normal foot development [12]. In addition, orthoses do not improve quality of life for children with flexible flat feet [13]. The most recent Cochrane Review found no evidence supporting the use of orthoses for flexible flat foot in children [14]. Less expensive, over-the-counter inserts don't make a difference either. Comparison of over-the-counter inserts to custom foot orthoses and controls demonstrates no difference across all groups on arch development or pain [11]. The American Academy of Pediatrics and the Pediatric Orthopedic Society of North America have recommended against the "routine use of custom orthotics and shoe inserts for a child with minimally or asymptomatic flat feet" as part of their 2018 Choosing Wisely Guidelines [15].

One Possible Exception

One possible exception to the lack of benefit of orthoses involves children with Trisomy 21. Progressive foot deformity and pain are common in adolescents and adults with Trisomy 21 [16]. However, similar to children without Trisomy 21, research on prevention and proactive treatment is lacking. Foot orthoses have been shown to improve gait mechanics in adolescents and adults with Trisomy 21 [17]. Supra-malleolar orthoses (SMOs) and foot orthoses can improve gait mechanics, walking, running, and jumping in young ambulatory children with Trisomy 21 [18, 19]. However, one study indicated that SMOs might inhibit the developmental progression of these same skills in children with Trisomy 21 who are pulling to stand but not yet walking [20]. It is also unclear whether this benefit extends to other children with flexible flat feet and gross motor delays (e.g., due to hypotonia or other hypermobility-related conditions), despite frequent nonevidence-based recommendations for such interventions, or prevents development of future foot deformity. In addition, the potential indirect benefit of orthoses on social and verbal development, such as interacting with peers, in children with Trisomy 21 has not been studied.

Surgery Infrequently Helpful

Surgery may be beneficial for children with painful, flexible flat feet with tight Achilles tendons. Several surgical procedures have been suggested for the treatment of symptomatic flexible flat feet, including Achilles lengthening, calcaneal osteotomy, and arthroereisis [21]. While these procedures can improve clinical motion, radiographic alignment, and reduce pain in symptomatic patients, especially with a tight Achilles tendon or rigid flat foot, surgery has no role in the treatment of *asymptomatic* children with flexible flat feet.

Case Example

A 4-year-old girl presented for evaluation of her feet. Her parents noticed that since she began standing and walking at 1 year, her arches collapsed, and her feet were flat. The feet were painless, and she was able to keep up with her peers. However, her parents were concerned that she may experience problems as an adult since her father has flat feet and foot pain.

On examination, her arches collapsed with weight-bearing. However, when she raised onto her tiptoes, her heels rolled into varus, and her arch reconstituted. When sitting, her arch was normal. When the ankles dorsiflexed to 20° the arch was normal. No radiographs were necessary.

The natural history of arch development and the low likelihood of future problems were discussed with the parents. The parents were encouraged to let her spend as much time barefoot as possible. When wearing shoes outside the home, they were advised to choose flexible footwear that allowed her feet to move as naturally as possible. The use of shoe inserts and orthotics were discouraged because these have not been shown to promote, and may even inhibit, normal arch development. The parents were advised to return for follow-up only if she experiences pain in the future.

Summary

The most recent Cochrane Review puts it best, concluding that there is no benefit to the use of orthoses and even recommending that additional research into asymptomatic flexible flat feet be "relegated to history" [14]. This may be one of the strongest statements regarding the management of flexible flat feet in children.

Author Pearls

- Children's feet are best allowed to develop naturally by being barefoot, and wearing flexible footwear only when required by activity or environment.
- Shoe inserts and orthoses have no role in the treatment of asymptomatic flexible flat feet.
- SMOs improve gait and gross motor development in ambulatory children with Trisomy 21 but may inhibit gross motor development in those with Trisomy 21 who have not yet begun walking.
- Surgery should not be performed in children with asymptomatic flexible flat feet, but may be considered in symptomatic flat feet when pain is associated with a tight Achilles tendon or a rigid flat foot.

Editors Comments

WLH

The American Academy of Pediatrics Orthopaedic Section and POSNA selected flexible flat feet as one of 5 topics for the Choosing Wisely campaign for good reason. Traditional treatment for flexible flat feet has been overdone with many nonevidence-based interventions. Dr. Nemeth's current elegant chapter sets the record straight on flexible flat foot. Less is more. Observe, reassure, and offer to follow is the best management strategy for most cases of asymptomatic flexible flat feet in children.

RMS

A conservative estimate is that 100s of millions of dollars are spent on custom shoe wear and orthotics for flexible flat feet in children. When evaluating flexible flat feet, first rule out a rigid foot, which may indicate an underlying tarsal coalition or other pathologic condition requiring further imaging or intervention. Additionally, assess for signs of generalized ligamentous laxity using the Beighton scoring system. In some cases, flexible flat feet may be a presenting feature of a systemic condition such as Marfan syndrome or Ehlers-Danlos syndrome. Recognizing these exceptions ensures that appropriate evaluation and care are provided, thereby avoiding misdiagnosis and enhancing value through targeted intervention.

References

1. Staheli LT, Chew DE, Corbett M. The longitudinal arch: a survey of eight hundred and eighty-two feet in normal children and adults. J Bone Joint Surg. 1987;69-A(3):426–8.

2. Rao UB, Joseph B. The influence of footwear on the prevalence of flat foot. A survey of 2300 children. J Bone Joint Surg Br. 1992;74(4):525–7.
3. Pfeiffer M, Kotz R, Ledl T, Hauser G, Sluga M. Prevalence of flat foot in preschool-aged children. Pediatrics. 2006;118(2):634–9.
4. Harris RI, Beath T. Hypermobile flat-foot with short tendo achillis. J Bone Joint Surg. 1948;30-A(1):116–40.
5. Echarri JJ, Forriol. The development in footprint morphology in 1851 Congolese children from urban and rural areas, and the relationship between this and wearing shoes. J Pediatr Orthop B. 2003;12(2):141–6.
6. Mosca VS. Flexible flatfoot in children and adolescents. J Child Orthop. 2010;4:107–21.
7. Moraleda L, Mubarak SJ. Flexible flatfoot: differences in the relative alignment of each segment of the foot between symptomatic and asymptomatic patients. J Pediatr Orthop. 2011;31(4):421–8.
8. Banwell HA, Paris ME, Mackintosh, Williams CM. Paediatric flexible flat foot: how are we measuring it and are we getting it right? A systematic review. J Foot Ankle Res. 2018;11:21.
9. Wenger DR, Mauldin D, Speck G, Morgan D, Lieber RL. Corrective shoes and inserts as treatment for flexible flatfoot in infants and children. J Bone Joint Surg. 1989;71-A(6):800–10.
10. Kanatli U, Aktas E, Yetkin H. Do corrective shoes improve the development of the medial longitudinal arch in children with flexible flat feet? J Orthop Sci. 2016;21:662–6.
11. Whitford D, Eseterman A. A randomized controlled trial of two types of in-shoe orthoses in children with flexible excess pronation of the feet. Foot Ankle Int. 2007;28(6):715–23.
12. Riccio I, Gimigliano F, Gimigliano R, Porpora G, Iolascon G. Rehabilitative treatment in flexible flatfoot: a perspective cohort study. Musculoskelet Surg. 2009;93:101–7.
13. Camurcu Y, Ucpunar H, Karakose R, Ozcan S, Sahin V. Foot orthoses use for pediatric flexible flatfoot: comparative evaluation of quality of life for children and parents. J Pediatr Orthop B. 2020;30(3):282–6.
14. Evans AM, Rome K, Carroll M, Hawke F. Foot orthoses for treating paediatric flat feet. Cochrane Database Syst Rev. 2022;1:CD006311.
15. https://publications.aap.org/aapnews/news/9893/FYI-5-things-to-question-in-orthopedics?autologincheck=redirected. Accessed 15 May 2025.
16. Lim PQ, Shields N, Nikolopoulos N, Barrett J, Evans AM, Taylor NF, Munteanu SE. The association of foot structure and footwear fit with disability in children and adolescents with Down syndrome. J Foot Ankle Res. 2015;8:4.
17. Galafate D, Pournajaf S, Condoluci C, Gofredo M, Di Girolamo G, Manzia CM, Pellicciari L, Franceschini M, Galli M. Bilateral foot orthoses elicit changes in gait kinematics of adolescents with Down syndrome with flatfoot. Int J Environ Res Public Health. 2020;17:4994.
18. Martin K. Effects of supramalleolar orthoses on postural stability in children with Down syndrome. DevMed Child Neurol. 2004;46:406–11.
19. Selby-Silverstein L, Hillstrom HJ, Palisano RJ. The effect of foot orthoses on standing foot posture and gait of young children with Down Syndrome. Neuro Rehabilitation. 2001;16(3):183–93.
20. Looper J, Ulrich DA. Effect of treadmill training and supramalleolar orthosis use on motor skill development in infants with Down syndrome: a randomized clinical trial. Phys Ther. 2010;90(3):382–90.
21. Chong DY, Macwilliams BA, Hennessey TA, Teske N, Stevens PM. Prospective comparison of subtalar arthroereisis with lateral column lengthening for painful flatfeet. J Pediatr Orthop B. 2015;24(4):345–53.

10 Osteogenesis Imperfecta: Weak Bones, Strong Children, and Value Care

Emily Elmore and Kelsie Coe

Introduction

Osteogenesis imperfecta (OI) is a heritable connective tissue disorder caused by mutations in type I collagen, with an incidence ranging from 1 in 15,000 to 20,000 [1]. OI is most commonly associated with autosomal dominant mutations in the COL1A1 or COL1A2 genes and has traditionally been classified into four types (I–IV) according to the Sillence criteria [1–3].

The Sillence criteria is described as follows:

- Type I: Absence of bone deformities, near-normal-to-normal stature, intermittent fractures
- Type II: Severe fractures and deformity, perinatally lethal
- Type III: Significant bone and spinal deformities, short stature, most severe postnatally
- Type IV: Mild-moderate bone deformities with variation in stature

Advancements in genetic testing have identified up to 13 mutations contributing to the various phenotypes of osteogenesis imperfecta, each associated with a spectrum of skeletal manifestations. These include chest wall deformities, frequent long bone fractures, scoliosis, kyphosis, and limb bowing [1, 2]. Extra-skeletal manifestations may also be present, such as odontogenesis imperfecta, hearing loss, blue sclerae, and cardiac valvular disease [1].

E. Elmore
Penn State College of Medicine, Hershey, PA, USA
e-mail: eelmore@pennstatehealth.psu.edu

K. Coe (✉)
Department of Orthopaedics, Penn State College of Medicine, Hershey, PA, USA
e-mail: kcoe@pennstatehealth.psu.edu

W. L. Hennrikus, R. M. Schwend (eds.), *Value in Pediatric Orthopaedics*,
https://doi.org/10.1007/978-3-032-19570-8_10

Despite the variability in disease presentation, the primary goal of osteogenesis imperfecta management is to reduce fracture frequency and improve mobility through both nonpharmacologic and pharmacologic therapies [2, 4]. Nonpharmacologic interventions include orthopedic surgery, physical and occupational therapy, safe handling practices, and avoidance of high-impact activities [2, 4]. In contrast, bisphosphonates have been the cornerstone of pharmacologic treatment for pediatric OI patients since the 1990s, leading to significant reductions in fracture rates and improvements in mobility and walking [2–4].

Concerns about cost-effective care for patients with osteogenesis imperfecta stem from the frequent fractures that often require emergency department visits, hospitalizations, imaging, and potentially additional surgical interventions [4]. Depending on the severity of OI, secondary costs may include surgical correction of limb and spinal deformities, diagnostic testing, bisphosphonate infusions, rehabilitation services, assistive devices, and home modifications [4, 5]. For adult patients, the financial burden also includes the cost of unemployment and the indirect costs associated with missed workdays [5].

Effective value-based care for patients with osteogenesis imperfecta requires a coordinated, multidisciplinary approach that integrates both pharmacologic and nonpharmacologic strategies to reduce fractures and improve quality of life [6].

Value-Based Themes

Benefits of Genetic Testing

With the advent of next-generation sequencing (NGS) technologies, genetic testing has become more affordable and efficient compared to earlier methods [7]. This increased accessibility allows families to identify specific disease-causing mutations and facilitates the diagnosis of new or rare variants of OI [7, 8]. While identifying genotypes may not change clinical outcomes, it can offer valuable insights for both patients and parents, particularly in predicting disease progression and informing management strategies.

Interdisciplinary Approach

Many patients with OI require care from a range of medical and surgical specialists, including orthopedic surgeons, endocrinologists, rheumatologists, and primary care physicians [9]. Establishing a coordinated interdisciplinary care team including physicians, nurses, and therapy staff can improve the cost-effectiveness and overall care of patients with OI [10]. Challenges in providing interdisciplinary care for OI can stem from clinicians who lack familiarity with the condition or do not fully understand the specific needs of OI patients [11]. These difficulties may be mitigated through improved communication and collaboration among specialists. The use of telehealth may also be helpful.

Caregiver Education and Experience

Caregivers should be educated in safe-handling techniques, initial fracture management, home environment adaptations, pain management, basic rehabilitation, daily activity routines, safe play methods, and the avoidance of high-impact sports [11, 12]. Patient transfers, including to and from beds, vehicles, and toilets, pose challenges due to the risk of fractures [11]. In addition, coordinating transportation, medical appointments, and surgical procedures can be difficult for caregivers [11]. Caregiver involvement should also be considered in the evaluation of extra-skeletal manifestations of OI, particularly during specialist appointments for dental, cardiac, pulmonary, sleep, auditory, gynecologic, and psychiatric concerns [13].

Pharmacologic Management and Benefits of Home Infusions

Pharmacologic management of OI involves the use of bisphosphonates, typically pamidronate, which has been shown to reduce fracture incidence and improve ambulation, chronic pain, and fatigue [3, 14]. Moreover, initiating bisphosphonate therapy during infancy increases vertebral height, improves vertical growth, and reduces fracture frequency during childhood [3].

Other studies have reported on alternative therapies such as calcitonin nasal spray and denosumab, a monoclonal antibody that inhibits Receptor Activator of Nuclear Factor B Ligand (RANKL), for their potential to reduce fractures. However, at this time, these treatments are not considered first-line and are reserved for patients who respond poorly to bisphosphonates [14, 15]. In addition, ongoing research is investigating the potential benefits of mesenchymal stem cells and induced pluripotent stem cells for OI [15].

The administration of bisphosphonates via infusion can pose a financial burden for some families [16]. However, infusions given in the patient's home lower costs compared to infusions given at the hospital or infusion center, particularly for those patients receiving multiday infusions [16]. Although home infusions are convenient and less expensive, home infusions also require proper training for caregivers or home health nurses and reliable access to necessary supplies.

Surgical Management of Fractures and Deformities: Telescoping Versus Static Rods

Patients with OI commonly experience long-bone fractures involving the radius, ulna, humerus, femur, tibia, and fibula. Most fractures typically occurs within the first 20 years of life, with peak fracture rates observed between ages 11 and 15, coinciding with periods of rapid growth [17]. Intramedullary (IM) rodding of the humerus, femur, and tibia are commonly performed to prevent and treat long bone fractures and deformities in patients with OI [18, 19]. Static intramedullary rods, while easier to place and effective for managing fractures and deformities, are associated with higher rates of reoperations [20]. In contrast, IM telescoping rods offer longer durability and require fewer follow-up visits. Regardless of disease severity or presentation, comprehensive medical and surgical management of OI can lead to reduced fracture frequency and help prevent long bone deformities. A range of interventions can enhance mobility, independence, and overall quality of life. In addition, fewer fractures enhance value with reduced hospital admissions, fewer surgical procedures, and decreased need for diagnostic imaging and postinjury rehabilitation or future revision surgeries [20]. The choice between static and telescoping rods should be guided by the patient's age, disease severity, and anticipated growth.

Management of Humerus Fractures and Deformities

Humerus fractures are common in patients with OI and vary with disease severity. Humerus fractures often lead to deformities that can lessen independence and quality of life [21]. Humeral deformities between 30° and 60° can limit a patient's ability to perform activities of daily living, such as dressing, toileting, and working [21]. IM rodding of the humerus may be performed using either telescoping or static rods, depending on the patient's size and anticipated growth [18]. Traditionally, IM rodding of the humerus has been performed using an antegrade approach through the rotator cuff; however, this technique can be associated with rotator cuff injury and chronic shoulder pain [21]. Alternatively, the retrograde approach can be used for acute fractures or deformity correction. In the retrograde approach, the nails are inserted through the medial and lateral condyles and result in comparable efficacy in fracture reduction and stability, a low complication rate, and high implant longevity [21]. Distal humeral deformities may potentially develop via the retrograde approach [21].

Management of Lower Extremity Fractures and Deformities

Patients with lower extremity fractures and deformities may choose static rod or telescoping rod placement to achieve fracture stabilization [19]. While telescoping rods, such as the Bailey-Dubow rod, allow growth through passive telescoping, they may pose a risk of injury to the physis [19]. The Fassier-Duval (FD) telescoping rod is among the most widely used implants for long bone fractures in OI. The FD rod allows for less invasive placement through a single entry point and is associated with shorter operative times, reduced implant migration, and less joint surface damage [19, 22]. Despite these advantages, FD rods can lead to complications such as rotational malalignment, and FD rods may be difficult to place in young children with narrow medullary canals [22].

Recent studies demonstrate that the sliding double flexible intramedullary nail (SDFIN) may offer benefits in reducing lower extremity long bone fractures and deformities in patients with OI [22]. This technique may be preferred due to the greater availability and cost-effectiveness of SDFIN compared to more expensive

FD rods [22]. Early outcomes using the SDFIN demonstrate favorable results at a lower cost [22].

Spinal Deformity

Scoliosis and kyphosis are common in patients with OI, with a higher incidence observed in those with more severe phenotypes [23]. Bracing is used selectively due to thoracic fragility in OI patients. However, spinal fusion may be indicated for individuals with significant spinal deformity and/or respiratory compromise [23]. Some studies also support the use of preoperative halo gravity traction to improve curve correction prior to instrumented posterior spinal fusion [24]. Cost concerns related to spinal fusion in patients with OI stem from the technical challenges of implanting spinal instrumentation, the risk of significant intraoperative bleeding requiring transfusion, and the need for prolonged postoperative hospitalization [23, 24]. OI patients typically experience hospital stays that are 2–3 days longer and often require fusion of a greater number of vertebrae, resulting in higher overall costs compared to other patient populations [23].

Prevention of Iatrogenic Fractures

Patients with OI are at high risk for accidental iatrogenic fractures even within hospital settings [25]. Extra caution is essential in the newborn nursery during activities such as bathing, dressing, feeding, and diapering to prevent fractures in infants [26]. Medical and nursing staff should be particularly careful when applying devices like blood pressure cuffs and tourniquets, and adopt gentler techniques when handling, moving, or transporting OI patients [25]. Unfortunately, intraoperative iatrogenic fractures can occur in patients with OI during limb manipulation, traction application, implant removal, or osteotomies [25]. Orthopedic surgeons should be mindful to minimize the risk of these fractures and remain vigilant to identify and treat iatrogenic fractures early [25].

Benefits of Physical Rehabilitation

Physical and occupational therapy are beneficial for patients with OI by improving mobility, self-care, and functional independence, with an emphasis on developing both fine and gross motor skills [26, 27]. Maintaining muscle mass and aerobic capacity supports bone formation and enhances strength and confidence with movement [27]. Therapist evaluations provide a needs-based approach to acquiring adaptive equipment for the home and car and access to assistive devices such as canes, crutches, and manual or power wheelchairs [26].

Pain Management

Patients with OI experience both acute and chronic pain. The pain can be localized to specific injury sites or present as diffuse discomfort throughout the body [28]. This pain can affect daily activity levels, sleep, self-care, mobility, school attendance, and work performance [28].

Research on pain management strategies for OI is limited. Interestingly, bisphosphonate infusions can reduce pain; however, they are not administered solely for this purpose [29]. Physical and occupational therapy also contribute to partial pain relief by improving strength and reducing fracture risk [29].

Advantages of Telehealth

Few studies have assessed the benefits of telehealth for managing acute fractures or conducting follow-up appointments in patients with OI. Theoretically, telehealth can reduce costs by lessening the need for expensive and time-consuming transportation and improving access to specialists who practice in nonlocal locations. The benefits of telehealth extend beyond patient care to include the education of medical clinicians in the management of rare bone diseases [30]. For example, the Rare Bone Disease Alliance hosts monthly video teleconferences that facilitate learning and discussion among healthcare professionals [30]. Telehealth can serve as a cost-effective tool to promote physician collaboration and value-based care [30].

First Aid

Currently, there is no research on the benefits of first aid management for OI. However, initial at-home care, such as splinting uncomplicated fractures, may be beneficial and cost-effective. Proper first aid can potentially reduce the need for imaging, emergency department visits, and office consultations, particularly when the management of an acute minor fracture would be managed by the same treatment method at the office or emergency department. Effective at-home fracture management requires that caregivers are properly trained and have access to appropriate supplies for splinting and pain control. Telehealth may serve as a valuable and cost-effective tool in these situations, allowing clinicians to provide guidance on splinting and acute fracture care. The patient must be followed carefully for potential complications such as a limb deformity that may need subsequent surgery. Overall, further research is needed to establish safe, effective first aid protocols and follow-up for managing fractures at home in patients with osteogenesis imperfecta.

Case Example

A 14-year-old ambulatory female with suspected type I or type IV osteogenesis imperfecta presented with a history of frequent femur fractures and progressive scoliosis. From infancy through childhood, her family, caregivers, and medical team emphasized safe handling practices and encouraged participation in low-impact activities such as swimming and dance. A safety plan was established with her school, and both teachers and classmates were educated on the importance of being mindful of her physical safety. She began receiving pamidronate infusions every 8 weeks, starting at 7 months of age until the age of 3, and then continuing twice per year until 12 years old. She was followed by OI specialists at a referral hospital, where she underwent regular DEXA scans and received her pamidronate treatments. In addition, a local pediatric orthopedic surgeon managed her surgical interventions for fractures as needed.

Despite precautions, she experienced multiple femur fractures during infancy and early childhood, treated with closed reduction and spica casting. Later fractures were treated with static IM rodding, with rods replaced following acute fractures in early adolescence. At age 10, she received a Fassier-Duval rod in the left femur, and at 13, a static rod was placed in the right femur after an acute fracture (Figs. 10.1 and 10.2).

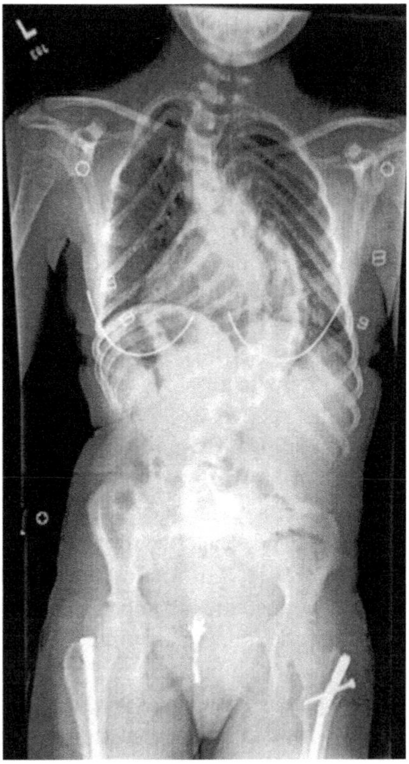

Fig. 10.1 Posteroanterior radiograph prior to posterior thoracic spinal fusion with view of bilateral intramedullary rodding of the femurs

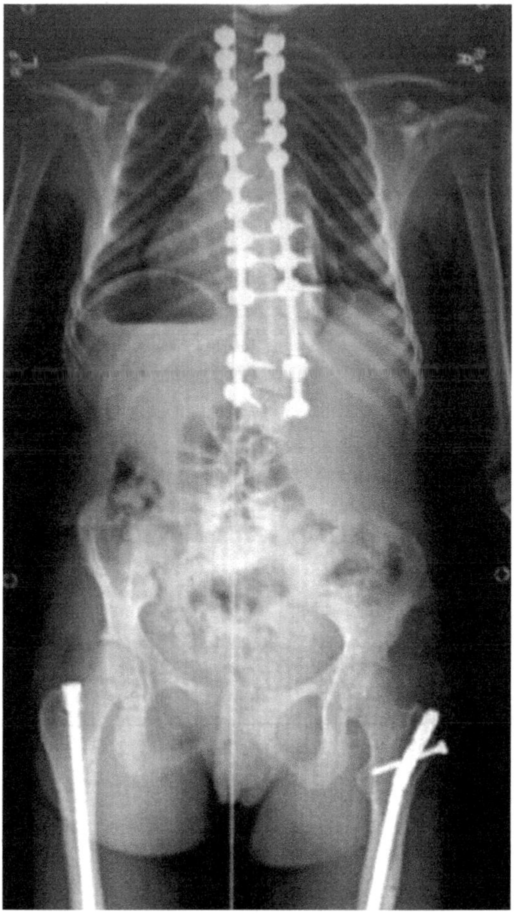

Fig. 10.2 PA radiograph following posterior thoracic spinal fusion with instrumentation

Throughout adolescence, she developed progressive scoliosis and bracing was attempted. Despite bracing, she developed rib cage deformities and worsening spinal curvature. At 14 years of age, she underwent posterior spinal fusion and required a blood transfusion. She subsequently received physical therapy and rehabilitation during her recovery.

IM rodding was performed following the acute fractures. This approach may have contributed to higher overall costs, such as expenses related to ambulance transport, emergency department visits, surgery, and prolonged hospital stays. On the other hand, once the initial static rods were outgrown, proactive replacement of the static rods with a telescoping rod may have minimized additional costs and complications. She did not experience upper extremity fractures or long bone deformities of the humerus or tibia. No home or car modifications were necessary. She was typically ambulatory without assistive devices, though she intermittently used a mechanical wheelchair, walker, or crutches following acute fractures. Physical therapy was conducted at home, helping to minimize outpatient rehabilitation expenses. She maintained muscle strength and endurance through low-impact activities such as swimming, walking, and dancing.

Summary

Providing standardized care for patients with OI is challenging due to the variability in disease presentation. However, individualized cost-effective care can still be achieved through tailored approaches. A multidisciplinary strategy offers numerous benefits, including optimized fracture and deformity management, improved mobility and function through physical and occupational therapy, and increased access to assistive devices—ultimately enhancing the patient's quality of life. Regardless of the disease's severity or presentation, comprehensive medical and surgical management of OI can reduce fracture frequency and prevent long bone deformities. Reducing fracture frequency improves value by leading to fewer hospital admissions, surgical procedures, diagnostic imaging, and postinjury rehabilitation.

Author Pearls

- Advancements in genetic testing have identified up to 13 mutations associated with osteogenesis imperfecta.
- Bisphosphonate infusions are the standard pharmacologic treatment for OI. Home infusions can reduce both patient and hospital costs and enhance value.
- Decisions on static versus telescoping intramedullary rods for deformities and fractures should be based on the patient's size and expected growth.
- A retrograde approach to intramedullary rodding of the humerus may reduce chronic shoulder and rotator cuff injuries compared to an antegrade approach.
- Being mindful of fracture risk in hospital and operating room settings can help prevent costly iatrogenic fractures.
- Physical and occupational rehabilitation can improve strength, mobility, and confidence in movement.
- Telehealth and first aid management offer opportunities to reduce costs for both patients and hospitals.
- An interdisciplinary, team-based approach can optimize both pharmacologic and nonpharmacologic treatments, reducing fracture rates, increasing mobility, and improving quality of life.

Editors Comments

WLH

Unfortunately, there is no cure for OI; however, various treatments can help manage symptoms, prevent and treat fractures, improve mobility and independence, and enhance overall quality of life. A multidisciplinary team approach incorporating orthopedic surgeons, pediatric specialists, therapists, and other healthcare professionals can optimize patient outcomes. The authors of the current comprehensive chapter emphasize practical methods to enhance value in the care of children with OI, including: utilizing home infusions of Pamidronate, employing sliding double flexible intramedullary (IM) nails for long bone fractures, using telehealth services when feasible, and encouraging initial at-home management for minor fractures.

RMS

Value-based care in osteogenesis imperfecta focuses on preventing fractures, maintaining mobility, and reducing costly interventions. This chapter highlights high-impact strategies such as early bisphosphonate use, timely intramedullary rodding for prophylaxis and fracture management, home infusions, and telehealth-guided fracture care. Globally, value is maximized by empowering caregivers in first aid management of fractures, using durable low-cost implants, and coordinating care through telemedicine and interdisciplinary teams.

References

1. Deguchi M, Tsuji S, Katsura D, Kasahara K, Kimura F, Murakami T. Current overview of osteogenesis imperfecta. Medicina (Kaunas). 2021;57(5):464. https://doi.org/10.3390/medicina57050464. PMID: 34068551; PMCID: PMC8151368.
2. Thomas IH, DiMeglio LA. Advances in the classification and treatment of osteogenesis imperfecta. Curr Osteoporos Rep. 2016;14:1–9. https://doi.org/10.1007/s11914-016-0299-y.
3. Zeitlin L, Fassier F, Glorieux FH. Modern approach to children with osteogenesis imperfecta. J Pediatr Orthop B. 2003;12(2):77–87. https://doi.org/10.1097/01.bpb.0000049567.52224.fa. PMID: 12584489.
4. Rapoport M, Bober MB, Raggio C, Wekre LL, Rauch F, Westerheim I, Hart T, van Welzenis T, Mistry A, Clancy J, Booth L, Prince S, Semler O. The patient clinical journey and socioeconomic impact of osteogenesis imperfecta: a systematic scoping review. Orphanet J Rare Dis. 2023;18(1):34. https://doi.org/10.1186/s13023-023-02627-3. PMID: 36814274; PMCID: PMC9945474.
5. Hart T, Westerheim I, van Welzenis T, Semler O, Raggio C, Rauch F, Dadzie R, Prince S, Wekre LL. The IMPACT survey: the economic impact of osteogenesis imperfecta in adults. Orphanet J Rare Dis. 2024;19(1):222. https://doi.org/10.1186/s13023-024-03218-6. PMID: 38831282; PMCID: PMC11149192.

6. Cho TJ, Ko JM, Kim H, Shin HI, Yoo WJ, Shin CH. Management of osteogenesis imperfecta: a multidisciplinary comprehensive approach. Clin Orthop Surg. 2020;12(4):417–29. https://doi.org/10.4055/cios20060. Epub 2020 Nov 18. PMID: 33274017; PMCID: PMC7683189.
7. Pedrini E, Negro A, Di Brino E, Pecoraro V, Sculco C, Abelli E, Gnoli M, Magrelli A, Sangiorgi L, Cicchetti A. Real-world data and budget impact analysis (BIA): evaluation of a targeted next-generation sequencing diagnostic approach in two orthopedic rare diseases. Front Pharmacol. 2022;13:785705. https://doi.org/10.3389/fphar.2022.785705. PMID: 35734413; PMCID: PMC9207266.
8. Garg B, Tomar N, Biswas A, Mehta N, Malhotra R. Understanding musculoskeletal disorders through next-generation sequencing. JBJS Rev. 2022;10(4):e21.00165. https://doi.org/10.2106/JBJS.RVW.21.00165. PMID: 35383688.
9. Kolovos S, Javaid MK, Pinedo-Villanueva R. Hospital admissions of patients with osteogenesis imperfecta in the English NHS. Osteoporos Int. 2021;32(6):1207–16. https://doi.org/10.1007/s00198-020-05755-9. Epub 2021 Jan 7. PMID: 33411004; PMCID: PMC8128734.
10. Aubry-Rozier B, Richard C, Unger S, Hans D, Campos-Xavier B, Schneider P, Paquier C, Pasche J, Bonafé L, Bregou A. Osteogenesis imperfecta: towards an individualised interdisciplinary care strategy to improve physical activity and quality of life. Swiss Med Wkly. 2020;150:w20285. https://doi.org/10.4414/smw.2020.20285. PMID: 32667677.
11. Castro AR, Marinello J, Chougui K, Morand M, Bilodeau C, Tsimicalis A. The day-to-day experiences of caring for children with osteogenesis imperfecta: a qualitative descriptive study. J Clin Nurs. 2020;29(15–16):2999–3011. https://doi.org/10.1111/jocn.15310. Epub 2020 May 22. PMID: 32350946.
12. Wang X, Li Y, Zhong Y, Wang M, Liu X, Han W, Chen H, Ji J. Home care needs assessment among caregivers of children and adolescents with osteogenesis imperfecta: a cross-sectional study. BMC Prim Care. 2024;25(1):119. https://doi.org/10.1186/s12875-024-02367-8. PMID: 38641795; PMCID: PMC11027538.
13. Westerheim I, Hart T, van Welzenis T, Wekre LL, Semler O, Raggio C, Bober MB, Rapoport M, Prince S, Rauch F. The IMPACT survey: a mixed methods study to understand the experience of children, adolescents and adults with osteogenesis imperfecta and their caregivers. Orphanet J Rare Dis. 2024;19(1):128. https://doi.org/10.1186/s13023-024-03126-9. PMID: 38515144; PMCID: PMC10956293.
14. Hidalgo Perea S, Green DW. Osteogenesis imperfecta: treatment and surgical management. Curr Opin Pediatr. 2021;33(1):74–8. https://doi.org/10.1097/MOP.0000000000000968. PMID: 33278111.
15. Botor M, Fus-Kujawa A, Uroczynska M, Stepien KL, Galicka A, Gawron K, Sieron AL. Osteogenesis imperfecta: current and prospective therapies. Biomolecules. 2021;11(10):1493. https://doi.org/10.3390/biom11101493. PMID: 34680126; PMCID: PMC8533546.
16. Rush ET, DeHaai K, Kreikemeier RM, Lutz RE. Evaluation and comparison of safety, convenience and cost of administering intravenous pamidronate infusions to children in the home and ambulatory care settings. J Pediatr Endocrinol Metab. 2012;25(5–6):493–7. https://doi.org/10.1515/jpem-2011-0498. PMID: 22876544.
17. Folkestad L, Hald JD, Ersbøll AK, Gram J, Hermann AP, Langdahl B, Abrahamsen B, Brixen K. Fracture rates and fracture sites in patients with osteogenesis imperfecta: a nationwide register-based cohort study. J Bone Miner Res. 2017;32(1):125–34. https://doi.org/10.1002/jbmr.2920. Epub 2016 Aug 29. PMID: 27448250.
18. Rosemberg DL, Goiano EO, Akkari M, Santili C. Effects of a telescopic intramedullary rod for treating patients with osteogenesis imperfecta of the femur. J Child Orthop. 2018;12(1):97–103. https://doi.org/10.1302/1863-2548.12.170009. PMID: 29456761; PMCID: PMC5813132.
19. Musielak BJ, Woźniak Ł, Sułko J, Oberc A, Jóźwiak M. Problems, complications, and factors predisposing to failure of Fassier-Duval rodding in children with osteogenesis imperfecta: a double-center study. J Pediatr Orthop. 2021;41(4):e347–52. https://doi.org/10.1097/BPO.0000000000001763.

20. Nguyen CV, Makarewich CA, Poon SC, Cho RH, Hennessey TA. Long-term outcomes of intramedullary nails in osteogenesis imperfecta: fewer surgeries and longer survival times with telescoping rods in patients with over ten years follow-up. J Pediatr Orthop. 2025;45(1):51–5. https://doi.org/10.1097/BPO.0000000000002810.
21. Marwan Y, Abu Dalu K, Hamdy RC, Janelle C, Fassier F. Retrograde application of humerus Fassier-Duval rod in osteogenesis imperfecta: a new surgical technique. J Pediatr Orthop. 2022;42(2):e224–8. https://doi.org/10.1097/BPO.0000000000002023.
22. Karami M, Minator Sajjadi M, Fakhrzadegan M, Ehsani A. A novel sliding double flexible intramedullary nail technique for the management of lower extremity long bone fractures and deformities in osteogenesis imperfecta. J Pediatr Orthop B. 2025;34(3):257–63. https://doi.org/10.1097/BPB.0000000000001178. Epub ahead of print. PMID: 38547191.
23. Belyea CM, Knox JB. Spinal fusion in children with osteogenesis imperfecta: a nationwide retrospective comparative cohort study over a 12-year period. Curr Orthop Pract. 2020;31(1):72–5. https://doi.org/10.1097/BCO.0000000000000805.
24. Ito M, Kakutani K, Miyamoto H, Suzuki T, Yurube T, Uno K. Surgical outcome of spinal fusion for osteogenesis imperfecta with scoliosis: is the hybrid system with pedicle screws applicable to weak, tiny, and fragile vertebrae? J Pediatr Orthop. 2021;41(6):368–73. https://doi.org/10.1097/BPO.0000000000001829.
25. Georgiadis AG, Pottinger TJ, Sigrist EJ, Truong WH. Iatrogenic intraoperative fracture in patients with osteogenesis imperfecta. J Pediatr Orthop. 2024;44(10):e945–50. https://doi.org/10.1097/BPO.0000000000002778.
26. Donohoe M. Therapy, orthotics and assistive devices for osteogenesis imperfecta. In: Kruse R, editor. Osteogenesis imperfecta. Cham: Springer; 2020. https://doi.org/10.1007/978-3-030-42527-2_3.
27. Mueller B, Engelbert R, Baratta-Ziska F, et al. Consensus statement on physical rehabilitation in children and adolescents with osteogenesis imperfecta. Orphanet J Rare Dis. 2018;13:158. https://doi.org/10.1186/s13023-018-0905-4.
28. Nghiem T, Louli J, Treherne SC, Anderson CE, Tsimicalis A, Lalloo C, Stinson JN, Thorstad K. Pain experiences of children and adolescents with osteogenesis imperfecta: an integrative review. Clin J Pain. 2017;33(3):271–80. https://doi.org/10.1097/AJP.0000000000000395. PMID: 27258996.
29. Dlesk TE, Larimer K. Multimodal pain management of children diagnosed with osteogenesis imperfecta: an integrative literature review. Pain Manag Nurs. 2023;24(1):102–10. https://doi.org/10.1016/j.pmn.2022.08.014. Epub 2022 Oct 4. PMID: 36207231.
30. Tosi LL, Rajah EN, Stewart MH, Gillies AP, Hart TS, Lewiecki EM. The rare bone disease TeleECHO program: leveraging telehealth to improve rare bone disease care. Curr Osteoporos Rep. 2020;18(4):344–9. https://doi.org/10.1007/s11914-020-00595-2. PMID: 32514667; PMCID: PMC7419447.

Infants to 1 Year Old with Developmental Dysplasia of the Hip: Follow the AAP Guidelines

11

Breanna Alexa Polascik and John Francis Sarwark

Introduction

Developmental dysplasia of the hip (DDH) is a common orthopedic condition in newborns, with approximately 1 in 1,000 having a clinical dislocation and about 1 in 100 having evidence of hip dysplasia [1]. Early detection and appropriate treatment are essential for achieving optimal outcomes. Value in healthcare is defined as maximizing outcomes while minimizing cost [2]. In this chapter, we explore strategies to improve value in the diagnosis and management of DDH in infants under 1 year of age.

Value-Based Themes

Targeted Screening Is Superior to Universal Screening

The value of universal screening for DDH is controversial [3–5]. A successful screening strategy should facilitate early detection to reduce the incidence of complex presentations, the need for more invasive interventions associated with delayed diagnosis, and complications. DDH is typically identified through a combination of physical exams and selective imaging. In infants under 3 months of age, screening

B. A. Polascik
Division of Orthopaedic Surgery, Ann & Robert H. Lurie Children's Hospital of Chicago, Chicago, IL, USA

Department of Orthopaedic Surgery, Northwestern Memorial Hospital, Chicago, IL, USA

J. F. Sarwark (✉)
Division of Orthopaedic Surgery, Ann & Robert H. Lurie Children's Hospital of Chicago, Chicago, IL, USA

W. L. Hennrikus, R. M. Schwend (eds.), *Value in Pediatric Orthopaedics*,
https://doi.org/10.1007/978-3-032-19570-8_11

with the Ortolani, Barlow, and Galeazzi tests is performed to palpate hip clunks. Hip clicks are considered nonspecific finding [6]. Between 3 months and 1 year of age, limited or asymmetric hip abduction becomes the primary clinical sign of DDH. In cases of dislocation, leg length discrepancy may also be observed. Up to about 6 months of age, treatment of reducible hips is typically managed nonoperatively using a Pavlik harness or another brace. Beyond this age, closed or open surgical reduction and spica casting are often required. Therefore, early detection adds value by reducing the likelihood of late diagnosis and the need for surgical intervention.

Current literature demonstrates that universal ultrasound (US) screening does not improve the overall value of DDH treatment. For example, A 2022 systematic review and meta-analysis of 76 studies involving 16,901,079 infants found that universal US screening increased early detection (before 12 weeks of age) and the use of nonoperative treatment. However, universal US screening did not reduce the incidence of late detection (after 12 weeks) or the need for operative intervention compared to clinical examination combined with targeted ultrasonography for high-risk infants [7]. Therefore, to enhance value by maximizing cost-effectiveness and optimizing resource utilization without compromising outcomes, targeted US screening is recommended.

Targeting patients in high-risk groups for DDH with a US exam adds value. Per American Academy of Pediatrics (AAP) guidelines, high-risk infants include females, those with a positive family history of DDH, and those in breech position during the third trimester of pregnancy [8]. One study (1995) compared the cost-effectiveness of universal US screening, targeted US screening, and no US screening in a randomized study of 11,925 newborns [9]. The study tabulated the costs of screening, treatment of early and late DDH diagnoses, and follow-up. Although total costs were similar across all 3 screening strategies, late-diagnosis treatment represented 65% of costs in the targeted and no US groups, compared to only 22% in the universal US screening group. The authors concluded that screening all girls and at-risk boys may be the most cost-effective approach. Despite these findings, such screening is not currently standard practice in the United States.

According to AAP guidelines, all newborns should undergo a hip exam at every well-child visit from birth until independent walking [8]. In addition, per the 2016 AAP update by Shaw and Segal, consider imaging before 6 months of age for female or male infants with normal findings on physical examination and the following risk factors:

1. Breech presentation in the third trimester (regardless of cesarean or vaginal delivery)
2. Positive family history
3. History of previous clinical instability
4. Parental concern
5. History of improper swaddling
6. Suspicious or inconclusive physical examination

Imaging before 6 weeks of age is not recommended due to a high false-positive rate on the US exam. If DDH is suspected or confirmed, prompt referral to a pediatric orthopedic surgeon is indicated [8].

Optimizing Imaging Modalities

The two primary imaging modalities used for screening and monitoring DDH are US and X-rays. Due to the cartilaginous nature of the infant hip, from 6 weeks to 4 months of age, US is the preferred modality for targeted screening or to monitor hip reduction during Pavlik harness treatment [9]. In this age group, US has demonstrated a sensitivity of 88%, specificity of 97%, positive predictive value of 62%, and negative predictive value of 99% [10]. After 4 months of age, as the femoral heads begin to ossify, anteroposterior (AP) pelvis radiographs with abduction and internal rotation become the preferred imaging method [11]. In terms of cost-effectiveness, US is more expensive than X-rays.

Arthrography, computed tomography (CT), and magnetic resonance imaging (MRI) are not used for primary detection of DDH, but are valuable for assessing hip reduction during or after intervention. Arthrography involves injecting contrast dye into the joint under fluoroscopic guidance in the operating room to identify obstacles to reduction and confirm concentric reduction after a closed reduction and spica casting procedure. Arthrography costs about $1,600 [12]. Postoperative imaging to confirm reduction can be performed with CT or MRI. MRI's higher cost ($2,400) and the need for sedation or general anesthesia in infants are drawbacks. If CT ($1,600) is used, a low-dose protocol is recommended to minimize radiation exposure [12].

Effective Family Education Is Essential

The Pavlik harness is the preferred brace for treatment of DDH in infants under 6 months of age in most centers in the United States. The success rate of the Pavlik harness is approximately 90% [1]. Since Pavlik harness treatment is conducted at home, family education is essential to ensure proper use, optimize outcomes, and reduce the likelihood of more invasive and costly interventions later.

Value can be enhanced by achieving family cooperation through education on the benefits of Pavlik harness treatment and proper harness application. Caregivers should be instructed on maintaining the harness for 23 hours per day to ensure treatment success. Simulated training modules have been shown to significantly improve caregiver confidence and skill in applying the harness correctly [13]. Improper application and inadequate follow-up can lead to complications, including femoral nerve palsy if the harness is applied with >60° of flexion, avascular necrosis (AVN) of the femoral head if the harness is applied with >100° of abduction, and inadequate acetabular development with improper harness position. A study by Hassan (2009) involving 160 parents over 3.5 years identified common challenges such as dressing, handling the infant, reapplying the harness after bathing, skin-crease dermatitis, and feet slipping from stirrups [14]. Compliance may be influenced by cultural norms and practices [15].

Preventative Measures

An important preventative practice that enhances value in DDH care is avoiding improper swaddling; instead practice "safe swaddling," in which the hips are allowed to move freely [15]. Traditional Mongolian swaddling, which tightly wraps the infant with the hips in extension and adduction, has been associated with an increased risk of DDH. In a randomized controlled trial by Ulziibat et al. (2021), 80 newborns at risk for DDH were randomized to swaddling versus nonswaddling groups. The swaddled group showed a higher incidence of DDH, with risk strongly correlated to the number of swaddling hours per day and total swaddling days [16]. Promoting simple alternative practices, such as carrying the baby in a position that places the hips in an abducted position, can reduce the incidence of DDH and enhance value. Education about safe swaddling techniques should be included in routine guidance provided by family medicine practitioners, pediatricians, and obstetricians.

Telemedicine and Remote Monitoring in a Post-COVID Era

DDH, when managed with a Pavlik harness, requires close monitoring and frequent early follow-up. Recent studies support the use of telemedicine and digital monitoring to provide follow-up for DDH patients. Telemedicine can potentially reduce costs, maintain continuity of care, and monitor brace compliance. For example, Murphy et al. (2021) developed and prospectively evaluated a virtual DDH clinic, demonstrating that telemedicine offers improved value, efficiency, and cost savings [17]. On average, families saved approximately $200 per visit, and total cost savings across the cohort reached nearly $700,000. This model is especially beneficial for families in remote or underserved areas.

Enhancing Provider Training and Multidisciplinary Care

DDH outcomes can be improved with interdisciplinary collaboration. For example, risk awareness for DDH should begin during pregnancy, with patient education about DDH provided by family medicine, pediatric, or obstetrics doctors. After birth, pediatricians, family medicine doctors, and radiologists must be well-versed in identifying clinical and imaging findings that warrant referral to an orthopedic specialist [18]. Training of primary care physicians can facilitate timely recognition and referral of DDH cases, thereby enhancing value.

A 2022 study revealed variation in DDH screening practices among 126 pediatricians across the country [19]. Notably, half lacked standardized care pathways for DDH, and 10% were unfamiliar with key physical exam maneuvers. Prior research has shown that targeted education for primary care doctors leads to more accurate and timely referrals to orthopedic specialists [20]. Therefore, implementing standardized guidelines for DDH screening, imaging, and referral among primary care doctors would represent a high-value intervention to improve early detection and outcomes for affected children [19].

Case Example

A 6-week-old female was referred to the pediatric orthopedic clinic by her primary care physician following an abnormal hip US. Although her physical exam was normal and there was no family history of hip dysplasia, screening was performed due to her status as a first-born female and history of breech positioning prior to cesarean delivery at 37 weeks gestation. She had not received any prior treatment. On examination, the infant was alert and interactive with normal tone, a supple neck, and no midline spinal anomalies. Bilateral flexible calcaneo-valgus feet were noted.

Ortolani, Barlow, and Galeazzi tests were negative. Review of the initial hip US revealed bilaterally concentrically located femoral heads with immature acetabula. The alpha angle measured 31° on the right and 50° on the left (Fig. 11.1). The alpha angle is a key parameter in DDH evaluation, representing the slope of the bony

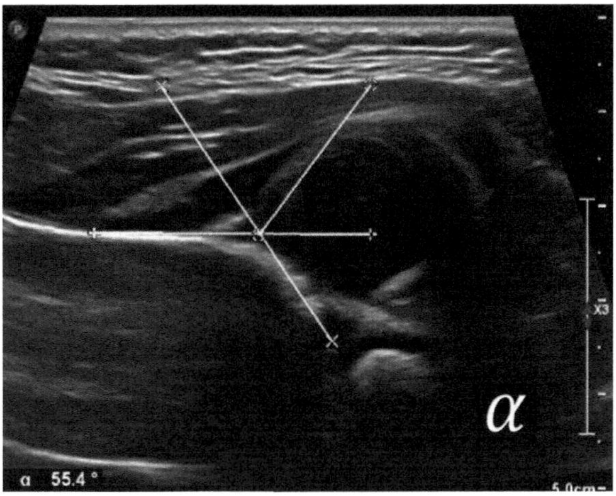

Fig. 11.1 Calculation of alpha angle

Type	Alpha Angle	Clinical Significance	Treatment
I	>60°	Normal	None
II		**Immature, mildly dysplasti chip**	
a	50-59°	a: Mildly shallow but stable AT b: Shallow AT,low risk of subluxation	Observation
b	>50-59°	**Dysplastic hip**	Observation +/- Pavlik
c	43-49°	c: Shallow AT, high risk of subluxation	Pavlik +/- surgery
d	43-49°	d: Veryshallow AT, high risk of dislocation	Surgery (closed vs. open)
III	<43°	Subluxated	Pavlik harness
IV	Cannot be determined	Dislocated	Closed reduction in Pavlik harness vs open reduction and spica casting

Fig. 11.2 Graf classification. AT acetabulum

acetabular roof. It is measured at the intersection of a line along the osseous acetabulum and a line along the ilium. This measurement is used to classify hips according to the Graf system: >60° indicates a normal hip (Graf type I), 50–59° denotes an immature or mildly dysplastic hip (Graf type II), and <50° reflects dysplasia (Graf type IIc or worse) (Fig. 11.2). We initiated treatment with a rigid hip abduction brace to be worn 24 hours per day. The brace was fitted in clinic, and the family received detailed education on its use. We also instructed the parents on hindfoot stretching exercises to address her bilateral calcaneo-valgus feet. Follow-up was scheduled for 2 weeks to reassess the physical exam, evaluate brace fit, and repeat US imaging.

At her 2-week follow-up visit, repeat US demonstrated a satisfactory left hip (alpha angle 58°) but persistent deficiency in the right hip (alpha angle 44°) (Fig. 11.3). Dynamic stress testing revealed mild bilateral instability. We elected to continue full-time use of the rigid abduction brace (24 hours/day). She returned 2–4 weeks later for repeat US, which showed improvement in alpha angles, and the same management plan was continued. At each visit, the brace fit was reassessed, and brace care instructions were reinforced with the family to ensure compliance and optimize outcomes.

At her 3-month visit, the patient continued to do well with brace treatment. At this age, the physical exam added the assessment of hip abduction symmetry, which was found to be normal. US demonstrated continued improvement in alpha angles. Brace wear was adjusted to 18–20 hours per day. She returned 6 weeks later with stable findings, and a similar management plan was continued.

At her 7-month visit, AP pelvis X-rays with abduction and internal rotation were obtained. At this age, the acetabular index (AI) becomes a key radiographic parameter used to monitor DDH. The AI is measured at the intersection of Hilgenreiner's line—a horizontal line connecting the superior edges of the bilateral triradiate cartilages—and a line drawn from the superolateral edge of the triradiate cartilage to the lateral margin of the acetabulum. In children over 6 months of age, a normal AI is <25°. Our patient's AI measurement demonstrated continued residual dysplasia with an AI of 35° on the right and 28° on the left (Fig. 11.4). The brace wear was

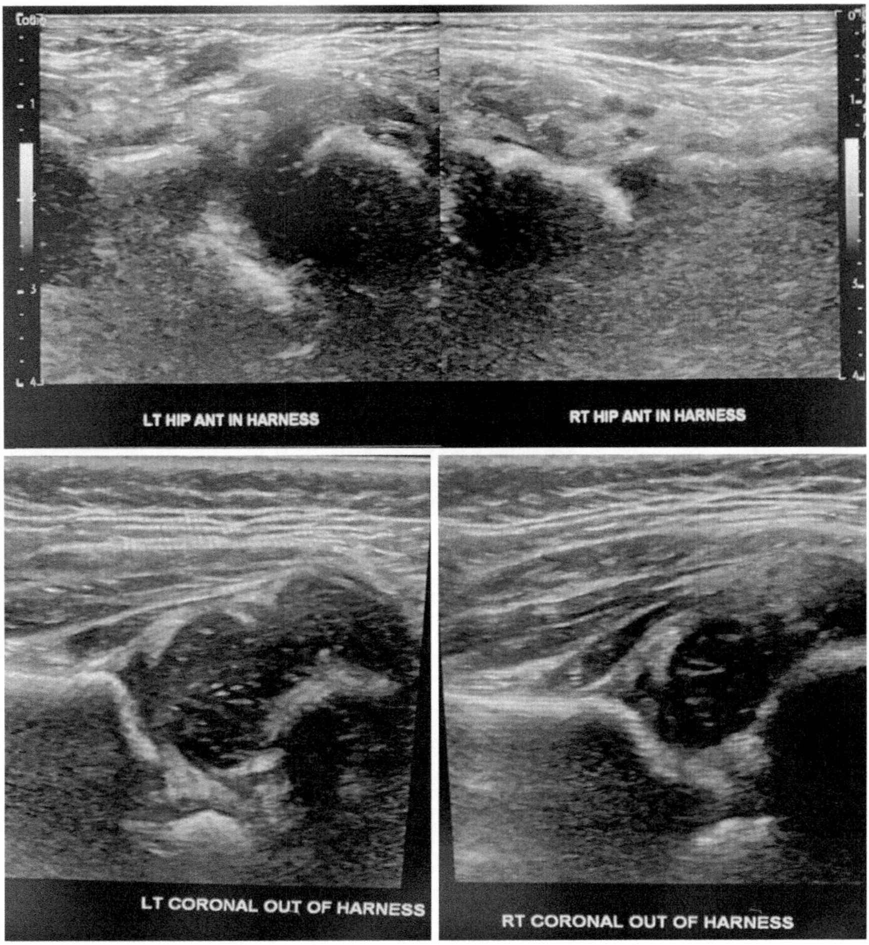

Fig. 11.3 Ultrasound of bilateral hips at 8 weeks old

continued at 12 hours per day with plans for follow-up in 2–3 months. The next two follow-up appointments showed continued improvement, and the current management plan was maintained.

At her 14-month follow-up, the patient was walking and running independently with age-appropriate developmental milestones. She was using the abduction brace only at night 8 hours per day. X-rays at that time revealed a right acetabular index (AI) of 29° and a left AI of 25°. The plan was to continue the brace at night. At her next follow-up, 6 months later, both AIs were near normal (Fig. 11.5). The brace was continued at night until 24 months of age and then discontinued. Ongoing surveillance will include clinical and radiographic evaluations every 6–12 months until age 6.

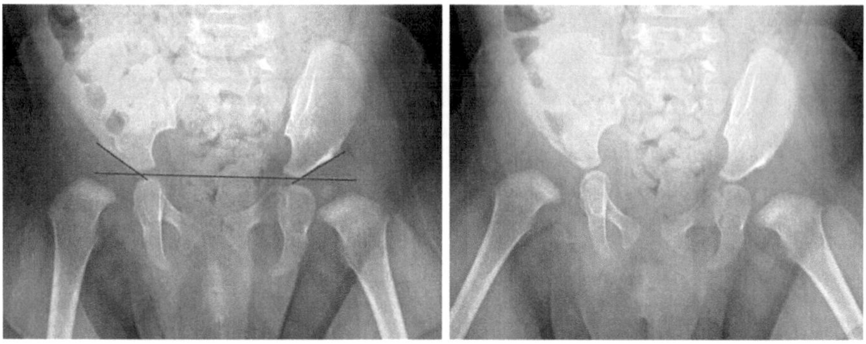

Fig. 11.4 Acetabular index. AP pelvis radiographs with abduction and internal rotation

Fig. 11.5 AP Pelvis XR at 21 months old. Mild right residual acetabular dysplasia. Under observation and q6mo follow-up

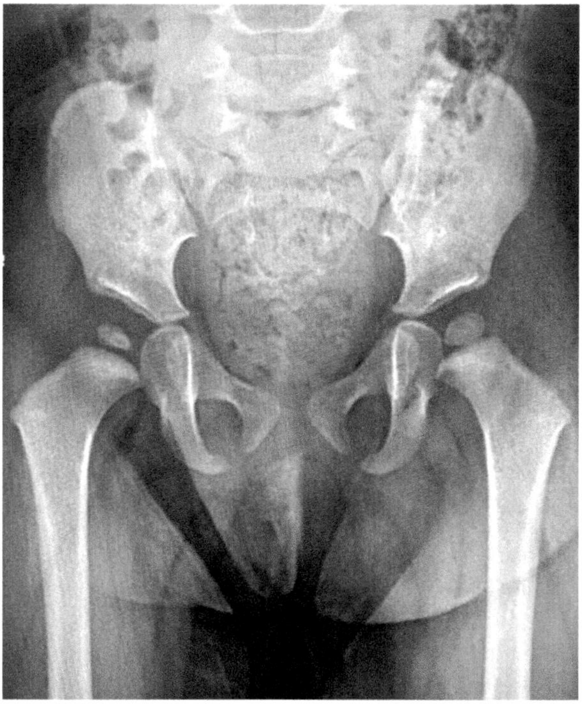

Summary

DDH is a common orthopedic condition in newborns. Value-driven care is essential. Strategies to optimize value include targeted screening, appropriate imaging utilization, effective education for families, implementation of preventive measures, collaborative multidisciplinary training, and the use of telemedicine on a case-by-case basis for follow-up. This chapter offers practical recommendations to enhance value in the management of DDH in infants under 1 year of age.

Chapter Pearls

- Targeting US screening adds value compared to universal US screening.
- US is the best imaging test for infants between 6 weeks and 4 months of age. After this age, X-rays are preferred due to the natural ossification of the femoral head and lower cost.
- During closed reduction and spica casting, arthrograms are useful for identifying barriers to reduction and confirming successful intraoperative reduction.
- Either CT or MRI can be used to confirm reduction following closed reduction and spica casting.
- Family education is important to the success of Pavlik harness treatment.
- Safe swaddling should be emphasized. In addition, parents should be encouraged to hold their infant in a position where their hips are flexed and abducted, such as when straddling the parent's hip.
- Telemedicine offers a cost-effective alternative to in-person monitoring for DDH and brace treatment.

Editors Comments

WLH

DDH is a pediatric condition in which the ball-and-socket hip joint fails to develop properly during infancy. This abnormal joint formation can result in mechanical stress that increases the risk of early-onset osteoarthritis in adulthood. Early diagnosis through physical examination and imaging is critical to achieving optimal outcomes. The current chapter emphasizes the value of US as a diagnostic tool in infants under 4 months of age. However, a "normal" ultrasound at 6 weeks does not eliminate the risk of developing dysplasia later in childhood. Follow-up should not be assumed to be unnecessary. Unfortunately, hips may still become dysplastic or dislocate despite an initially normal ultrasound (Pan T, et al. Late presenting developmental dysplasia of the hip after a normal hip ultrasound at 6 weeks of age: A report of two cases. *J Paediatr Child Health.* 2022;58(10):1887–9). An exam and x-ray at 6 months and 1 year may still be needed.

RMS

In the context of value-based care for newborns and infants, two impactful practices stand out: avoiding tight swaddling and ensuring proper, consistent performance of the Ortolani maneuver. The concept of "safe swaddling," as endorsed by the POSNA/AAOS/International Hip Dysplasia Institute joint statement (Swaddling Position Statement, April 2015), should be emphasized both in the newborn nursery and during pediatric visits. Improper swaddling remains a modifiable risk factor for DDH. Also important is training pediatric and family practice clinicians to competently perform the Ortolani maneuver. This allows for early identification of hip instability, timely referral, and value-enhanced care. We do not recommend repeated use of the Barlow maneuver because the Barlow maneuver may exacerbate instability if performed forcefully and repeatedly.

References

1. Ahn L, Souder C. Developmental dysplasia of the hip (DDH) Internet. Orthobullets; 2023.
2. Porter ME. What is value in health care? N Engl J Med. 2010;363(26):2477–81.
3. Biedermann R, Eastwood DM. Universal or selective ultrasound screening for developmental dysplasia of the hip? A discussion of the key issues. J Child Orthop. 2018;12(4):296–301.
4. Rosendahl K, Markestad T, Lie RT. Ultrasound screening for developmental dysplasia of the hip in the neonate: the effect on treatment rate and prevalence of late cases. Pediatrics. 1994;94(1):47–52.
5. Holen KJ, Tegnander A, Bredland T, Johansen OJ, Saether OD, Eik-Nes SH, et al. Universal or selective screening of the neonatal hip using ultrasound? A prospective, randomised trial of 15,529 newborn infants. J Bone Joint Surg Br. 2002;84(6):886–90.
6. Bond C, Hennrikus W, DellaMaggiorie E. Prospective evaluation of newborn soft-tissue hip clicks with ultrasound. J Pediatr Orthop. 1997;17:199–201.
7. Kuitunen I, Uimonen MM, Haapanen M, Sund R, Helenius I, Ponkilainen VT. Incidence of neonatal developmental dysplasia of the hip and late detection rates based on screening strategy: a systematic review and meta-analysis. JAMA Netw Open. 2022;5(8):e2227638.
8. Shaw BA, Segal LS, Section on Orthopaedics. Evaluation and referral for developmental dysplasia of the hip in infants. Pediatrics. 2016;138(6):e20163107.
9. Lee J. Developmental dysplasia of the hip: universal or selective ultrasound screening? Ann Acad Med Singap. 2008;37(12 Suppl):101–3.
10. Roovers EA, Boere-Boonekamp MM, Castelein RM, Zielhuis GA, Kerkhoff TH. Effectiveness of ultrasound screening for developmental dysplasia of the hip. Arch Dis Child Fetal Neonatal Ed. 2005;90(1):F25–30.
11. Woolacott NF, Puhan MA, Steurer J, Kleijnen J. Ultrasonography in screening for developmental dysplasia of the hip in newborns: systematic review. BMJ. 2005;330(7505):1413.
12. Grissom L, Harcke HT, Thacker M. Imaging in the surgical management of developmental dislocation of the hip. Clin Orthop Relat Res. 2008;466(4):791–801.
13. Gargan KE, Bradley CS, Maxwell A, Moktar J, Wedge JH, Murnaghan ML, et al. Education of parents in Pavlik harness application for developmental dysplasia of the hip using a validated simulated learning module. J Child Orthop. 2016;10(4):289–93.
14. Hassan FA. Compliance of parents with regard to Pavlik harness treatment in developmental dysplasia of the hip. J Pediatr Orthop B. 2009;18(3):111–5.
15. Omeroglu H. Treatment of developmental dysplasia of the hip with the Pavlik harness in children under six months of age: indications, results and failures. J Child Orthop. 2018;12(4):308–16.
16. Ulziibat M, Munkhuu B, Bataa AE, Schmid R, Baumann T, Essig S. Traditional Mongolian swaddling and developmental dysplasia of the hip: a randomized controlled trial. BMC Pediatr. 2021;21(1):450.
17. Murphy EP, Fenelon C, Kennedy JF, O'Sullivan MD, Noel J, Kelly PM, et al. Establishing a virtual clinic for developmental dysplasia of the hip: a prospective study. J Pediatr Orthop. 2021;41(4):209–15.
18. Agostiniani R, Atti G, Bonforte S, Casini C, Cirillo M, De Pellegrin M, et al. Recommendations for early diagnosis of Developmental Dysplasia of the Hip (DDH): working group intersociety consensus document. Ital J Pediatr. 2020;46(1):150.

19. Taylor IK, Burlile JF, O'Brien K, Schaeffer EK, Mulpuri K, Shea KG. Developmental dysplasia of the hip: an examination of care practices of pediatricians. J Pediatr. 2022;246:179–83 e2.
20. Humphry S, Thompson D, Evans R, Price N, Williams P. Newborn and infant physical examination standards in a dedicated clinic for developmental dysplasia of the hip. Ann R Coll Surg Engl. 2018;100(7):566–9.

Removing Metal Implants in Children: Value Matters

12

Grant M. Quilling, Troy T. Lenz, and Alex Burton

Introduction

Hardware removal is a common procedure that accounts for up to 30% of elective case volumes [1, 2]. "Implant" is technically a more appropriate term than "hardware," although in discussions with patients, the term "hardware removal" is understood and frequently used. The most common reasons for implant removal include patient/parent preference, irritation, possible functional limitation, and concerns for future growth deformity [1]. In a survey of over 250 pediatric orthopedic surgeons, over 40% indicated that they remove asymptomatic implants nearly all the time, while only 21% said they almost never remove asymptomatic implants [3]. Although often considered a routine procedure, hardware removal is not free of risks. Removal of metallic implants is associated with a complication rate of 2–40% [4, 5], and thus, before metal removal, a surgeon should always consider the risks of anesthesia, infection, neurovascular injury, and incomplete removal.

A value-based approach to implant removal in pediatric patients is especially important due to the high frequency of these procedures. Although outcomes are generally favorable and complication rates are low [2], the associated costs are multifaceted. These include expenses related to returning to the operating room, surgical and anesthetic risks, and the potential for postoperative complications. In one study of orthopedic implant removal, the average cost of hospitalization was $11,792, while the procedure itself ranged from $9000 to over $13,000 [6]. In addition, costs are often higher when removal is necessitated by implant-related complications. The aim of this chapter is to equip surgeons with practical strategies to optimize value in implant removal in children.

G. M. Quilling · T. T. Lenz · A. Burton (✉)
Medical College of Wisconsin, Milwaukee, WI, USA
e-mail: gquilling@mcw.edu; tlenz@mcw.edu

W. L. Hennrikus, R. M. Schwend (eds.), *Value in Pediatric Orthopaedics*,
https://doi.org/10.1007/978-3-032-19570-8_12

Value-Based Themes

Costs of Implant Removal

As all surgeons are aware, every decision to bring a patient to the operating room carries costs, including time and resource utilization. Even a seemingly straightforward procedure like implant removal is not exempt from these burdens. For example, there are costs associated with the preoperative optimization process. Although not specific to orthopedic surgery, the average pediatric patient incurs over $2000 in preoperative testing during preparation for elective surgery [7]. In addition, the procedure itself contributes to overall costs. According to a recent meta-analysis, even when excluding anesthesia and implant expenses, the cost for time spent in the operating room is approximately $46 per minute [8].

The average pediatric hospitalization costs about $13,400 [9]. In addition, postoperative care also contributes to the overall cost burden. For example, the estimated cost for patients after a hospital admission is approximately $1300, with many cases exceeding $3000 [10]. Elective hardware removal adds to system-wide costs through follow-up visits and radiographic imaging.

A surgeon must also consider the hidden costs associated with every surgical procedure. These costs impact both the patient and the surgeon. For the patient, hidden costs include the risk of complications, cosmetic concerns, and time away from school, sports, or other activities during the recovery period. Prior to elective hardware removal, it is important that surgeons explain these costs to the parent and child. From the surgeon's perspective, hidden costs also involve the limited availability of operating room time. One retrospective study found that elective implant removal is one of the most common orthopedic procedures [11]. Each elective implant removal occupies time that could otherwise be used for patients with more urgent needs. This may result in surgeons working extended hours, often at the expense of personal time with family or friends, or in delays to care for patients requiring time-sensitive interventions.

True Indications for Implant Removal

The goal of the current chapter is not to suggest that all implant removal should be avoided. Clear indications exist, such as infection or persistent pain caused by implant prominence. In pediatric patients, there are additional scenarios where implant removal may be appropriate. One example is the potential for soft tissue irritation by the retained metal as the child grows. In adults, the bone–soft tissue relationship remains fixed. However, in children with open growth plates, this relationship is dynamic. As the bone grows, its spatial relationship to surrounding soft tissues, including neurovascular structures and muscle attachments, changes potentially leading to hardware irritation [12, 13].

Another key indication for implant removal is in cases in which the metal implant crosses the physis, whether a plate, screw, or Kirschner wire. Retained implants should not lead to avoidable limb length discrepancies or angular deformities. Once the fracture has healed or growth modulation has done its job, it is important to assess the potential future impact of the retained metal on the physis and remove the implant when necessary.

A retained implant may need to be removed if prominent, such as long screws causing patient discomfort. Anterior tibial screws used in tibial tubercle transfers or fractures are commonly associated with pain from the screwheads during kneeling, so they are frequently removed. Intraarticular screws may cause abrasive injury to joint surfaces over time. A screw used to fix a pediatric tibial spine fracture could loosen or back out, eventually leading to wear on the femoral condyles during joint movement. Another indication for removal is to restore native anatomy for potential later adult reconstruction surgery [14].

There are several areas of pediatric implant removal where consensus among surgeons is lacking. It is unclear whether implant removal or retention impacts long-term fracture risk [12]. Some case reports have documented subtrochanteric fractures occurring both with retained implants and following elective removal [15–17]. Additionally, there is no agreement on whether certain implant materials pose a higher long-term risk of diseases such as cancer when retained in pediatric patients [12].

Understanding the Risks of Hardware Removal

The process of hardware removal itself carries risks, with the overall complication rate in pediatric patients exceeding 10% [5, 14, 18]. Fracture rates following implant removal in pediatric patients vary, ranging from 0% to 15% [19]. Specifically, following internal fixation of forearm fractures, the postremoval fracture rate was 5% [20]. Another study found refracture rates of 10% after plating and 17% following treatment with elastic nails [21]. Comparable refracture rates have been reported across other pathologies using metal implants as well [19, 22].

Impaired wound healing (2.1%) and infection (1.6%) are additional risks following elective implant removal in pediatric patients [18]. Incisional healing issues and infections are common complications, exceeding 10% after implant removal [23, 24]. Failure to remove all the hardware is a frequent and frustrating complication. This complication can be especially problematic if the family was not counselled of this possibility beforehand. Lastly, the surgeon should always carefully inspect the radiographs before implant removal surgery for subtle cracks in the metal, indicating a broken implant.

Smart Implant Selection During the Index Procedure to Minimize Need for Future Removal

Important decisions made before the index procedure can impact the need for potential future implant removal. These decisions center on the type of implant selected.

When two implant options offer equivalent clinical outcomes, we recommend choosing the one that is less likely to require removal. If implant removal is anticipated with either option, preference should be given to the implant that allows for a simpler, lower-risk removal procedure.

Even within similar fixation strategies, implant selection can influence the likelihood of future removal. For example, using low-profile implants, such as headless compression screws, can reduce the need for removal, particularly in anatomically sensitive areas where implant prominence may lead to discomfort or injury to tendons and ligaments [25–28]. Despite concerns about the higher initial cost of headless screws, their use may be more cost-effective in the long term. Although not specific to pediatric populations, one recent study reported that headed screws required removal 8.5 times more often than headless screws, with overall costs favoring the headless screws when return-to-operating-room expenses were included [29]. A headless screw to fix a medial epicondyle or a tibia tubercle fracture are good examples of placing an implant that can remain implanted, compared to traditional screw fixation that may be prominent and need later removal.

In some cases, implant removal may be necessary, regardless of the fixation method used. When this is anticipated, the ease of future removal should be considered during the implant selection. It's important to use implants that can be removed through smaller incisions and can lead to shorter recovery times. For example, plates often cause more soft tissue disruption during removal compared to flexible nails or screws. Larger implants such as plates, which require expensive soft tissue dissection, can prolong recovery and delay the return to normal activities. Another example, fully threaded screws, especially those that are not cannulated, are stronger and do not require a path to be cut for removal. This makes them less likely to break during removal compared to partially threaded cannulated screws. However, any screw that has been in place for a long time may be more difficult to remove, and there's a risk of stripping the hex screw head. To prevent this, initially turning the screw clockwise can help loosen the bone-screw interface before turning it counterclockwise to remove the screw. This maneuver reduces the likelihood of stripping the hex-head.

Discussion of Implant Expectations Preoperatively

In keeping with the goal of maximizing the value of hardware removal, discussions about the potential need for removal should take place with the family before the index procedure. Addressing this topic during the initial surgical consultation allows the care team to provide families with a clear understanding of whether a second operation is likely and what clinical factors may warrant eventual hardware removal. Presenting a complete care plan from the outset helps set realistic expectations.

When placing an implant, the surgeon should consider how and when the metal will be removed. Over time, screws can undergo cycles of stress and may eventually break. This possibility should be discussed with the family prior to removal, so they are not surprised if an implant cannot be completely removed. One reason for considering earlier removal is the risk of screw breakage, which may not always be visible on radiographs. Fully threaded screws, unlike partially threaded screws, do not require a path to be cut during removal. This should be a factor in the decision-making process during the initial surgery. Furthermore, during the preremoval discussion and consent process, parents should always be informed that some or all of the implant may not be removable and could potentially be left in place.

Timing of Implant Removal and Shared Decision-Making

Another decision in implant removal is determining the optimal timing. Removing implants too early, before sufficient bony healing has occurred, increases the risk of refracture. Conversely, leaving implants in longer than necessary can lead to complications such as infection, stress shielding, growth arrest or imbalance, and increased bony overgrowth, which may result in a more difficult removal or even incomplete removal [30, 31].

The type of implant is also a key factor in determining the appropriate timing for removal. Exposed pins and wires—particularly those that are intra-articular—are recommended for removal within 4 weeks to minimize the risk of infection and/or soft tissue irritation. Flexible nails are typically placed with the intention of later removal following fracture healing. Most surgeons plan or offer flexible nail removal from 3 to 12 months postoperatively. Plate and screw fixation is usually removed at about 12 months. Rigid intramedullary nails are not routinely removed unless there is a clear indication. In such cases, removal is typically recommended between 1 and 2 years postoperatively, once fracture healing is complete and before bony overgrowth at the nail tip has occurred [31].

Intraoperative Cost Savings

Intraoperative cost savings play a role in the overall cost-effectiveness of metal removal procedures, and many of these opportunities begin even before the first incision is made.

For example, standardization of draping can enhance value. Surgeons often base draping techniques on personal preference or tradition rather than evidence-based practice. However, studies have shown no advantage of using 1000, 1010, or 1015 drapes (3M™ Minnesota) over more affordable split drapes, which can yield cost savings without compromising sterility. Similarly, there is no evidence that a sterile stockinette reduces infection rates compared to Coban (3M™ Minnesota) alone, representing another opportunity for savings. Simply prepping the hand or foot and using no covering is another cost-savings option. Simple limb elevation for limb exsanguination is as effective as using an Esmarch bandage and is less expensive [32].

Patient positioning equipment represents another hidden cost. In many cases, inexpensive and reusable blankets and tape can effectively replace specialized positioning equipment without sacrificing patient safety or surgical efficiency. While each of these adjustments may offer only modest savings per case, the cumulative impact is substantial, given that implant removal accounts for so many elective orthopedic procedures.

Additional cost savings can be achieved through ambulatory surgery center utilization. Since many pediatric implant removal procedures are performed on an outpatient basis, they are well-suited for ambulatory surgery centers (ASCs). One study demonstrated up to a 43% cost savings when procedures were performed at an ASC compared to a university hospital [33]. Most implant removals can be safely and effectively performed at ASCs, resulting in cost reductions.

Limiting the use of surgical instruments to only those that are necessary can save cost and time. Optimizing surgical instrument trays not only reduces expenses but also minimizes errors and decreases surgical delays. In one study, a targeted effort by surgeons and staff to streamline instrument trays led to a 55% reduction in the number of instruments, resulting in over $270,000 in annual savings [34].

Cost savings can also be realized during incision closure. Many new closure options exist, including barbed sutures, suture-less systems, and knotless wound closure devices. However, there is no evidence demonstrating the superiority of new closure options over traditional nylon or monofilament skin sutures. For example, a single 2-0 barbed suture can cost up to $24, whereas nylon sutures typically cost around $2 each. Finally, implant removal cases should not be relegated to the most junior residents [2].

Maximize Value of Care During the Postoperative Period

Postoperative care can also impact value. One example of this is the tradition of obtaining postimplant removal radiographs. While sequential radiographs are essential after initial fixation to ensure proper healing and alignment, the routine use of radiographs following implant removal warrants reconsideration. Intraoperative imaging can and should confirm complete removal of targeted implants. Routine postoperative radiographs are not necessary. We recommend limiting radiographs in the clinic after metal removal surgery to cases in which the patient has a specific complaint that could indicate a potential complication.

It is also important to carefully consider the number of follow-up visits. If the patient is recovering well and the incisions are healing as expected, follow-up appointments can be spaced out, or the patient can be discharged to as-needed follow-up after suture removal. For reliable patients or those with small incisions, using absorbable sutures that don't require in-clinic removal can enable virtual visits to assess healing and discuss progress. Unnecessary follow-up appointments after hardware removal place a strain on healthcare resources by occupying clinic time that could be allocated to patients with more urgent needs. Additionally, these visits impose indirect costs on patients and their families, including missing school and the parents needing to take time off work.

Case Example

A 12-year-old boy with a history of Duchenne muscular dystrophy sustained a multiple-stair fall, landing directly on his knees. He presented to the clinic the next day and a patellar sleeve avulsion fracture was identified. Due to his medical comorbidities, he was admitted to the hospital and underwent multidisciplinary optimization prior to surgery. This included multiple specialty consultations and preoperative evaluation with echocardiography, electrocardiogram, and comprehensive laboratory testing.

He had surgery 2 days after admission. Intraoperatively, implant options that could be removed in clinic were not feasible. As a result, a buried Kirschner wire and suture fixation was utilized, and he was placed in a long leg cast and was discharged on postoperative day 2. Postoperative follow-up was in clinic at 2, 4, and 8 weeks.

At the 8-week follow-up visit, radiographs confirmed appropriate healing of the fracture and implant removal was planned (Fig. 12.1). Several steps were taken to maximize the value of the implant removal procedure. After communication with the anesthesia team and the muscular dystrophy specialists, they recommended that since the procedure would be performed within 3 months of his most recent evaluations, no additional preop testing would be required, and the procedure could be performed as an outpatient in the ambulatory surgery center.

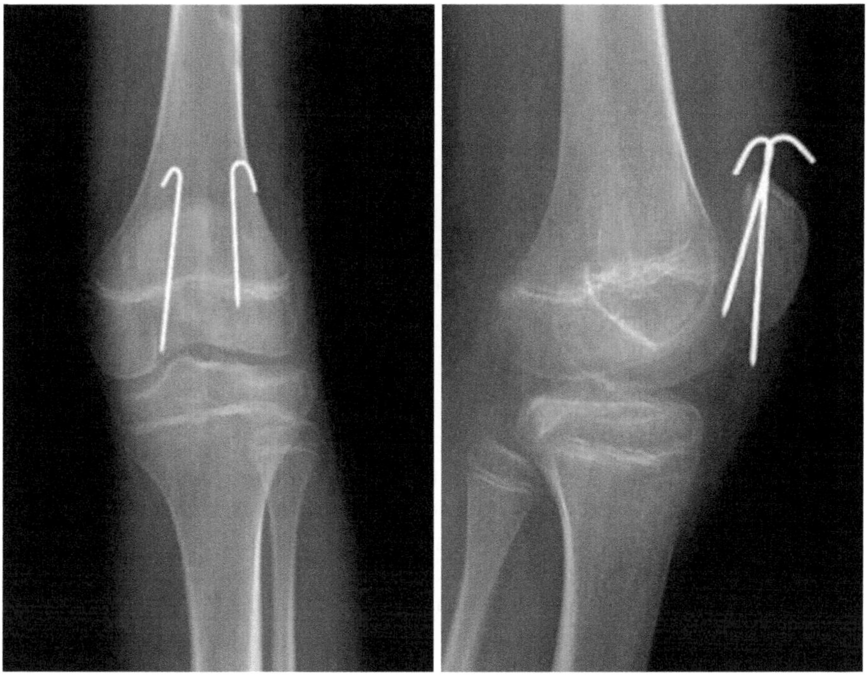

Fig. 12.1 Healed patella fracture with retained metal implants: AP and Lat X-rays

At 11 weeks postoperatively, he underwent implant removal. The surgical team was informed about the specific equipment required, since the goal was simply to remove a pair of Kirschner wires. The setup included a small set of retractors, 2 split drapes, a scalpel, needle drivers for K-wire removal, and suture material. A mini-C-arm was utilized to confirm complete implant removal. Absorbable sutures were used, and no postoperative immobilization was necessary. He recovered uneventfully in the postanesthesia care unit (PACU). A single postoperative visit at 4 weeks showed that the incision had healed and he had returned to his regular activities. He was discharged at that visit and resumed routine care through the muscular dystrophy clinic.

Summary

In this chapter, we explored various strategies to optimize value in implant removal for pediatric patients, including selection of fixation strategy and implant materials, planning the appropriate setting for hardware removal (e.g., ambulatory surgery center vs. hospital), minimizing the number of instrument trays, and reducing unnecessary follow-up visits and radiographs. Rather than falling into the mindset of "it's just a hardware removal," surgeons must remain mindful of the inherent risks and costs associated with any trip to the operating room. A thoughtful, value-based approach ultimately leads to safer, more efficient, and more cost-effective treatment.

Editors Comments

WLH

Despite the challenging and historically troublesome nature of deep metal implant removal, the current chapter nicely reviews multiple value-based strategies to ensure that implant removal in children is safe and effective.

RMS

The term "hardware removal" is used frequently to describe the surgical extraction of orthopedic metal implants. While this terminology is widely used, readers should be aware that the more professionally accepted term is "implant removal." "Implant" aligns with terminology used in procedural coding (such as CPT and ICD). Implant specifically refers to devices placed inside the body to support healing or function, whereas "hardware" is a more informal, nonspecific term. As such, readers are encouraged to adopt "implant removal" in academic writing, documentation, coding, and formal communication.

References

1. Böstman O, Pihlajamäki H. Routine implant removal after fracture surgery: a potentially reducible consumer of hospital resources in trauma units. J Trauma. 1996;41(5):846–9.
2. Ryan C, Dunleavy M, Burton A, Hennrikus W. Outcomes of hardware removal in children. Orthopaedics. 2022;46:e91–5.
3. Loder RT, Feinberg JR. Orthopaedic implants in children: survey results regarding routine removal by the pediatric and nonpediatric specialists. J Pediatr Orthop. 2006;26(4):510.
4. Peterson HA. Metallic implant removal in children. J Pediatr Orthop. 2005;25(1):107.
5. Raney EM, Freccero DM, Dolan LA, Lighter DE, Fillman RR, Chambers HG. Evidence-based analysis of removal of orthopaedic implants in the pediatric population. J Pediatr Orthop. 2008;28(7):701–4.
6. Boulos A, DeFrofa S, Kleinier J, Thomas N, Gil J, Cruz A. Inpatient orthopaedic hardware removal in children. J Clin Orthop Trauma. 2017;8:270–5.
7. Nieto RM, De León LE, Diaz DT, Krauklis KA, Fraser CD. Routine preoperative laboratory testing in elective pediatric cardiothoracic surgery is largely unnecessary. J Thorac Cardiovasc Surg. 2017;153(3):678–85.
8. Smith T, Evans J, Moriel K, Tihista M, Bacak C, Dunn J, et al. The cost of OR time is $46.04 per minute. J Orthop Bus. 2022;2(4):10–3.
9. Costs of Pediatric Hospital Stays, 2016 #250 [Internet]. [zitiert 26. Februar 2025]. Verfügbar unter: https://hcup-us.ahrq.gov/reports/statbriefs/sb250-Pediatric-Stays-Costs-2016.jsp.
10. Galbraith AA, Gaye M, Sinaiko AD. The Price of admission—the financial burden of out-of-pocket hospital costs for children. JAMA Pediatr. 2023;177(5):456–8.
11. Kellam PJ, Harrast J, Weinberg M, Martin DF, Davidson NP, Saltzman CL. Complications of hardware removal. J Bone Joint Surg. 2021;103(22):2089–95.
12. Hanson B, van der Werken C, Stengel D. Surgeons' beliefs and perceptions about removal of orthopaedic implants. BMC Musculoskelet Disord. 2008;9(1):73.
13. Barr ML, Jain NS, Bunting H, Benhaim P. Proximal plate migration after internal fixation of a pediatric distal radius fracture. Hand. 2023;18(4):NP1.
14. Desai VM, Mahon SJ, Pang A, Hauth L, Shah AS, Anari JB. Complications of hardware removal in pediatric orthopaedic surgery. J Pediatr Orthop. 2024;44(10):e957.
15. Song KS, Lee SW. Subtrochanteric femur fracture after removal of screws for femoral neck fracture in a child. Am J Orthop Belle Mead NJ. 2015;44(1):40–2.
16. Bryant J, Butler L, Green B, Krenk D. Complications in a young adult attributable to a retained pediatric dynamic hip screw. Case Rep Orthop. 2019;2019:6814375.
17. Montufar Wright PE, da Almeida Silva LC, Howard JJ, Raab S, Rogers KJ, Lindgren A, et al. Incidence of femur fracture post hardware removal in children with cerebral palsy who have undergone varus derotational osteotomy. J Pediatr Orthop. [zitiert 3. März 2025]. Verfügbar unter: https://journals.lww.com/pedorthopaedics/abstract/9900/incidence_of_femur_fracture_post_hardware_removal.773.aspx.
18. Kellam PJ, Harrast J, Weinberg M, Martin DF, Davidson NP, Saltzman CL. Complications of hardware removal. J Bone Joint Surg Am. 2021;103(22):2089.
19. Padgett AM, Howie CM, Sanchez TC, Cimino A, Williams KA, Gilbert SR, et al. Pediatric fractures following implant removal: a systematic review. J Child Orthop. 2022;16(6):488–97.
20. Kelly BA, Miller P, Shore BJ, Waters PM, Bae DS. Exposed versus buried intramedullary implants for pediatric forearm fractures: a comparison of complications. J Pediatr Orthop. 2014;34(8):749.
21. Makki D, Kheiran A, Gadiyar R, Ricketts D. Refractures following removal of plates and elastic nails from paediatric forearms. J Pediatr Orthop B. 2014;23(3):221.
22. Ding J, Dai ZZ, Liu Z, Wu ZK, Zhang ZM, Li H. Risk factors for implant-related fractures after proximal femoral osteotomy in children with developmental dysplasia of the hip: a case-control study. Acta Orthop. 2021;92(2):228–34.

23. Reith G, Schmitz-Greven V, Hensel KO, Schneider MM, Tinschmann T, Bouillon B, et al. Metal implant removal: benefits and drawbacks – a patient survey. BMC Surg. 2015;15:96.
24. Backes M, Schep NWL, Luitse JSK, Goslings JC, Schepers T. High rates of postoperative wound infection following elective implant removal. Open Orthop J. 2015;31(9):418–21.
25. Assari S, Darvish K, Ilyas AM. Biomechanical analysis of second-generation headless compression screws. Injury. 2012;43(7):1159–65.
26. Fowler JR, Ilyas AM. Headless compression screw fixation of scaphoid fractures. Hand Clin. 2010;26(3):351–61.
27. Wegner AM, Wolinsky PR, Robbins MA, Garcia TC, Maitra S, Amanatullah DF. Headless compression screw fixation of vertical medial malleolus fractures is superior to unicortical screw fixation. Am J Orthop [Internet]. 2018 [zitiert 5. April 2025];47(8). Verfügbar unter: https://www.amjorthopedics.com/article/headless-compression-screw-fixation-vertical-medial-malleolus-fractures-superior-unicortical.
28. Bulut T, Gursoy M. Isolated medial malleolus fractures: conventional techniques versus headless compression screw fixation. J Foot Ankle Surg. 2018;57(3):552–6.
29. Boren M, Steginsky B, Suhling M, Vora A. Cost of headless vs headed screw fixation for calcaneal osteotomy and subtalar arthrodesis. Foot Ankle Orthop. 2021;6(1):2473011420977864.
30. Kellam PJ, Harrast J, Weinberg M, Martin DF, Davidson NP, Saltzman CL. Complications of hardware removal. PubMed [Internet]. 2021 [zitiert 18. Februar 2025]. Verfügbar unter: https://pubmed.ncbi.nlm.nih.gov/34398858/.
31. Montgomery BK, Gamble JG, Kha ST, Hecht GG, Vorhies JS, Lucas JF. Indications for and risks associated with implant removal after pediatric trauma. JAAOS Glob Res Rev. [zitiert 26. Februar 2025]. Verfügbar unter: https://journals.lww.com/jaaosglobal/fulltext/2022/04000/indications_for_and_risks_associated_with_implant.16.aspx.
32. Gurnea TP, Frye WP, Althausen PL. Operating room supply costs in orthopaedic trauma: cost containment opportunities. J Orthop Trauma. [zitiert 15. April 2025]. Verfügbar unter: https://journals.lww.com/jorthotrauma/fulltext/2016/12001/Operating_Room_Supply_Costs_in_Orthopaedic_Trauma_.5.aspx%23.
33. Fabricant PD, Seeley MA, Rozell JC, Fieldston E, Flynn JM, Wells LM, et al. Cost savings from utilization of an ambulatory surgery center for orthopaedic day surgery. JAAOS – J Am Acad Orthop Surg. [zitiert 15. April 2025]. Verfügbar unter: https://journals.lww.com/jaaos/FullText/2016/12000/Cost_Savings_From_Utilization_of_an_Ambulatory.7.aspx.
34. Cichos KH, Hyde ZB, Mabry SE, Ghanem ES, Brabston EW, Hayes LW, et al. Optimization of orthopedic surgical instrument trays: lean principles to reduce fixed operating room expenses. J Arthroplasty. 2019;34(12):2834–40.

Pediatric Intoeing: Patience, Education, Reassurance

13

Brian Piazza and Jon Raso

Introduction

Intoeing is a common gait finding observed in children, affecting approximately 10–20% during early childhood [1, 2]. Most cases are attributed to one of three etiologies: metatarsus adductus, internal tibial torsion, and femoral anteversion [3, 4]. Historically, evaluation and treatment have often included the use of orthotic devices, physical therapy, advanced imaging, orthopedic consultation, and, in some instances, surgical intervention [5]. Optimizing the use of orthopedic referrals can reduce healthcare costs associated with intoeing. Value can be enhanced through a clear understanding and classification of the common causes of intoeing, the use of appropriate examination techniques, recognition of normal anatomic variations, and adherence to evidence-based guidelines [6, 7].

Value-Based Themes

Educating Primary Care Doctors About Age-Expected Normal Alignment, Natural History of Intoeing, and Physical Exam Findings

Understanding the primary causes and natural history of intoeing by the primary care physician is essential to make appropriate referrals to an orthopedic surgeon. The etiology of intoeing can be anatomically localized to three regions: the foot, the leg, and the hip. Metatarsus adductus (MA) is a cause of intoeing at the level of the

B. Piazza (✉)
Children's Orthopaedic and Scoliosis Surgery Associates, St. Petersburg, FL, USA

J. Raso
University of South Florida, Tampa, FL, USA

W. L. Hennrikus, R. M. Schwend (eds.), *Value in Pediatric Orthopaedics*, https://doi.org/10.1007/978-3-032-19570-8_13

foot. MA typically affects newborns and infants up to 12 months of age, with an incidence of approximately 1 in 1000 live births. MA occurs equally in males and females, with bilateral involvement seen in about 50% of cases [1, 8]. MA is characterized by medial deviation of the forefoot while the hindfoot remains normally aligned. The forefoot appears adducted, and the lateral border of the foot is curved rather than straight. This condition is believed to result from intrauterine positioning that leads to adduction at the tarsometatarsal joint. Consequently, MA is more commonly observed in late-term pregnancies, first pregnancies, twin gestations, and cases of oligohydramnios [8, 9]. Given the association of MA with "packaging disorders," patients with MA may also present with developmental dysplasia of the hip (DDH) or congenital muscular torticollis [9].

The treatment and outcome of metatarsus adductus (MA) depend on the severity and flexibility of the deformity. About 90% of cases of MA are flexible and spontaneously resolve without treatment by the age of 4 years [1, 8, 9]. In contrast, rigid or severe deformities that persist beyond infancy may be indicated for treatment. For example, serial casting in rigid cases of MA identified before the age of 2 years old can be helpful. For rigid MA deformities unresponsive to conservative management at older ages, surgical intervention may be indicated. Surgical options include tarsometatarsal capsulotomy, lateral column shortening, medial column opening osteotomies, and, in some cases, multiple metatarsal osteotomies [10–15].

Tibial torsion (TT) affects toddlers in the age range of 1 to 3 years [16, 17]. Staheli et al. reported an incidence of internal tibial torsion in up to 30% of children as they begin walking [5]. TT is characterized by inward rotation of the tibia relative to the ipsilateral femur and is often bilateral. Similar to MA, TT is believed to result from intrauterine positioning and molding [1, 16]. Parents commonly report increased tripping or falling as children begin to walk, along with visible inward rotation of the legs. TT often resolves spontaneously without treatment by around 4 years of age. Management is observation in younger children. Surgical intervention is reserved for children older than 8 years who have persistent torsion causing functional gait problems [16, 17]. Surgical treatment is rotational osteotomy of the tibia [18–20].

Lastly, internal femoral anteversion (torsion) (FA) is the most common cause of intoeing in the older child and typically affects preschool and early school-age range (3–8 years old). In FA, the anatomic site of intoeing is localized to the proximal femur, where excessive femoral neck torsion results in increased internal hip rotation and an intoeing gait [1].

Children with FA often sit in a "W" position and may exhibit a circumduction or "eggbeater" pattern while running [16, 17]. FA usually improves with growth and often resolves spontaneously by around 10 years of age. Management is primarily observation and reassurance. However, in children older than 10 years who have persistent FA associated with functional limitations or notable cosmetic concerns, femoral derotation osteotomy is a consideration [16].

Physical Examination for Intoeing

Physical examination distinguishes normal anatomical variation from pathological conditions. Intoeing may originate from one of three primary anatomical locations: the forefoot (MA), the tibia (TT), or the proximal femur (FA). A careful examination of each of these three areas can identify the underlying cause of intoeing. An intoeing evaluation should include observation of the patient's gait, rotational profile, limb flexibility, and lower extremity alignment [1].

When assessing a patient's gait, observe for asymmetry, abnormal arm swing, and tripping. A useful clinical tool in gait evaluation is the foot progression angle (FPA). The FPA is the angle formed between the direction of the child's foot and a straight line representing the path of forward motion [1] (Fig. 13.1). More specifically, the FPA is measured by drawing a line from the calcaneus to the second metatarsal and comparing it to the axis along which the patient is walking. A normal FPA is approximately +10° (external) during walking. A negative angle indicates intoeing [21, 22]. It is important to note that the FPA may appear normal in patients with offsetting internal and external torsional deformities of the femur and tibia [21]. An example of this is "miserable malalignment," in which there is increased femoral torsion and external tibia torsion, but a normal FPA.

Examination for MA should begin by assessing the lateral border of the foot for a curve and adduction of the forefoot. An additional useful tool is the heel bisector line, as described by Bleck et al. (Fig. 13.2), which helps determine the severity of

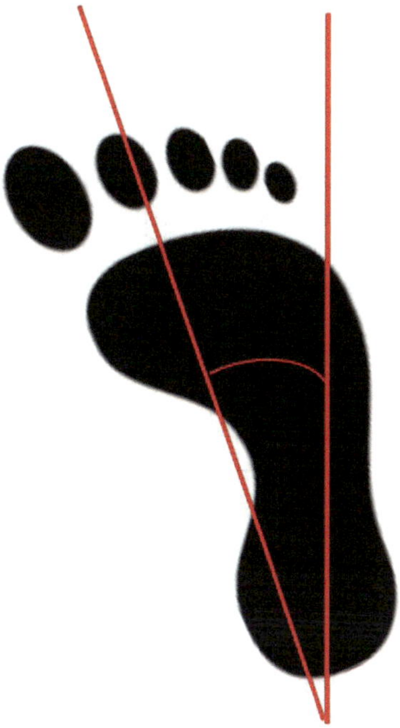

Fig. 13.1 Foot progression angle = angle between longitudinal axis of the foot and line of gait progression

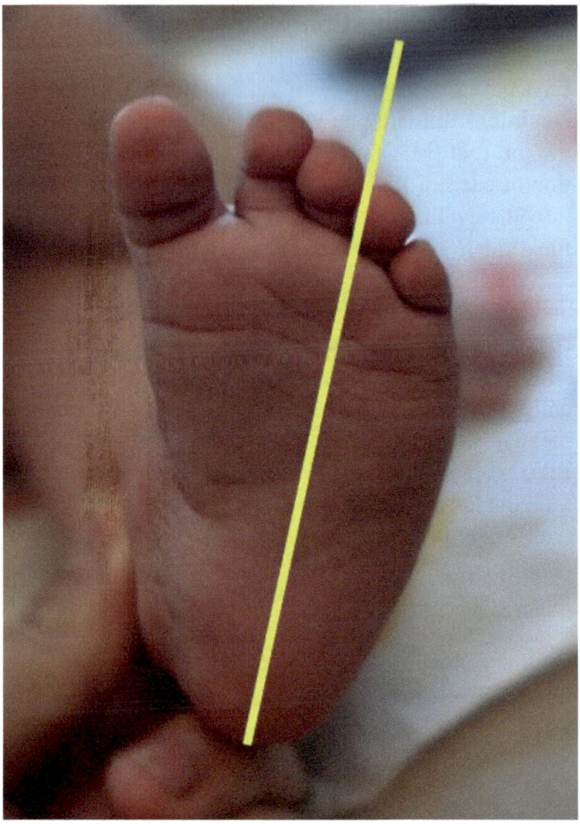

Fig. 13.2 Heel bisector line. The Bleck classification uses the position of this bisector line drawn from the heel through the forefoot to classify the severity of MA

the deformity [8]. Severity ranges from normal to severe, based on an increasing lateral deviation of the line across the forefoot.

The flexibility of the MA deformity offers insight into both the likelihood of spontaneous resolution and the need for intervention [12]. Flexible deformities that can be actively corrected to the midline do not require treatment and can be observed. Occasionally, some physicians will prescribe stretching exercises for the parents to do at home. In contrast, rigid MA deformities demonstrating a medial skin crease benefit from serial casting to achieve a straight lateral border of the foot [16].

The thigh-foot angle (TFA) is a helpful clinical measurement for assessing internal tibial torsion. TPA is measured with the child in the prone position, with the knees flexed to 90°. The angle between the long axis of the thigh and the long axis of the foot is measured [1]. A normal TFA ranges from 0° to 30° of external rotation [23] (Fig. 13.3). An additional useful clinical measurement is the transmalleolar axis viewed from a superior-to-inferior perspective. TT is present when the medial malleolus appears posterior to the lateral malleolus.

In patients with FA, examination of the hips reveals increased internal rotation and decreased external rotation, often accompanied by a preference for W-sitting. To assess for femoral anteversion, the patient is positioned prone, with hips in a

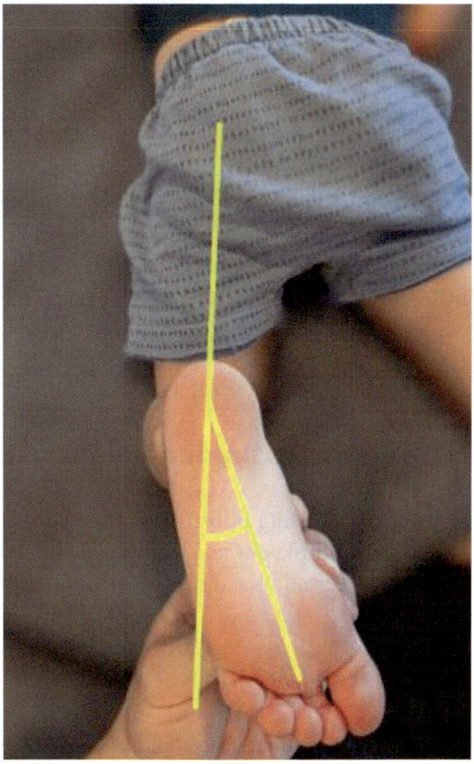

Fig. 13.3 Thigh foot angle

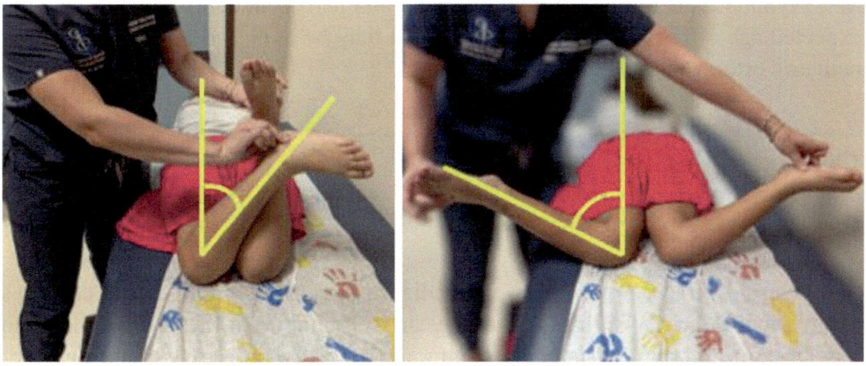

Fig. 13.4 Assessment of hip external rotation and hip internal rotation

neutral position and knees flexed to 90° [1]. The clinician then evaluates the range of motion of the hips. Internal rotation greater than 70° and external rotation less than 20° indicates FA [3] (Fig. 13.4).

In some cases, intoeing may be associated with underlying systemic or neuromuscular conditions such as cerebral palsy or spina bifida. During the physical examination, assess for neurologic abnormalities by checking for hyperreflexia, clonus, or asymmetries in muscle strength or tone. Additionally, the presence of a leg length discrepancy warrants further evaluation for an underlying pathological cause [3].

When to Refer to a Pediatric Orthopedic Surgeon?

Referral to an orthopedic surgeon for intoeing should be reserved for unusual cases presenting functional impairments of gait, rigid MA, marked asymmetry, neurological findings, pain, and persistent deformities beyond the expected age of resolution for each condition [5].

Is There Value in Bracing and Orthotics?

Historically, bracing or orthotics were commonly used in the treatment of intoeing. However, multiple clinical trials have shown no benefit of braces or orthotics compared to observation and parental reassurance [24–26].

Is Advanced Imaging Necessary?

Most cases of intoeing are benign and self-limiting, and imaging is not indicated. However, select patients presenting with functional impairments affecting gait, rigid MT, asymmetry, neurological findings, pain, and persistent deformities beyond the expected age of resolution for each condition may be indicated for imaging by the pediatric orthopedic surgeon [16].

Case Examples

Case 1

A 6-year-old girl was referred to the pediatric orthopedic clinic due to concerns about tripping and W-sitting. At her 5-year well-child visit, her pediatrician had reassured the family that intoeing commonly resolves with growth and development. However, the patient was referred for further evaluation after her parents reiterated their concerns at her 6-year well-child visit. Examination revealed a bilateral FPA of +10° of intoeing, a neutral heel bisector line, and a neutral thigh-foot axis. The patient demonstrated hip internal rotation of 60° and external rotation of 40°. The diagnosis of mild FA was made. The parents were reassured that FA is a common, age-appropriate variation that typically resolves with growth. Imaging was not indicated. The patient was seen at age 11 years for a sport physical examination, where it was noted that her intoeing and femoral anteversion had resolved.

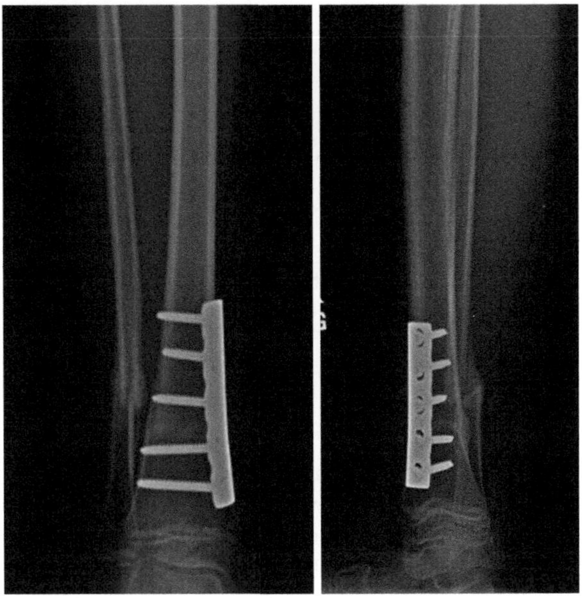

Fig. 13.5 AP and lateral radiographs of right distal tibia and fibula osteotomy

Case 2

A 9-year-old girl was referred to the pediatric orthopedic clinic for evaluation of asymmetric intoeing, with functional concerns including tripping and difficulty participating in sports. There was no relevant past medical history or history of injury. Examination demonstrated a foot progression angle of +25° on the right and +10° on the left, bilateral neutral heel bisector lines, a thigh-foot axis neutral on the left and +30° inward on right, and bilateral hip internal rotation of 35° and external rotation of 60°. A diagnosis of right TT was made. Given the patient's age and the degree of asymmetry, spontaneous correction with further growth was unlikely. After a thorough discussion of the risks and benefits of surgical correction, the parents and child elected to proceed with a tibial osteotomy (Fig. 13.5). She underwent a distal tibia and fibula osteotomy with good correction of her rotational alignment and recovered well.

Author Pearls

- Intoeing is most often a normal developmental variation.
- Physical examination is the key to identifying the underlying cause of intoeing.
- Braces and orthotics are not indicated.
- Imaging is rarely necessary.
- Referral to a pediatric orthopedic surgeon is indicated for asymmetry, pain, rigid MA, functional impairments affecting gait, neurological findings, or deformities that persist beyond the expected age of resolution.

Editors Comments

WLH

In most cases, intoeing is a normal developmental variation that can be managed by the primary care physician through counseling and observation. Imaging, braces, and orthotics are generally not indicated. Referral to a pediatric orthopedic surgeon is warranted in rare cases involving pain, functional gait impairments, neurological findings, deformities that fail to resolve with growth, or rigid metatarsus adductus requiring potential intervention.

RMS

A classic example of pathological outtoeing gait is an adolescent who was previously normal and then develops a painful limp and an external rotation foot progression angle. Based on this history and observation alone, it is most important to suspect hip pathology. They may be obese and have a history of an injury, but not always. Physical examination reveals painful and limited passive internal hip rotation compared to the normal side. An AP and frog lateral pelvic radiograph often reveal early signs of a slipped capital femoral epiphysis. This is one of the most missed serious orthopedic conditions, typically because the physician or practitioner never considers it as a possibility.

References

1. Sielatycki J, Hennrikus W, Swenson R, et al. Intoeing is often a primary care orthopaedic condition. J Pediatr. 2016;177:297–301.
2. Dormans JP. Pediatric orthopaedics: core knowledge in orthopaedics. Mosby; 2005.
3. Rerucha CM, Dickison C, Baird DC. Lower extremity abnormalities in children. Am Fam Physician. 2017;96:226–33.
4. Faulks S, Brown K, Birch JG. Spectrum of diagnosis and disposition of patients referred to a pediatric orthopaedic center for a diagnosis of intoeing. J Pediatr Orthop. 2017;37:e432–5.
5. Staheli LT, Corbett M, Wyss C, King H. Lower-extremity rotational problems in children. Normal values to guide management. J Bone Joint Surg Am. 1985;67:39–47.
6. Reeder BM, Lyne ED, Patel DR, Cucos DR. Referral patterns to a pediatric orthopedic clinic: implications for education and practice. Pediatrics. 2004;113:e163–7.
7. Sabharwal S, Zhao C, McClemens E, Edmonds EW. Do referral guidelines improve the quality of pediatric orthopedic consultations? J Pediatr Orthop. 2007;27:310–4.
8. Bleck EE. Metatarsus adductus: classification and relationship to outcomes of treatment. J Pediatr Orthop. 1983;3(1):2–9.
9. Herring JA. Tachdjian's pediatric orthopaedics: from the Texas Scottish Rite Hospital for Children e-book: 2-volume set. Elsevier Health Sciences; 2020.
10. Schoenecker PL, Anderson DJ, Blair VP, Capelli-Anderson AM. Combined lateral column shortening and medial column lengthening in the treatment of severe forefoot Adductus. In: Simons GW, editor. The clubfoot. New York: Springer; 1994. p. 412–6.

11. Berman A, Gartland JJ. Metatarsal osteotomy for the correction of adduction of the fore part of the foot in children. J Bone Joint Surg Am. 1971;53:498–506.
12. Kendrick RE, Sharma NK, Hassler WL, Herndon CH. Tarsometatarsal mobilization for resistant adduction of the fore part of the foot. A follow-up study. J Bone Joint Surg Am. 1970;52:61–70.
13. Lincoln CR, Wood KE, Bugg EI. Metatarsus varus corrected by open wedge osteotomy of the first cuneiform bone. Orthop Clin North Am. 1976;7:795–8.
14. McHale KA, Lenhart MK. Treatment of residual clubfoot deformity--the "bean-shaped" foot--by opening wedge medial cuneiform osteotomy and closing wedge cuboid osteotomy. Clinical review and cadaver correlations. J Pediatr Orthop. 1991;11:374–81.
15. Stark JG, Johanson JE, Winter RB. The Heyman-Herndon tarsometatarsal capsulotomy for metatarsus adductus: results in 48 feet. J Pediatr Orthop. 1987;7:305–10.
16. Lincoln TL, Suen PW. Common rotational variations in children. J Am Acad Orthop Surg. 2003;11:312–20.
17. Mooney JF. Lower extremity rotational and angular issues in children. Pediatr Clin N Am. 2014;61:1175–83.
18. Walton DM, Liu RW, Farrow LD, Thompson GH. Proximal tibial derotation osteotomy for torsion of the tibia: a review of 43 cases. J Child Orthop. 2012;6:81–5.
19. Savva N, Ramesh R, Richards RH. Supramalleolar osteotomy for unilateral tibial torsion. J Pediatr Orthop B. 2006;15:190–3.
20. Krengel WF, Staheli LT. Tibial rotational osteotomy for idiopathic torsion. A comparison of the proximal and distal osteotomy levels. Clin Orthop Relat Res. 1992;283:285–9.
21. Talley W, Goodemote P, Henry SL. Managing intoeing in children. Am Fam Physician. 2011;84:937–44.
22. Cibulka MT, Winters K, Kampwerth T, McAfee B, Payne L, Roeckenhaus T, Ross SA. Predicting foot progression angle during gait using two clinical measures in healthy adults, a preliminary study. Int J Sports Phys Ther. 2016;11:400–8.
23. Stuberg W, Temme J, Kaplan P, Clarke A, Fuchs R. Measurement of tibial torsion and thigh-foot angle using goniometry and computed tomography. Clin Orthop Relat Res. 1991;272:208–12.
24. Heinrich SD, Sharps CH. Lower extremity torsional deformities in children: a prospective comparison of two treatment modalities. Orthopedics. 1991;14:655–9.
25. Fabry G, MacEwen GD, Shands AR. Torsion of the femur. A follow-up study in normal and abnormal conditions. J Bone Joint Surg Am. 1973;55:1726–38.
26. Knittel G, Staheli LT. The effectiveness of shoe modifications for intoeing. Orthop Clin N Am. 1976;7:1019–25.

Pediatric Popliteal Cysts: Let It Be 14

Dale Jarka

Introduction

Pediatric popliteal cysts (PPCs) are an infrequent clinical finding in children, despite a reported prevalence of 6.3% on pediatric knee magnetic resonance imaging (MRI) studies [1]. This discrepancy reflects the identification of cysts on MRI that are too small to be detected clinically. Most PPCs are minimally symptomatic, if at all, and typically resolve spontaneously.

Popliteal cysts are sometimes referred to as Baker cysts, named after the nineteenth-century British surgeon William Morrant Baker. Unlike in adults, in whom popliteal cysts typically arise secondary to intraarticular pathology such as meniscal tears or degenerative arthritis, in children, cysts are considered a primary process. PPCs generally present before the age of 15 and are located posteromedially [3] (Fig. 14.1), and rarely communicate with the knee joint [2]. The most common PPC is thought to represent a distension of the preexisting gastrocnemio-semimembranosus bursa, or less commonly, the subgastrocnemius bursa (Type I) [2]. Pain may result from expansion into both bursae (Type II).

Value-Based Themes

Natural History

PPCs are more common in boys, with a mean age of presentation around 6 years. These cysts are typically asymptomatic, and when symptoms do occur, they generally resolve with time. In one study, 85% of PPCs resolved spontaneously, with the average time for complete resolution being 3.6 years [2]. If the cyst is present in the

D. Jarka (✉)
Department of Orthopaedics, Children's Mercy Hospital, Kansas City, MO, USA

W. L. Hennrikus, R. M. Schwend (eds.), *Value in Pediatric Orthopaedics*,
https://doi.org/10.1007/978-3-032-19570-8_14

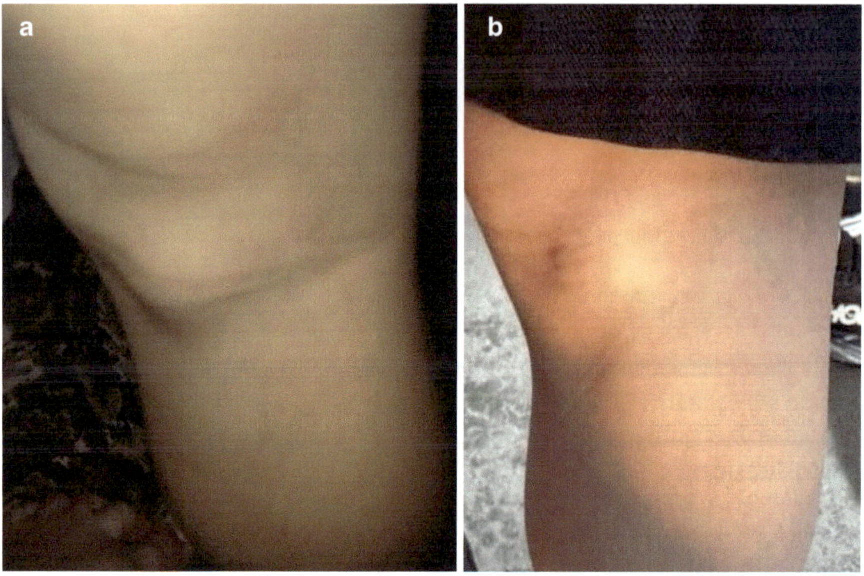

Fig. 14.1 (**a**) Popliteal cyst in a 3-year-old boy. (**b**) Popliteal cyst in the same boy, 5 years later at age 8 years

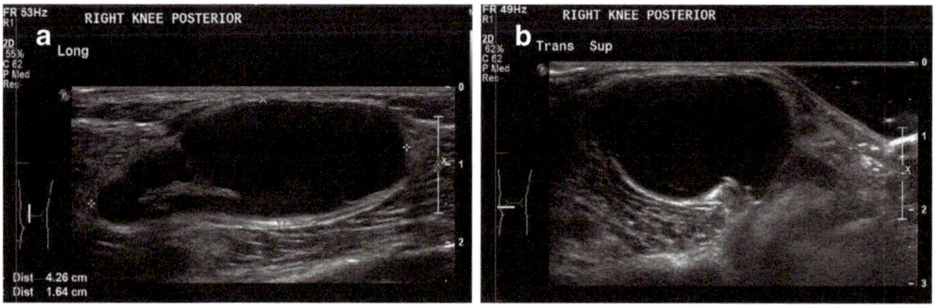

Fig. 14.2 (**a**) Longitudinal ultrasound image in a 7-year-old boy. (**b**) Transverse ultrasound image in a 7-year-old boy

posteromedial popliteal fossa, transilluminates clearly with a narrow light source, such as a penlight or otoscope, and there is no joint effusion, MRI is not necessary [2]. A plain X-ray may be performed, but it is typically normal if the clinical exam is consistent with a PPC. Ultrasound can be considered to confirm the clinical diagnosis, showing a well-circumscribed, anechoic, and fluid-filled cyst (Fig. 14.2). Routine follow-up imaging, including repeat ultrasound or MRI, does not influence management and only adds unnecessary costs to care. About half of the cases experience clinical resolution without intervention [2, 4]. Simple aspiration of the gelatinous contents is not recommended, as recurrence and refilling of the cyst are common.

Persistent Symptoms

In cases of persistent pain and/or concerning posterior knee fullness, families may be reluctant to wait for spontaneous improvement. Following shared decision-making, surgical excision may be rarely considered.

Surgical Excision

Although cyst recurrence following excision has been frequently reported, this has not been the author's experience. The procedure is typically performed on an outpatient basis. The patient is positioned prone, with critical pressure points appropriately padded. A curvilinear incision is made starting vertically on the medial side and directed laterally in its distal extent. Although some authors describe dissecting around and mobilizing an intact cyst, the author has found it easier to first aspirate the contents using an 18-gauge needle attached to a large syringe. This reduces the bulk of the cyst, which can obstruct deep dissection and often ruptures during the procedure (Fig. 14.3). Applying an Allis clamp to the deflated cyst wall provides traction and improves visualization. PPCs typically do not communicate with the knee joint, and closing the knee capsule is not necessary in such cases to potentially reduce the risk of recurrence. The incision is closed using deep dermal sutures and a running subcuticular absorbable Monocryl suture. Postoperative immobilization is generally unnecessary in younger patients, though older children may benefit from a knee immobilizer for the first few days. Patients may bear weight as tolerated and return to activity when comfortable. Unless the cyst recurs, routine long-term follow-up is not required. A recurrent cyst is only treated with repeat surgery if symptomatic.

Author Pearls

- PPCs are rarely symptomatic, and when symptoms do occur, they typically resolve spontaneously.
- More than half will resolve within 18 months; however, the average time to complete resolution is 3.6 years, so families should be counseled to remain patient.
- Persistence of the cyst alone does not indicate a need for excision.
- If surgery is considered following shared decision-making, the procedure is technically easier after aspirating the cyst contents. The parents should be counseled about the risk of recurrence even after surgery.

Editors Comments

WLH

PPCs in children are usually harmless. Value is enhanced by leaving these cysts alone and resisting the urge to operate. Transillumination and, if needed, ultrasound

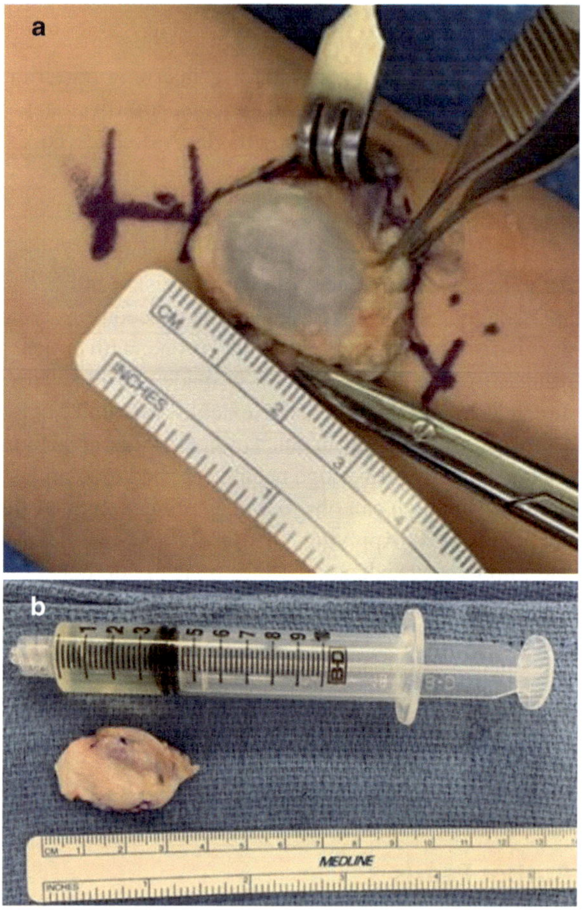

Fig. 14.3 (**a**) Surgically exposed popliteal cyst. (**b**) Aspirated cyst contents and the excised deflated cyst

are helpful diagnostic tests. MRI is not needed. Parents can be reassured that the cyst is not dangerous and is rarely associated with other knee problems in children. Second opinions can be helpful when parents need more reassurance.

RMS

Popliteal cysts are common and may persist for years. They can coexist with more concerning knee pathology, making a thorough physical examination essential. The entire limb, including the foot, should be assessed. Carefully evaluate the knee for effusion, tenderness, range of motion, and stability. An associated knee effusion warrants further evaluation for arthritis or intraarticular pathology. Lyme disease has been reported in cases of knee effusion with a popliteal cyst. In rare cases, a firm posterior knee mass with a cavus foot may represent tibial nerve fibromatosis in the popliteal fossa. Persistent deep pain, night pain, or swelling should prompt radiographic imaging to rule out bone lesions such as osteosarcoma.

References

1. De Maeseneer M, Debaere C, Desprechins B, Osteaux M. Popliteal cysts in children: prevalence, appearance and associated findings at MR imaging. Pediatr Radiol. 1999;29(8):605–9.
2. Akagi R, Saisu T, Segawa Y, Sasho T, Moriya H, Takahashi K, Kamegaya M. Natural history of popliteal cysts in the pediatric population. J Pediatr Orthop. 2013;33(3):262–8.
3. Fritschy D, Fasel J, Imbert J-C, Bianchi S, Verdonk R, Wirth CJ, O'Connor D, Clark NMP, Hegarty SE, Fairhurst JJ. The natural history of popliteal cysts in children: an ultrasound study. Knee. 1998;5(4):249–51.
4. Harcke HT, Niedzielski A, Thacker MM. Popliteal cysts in children: another look. J Pediatr Orthop B. 2016;25(6):539–42.

15 Pediatric Musculoskeletal Infection: Treat Early and Monitor Response

Michael Benvenuti

One in ten hospital consultations are related to concerns about musculoskeletal infection (MSKI). Unfortunately, only 37% of work ups for a possible infection result in positive cultures. Therefore, it can be challenging to distinguish between infections that require surgical treatment and conditions like transient synovitis or other benign conditions that mimic MSKI but can be treated without surgery [1]. The response to treatment in an MSKI can be unpredictable; therefore, ongoing monitoring and careful reevaluation are essential.

Value can be enhanced when managing pediatric MSKI by avoiding complications from missed or inadequately treated infections. Poorly treated infections can lead to sepsis, organ failure, arthritis, and long-term disability. Outcomes can be optimized by using appropriate lab tests and imaging, making a timely and accurate diagnosis, performing adequate surgical debridement, and carefully monitoring the treatment response with follow-up lab tests, imaging, and additional surgery as needed.

Value-Based Themes

Identify Sick Versus Not Sick

The first step in care is distinguishing between infectious and noninfectious conditions. The workup often remains costly and time-consuming.

Evaluation should begin with a thorough history and physical examination. Key aspects to explore include the onset of symptoms, any precipitating events or exposures, and the location of pain, all of which will help guide further workup and

M. Benvenuti (✉)
Children's Mercy Hospital, Kansas City, MO, USA
e-mail: mabenvenuti@cmh.edu

W. L. Hennrikus, R. M. Schwend (eds.), *Value in Pediatric Orthopaedics*,
https://doi.org/10.1007/978-3-032-19570-8_15

treatment. The physical exam can help identify the site(s) of possible infection by pain elicited during range of motion, pain with palpation, swelling, and overlying skin changes. The history and exam can, help to determine the severity of illness, and guide decisions about early antibiotics and intensive care unit (ICU) admission.

Use Systemic Inflammatory Markers for Diagnosis and Monitoring

Inflammatory markers help quantify tissue damage caused by infection. C-reactive protein (CRP) is the most widely available and well-established marker, though procalcitonin can serve a similar role [2–4]. Elevated inflammatory markers without another known source of tissue injury are concerning for infection and indicate the need for further workup. Moreover, significantly elevated inflammatory markers should raise suspicion for systemic complications and multiorgan dysfunction. In such severe cases, emergent surgical intervention to control the source of the infection may be needed. Failure of inflammatory markers to improve after initial debridement should prompt further investigation for other potential sites of infection and consideration for repeat debridement [2]. A small practical cost saving can be achieved by checking inflammatory markers every other day rather than daily.

Identify the Pathogen If Possible

Blood cultures should be obtained before initiating treatment in all patients with suspected MSKI [5]. Although several studies have shown that antibiotic administration may not significantly reduce tissue culture yields in MSKI; some authors still recommend obtaining tissue cultures before starting antibiotics if the cultures can be collected easily and promptly [6–9]. Empiric antibiotics should be started as soon as possible, particularly in patients who are systemically ill [10]. In endemic areas, testing for Lyme disease serology should also be performed, keeping in mind that Lyme results typically take several days to return [11, 12]. Lyme serology is valuable for determining the final diagnosis but may not be useful in guiding urgent treatment decisions.

A recent adjunct to traditional cultures and Lyme serology is PCR-based genetic identification of pathogenic bacteria, which can quickly identify the causative organism and guide antibiotic treatment. The rapid identification of pathogens and the ability to detect septic arthritis help save resources. Timely pathogen detection can speed up intervention and enhance patient outcomes. Negative results often allow for earlier patient discharge. Although PCR testing is more expensive than traditional cultures, PCR testings' increased sensitivity and ability to detect antibiotic resistance add value [13]. For example, in children, *Kingella kingae* is a common but difficult-to-culture pathogen that can be identified quickly using PCR methods [14].

Synovial fluid analysis for cell count can also aid in the diagnosis of infection. While a white blood cell (WBC) count of 50,000 WBC/mm^3 has been used as a threshold to differentiate septic from nonseptic conditions, this threshold number has limited sensitivity and specificity, even when combined with neutrophil count [15]. However, when considered alongside the history, physical exam, systemic lab results, and imaging, the synovial WBC count can serve as a useful data point, particularly if the count is extremely elevated or nearly normal.

Be Efficient But Thorough with Imaging

Imaging plays a crucial role in diagnosing and effectively treating infections, though it can increase the cost of care. X-rays and ultrasound (US) are relatively inexpensive and provide important information in the workup of potential MSKI. X-rays of the affected extremity can help rule out trauma and certain neoplasms, but X-rays are often insufficient for diagnosing acute infections.

Ultrasound can identify soft tissue fluid collections and swelling associated with cellulitis. US is also valuable in detecting joint effusions, particularly in deeper joints, such as the shoulder and hip [16]. For example, a child with elevated CRP, inability to bear weight, and a hip effusion on US should raise significant concern for septic arthritis.

Computed tomography (CT) and magnetic resonance imaging (MRI) are the most sensitive and specific imaging modalities for pediatric MSKI. Due to the radiation risk of CT, MRI is often the preferred diagnostic imaging method in children. However, MRI in children can require sedation or general anesthesia. The added cost of anesthesia reduces value. Recent efforts to develop rapid MRI protocols have shown promise. These protocols allow for near-equivalent sensitivity and specificity in diagnosing acute infections without the need for sedation/anesthesia and with less time spent in the MRI scanner [17–19]. Rapid MRIs can enhance value by enabling faster diagnoses, earlier discharge for patients without evidence of infection, and more timely intervention for those requiring surgical debridement.

MRI provides additional value when identifying multiple sites of infection and guiding surgical intervention. Due to the heterogeneity of pediatric infections, it is crucial to determine which tissues require debridement before surgery [20]. In cases of *S. aureus* infection, intra-articular and extra-articular involvement is common and best identified using MRI imaging to guide accurate surgical debridement and minimize the need for repeat procedures. Additionally, MRI is helpful in differentiating Lyme arthritis from septic arthritis when other clinical indicators and patient history are inconclusive [21, 22]. In these cases, MRI helps prevent unnecessary surgeries for Lyme arthritis while ensuring timely debridement for septic arthritis.

Algorithms have been developed to predict the likelihood of concurrent osteomyelitis in septic arthritis. However, attempts to validate these algorithms at different institutions have failed, likely due to regional and institutional variations in pathology [23–26].

Treatment

Give Antibiotics Early and Involve Infectious Disease Colleagues for Difficult Cases

Early debridement, coupled with appropriate antibiotic treatment, is key to optimizing outcomes, minimizing length of stay, and reducing the need for multiple surgical interventions. Collaboration with an infectious disease (ID) colleague plays an important role in achieving successful outcomes for some MSKI. Understanding the local antimicrobiogram is helpful for determining initial empiric treatment, especially before cultures or PCR results are known. Additionally, utilizing a protocol that includes collaboration with ID can potentially improve outcomes and reduce costs [27].

Antibiotic therapy should be initiated as soon as possible, particularly in cases of systemic infection. Early administration of antibiotics has been shown to shorten hospital length of stay and reduce complications [6, 9, 28–30]. Especially in cases of severe MSKI, early antibiotic treatment can reduce costs and improve value.

Multiple studies have examined the optimal duration of both intravenous and oral antibiotic therapy to maximize outcomes while minimizing antibiotic-related complications and costs. Some studies have suggested using CRP levels to guide the transition from IV to oral antibiotics, although results have been mixed [31–33]. Rather than relying on specific CRP cutoffs, an improving clinical picture coupled with decreasing inflammatory markers is likely a more practical guide for antibiotic transition. In addition, some studies indicate that shorter durations of antibiotics are noninferior for treating septic arthritis, myositis, and osteomyelitis, with 2–3 weeks of therapy often being sufficient. This approach improves value compared to traditional prolonged 6-week antibiotic regimens [34].

Adjuncts to antibiotic therapy have the potential to add value in the management of MSKI, though their use remains controversial. Two studies have demonstrated that corticosteroids can improve symptoms, shorten the time to transition to oral antibiotics, reduce treatment duration, minimize complications, and hasten discharge [35, 36]. In children with severe MSKI, corticosteroids may help modulate the dysregulated inflammatory response, but their use remains debated. For example, while corticosteroids have been shown to reduce mortality in adults with septic shock, evidence in children is less clear, with one study suggesting an increased risk of complications [37]. However, other research indicates that corticosteroids are beneficial in children with shock that is refractory to fluid resuscitation and vasopressor therapy [38, 39].

Perform Effective Surgical Intervention

Surgical debridement is essential in managing many MSKIs by controlling the source of infection. Surgery should not be delayed for imaging in children with necrotizing fasciitis or other severe systemic infections. Surgery can be performed urgently after imaging for most cases of septic arthritis. Surgical debridement can prevent death, prevent arthritis, reduce long-term disability, reduce morbidity, and promote faster recovery. Well-done and well-timed surgery adds value.

One potential, but controversial, lower-cost alternative to open or arthroscopic debridement of a septic joint is serial needle aspiration and/or needle lavage [40–43]. Single or repeat needle aspiration and lavage, combined with appropriate antibiotics, can treat select cases of septic arthritis. However, research is ongoing to identify which children would benefit most from this approach without risking increased complications. In patients with septic arthritis who are too ill for surgery, serial needle lavage can also be performed.

Prevent Postoperative Infections

Strategies to reduce postoperative infection risk while avoiding overtreatment add value for elective pediatric orthopedic surgical cases. Cefazolin is the first-line antibiotic for prophylaxis in most cases, with additional antibiotic coverage indicated for contaminated wounds and neuromuscular scoliosis surgery [44]. Adhering to the recommendation of cefazolin over less effective and more expensive alternative antibiotics can reduce infection rates, reduce costs, and enhance value. Administering a small initial test dose of cefazolin for patients with a remote history of penicillin allergy is an inexpensive method to enable more patients to receive cefazolin. Other simple, practical, and cost-effective interventions to reduce infection risk include proper handwashing, using strict sterile techniques, and limiting operating room traffic.

Case Example

A 5-month-old male presented with 1 week of shoulder discomfort and worsening erythema over his clavicle. On examination, he was fussy with any manipulation of his arm and had swelling over the midshaft clavicle. Radiographs were obtained, which did not show a fracture or lesion. Laboratory tests revealed a CRP of 6.8 mg/dL (normal <1), erythrocyte sedimentation rate (ESR) of 35, and anemia with a hemoglobin (Hgb) of 9.0. A rapid MRI was performed (Fig. 15.1) showing a large subperiosteal fluid collection around the clavicle with intraosseous edema, consistent with osteomyelitis and abscess. Cefazolin was initiated based on the local antimicrobiogram, and surgical treatment with irrigation and debridement was carried out. Intraoperative cultures grew methicillin-susceptible staphylococcus aureus (MSSA). On postoperative day 2, the drain was removed, and the CRP had decreased to 2.4. The patient was discharged on oral cephalexin for 5 weeks. Follow-up at 2 weeks showed improved clinical examination, no apparent discomfort, and normalization of both ESR and CRP.

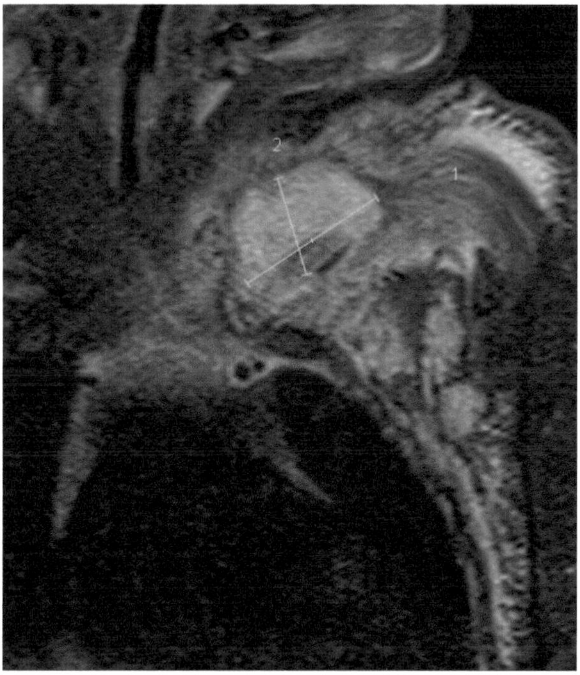

Fig. 15.1 Left shoulder MRI demonstrates clavicle osteomyelitis with subperiosteal abscess

Summary

MSKI can be unpredictable. Value is enhanced by preventing long-term morbidity. A thorough history and physical, accurate diagnosis, timely treatment, and careful monitoring are key to optimizing outcomes. Rapid protocol MRI and consultation with an ID specialist can also add value. Because MSKIs are a heterogeneous group of diseases, highly regimented treatment protocols are not recommended. Instead, each MSKI case is treated on a case-by-case basis.

Author Pearls

- Perform a comprehensive history and physical examination.
- Obtain inflammatory markers and blood cultures early.
- Perform X-rays of the affected area and obtain a rapid protocol unsedated MRI if available.
- Initiate antibiotics promptly and perform surgical irrigation and debridement.
- Monitor the patient's response to treatment closely and consider a second debridement if no improvement is observed within 2–3 days.
- Follow proper sterile procedures and adhere to antibiotic prophylaxis protocols.

Editors Comments

WLH

In children with suspected MSKI, obtain immediate blood cultures, a CRP, and a PCR. Once blood cultures are obtained, start empiric antibiotics based on local susceptibility data and the patient's history (if any) of prior infections. Modify the antibiotics based on culture and PCR results. X-rays should be performed, partly, to rule out other diagnoses. In select cases of suspected hip infection a US can be obtained, and in all cases of suspected hip infection, a hip aspiration and irrigation/debridement should be performed. In uncomplicated cases of suspected osteomyelitis, a biopsy, followed by irrigation and debridement, can be performed. In cases suspected to be complicated osteomyelitis, a fast MRI should be obtained, followed by biopsy, irrigation, and debridement. Careful follow-up of all MSKI cases is warranted. If no improvement in symptoms occurs at 48 hours, consider a second debridement or a more complete MRI.

RMS

Before the advent of antibiotics, the mortality rate from musculoskeletal infections (MSKI) was approximately 40%. While there have been significant improvements in developed nations, globally, acute MSKI and its sequelae remain among the most poorly treated conditions in primary care. The greatest opportunity for improvement lies in raising awareness and fostering clinical suspicion to enable early diagnosis. Eradicating a bone infection may necessitate multiple surgeries, and parents should be informed about this possibility before the first surgery is performed. In children with infections near the growth plate (physis), long-term follow-up is essential to monitor for potential growth disturbances. The severity of the infection often correlates with the severity of its sequelae.

References

1. Koehler RJ, et al. Defining the volume of consultations for musculoskeletal infection encountered by pediatric orthopaedic services in the United States. PLoS One. 2020;15(6):e0234055.
2. Moore-Lotridge SN, et al. CRP predicts the need to escalate care after initial debridement for musculoskeletal infection. J Pediatr Orthop. 2024;44(3):188–96.
3. van der Laan L, et al. Comparison of procalcitonin with commonly used biomarkers and algorithms for evaluating suspected pediatric musculoskeletal infection in the emergency department. J Pediatr Orthop. 2023;43(2):e168–73.
4. Benvenuti MA, et al. A clinical prediction algorithm to stratify pediatric musculoskeletal infection by severity. J Pediatr Orthop. 2019;39(3):153–7.
5. Scheer CS, et al. Impact of antibiotic administration on blood culture positivity at the beginning of sepsis: a prospective clinical cohort study. Clin Microbiol Infect. 2019;25(3):326–31.
6. Benvenuti MA, et al. Effects of antibiotic timing on culture results and clinical outcomes in pediatric musculoskeletal infection. J Pediatr Orthop. 2019;39(3):158–62.

7. Gramberg M, et al. Effect of prior antibiotic use on culture results in people with diabetes and foot osteomyelitis. Antibiotics (Basel). 2023;12(4):684.
8. Marschall J, et al. The impact of prebiopsy antibiotics on pathogen recovery in hematogenous vertebral osteomyelitis. Clin Infect Dis. 2011;52(7):867–72.
9. Section J, et al. Microbiological culture methods for pediatric musculoskeletal infection: a guideline for optimal use. J Bone Joint Surg. 2015;97(6):441–9.
10. Ferrer R, et al. Empiric antibiotic treatment reduces mortality in severe sepsis and septic shock from the first hour: results from a guideline-based performance improvement program*. Crit Care Med. 2014;42(8):1749–55.
11. Lyons TW, et al. A clinical prediction rule for bacterial musculoskeletal infections in children with monoarthritis in Lyme endemic regions. Ann Emerg Med. 2022;80(3):225–34.
12. Cruz AI Jr, et al. Distinguishing pediatric Lyme arthritis of the hip from transient synovitis and acute bacterial septic arthritis: a systematic review and meta-analysis. Cureus. 2018;10(1):e2112.
13. Esteban J, et al. Multicenter evaluation of the BIOFIRE Joint Infection Panel for the detection of bacteria, yeast, and AMR genes in synovial fluid samples. J Clin Microbiol. 2023;61(11):e0035723.
14. Yagupsky P. The past, present, and future of Kingella kingae detection in pediatric osteoarthritis. Diagnostics (Basel). 2022;12(12):2932.
15. Eren TK, Aktekin CN. How reliable are the synovial cell count and blood parameters in the diagnosis of septic arthritis? Joint Dis Relat Surg. 2023;34(3):724–30.
16. Alamdaran SA, et al. Role of ultrasound and inflammatory factors in the management of pediatric hip joint effusion. Pediatr Rheumatol Online J. 2023;21(1):146.
17. Chan KS, et al. A rapid MRI protocol for the evaluation of acute pediatric musculoskeletal infections: eliminating contrast and decreasing anesthesia, scan time, and hospital length of stay and charges. J Bone Joint Surg Am. 2024;106(8):700–7.
18. Ojeaga PO, et al. Quality improvement of magnetic resonance imaging for musculoskeletal infection in children results in decreased scan duration and decreased contrast use. J Bone Joint Surg. 2019;101(18):1679–88.
19. Markhardt BK, Woo K, Nguyen JC. Evaluation of suspected musculoskeletal infection in children over 2 years of age using only fluid-sensitive sequences at MRI. Eur Radiol. 2019;29(10):5682–90.
20. Gibian JT, et al. The heterogeneity of pediatric knee infections: a retrospective analysis. J Pediatr Orthop. 2020;40(6):314–21.
21. Ecklund K, et al. MRI features of Lyme arthritis in children. AJR Am J Roentgenol. 2005;184(6):1904–9.
22. Powell JE, et al. MRI features distinguishing pediatric Lyme arthritis from septic arthritis. Skeletal Radiol. 2024;54:1043.
23. Montgomery CO, et al. Concurrent septic arthritis and osteomyelitis in children. J Pediatr Orthop. 2013;33(4):464–7.
24. Rosenfeld S, et al. Predicting the presence of adjacent infections in septic arthritis in children. J Pediatr Orthop. 2016;36(1):70–4.
25. Hunter S, Kennedy J, Baker JF. External validation of an algorithm to predict adjacent musculoskeletal infection in pediatric patients with septic arthritis. J Pediatr Orthop. 2020;40(10):e999–e1004.
26. Refakis CA, et al. Predicting periarticular infection in children with septic arthritis of the hip: regionally derived criteria may not apply to all populations. J Pediatr Orthop. 2019;39(5):268–74.
27. Spruiell MD, et al. Clinical care guideline for improving pediatric acute musculoskeletal infection outcomes. J Pediatr Infect Dis Soc. 2017;6(3):e86–93.
28. McNeil JC, et al. Role of operative or interventional radiology-guided cultures for osteomyelitis. Pediatrics. 2016;137(5):e20154616.
29. Lansell A, et al. Impact of antibiotic pretreatment on cultures in children with osteomyelitis and septic arthritis: a retrospective review. BMC Pediatr. 2021;21(1):342.

30. Yi J, et al. Clinical epidemiology and outcomes of pediatric musculoskeletal infections. J Pediatr. 2021;234:236–244.e2.
31. Bouchard M, Shefelbine L, Bompadre V. C-reactive protein level at time of discharge is not predictive of risk of reoperation or readmission in children with septic arthritis. Front Surg. 2019;6:68.
32. Pääkkönen M, et al. Sensitivity of erythrocyte sedimentation rate and C-reactive protein in childhood bone and joint infections. Clin Orthop Relat Res. 2010;468(3):861–6.
33. Pääkkönen M, Peltola H. Management of a child with suspected acute septic arthritis. Arch Dis Child. 2012;97(3):287–92.
34. Huang C-Y, et al. Short- versus long-course antibiotics in osteomyelitis: a systematic review and meta-analysis. Int J Antimicrob Agents. 2019;53(3):246–60.
35. Harel L, et al. Dexamethasone therapy for septic arthritis in children: results of a randomized double-blind placebo-controlled study. J Pediatr Orthop. 2011;31(2):211–5.
36. Qin YF, Li ZJ, Li H. Corticosteroids as adjunctive therapy with antibiotics in the treatment of children with septic arthritis: a meta-analysis. Drug Des Devel Ther. 2018;12:2277–84.
37. Chaudhuri D, et al. 2024 Focused update: guidelines on use of corticosteroids in sepsis, acute respiratory distress syndrome, and community-acquired pneumonia. Crit Care Med. 2024;52(5):e219–33.
38. Annane D, et al. Corticosteroids for treating sepsis in children and adults. Cochrane Database Syst Rev. 2019;12(12):CD002243.
39. Bline KE, et al. Hydrocortisone treatment is associated with a longer duration of MODS in pediatric patients with severe sepsis and immunoparalysis. Crit Care. 2020;24(1):545.
40. Journeau P, et al. Hip septic arthritis in children: assessment of treatment using needle aspiration/irrigation. Orthop Traumatol Surg Res. 2011;97(3):308–13.
41. Weigl DM, et al. Percutaneous aspiration and irrigation technique for the treatment of pediatric septic hip: effectiveness and predictive parameters. J Pediatr Orthop B. 2016;25(6):514–9.
42. Pääkkönen M, et al. Pediatric septic hip with or without arthrotomy: retrospective analysis of 62 consecutive nonneonatal culture-positive cases. J Pediatr Orthop B. 2010;19(3):264–9.
43. Cohen E, et al. Surgical treatment of septic arthritis of the hip in children: arthrotomy compared with repeated aspiration-lavage. Int Orthop. 2023;47(6):1609–18.
44. Opri F, et al. Surgical antimicrobial prophylaxis in patients of neonatal and pediatric age undergoing orthopedic and hand surgery: a RAND/UCLA appropriateness method consensus study. Antibiotics (Basel). 2022;11(3):289.

Limb Deficient Child—The Value of Adaptability

16

Julia L. Conroy, Jeffery E. Brooks, Adam Kohn, Jorgen Post, and Joshua M. Abzug

Introduction

Congenital limb deficiencies can result from a variety of causes, including genetic variations, environmental teratogen exposure, or gene–environment interactions [1]. The incidence has remained stable over time and is consistent across countries and studies [1]. Reported incidence rates range from 2 to 7 per 10,000 live births, with upper extremity deficiencies occurring two to three times more frequently than lower extremity deficiencies [1].

The management of congenital limb deficiencies is multifaceted and benefits from a multidisciplinary approach. This team typically includes physicians, occupational and physical therapists, prosthetists, social workers, and psychological counselors, as well as the patient and their family. Care is individualized, often incorporating prosthetic use when appropriate, surgical intervention when indicated, and rehabilitation programs aimed at enhancing function, independence, and quality of life.

Because congenital limb deficiencies are present at birth and persist throughout all stages of development, the growth of the child presents management challenges not seen in the adult amputee population. These include the cost of the initial prosthesis and the need for multiple replacements over time, and the time and cost of follow-up visits. These visits may involve travel and lost wages for parents.

J. L. Conroy · J. M. Abzug (✉)
Department of Orthopaedics, University of Maryland School of Medicine, Baltimore, MD, USA
e-mail: jconroy@som.umaryland.edu; jabzug@som.umaryland.edu

J. E. Brooks · A. Kohn · J. Post
D & J Medical, Orthotics & Prosthetics, Baltimore, MD, USA
e-mail: jbrooks@dandjmedical.com; akohn@dandjmedical.com; jorgen@dandjmedical.com

W. L. Hennrikus, R. M. Schwend (eds.), *Value in Pediatric Orthopaedics*,
https://doi.org/10.1007/978-3-032-19570-8_16

Additional challenges include the psychological impact of a visible limb difference in comparison to peers.

Value-based care for children with limb deficiencies aims to optimize outcomes while minimizing costs and treatment burden. The current chapter explores both functional and psychological outcomes for children and their parents, as well as the direct and indirect financial and time-related costs associated with care.

Value-Based Themes

Upper Extremity Limb Deficiencies: Is a Prosthesis Always Necessary?

Children typically use an upper extremity prosthesis only if it enhances their function. Among those with unilateral congenital below-elbow deficiency (UCBED), prosthesis rejection rates are high, ranging from 49% to 75% [2, 3]. Nonwearers often demonstrate functional abilities and quality of life comparable to those of prosthesis users. In one study, prosthesis wearers aged 11–20 performed tasks more effectively without their device, whereas younger children performed better with it [4]. James and colleagues found that although functional scores in children with UCBED were slightly lower than those in the general population, they remained within the normal range [4]. In some cases, children with UCBED reported even higher quality of life scores than their peers [4].

Children with UCBED are often able to perform most activities without the use of adaptive equipment. The residual limb is incorporated into bimanual tasks and provides valuable sensory feedback. When a prosthetic device is used, this sensory input is inhibited, which contributes to prosthesis rejection in some children [3]. In addition, users report that their prosthesis is helpful in only 39% of daily activities [3]. As a result, activity-specific prostheses may offer greater usefulness and lead to increased wear time (see case example). Choosing to forgo a prosthesis altogether or to use only an activity-specific device can lead to both direct and indirect cost and time savings for the child and their family by reducing or eliminating the need for frequent prosthetist visits.

Upper Extremity Limb Deficiencies: Prosthetic Management

Although many children with UCBED function well without an adaptive device, up to 51% report a successful prosthesis outcome. Success is defined as continued participation in a longitudinal clinic and any degree of prosthesis use [2]. Davids and colleagues proposed a staged prosthetic management strategy, beginning with the introduction of a passive device once the child can walk independently around 1 year of age [2]. If the child continues to use the device daily and/or the parents express interest in a more advanced option, the child may then be fitted with a body-powered or myoelectric device between the ages of 2 and 4 years. This stepwise approach allows for an initial trial period, helping to reduce financial barriers and potential losses if the child does not tolerate or benefit from the device.

Several factors have been associated with improved prosthesis outcomes, including fitting the prosthesis before the age of 3, providing training with an occupational therapist when an active terminal device is introduced, and utilizing a variety of prosthetic designs as the child grows [2]. Awareness of these factors can help guide prosthetic management.

Three-Dimensional (3D) Printed Transitional Prostheses May Be a Cost-Effective Alternative for Children with Congenital Upper Extremity Deficiencies

Conventional prosthetic devices can be prohibitively expensive. Body-powered prostheses typically range from $3800 to $7700, while myoelectric prostheses are even more costly, ranging from $23,800 to $47,600 [5]. For children with congenital limb deficiencies, growth necessitates prosthetic refittings and replacements, placing a financial burden on families. In contrast, 3D-printed prostheses offer a cost-effective alternative. These devices are lighter, stronger, easier to customize, and have shorter production times compared to traditional prostheses. A 3D-printed prosthesis can be produced for just $50 and takes 5–10 hours to construct [6]. A recent pilot study found that after 6 months of training, children with upper extremity deficiencies showed improved manual gross dexterity using 3D-printed prostheses; however, there was limited success with lateral and tripod pinch functions [6].

Lower Limb Deficiencies: Amputation and Prosthetic Management Versus Limb Lengthening Procedures

The primary goals of managing lower limb deficiencies are to achieve limb length equality, a normal gait, and normal weight-bearing function. Patients with mild deficiencies who have a functional, plantigrade foot and less than 6% limb length inequality (LLI) can often be managed with a shoe lift and foot orthosis [7]. In more severe cases, operative management is recommended. Amputation and prosthetic rehabilitation are appropriate when there is significant foot deformity (absence of three or more rays), a predicted LLI of ≥30% at skeletal maturity, or an LLI greater than 5 cm at birth [8–10]. Patients with less severe foot deformities and an expected LLI of <30% are candidates for limb preservation and lengthening procedures [7].

Multiple studies have compared the long-term outcomes of amputation versus limb preservation and lengthening procedures [11–14]. Findings consistently show that patients who undergo amputation followed by prosthetic rehabilitation experience fewer hospitalizations, fewer surgical interventions, lower readmission rates, fewer complications, and improved functional outcomes compared to those treated with limb lengthening. In addition, a recent study by Birch and colleagues found no significant differences in functional or psychological outcomes between patients who underwent amputation and those who received limb reconstruction. Both groups reported satisfaction with their outcomes by mid-childhood [15]. Although advancements in limb lengthening and reconstructive techniques show promise for improving outcomes and preserving the limb, long-term data supporting their efficacy remain limited. In contrast, amputation and prosthetic rehabilitation have demonstrated positive long-term outcomes, including fewer complications and reduced healthcare utilization. Ultimately, the decision between amputation and limb preservation should be individualized, with shared decision-making involving the child, their family, and the care team.

A Multifactorial Approach Can Improve Psychological Outcomes Among Children and Adolescents with Congenital Limb Differences

Congenital limb differences are often visibly apparent, which can pose challenges for psychosocial adjustment in affected children [16, 17]. In an online focus group study by de Jong and colleagues, children and adolescents with unilateral congenital below-elbow deficiencies reported mixed emotions regarding their condition [18]. Feelings of shame or of being different were often linked to negative social experiences, such as being stared at or receiving unwanted attention from strangers. Adolescents aged 13–16 were particularly vulnerable to negative emotions, likely due to the heightened social sensitivity of the pubescent period. In contrast, older participants reported greater acceptance and even pride in their limb difference, often influenced by positive social interactions. Support from family and peers, opportunities for peer-to-peer contact, and wearing a prosthesis were identified as effective coping mechanisms [18].

Parental support has a major influence on how children perceive their limb difference [18]. When parents maintain a positive attitude and speak optimistically about their child's condition, children are more likely to develop positive feelings about themselves. Therefore, it is essential that physicians and the rehabilitation team educate parents about their role in shaping their child's self-perception. Clinicians should also recognize that parents may experience feelings of shame, grief, or guilt following the birth of a child with a limb difference [18]. Resources such as peer groups for children with limb differences, support groups for parents, and community-based activities such as camps for children with limb differences can provide education, emotional support, and social support for both children and their parents.

Case Example of a Task-Specific Prosthesis Designed for Upper Extremity Function

Background

A 10-year-old girl presented with a congenital transverse deficiency of the left upper extremity, approximately 4 inches distal to the elbow. There was no history of prior surgeries or trauma to the residual limb. She enjoyed dancing, ballet, acting, and playing the keyboard. Physical examination revealed full range of motion at the shoulder and elbow, intact skin integrity, and no tenderness. Her primary goal was to learn to play the viola using a body-powered prosthesis to control the bow.

Prosthesis Planning, Casting, and Fitting

The prosthetic fitting process began with an evaluation and casting of the residual limb. Due to the shortened limb length, a Muenster-style casting technique was utilized to achieve a secure fit proximal to the elbow, enhancing suspension during activities (Fig. 16.1a, b). Special attention was given to relieving pressure over the biceps tendon within the socket to ensure comfort and maintain full elbow flexion.

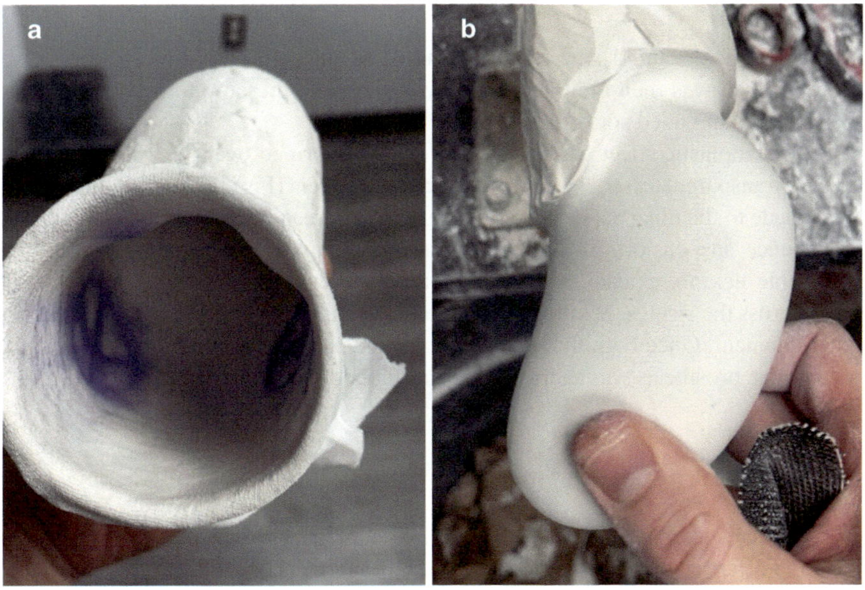

Fig. 16.1 The Muenster-style casting procedure (**a**). The cast is removed from the patient, and then the inside of the cast is filled with plaster to create a positive mold that the prosthetist will modify by applying plaster buildups over bony anatomy and removing plaster in strategic areas to apply proper pressures to the soft tissue based on the socket design (**b**). (Courtesy of Joshua M. Abzug, MD)

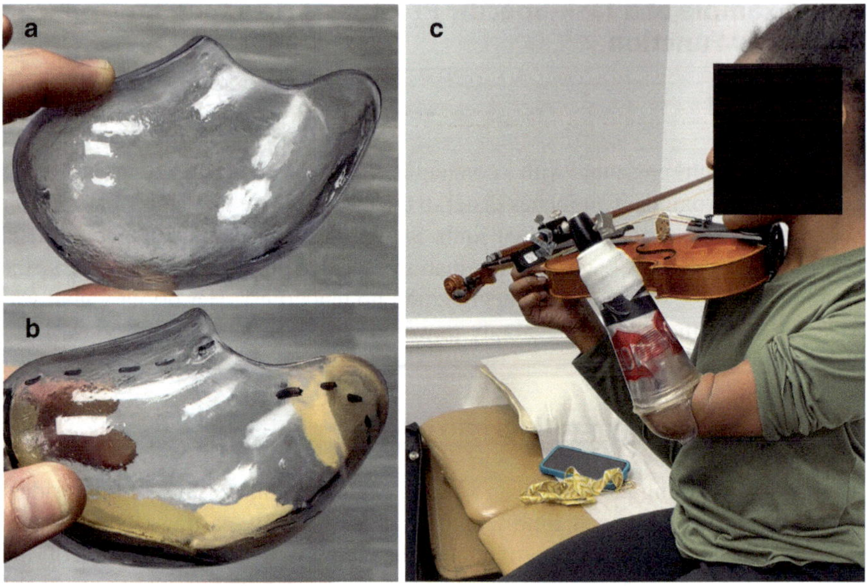

Fig. 16.2 Photographs depicting a thermoplastic sheet that has been heated and vacuum-formed to produce a transparent test socket. Images of the test socket alone (**a**, **b**) as well as in use (**c**) to assess fit and function while playing the viola are presented. (Courtesy of Joshua M. Abzug, MD)

After casting, the mold was removed and filled with plaster to create a positive model, which was then modified to apply appropriate pressure to soft tissue areas based on the intended socket design.

A thermoplastic sheet was heated and vacuum-formed over the plaster mold to create a transparent test socket to assess fit and alignment (Fig. 16.2a–c). Adjustments were made to the ulnar aspect of the socket and the area proximal to the epicondyles to enhance suspension. To accommodate viola playing, a terminal device with adjustable flexion, extension, and rotation was selected, allowing the bow to rest flatly across the strings. Multiple test sockets were trialed to ensure optimal comfort and alignment. Once both the prosthetist and the patient were satisfied with the fit, a definitive prosthesis was fabricated for use in her daily activities (Fig. 16.3).

Summary

Clinical management of children with limb deficiencies is long-term and multifaceted and offers several opportunities to enhance value. These opportunities include individualized prosthetic management, including in some cases the decision to forgo prosthetic use; 3D-printed transitional prostheses; and, for children with lower limb deficiencies, considering amputation and prosthetic rehabilitation as an alternative to multiple limb lengthening procedures. Equally important is a focus on psychological well-being and quality of life for both the child and their family.

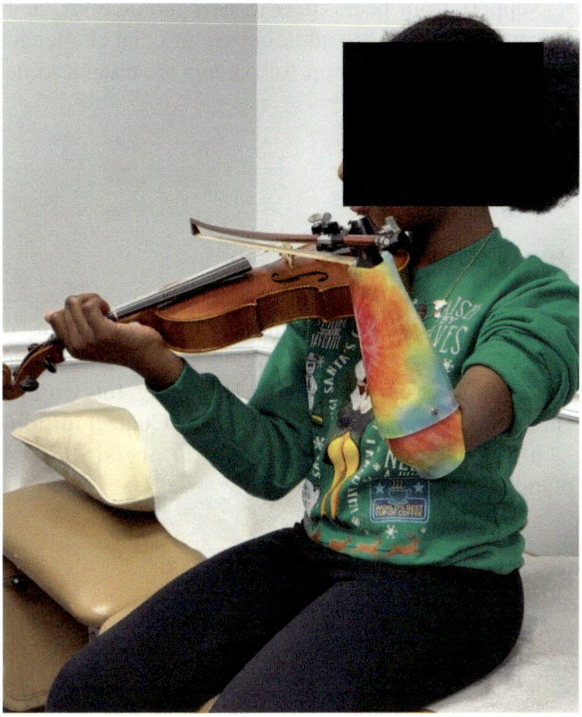

Fig. 16.3 A photograph showing the patient utilizing the finalized body-powered, activity-specific prosthesis is presented. (Courtesy of Joshua M. Abzug, MD)

Supportive interventions such as peer-to-peer interaction, social support, and the use of prostheses for cosmetic or functional purposes can improve outcomes. The parents should also receive ongoing support and education, recognizing the essential role of the parents in helping their child thrive.

Author Pearls

- Prostheses are not always necessary or accepted by children with upper extremity limb deficiencies.
- Activity-specific prostheses may be more beneficial than general-use devices for children with upper extremity limb deficiencies.
- A staged approach to prosthesis management is recommended for children with upper extremity limb deficiencies.
- Early fitting around the age of independent walking, occupational therapy training, and exposure to a variety of prosthetic devices can improve outcomes.
- 3D-printed transitional prostheses offer a novel, cost-effective option to reduce the financial burden.
- Children with lower limb deficiencies may benefit more from amputation and prosthetic rehabilitation than from limb lengthening and reconstruction; however, this decision should be individualized.

- Support from peers, peer-to-peer interactions, and prosthesis use are effective coping strategies to address psychosocial challenges.
- Education and support for parents are crucial to help both parents and children cope effectively.

Editors Comments

WLH

If you would like to learn more or get involved in supporting children with limb deficiencies, consider volunteering as a camp counselor at *Camp Open Arms*. Now in its 12th year and directed by Dr. Abzug, this camp provides an enriching experience for children and volunteers alike. Contact information can be found below:

https://secure.ummsfoundation.org/site/SPageServer?pagename=CampOpenArms

RMS

One practical innovation in the care of children with limb deficiencies is the use of simple, locally available materials, such as thermoplastic and PVC pipe, to fabricate temporary below-knee prostheses. This approach proved especially valuable following the 2010 earthquake in Haiti, where conventional prosthetic services were disrupted. These low-cost devices can be assembled quickly, providing immediate mobility and restoring a sense of dignity to children in need. Importantly, the utility of such interim prostheses extends beyond Haiti and can be adapted for use in other disaster-stricken regions where access to traditional prosthetic care is limited. This underscores that value in pediatric orthopedics often lies in resourcefulness. Effective solutions do not always require advanced technology but rather practical innovations tailored to the context.

References

1. Ephraim PL, Dillingham TR, Sector M, Pezzin LE, Mackenzie EJ. Epidemiology of limb loss and congenital limb deficiency: a review of the literature. Arch Phys Med Rehabil. 2003;84(5):747–61.
2. Davids JR, Wagner LV, Meyer LC, Blackhurst DW. Prosthetic management of children with unilateral congenital below-elbow deficiency. J Bone Joint Surg Am. 2006;88(6):1294–300.
3. Huizing K, Reinders-Messelink H, Maathuis C, Hadders-Algra M, van der Sluis CK. Age at first prosthetic fitting and later functional outcome in children and young adults with unilateral congenital below-elbow deficiency: a cross-sectional study. Prosthetics Orthot Int. 2010;34(2):166–74.
4. James MA, Bagley AM, Brasington K, Lutz C, McConnell S, Molitor F. Impact of prostheses on function and quality of life for children with unilateral congenital below-the-elbow deficiency. J Bone Joint Surg Am. 2006;88(11):2356–65.

5. Resnik L, Meucci MR, Lieberman-Klinger S, Fantini C, Kelty DL, Disla R, et al. Advanced upper limb prosthetic devices: implications for upper limb prosthetic rehabilitation. Arch Phys Med Rehabil. 2012;93(4):710–7.
6. Bhat AK, Vamsikrishna M, Acharya AM. Functional assessment of 3D printed prosthesis in children with congenital hand differences-a prospective observational study. J Hand Surg Asian-Pac Vol. 2021;26(4):535–44.
7. Hamdy RC, Makhdom AM, Saran N, Birch J. Congenital fibular deficiency. J Am Acad Orthop Surg. 2014;22(4):246–55.
8. Maffulli N, Fixsen JA. Management of forme fruste fibular hemimelia. J Pediatr Orthop Part B. 1996;5(1):17–9.
9. Birch JG, Walsh SJ, Small JM, Morton A, Koch KD, Smith C, et al. Syme amputation for the treatment of fibular deficiency. An evaluation of long-term physical and psychological functional status. J Bone Joint Surg Am. 1999;81(11):1511–8.
10. Changulani M, Ali F, Mulgrew E, Day JB, Zenios M. Outcome of limb lengthening in fibular hemimelia and a functional foot. J Child Orthop. 2010;4(6):519–24.
11. Naudie D, Hamdy RC, Fassier F, Morin B, Duhaime M. Management of fibular hemimelia: amputation or limb lengthening. J Bone Joint Surg Br. 1997;79(1):58–65.
12. Choi IH, Kumar SJ, Bowen JR. Amputation or limb-lengthening for partial or total absence of the fibula. J Bone Joint Surg Am. 1990;72(9):1391–9.
13. McCarthy JJ, Glancy GL, Chnag FM, Eilert RE. Fibular hemimelia: comparison of outcome measurments after amputation and lengthening. J Bone Joint Surg Am. 2000;82(12):1732–5.
14. Walker KO, Moreno G, Grumbach K. The association among specialty, race, ethnicity, and practice location among California physicians in diverse specialties. J Natl Med Assoc. 2012;104(0):46–52.
15. Birch JG, Paley D, Herzenberg JE, Morton A, Ward S, Riddle R, et al. Amputation versus staged reconstruction for severe fibular hemimelia: assessment of psychosocial and quality-of-life status and physical functioning in childhood. JB JS Open Access. 2019;4(2):e0053.
16. Cadman D, Boyle M, Szatmari P, Offord DR. Chronic illness, disability, and mental and social well-being: findings of the Ontario Child Health Study. Pediatrics. 1987;79(5):805–13.
17. Wallander JL, Varni JW, Babani L, Banis HT, Wilcox KT. Children with chronic physical disorders: maternal reports of their psychological adjustment. J Pediatr Psychol. 1988;13(2):197–212.
18. de Jong IGM, Reinders-Messelink HA, Janssen WGM, Poelma MJ, van Wijk I, van der Sluis CK. Mixed feelings of children and adolescents with unilateral congenital below elbow deficiency: an online focus group study. PLoS One. 2012;7(6):e37099.

Cerebral Palsy: Quality of Life Value 17

Kimberly Spahn and Mark Katsma

Introduction

Cerebral palsy (CP) is the most common physical disability in children globally and represents a lifelong condition with significant personal, societal, and economic impact. In the United States, the prevalence of CP is approximately 3.2 per 1000 children, with higher rates observed among the poor [1]. CP is a nonprogressive neurologic disorder of the developing brain that results in persistent impairments in posture, movement, and motor control [2]. While CP most often originates during fetal development, CP can also arise from hypoxic or hemorrhagic brain injury in the perinatal or early postnatal period. Functional abilities in children with CP vary widely and are classified using the Gross Motor Function Classification System (GMFCS). The level of functional involvement is associated with healthcare utilization, the need for interventions, and long-term costs [2].

Annual expenditures associated with cerebral palsy (CP) care are substantial, encompassing direct medical costs such as surgeries, rehabilitation, assistive devices, and technologies and indirect costs borne by families and society. This economic burden is magnified at the Medicaid, state, and national levels, with global registry data reflecting similar trends [3, 4]. Value-based care that prioritizes improved outcomes while minimizing inefficiencies and avoidable expenditures is key.

K. Spahn (✉) · M. Katsma
Balboa Naval Medical Center San Diego, San Diego, CA, USA
e-mail: kimberly.m.spahn.mil@health.mil; mark.s.katsma.mil@health.mil

W. L. Hennrikus, R. M. Schwend (eds.), *Value in Pediatric Orthopaedics*,
https://doi.org/10.1007/978-3-032-19570-8_17

Value-Based Themes

Economic Impact of Cerebral Palsy

CP care imposes a considerable financial burden. Between 2013 and 2015, the average annual Medicaid expenditure per child with CP was $22,383; compared to $1,358 for a child without CP[3]. Costs rise linearly with increasing Gross Motor Function Classification System (GMFCS) level of need (Fig. 17.1); children with CP who were nonambulatory incurred average annual costs of $43,687, compared to $10,368 for those who remained ambulatory [3]. Interventions that delay or prevent children with CP from becoming nonambulatory, including bracing, spasticity management, and hip surveillance, have the potential to save costs and improve quality of life.

Early Diagnosis and Intervention with Multidisciplinary Support

Early recognition of cerebral palsy (CP) is important, as most children's functional trajectories are established by the age of 5. Management strategies range from conservative therapies to surgery and involve multidisciplinary teams providing lifelong care. This wide scope of needs highlights the challenge: children with CP benefit from sustained, coordinated, and resource-intensive support, which adds financial, emotional, and logistical burdens on families and hospital systems. Global efforts to improve access to prenatal and neonatal care are essential.

Early intervention includes services and resources that support children with developmental concerns and their families during the critical period from birth to 3 years of age. Timely diagnosis is essential for accessing these services. Standardized evaluation and assessment begin before 5 months of age, with

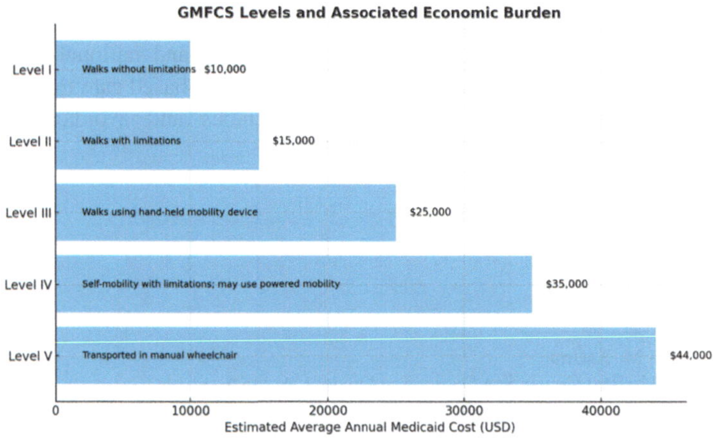

Fig. 17.1 Estimated annual Medicaid cost per child with CP according to GMFCS level [3]

ongoing surveillance and reassessment continuing through 24 months [5]. Identifying "at-risk" newborns and ensuring appropriate follow-up during the perinatal period is imperative, as 25–50% of children with CP may not exhibit clinical signs in the first few months of life [6]. Newborns considered at risk include those born preterm, those with neonatal encephalopathy, those requiring the Neonatal Intensive Care Unit (NICU) care, or those with birth defects. For infants under 5 months of corrected age, early diagnosis is best achieved using a combination of neonatal magnetic resonance imaging (MRI), the Prechtl Qualitative Assessment of General Movements (GMs), and the Hammersmith Infant Neurological Examination (HINE). After 5 months, recommended tools include MRI, HINE, and the Developmental Assessment of Young Children (DAYC). Early diagnosis enables prompt intervention, continued developmental surveillance, and ensures timely referrals to multidisciplinary subspecialty care [6].

Hip Surveillance Programs

Hip subluxation and dislocation affect approximately one in three patients with CP [7]. Hip dislocations result from muscle imbalance during growth and development, which generates abnormal forces across the hip joint. These muscle forces, combined with structural abnormalities including increased femoral anteversion, acetabular dysplasia, and valgus neck-shaft angles, cause the femoral head to migrate laterally, subluxate, and eventually dislocate. If left unaddressed, hip dislocation can lead to pain, impaired function, difficulties with sitting and positioning, and reduced quality of life [8]. The risk of hip displacement is higher in children with greater Gross Motor Function Classification System (GMFCS) levels and in those with hemiplegia exhibiting a Winters-Gage-Hicks gait pattern type IV [8]. In ambulatory children with CP, concentrically reduced hip joints provide stability during the stance phase of walking and help preserve hip cartilage [4]. In nonambulatory children, a reduced hip is helpful for standing, transfers, and caregiver access for perineal care. Maintaining hip reduction supports these functions and contributes to better quality of life into adulthood [9].

National hip surveillance programs in Australia, Scandinavia, and British Columbia have shown promising results in preventing hip dislocation in children with CP and reducing the need for salvage procedures [7, 8, 10]. The United States currently lacks a national screening program. However, both the American Academy for Cerebral Palsy and Developmental Medicine and the Pediatric Orthopaedic Society of North America have issued guidelines recommending hip surveillance from age 2 through skeletal maturity. The recommended screening frequency is based on the child's Gross Motor Function Classification System (GMFCS) level and hip migration percentage [11]. Referral to a pediatric orthopedic surgeon is advised when the migration percentage exceeds 30% (Fig. 17.2) [11]. Early identification and surgery are associated with improved functional outcomes and quality of life [8, 10] (Table 17.1).

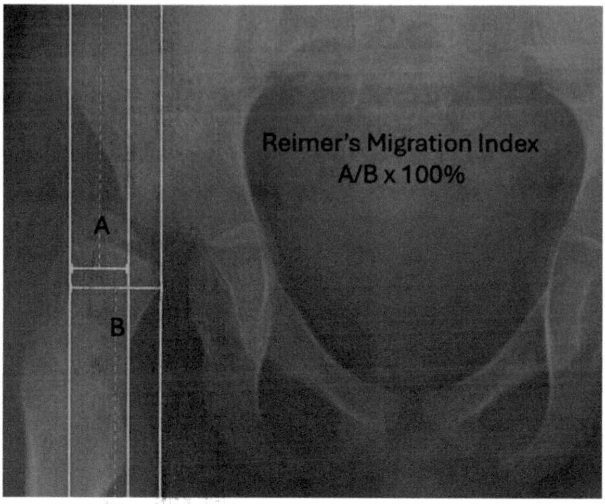

Fig. 17.2 Reimer's migration index measurement

Table 17.1 Summary of POSNA hip surveillance recommendations [11]

POSNA radiographic screening in cerebral palsy: Developing a POSNA wide consensus	
GMFCS I and II	Clinical exam and AP pelvis at ages 2, 6, and 10 years and skeletal maturity Discharge at skeletal maturity if stable MP under 30%
WGH Type IV	Clinical exam and AP pelvis at age 2, 6, and 10 years and then every 2 years until skeletal maturity Discharge at skeletal maturity if stable MP under 30%
GMFCS III	Clinical exam and AP pelvis every 12 months from age 2 to 10 years 10 years—skeletal maturity: Every 2 years if MP is stable over the previous 2 years After skeletal maturity: Frequency can decrease if MP is less than 30% and there is no change over 2 years after skeletal maturity
GMFCS IV and V	Age 2-skeletal maturity every 6–12 months until age 10 years 10 years—skeletal maturity: Decrease to yearly if MP is stable under 30% After skeletal maturity: Frequency can decrease if MP is less than 30% and there is no change over 2 years after skeletal maturity
Migration percentage guidelines	<30% continue to monitor >30% refer to pediatric orthopaedic surgeon

Screening for hip displacement involves a history, physical examination, and properly positioned anteroposterior (AP) pelvic radiographs. Clinical signs such as decreased hip abduction or pain with manipulation may indicate subluxation or dislocation. The AP radiograph is used to calculate the migration percentage (MP), which measures the proportion of the femoral head that is uncovered by the acetabulum. An MP greater than 30% is associated with an increased risk of dislocation, warranting referral for surgery [7, 8, 10]. Early detection and surgery can often prevent a hip dislocation, reducing the need for salvage procedures [11].

Optimizing Hip Interventions

Value in hip reconstructive surgery for CP patients lies in minimizing the number of surgeries and reducing costs associated with revision surgery and/or complications. Currently, reoperation rates range from 30% to 40% [12–14], with historical rates reported as high as 70% [15]. The most common reason for reoperation is hip resubluxation or dislocation [10, 16, 17]. Strategies to reduce this risk include optimizing the timing of reconstruction, implementing preventive measures to delay dislocation, adding a pelvic osteotomy, and performing bilateral hip procedures when appropriate. Hip surveillance programs have proven effective in identifying at-risk hips, reducing the number of surgeries performed, and avoiding salvage procedures, thereby increasing value [8, 10, 18]. Delaying hip preservation surgery until after 6–8 years of age results in a lower recurrence rate [12, 19]. In addition, performing a pelvic osteotomy concurrently with a varus derotation osteotomy (VDRO) lowers the rate of hip redislocation [20]. Indications for pelvic osteotomy include a migration percentage greater than 50%, an acetabular index over 30°, presence of the Gothic arch sign, or instability demonstrated on arthrogram [11, 21].

Proximal femoral guided growth is a new strategy to potentially delay primary hip reconstruction to a later age, optimizing both outcomes and value [22]. Additionally, secondary guided growth at the time of implant removal can be performed to maintain correction of the head–shaft angle and prevent redislocation [10].

Spine Surveillance Programs

Neuromuscular scoliosis is common in children with CP and shows a linear correlation with the GMFCS level. Scoliosis results from a combination of factors, including muscle imbalance, hypertonicity, and muscle weakness. Children classified as GMFCS levels I and II have a very low risk of developing neuromuscular scoliosis, whereas those at levels IV and V face a risk exceeding 50% [23, 24]. This form of scoliosis typically develops after the age of 8 and is often progressive, rigid, C-shaped, and associated with pelvic obliquity (Fig. 17.3). In children with CP, scoliosis can lead to a range of complications, including pain, decubitus ulcers, difficulty sitting, increased caregiver burden, and cardiopulmonary compromise [24]. Curve progression after skeletal maturity can still occur with larger curves at higher risk [25].

In idiopathic scoliosis, bracing is often used to slow curve progression and prevent the need for surgery. However, in children with CP, bracing is not typically indicated for this purpose. Instead, braces may be used to provide spinal support and help maintain sitting ability. These braces are expensive and are often poorly tolerated by patients. Curve flexibility should be assessed, and the choice of materials selected for use in brace fabrication is important to ensure effectiveness and comfort. In growing children, braces may need to be replaced annually to accommodate growth and to minimize skin complications from the brace; both add cost [26].

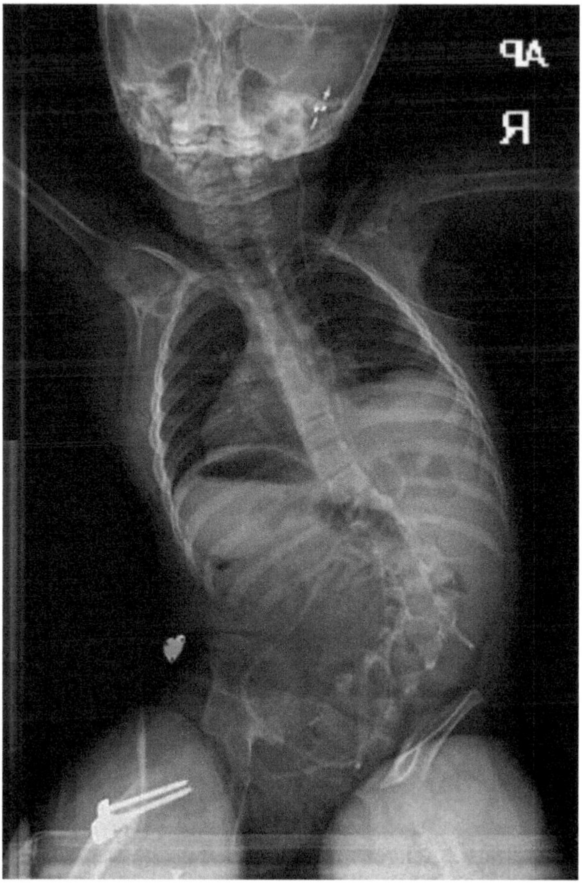

Fig. 17.3 8-year-old GMFCS IV female with neuromuscular scoliosis, pelvic obliquity, and difficulty sitting

Additional nonoperative interventions include spinal support with or without straps and custom wheelchair seating. These two interventions do not halt curve progression, but they can improve sitting tolerance.

Posterior spinal fusion and instrumentation is generally indicated when spinal curves reach 50°. Special considerations are necessary in this high-risk population. For example, a multidisciplinary team approach is helpful prior to surgery to optimize preoperative planning, obtain medical clearance, and improve safety and outcomes.

There is currently no national screening program for scoliosis in children with CP. However, curve progression in CP patients can be significant, and corrective surgeries are often complex and carry a higher risk of complications [27]. For CP patients classified as GMFCS levels IV and V, annual AP and lateral spine radiographs, beginning at age 8, or earlier if clinical signs of scoliosis are present, are recommended [24]. These X-rays help assess the magnitude of the primary curve and the degree of pelvic obliquity. Referral for surgical evaluation is indicated once the curve reaches 50°. Unlike idiopathic scoliosis, neuromuscular scoliosis may continue to progress after skeletal maturity, necessitating ongoing radiographic surveillance into adulthood [24].

The efficacy, benefits, and ethical considerations of spinal fusion in children with CP are controversial [25]. Preoperative evaluation is complex and requires the involvement of a multidisciplinary team, which has been shown to improve outcomes and reduce complications [28]. Comorbidities such as gastrostomy tubes, tracheostomies, and seizure disorders can impact surgical outcomes and postoperative quality of life [29]. Surgical decision-making represents an opportunity for establishing clear family-centered goals and engaging in shared decision-making. Additionally, factors such as prolonged hospitalization, ICU care, rehabilitation, and modifications to existing equipment, such as wheelchairs, contribute to the substantial costs associated with spinal fusion surgery in patients with CP.

Optimizing Spine Interventions

In patients with GMFCS Level V, scoliosis exceeding 40° occurs in over 75% of patients by the time they reach 20 years of age [23]. The complication rate for treating neuromuscular scoliosis in CP is high, approaching 40% [30]. Thirty-day readmission rates exceed 15%, and hospital costs are expensive, with stays lasting over 8 days and resulting in charges exceeding $110,000 [31]. Readmissions further drive costs up, increasing them by more than $70,000 [32]. Pulmonary complications are associated with increased risk, longer hospital stays, higher readmission rates, and elevated costs. Preoperative optimization through a multidisciplinary approach has been shown to reduce perioperative complications and risks. Key strategies include shared decision-making with the family, optimizing nutritional status, preoperative pulmonary evaluation and optimization, broad-spectrum infection prophylaxis, and the use of antifibrinolytics to minimize blood loss [33]. Standardized perioperative pathways are helpful in reducing length of stay and improving outcomes. Accelerated discharge protocols, with a target of 4 days, decrease hospital stay lengths, complication rates, pulmonary complications, and costs by nearly 20% [34, 35]. A two-surgeon team reduces operative time, estimated blood loss (EBL), length of stay, and perioperative complications [36, 37]. Infection prevention and early identification are key, as infection rates can be as high as 15% in CP spinal fusion cases [38]. When infections are promptly treated with systematic irrigation, debridement, and antibiotics, recurrence is rare, and outcomes remain favorable, with only mild changes in CPCHILD scores [39].

A proactive approach, involving early discussions with families when the major spinal curve reaches 50°, and intervening surgically before it progresses beyond 70°, can help reduce perioperative complications [24, 40]. Spinal deformities typically present by ages 8–10 years [24]. For early-onset cases, growth-friendly spine constructs are associated with significant complications and should be avoided in the CP population [41, 42]. Definitive spinal fusion and instrumentation are durable, safe, and effective, even in patients under 10 years of age [43, 44].

Bracing Management

Preventing contractures and limb deformities to maintain function is a primary goal of pediatric care for children with CP. Contractures typically develop in the hands, wrists, elbows, hips, knees, ankles, and feet due to abnormal motor control, increased muscle tone, and imbalances between agonist and antagonist muscle groups. Various modalities are employed to prevent contractures, including physical and occupational therapy, static and dynamic bracing, botulinum toxin injections, phenol injections, and surgery. Braces and orthoses, when used alongside therapy, can be utilized to prevent deformity. They also help improve balance and gait in ambulatory children [45]. Bracing may delay the need for surgery until the child is older. The type of brace prescribed depends on the child's GMFCS level and the specific goals of treatment. For nonambulatory children, a solid ankle-foot orthosis (AFO) can prevent contractures, facilitate shoe wear, and support use of a stander (Fig. 17.4). In some ambulatory children with a crouch gait, a ground reaction AFO can improve gait mechanics and reduce energy expenditure (Fig. 17.4) [46]. Consistent brace wear after surgery can also help prevent recurrence and the need for revision surgery.

Bracing, when combined with therapy, can lead to improvements in balance, energy expenditure, function, and ambulation. However, braces are expensive for growing children [47, 48]. The cost to the family may vary depending on insurance coverage. An

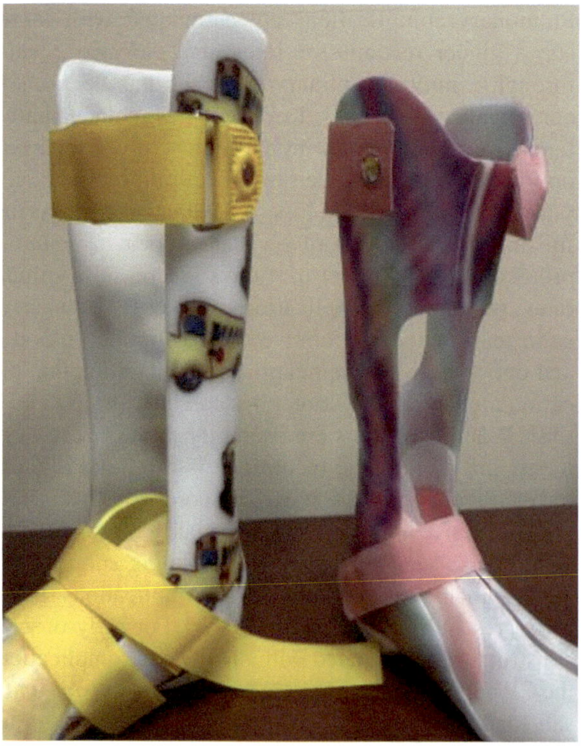

Fig. 17.4 Brace examples: Solid ankle-foot orthosis and ground reaction ankle-foot orthosis

internet search reveals a wide price range for braces, from $200 for off-the-shelf models to over $3000 for custom-made braces. As advancements are made in the field of orthotics and prosthetics, the cost of braces continues to rise. The selection of the most appropriate brace for a child is based on factors such as the pathology of the limb, the goals of treatment, and the effectiveness of the brace in addressing the child's unique needs.

Tone Management

Tone management is essential in preventing joint contractures. Baclofen plays a key role in reducing spasticity and muscle tone in children with CP. Studies have shown improvements in gait, reduced pain, and increased caregiver satisfaction with baclofen use [49]. Intrathecal baclofen (ITB) pumps provide an alternative to oral baclofen, helping mitigate side effects while offering effective spasticity control [50]. Although the ITB procedure carries risks, such as infection, wound complications, and the potential need for additional surgeries, it has been shown to be beneficial for patients with refractory spasticity or those who no longer respond to oral medication. The simultaneous implantation of an intrathecal baclofen pump during spinal fusion surgery carries minimal additional risk and can spare the child from needing a second operation [51].

Botulinum neurotoxin type A (BoNT-A) treats spasticity, prevents contractures, and improves range of motion in children with CP. Specific muscle groups are targeted with weight-based doses of BoNT-A, often in combination with physical therapy and bracing. BoNT-A improves muscle tone, motor function, and caregiver ease. However, these benefits are temporary and require repeated treatments. BoNT-A is expensive, with a market price of approximately $650 per 100-unit vial. The recommended dose for children is 12 units/kg, up to a maximum of 400 units. The effects typically last only about 3 months. A highly purified form of BoNT-A, incobotulinumtoxinA, has more recently been used in pediatric patients with cerebral palsy experiencing spasticity related pain, and has demonstrated effectiveness in reducing discomfort in these patients [52]. However, risks include short-lived benefits, skin reactions, unintended paralysis, gait difficulties, weakness, and, in rare cases, death [53]. Decisions regarding continued BoNT-A treatment should involve feedback from the patient, physical therapists, and parents. If the treatment no longer provides results, discontinuation is recommended. Alternatively, selective dorsal rhizotomy (SDR) offers a one-time surgical option for carefully selected children with predominantly spastic diplegia. When combined with rehabilitation, SDR can provide reductions in lower-limb spasticity and functional improvements, particularly in cases where repeated BoNT-A treatments are not possible.

Instrumented Gait Analysis

In ambulatory children with CP, computerized gait analysis (CGA) is used to assess gait abnormalities, guide surgical planning, and evaluate outcomes. Specifically, CGA helps address pathology at multiple levels before performing single-event multi-level surgery (SEMLS). SEMLS involves two or more soft-tissue or bony procedures at two or more levels during one operation. Gait analysis laboratories also provide insights into the efficacy of orthoses and inform surgical decision-making. CGA can influence surgical planning. For example, Kay et al. reported that preoperative gait analysis led to a change in the surgical plan for 89% of the 70 patients in their study [54]. The analysis provides objective data on multiple joints and muscle groups simultaneously, making it particularly helpful in planning SEMLS for children with CP. Use of preoperative CGA has led to more procedures being performed during the same surgery, resulting in a reduced rate of additional surgeries later on. While this may not translate into immediate cost savings due to the higher complexity of the index surgery, it benefits patients and families by minimizing the number of subsequent operations and anesthetics [55]. Additionally, postoperative CGA can measure surgical outcomes. Mobile phone-based gait analysis, a validated alternative to formal CGA, can also be utilized at much less cost [56].

Rehabilitation: Minimize Complications to Maximize Value

In some cases, postoperative immobilization using an abduction pillow, instead of a spica cast, offers easier management for the parents and helps avoid the complications associated with spica casts [57, 58]. All hip metal does not need to be removed [59, 60]. In fact, one study found that 80% of patients did not require implant removal when a reactive approach was used [60].

Maximal postoperative improvements can take up to 2 years [61]. Postoperative rehabilitation can safely be conducted in an outpatient setting [62]. Prehabilitation, which focuses on strengthening before surgery, enhances outcomes and accelerates the return to baseline function [62]. The therapy can be adjusted based on the scope of the surgery; for example, multiple osteotomies often benefit from more therapy sessions [61, 63].

Adult CP Care Paves the Way for the Future

Adults with CP represent an underserved population and a key area for future healthcare improvement. There is only a limited number of centers in the United States currently providing specialized services for adult CP patients. Transitional care from pediatric to adult services remains fragmented [64]. Adults with CP experience higher rates of cancer, chronic diseases, cardiovascular conditions, and epilepsy compared to the general population [65]. Identifying adult care centers or establishing coordinated care pathways within existing institutions for adults with CP is essential for monitoring preventable diseases and preserving health [66].

Case Example

A 6-year-old boy, born at 27 weeks gestation, with GMFCS Level V spastic quadriplegic CP secondary to neonatal intraventricular hemorrhage, presented after more than 3 years without orthopedic follow-up. His medical history is notable for short gut syndrome, requiring G-tube feeding as the primary nutritional source until approximately 5 years of age, as well as multiple courses of total parenteral nutrition (TPN). Initial orthopedic surveillance was performed during infancy (Fig. 17.5); however, the patient was lost to follow-up prior to age 3. At presentation, his weight was below the 10th percentile, and he continued to receive supplemental G-tube feeds. On examination, the Modified Ashworth Scale revealed 3+/4 spasticity in both upper and lower extremities, with hip adduction contractures. X-rays demonstrated bilateral hip subluxations with a migration index of 87% on the right and 52% on the left, as well as bilateral disruption of Shenton's line (Fig. 17.6). Frog-leg lateral views showed concentric reduction of both hips. Surgery was indicated, consisting of bilateral adductor releases, varus derotational femoral osteotomies, and pelvic osteotomies utilizing the San Diego technique.

The patient was initially referred for Botox injections, new orthotic bracing, and comprehensive preoperative optimization, including evaluations by pulmonology, primary care, and pediatric gastroenterology. His nutritional status was optimized over a 6-month period prior to surgery. He subsequently underwent bilateral hip reconstruction with a two-surgeon team without complications (Fig. 17.7). Postoperatively, he was admitted for 3 days, with hips immobilized using an abduction foam pillow to facilitate ease of care. Recovery progressed well, supported by outpatient physical therapy. At the 1-year follow-up, femoral implants remained

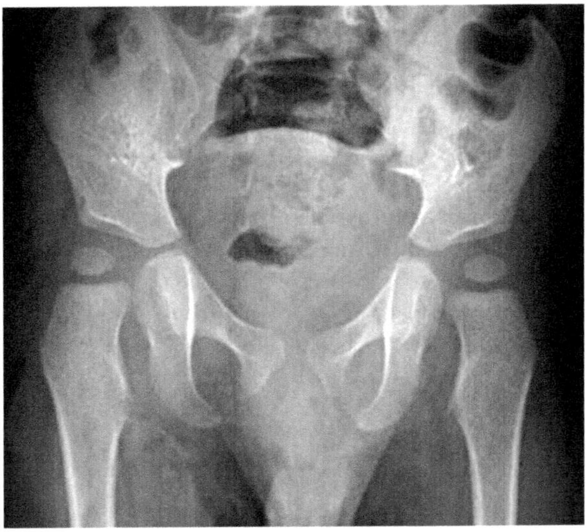

Fig. 17.5 AP pelvis radiograph at age 2 years at initial surveillance initiation

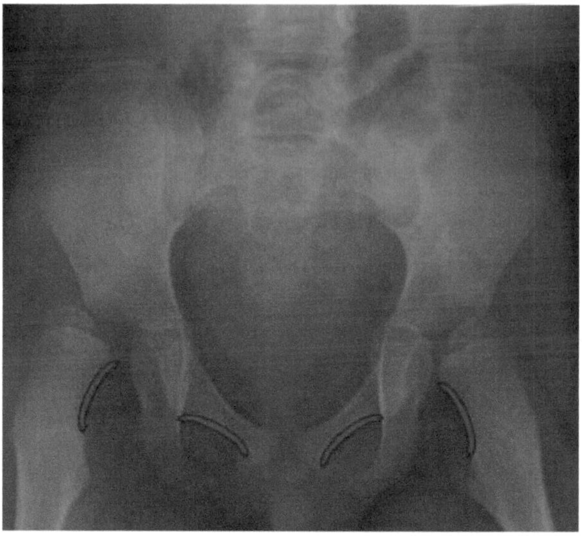

Fig. 17.6 AP pelvis radiograph at age 6 years after loss to surveillance with progression of bilateral hip subluxation. Note that Shenton line is broken bilaterally

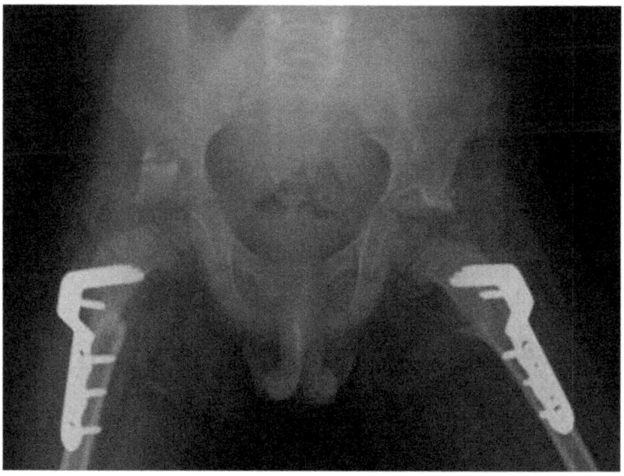

Fig. 17.7 AP pelvis radiograph 1-year postoperative from bilateral adductor tenotomy, VDRO, San Diego–type pelvic osteotomy

asymptomatic, appropriately positioned, and demonstrated stable concentric hip alignment. A reactive implant removal strategy was adopted, with ongoing monitoring every 6 months to assess for implant encroachment on the inferior femoral neck or the development of symptoms. Clinical spinal surveillance was recommended until age 8, after which annual radiographic screening will begin.

Summary

Value in the care of patients with cerebral palsy is enhanced by optimizing outcomes and minimizing the costs of chronic medical management and complications. Proactive surveillance, combined with prophylactic tone management and bracing, helps reduce the need for surgical intervention. Preventing complications, minimizing reoperations, and achieving long-term surgical success all contribute to lowering costs and maximizing value.

Author Pearls

- The GMFCS correlates with intervention needs, healthcare utilization, and associated costs.
- Value-based care emphasizes early diagnosis, surveillance, and prevention.
- Hip surveillance protocols should be integrated into clinical workflows.
- Identify children at risk for or showing early signs of cerebral palsy and establish timely referral pathways.
- Utilize proximal femoral guided growth proactively.
- Remove VDRO plates no earlier than 12 months postoperatively.
- Maintain a low threshold for adding pelvic osteotomy to reduce the risk of hip reconstruction failure.
- Refer GMFCS Level IV and V patients for preoperative medical clearance to optimize surgical recovery.
- Adopt a proactive spinal fusion strategy by beginning discussions when curves approach 50° and aim to fuse before reaching 70°.
- Develop standardized perioperative pathways for spine and hip procedures.
- Identify or establish a network of adult care doctors to support the transition of individuals with CP into adulthood.

Useful Websites

AACPDM care pathway—hip surveillance. Overview and downloadable PDF: https://www.aacpdm.org/publications/care-pathways/hip-surveillance-in-cerebral-palsy

Radiographic Hip Screening in Cerebral Palsy: Developing POSNA Wide Consensus. Hip Radiographic Screening for CP. Radiographic Hip Screening In Cerebral Palsy: Developing POSNA Wide Consensus

SEMLS explainer (family-facing) from Gillette Children's Hospital. Also, their spasticity/SEMLS pages: Single-Event Multilevel Surgery (SEMLS): What is SEMLS? | Gillette Children's

AHRQ Agency for Healthcare Research Quality. The SHARE Approach. AHRQ's SHARE Approach is a clinician-led shared decision-making model with five essential elements for meaningful dialogue with patients exploring benefits, harms, and risks of options and what matters most to them: The SHARE Approach | Agency for Healthcare Research and Quality

Goal Attainment Scaling (GAS) as a family-centered way to capture "the one goal," with a brief link to practical materials: goal-attainment-scaling.pdf

International Classification of Functioning, Disability, and Health (ICF): World Health Organization ICF

Editors Comments

WLH

As mentioned, but not fully explored in this excellent chapter on improving value when treating children with CP, salvage surgery may sometimes be necessary. Salvage surgery refers to procedures such as proximal femoral resection, subtrochanteric osteotomy, or hip arthrodesis, typically performed when preventive measures and other reconstructive surgeries have failed. The pediatric orthopaedic surgeon caring for children with CP must also be knowledgeable and facile at salvage surgery. As the authors note, the rate of hip redislocation following standard reconstructive surgery is high in children with CP. In these cases, salvage surgery offers a strategy to address chronic, painful hip dislocations or severe hip abnormalities when other surgical options are no longer viable.

RMS

Shared decision-making is potentially most successful when families and care teams can identify a single goal that meaningfully improves the child's daily life. Before any surgery, ask parents, caregivers, and the child to define the outcome that matters most to them—whether it's comfort in a wheelchair, easier transfers, improved sleep, or fewer pressure sores. For example, one child with painful scoliosis and hip subluxation had a simple goal: to travel on family road trips without discomfort. Surgery was aligned to this goal, and at the two-year follow-up, the child was traveling comfortably. Goal Attainment Scaling (GAS) translates the family's top priority into a structured 5-point scale (−2 to +2), enabling individualized goals to be measured alongside standardized outcomes such as the Gross Motor Function Measure (GMFM) and the Caregiver Priorities and Child Health Index of Life with Disabilities (CPCHILD). Integrating GAS into the WHO International Classification of Functioning, Disability and Health (ICF) framework keeps the focus on what matters most.

References

1. McGuire DO, Tian LH, Yeargin-Allsopp M, Dowling NF, Christensen DL. Prevalence of cerebral palsy, intellectual disability, hearing loss, and blindness, National Health Interview Survey, 2009–2016. Disabil Health J. 2019;12(3):443–51.
2. Bax M, Goldstein M, Rosenbaum P, Leviton A, Paneth N, Dan B, et al. Proposed definition and classification of cerebral palsy, April 2005. Dev Med Child Neurol. 2005;47(8):571–6.

3. Pulgar S, Bains S, Gooch J, Chambers H, Noritz GH, Wright E, et al. Prevalence, patterns, and cost of care for children with cerebral palsy enrolled in medicaid managed care. J Manag Care Spec Pharm. 2019;25(7):817–22.
4. Wynter M, Gibson N, Willoughby KL, Love S, Kentish M, Thomason P, et al. Australian hip surveillance guidelines for children with cerebral palsy: 5-year review. Dev Med Child Neurol. 2015;57(9):808–20.
5. Byrne R, Noritz G, Maitre NL. Implementation of early diagnosis and intervention guidelines for cerebral palsy in a high-risk infant follow-up clinic. Pediatr Neurol. 2017;76:66–71.
6. Novak I, Morgan C, Adde L, Blackman J, Boyd RN, Brunstrom-Hernandez J, et al. Early, accurate diagnosis and early intervention in cerebral palsy: advances in diagnosis and treatment. JAMA Pediatr. 2017;171(9):897–907.
7. Miller SD, Shore BJ, Mulpuri K. Hip surveillance is important to children with cerebral palsy: stop waiting, start now. JAAOS Glob Res Rev. 2019;3(4):e021.
8. Shrader MW, Wimberly L, Thompson R. Hip surveillance in children with cerebral palsy. J Am Acad Orthop Surg. 2019;27(20):760–8.
9. Viehweger E. Importance of hip problems in daily activities for cerebral palsy patients. J Child Orthop. 2013;7(5):401–6.
10. Howard JJ, Willoughby K, Thomason P, Shore BJ, Graham K, Rutz E. Hip surveillance and management of hip displacement in children with cerebral palsy: clinical and ethical dilemmas. J Clin Med. 2023;12(4):1651.
11. Shore BJ, Mulpuri K, Shrader MW. Radiographic hip screening in cerebral palsy: developing POSNA-wide consensus. J Pediatr Orthop Soc N Am. 2021;3(1):231.
12. Wimmer SP, Zusman NL, Wren TAL, Goldstein RY, Kay RM. An analysis of reoperations following proximal femoral varus derotational osteotomy in children with cerebral palsy. JBJS Open Access. 2025;10(1):e23.00159.
13. Kiapekos N, Broström E, Hägglund G, Åstrand P. Primary surgery to prevent hip dislocation in children with cerebral palsy in Sweden: a minimum 5-year follow-up by the national surveillance program (CPUP). Acta Orthop. 2019;90(5):495–500.
14. Shore BJ, Zurakowski D, Dufreny C, Powell D, Matheney TH, Snyder BD. Proximal femoral varus derotation osteotomy in children with cerebral palsy: the effect of age, gross motor function classification system level, and surgeon volume on surgical success. J Bone Joint Surg Am. 2015;97(24):2024–31.
15. Schmale GA, Eilert RE, Chang F, Seidel K. High reoperation rates after early treatment of the subluxating hip in children with spastic cerebral palsy. J Pediatr Orthop. 2006;26(5):617–23.
16. Valencia FG. Management of hip deformities in cerebral palsy. Orthop Clin North Am. 2010;41(4):549–59.
17. Davids JR. Management of neuromuscular hip dysplasia in children with cerebral palsy: lessons and challenges. J Pediatr Orthop. 2018;38:S21.
18. Dobson F, Boyd RN, Parrott J, Nattrass GR, Graham HK. Hip surveillance in children with cerebral palsy. Impact on the surgical management of spastic hip disease. J Bone Joint Surg Br. 2002;84(5):720–6.
19. Ayub A, Graff C, Horvat LM, Maizen C. Hip reconstruction in cerebral palsy: lessons from a single center and 137 hips. J Child Orthop. 2023;17(5):469–80.
20. Delbrück H, Gehlen Y, Hildebrand F, Brunner R. Redisplacement rate after bony hip reconstructive surgery in nonambulatory patients with cerebral palsy: a systematic review and meta-analysis. EFORT Open Rev. 2024;9(8):773–84.
21. Shore BJ, Graham HK. Management of moderate to severe hip displacement in nonambulatory children with cerebral palsy. JBJS Rev. 2017;5(12):e4.
22. Davids JR. Proximal femur guided growth for the management of hip dysplasia in children with cerebral palsy. J Pediatr Orthop Soc N Am. 2021;3(2):245.
23. Hägglund G, Pettersson K, Czuba T, Persson-Bunke M, Rodby-Bousquet E. Incidence of scoliosis in cerebral palsy: a population-based study of 962 young individuals. Acta Orthop. 2018;89(4):443–7.
24. Howard JJ, Sees JP, Shrader MW. Management of spinal deformity in cerebral palsy. J Pediatr Orthop Soc N Am. 2019;1(1):8.

25. Whitaker AT, Sharkey M, Diab M. Spinal fusion for scoliosis in patients with globally involved cerebral palsy: an ethical assessment. J Bone Joint Surg. 2015;97(9):782.
26. Kotwicki T, Jozwiak M. Conservative management of neuromuscular scoliosis: personal experience and review of literature. Disabil Rehabil. 2008;30(10):792–8.
27. Sponseller PD, Shah SA, Abel MF, Newton PO, Letko L, Marks M. Infection rate after spine surgery in cerebral palsy is high and impairs results: multicenter analysis of risk factors and treatment. Clin Orthop Relat Res. 2010;468(3):711.
28. Samdani AF, Belin EJ, Bennett JT, Miyanji F, Pahys JM, Shah SA, et al. Major perioperative complications after spine surgery in patients with cerebral palsy: assessment of risk factors. Eur Spine J. 2016;25(3):795–800.
29. Jain A, Sponseller PD, Shah SA, Samdani A, Cahill PJ, Yaszay B, et al. Subclassification of GMFCS level-5 cerebral palsy as a predictor of complications and health-related quality of life after spinal arthrodesis. J Bone Joint Surg. 2016;98(21):1821.
30. Rumalla K, Yarbrough CK, Pugely AJ, Koester L, Dorward IG. Spinal fusion for pediatric neuromuscular scoliosis: national trends, complications, and in-hospital outcomes. 2016 [cited 2025 Sept 5]. Available from: https://thejns.org/spine/view/journals/j-neurosurg-spine/25/4/article-p500.xml.
31. Lee NJ, Fields M, Boddapati V, Mathew J, Hong D, Sardar ZM, et al. Spinal deformity surgery in pediatric patients with cerebral palsy: a national-level analysis of inpatient and postdischarge outcomes. Glob Spine J. 2022;12(4):610–9.
32. Fields M, Lee NJ, McCormick K, Park PJ, Boddapati V, Cerpa M, et al. A national analysis on complications and readmissions for adult cerebral palsy patients undergoing primary spinal fusion surgery. Eur Spine J. 2022;31(3):718–25.
33. Belthur M, Bosch L, Wood W, Boan C, Miller F, Shrader MW. Perioperative management of patients with cerebral palsy undergoing scoliosis surgery: survey of surgeon practices. J Pediatr Rehabil Med. 2019;12(2):205–12.
34. Shaw KA, Heboyan V, Fletcher ND, Murphy JS. Comparative cost–utility analysis of postoperative discharge pathways following posterior spinal fusion for scoliosis in non-ambulatory cerebral palsy patients. Spine Deform. 2021;9(6):1659–67.
35. Bellaire LL, Bruce RW, Ward LA, Bowman CA, Fletcher ND. Use of an accelerated discharge pathway in patients with severe cerebral palsy undergoing posterior spinal fusion for neuromuscular scoliosis. Spine Deform. 2019;7(5):804–11.
36. Shrader MW, Wood W, Falk M, Segal LS, Boan C, White G. The effect of two attending surgeons on the outcomes of posterior spine fusion in children with cerebral palsy. Spine Deform. 2018;6(6):730–5.
37. McDonald TC, Gnam AL, Brooks JT, Sukkarieh H, Replogle WH, Wright PB. The value-added benefit of utilizing two attending surgeons for patients with scoliosis secondary to cerebral palsy. Spine Deform. 2021;9(4):1145–50.
38. Sebaaly A, El Rachkidi R, Yaacoub JJ, Saliba E, Ghanem I. Management of spinal infections in children with cerebral palsy. Orthop Traumatol Surg Res. 2016;102(6):801–5.
39. Jain A, Modhia UM, Njoku DB, Shah SA, Newton PO, Marks MC, et al. Recurrence of deep surgical site infection in cerebral palsy after spinal fusion is rare. Spine Deform. 2017;5(3):208–12.
40. Hollenbeck SM, Yaszay B, Sponseller PD, Bartley CE, Shah SA, Asghar J, et al. The pros and cons of operating early versus late in the progression of cerebral palsy scoliosis. Spine Deform. 2019;7(3):489–93.
41. McElroy MJ, Sponseller PD, Dattilo JR, Thompson GH, Akbarnia BA, Shah SA, et al. Growing rods for the treatment of scoliosis in children with cerebral palsy: a critical assessment. Spine. 2012;37(24):E1504.
42. Hariharan AR, Shah SA, Sponseller PD, Yaszay B, Glotzbecker MP, Thompson GH, et al. Definitive fusions are better than growing rod procedures for juvenile patients with cerebral palsy and scoliosis: a prospective comparative cohort study. Spine Deform. 2023;11(1):145–52.
43. Howard R, Sponseller PD, Shah SA, Miyanji F, Samdani AF, Newton PO, et al. Definitive fusion for scoliosis in late juvenile cerebral palsy patients is durable at 5 years postoperatively. Spine Deform. 2022;10(6):1423–8.

44. Sitoula P, Holmes LJ, Sees J, Rogers K, Dabney K, Miller F. The long-term outcome of early spine fusion for scoliosis in children with cerebral palsy. Clin Spine Surg. 2016;29(8):E406.
45. Stamp WG. Bracing in cerebral palsy. J Bone Joint Surg Am. 1962;44(7):1457.
46. Lintanf M, Bourseul JS, Houx L, Lempereur M, Brochard S, Pons C. Effect of ankle-foot orthoses on gait, balance and gross motor function in children with cerebral palsy: a systematic review and meta-analysis. Clin Rehabil. 2018;32(9):1175–88.
47. Miccinilli S, Santacaterina F, Della Rocca R, Sterzi S, Bressi F, Bravi M. Efficacy of lower limb orthoses in the rehabilitation of children affected by cerebral palsy: a systematic review. Child Basel Switz. 2024;11(2):212.
48. Betancourt JP, Eleeh P, Stark S, Jain NB. Impact of ankle-foot orthosis on gait efficiency in ambulatory children with cerebral palsy: a systematic review and meta-analysis. Am J Phys Med Rehabil. 2019;98(9):759.
49. Scannell B, Yaszay B. Scoliosis, spinal fusion, and intrathecal baclofen pump implantation. Phys Med Rehabil Clin. 2015;26(1):79–88.
50. McCormick ZL, Chu SK, Binler D, Neudorf D, Mathur SN, Lee J, et al. Intrathecal versus oral baclofen: a matched cohort study of spasticity, pain, sleep, fatigue, and quality of life. PM R. 2016;8(6):553–62.
51. Levy KH, Yaszay B, Abel MF, Shah SA, Samdani AF, Sponseller PD, et al. Baclofen pumps do not increase risk of complications following spinal fusion. Spine Deform. 2024;12(2):473–80.
52. Bonfert M, Heinen F, Kaňovský P, Schroeder AS, Chambers HG, Dabrowski E, et al. Spasticity-related pain in children/adolescents with cerebral palsy. Part 2: IncobotulinumtoxinA efficacy results from a pooled analysis. J Pediatr Rehabil Med. 2023;16(1):83–98.
53. Sapienza M, Kapoor R, Alberghina F, Maheshwari R, McCracken KL, Canavese F, et al. Adverse effects following botulinum toxin A injections in children with cerebral palsy. J Pediatr Orthop B. 2023;32(5):435.
54. Kay RM, Dennis S, Rethlefsen S, Reynolds RA, Skaggs DL, Tolo VT. The effect of preoperative gait analysis on orthopaedic decision making. Clin Orthop. 2000;(372):217–22.
55. Wren TAL, Kalisvaart MM, Ghatan CE, Rethlefsen SA, Hara R, Sheng M, et al. Effects of preoperative gait analysis on costs and amount of surgery. J Pediatr Orthop. 2009;29(6):558.
56. Kulkarni VA, Kephart DT, Olleac R, Davids JR. Enhancing observational gait analysis – techniques and tips for analyzing gait without a gait lab. J Pediatr Orthop Soc N Am. 2020;2(3):135.
57. Vasconcellos AL, Tagawa AS, Rhodes JT, Silveira LJ, Skinner AA, Frumberg DB. Postoperative immobilization after hip reconstruction in cerebral palsy: no difference between hip spica and abduction pillow. Front Surg. 2022;9:863287.
58. Stasikelis PJ, Lee DD, Sullivan CM. Complications of osteotomies in severe cerebral palsy. J Pediatr Orthop. 1999;19(2):207.
59. Montufar Wright PE, da Almeida Silva LC, Howard JJ, Raab S, Rogers KJ, Lindgren A, et al. Incidence of femur fracture post hardware removal in children with cerebral palsy who have undergone varus derotational osteotomy. J Pediatr Orthop. 2025;45(6):e575–80.
60. Truong WH, Novotny SA, Novacheck TF, Shin EJ, Howard A, Narayanan UG. Should proximal femoral implants be removed prophylactically or reactively in children with cerebral palsy? J Pediatr Orthop. 2019;39(8):e629–35.
61. Church C, Biermann I, Lennon N, Henley JD, Butler S, Niiler T, et al. Walking activity after multilevel orthopedic surgery in children with cerebral palsy. Dev Med Child Neurol. 2022;64(10):1289–96.
62. Shami AA. A comprehensive review of rehabilitation strategies post-orthopedic intervention in pediatric cerebral palsy. J Musculoskelet Surg Res. 2025;9(1):42–8.
63. Lennon N, Gerry G, Biermann I, Beaman J, Mamula N, Gilmore A, et al. Factors associated with short-term recovery following single-event multilevel surgery for children with cerebral palsy. Pediatr Phys Ther. 2023;35(1):93.
64. Mitchell DL, Shlobin NA, Winterhalter E, Lam SK, Raskin JS. Gaps in transitional care to adulthood for patients with cerebral palsy: a systematic review. Childs Nerv Syst. 2023;39(11):3083–101.

65. Murphy KP. The adult with cerebral palsy. Orthop Clin North Am. 2010;41(4):595–605.
66. Manikandan M, Kerr C, Lavelle G, Walsh M, Walsh A, Ryan JM. Health service use among adults with cerebral palsy: a mixed-methods systematic review. Dev Med Child Neurol. 2022;64(4):429–46.

Clubfoot Treatment: Dr. Ponseti Knew Value

18

Li Zhao, Xiaotang Sun, and Richard M. Schwend

Introduction

The estimated prevalence of clubfoot is 1.2 per 1000 births, with the highest rates observed in low- and middle-income countries [1]. Congenital clubfoot has ranked among the top ten birth defects in China [2]. If left untreated, clubfoot can result in lifelong disability, chronic pain, social disadvantages, and poverty for the affected child, while adding a burden on the family and society in general [3]. Therefore, improved access to effective treatment is a global health priority [1, 4, 5]. In the latter part of the twentieth century, extensive surgery for infants with clubfoot was the main treatment approach emphasized in medical textbooks [6].

Congenital clubfoot is classified as either primary (idiopathic) or secondary, associated with neuromuscular or syndromic conditions such as spina bifida, myelomeningocele, and arthrogryposis [7–11]. The goal of orthopedic treatment is to correct deformity and restore functional mobility. Achieving this outcome often requires collaboration with pediatricians, neurosurgeons, and rehabilitation physicians. Today, for infants with clubfoot, the Ponseti casting method is preferred rather than extensive surgery.

Three current treatment methods for clubfoot have been reported, including the French method [12], the Ponseti method [10, 11, 13], and a "hybrid method" [14]. The French method involves daily clinic visits and routine radiographic evaluations.

L. Zhao
Ying-Hua Medical Group of Children's Bone and Joint Healthcare, Shanghai, China

X. Sun
Department Orthopaedics, Dongfang Hospital Affiliated to Xiamen University, Fuzhou, China

R. M. Schwend (✉)
Children's Mercy Hospital, Kansas City, MO, USA
e-mail: rmschwend@cmh.edu

W. L. Hennrikus, R. M. Schwend (eds.), *Value in Pediatric Orthopaedics*,
https://doi.org/10.1007/978-3-032-19570-8_18

In contrast, the Ponseti method requires only weekly clinic visits and typically does not involve radiographs. In addition, early parental education improves compliance with casting and bracing, reduces relapses, and increases the success of treatment [11, 13, 15–17].

Value-Based Themes

Prenatal Counseling

With the use of prenatal ultrasound and fetal screening, clubfoot is often detected between the first trimester and the 28th week of pregnancy [9–11, 18]. Prenatal detection does not determine the specific treatment indicated [19]. Treatment decisions rely on the postnatal physical examination of the newborn by the orthopedic surgeon.

Prenatal identification of a clubfoot requires an assessment to identify any additional findings that may suggest a syndromic or neurogenic etiology, including, in some cases, genetic testing [11]. Fetuses with syndromic or neurogenic clubfoot have higher rates of associated genetic abnormalities. The prognosis for clubfoot associated with neuromuscular or syndromic conditions is influenced by the underlying diagnosis [9, 20].

Information gathered during the prenatal visit can aid in counseling the family. However, a prenatal diagnosis may also lead to anxiety and concern [21]. It is important to inform the family that clubfoot can only be definitively diagnosed after birth and that treatment is typically effective. Maternal attitudes toward prenatal diagnosis vary across different cultural backgrounds [22], and the obstetrician can play a key role in shaping the family's response and understanding [23]. Lastly, telemedicine can save time and reduce costs for prenatal consultations and follow-up visits [24, 25]. Telemedicine must adhere to established regulatory guidelines and legal requirements for patient safety and compliance [26, 27].

Diagnosis

The decision to utilize the Ponseti method treatment is based on an accurate diagnosis [9–11]. Clubfoot diagnosis is made by visual assessment and exam. Clubfoot consists of four primary components, commonly remembered by the mnemonic "CAVE": cavus, adductus, varus, and equinus (Fig. 18.1).

Occasionally, a postural foot deformity is mistaken for an idiopathic clubfoot. A postural or positional clubfoot is a self-resolving packaging condition that resolves with observation (Fig. 18.2) [28]. In such cases, follow-up exams may be needed over time to better understand the underlying foot pathology before starting treatment [7–11].

A medical history and a careful physical examination that assesses the baby's spine, upper extremities, hips, and feet are key. Radiographs are not required for diagnosing clubfoot or assessing the severity of the deformity. However,

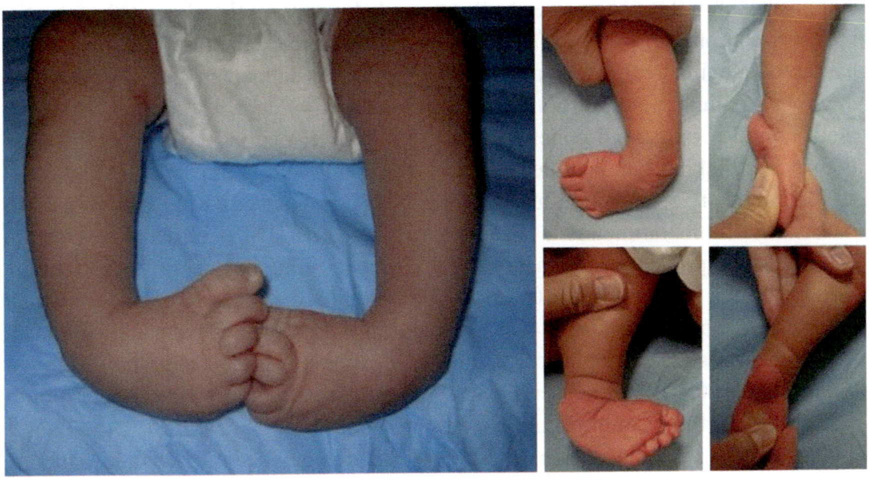

Fig. 18.1 The four components of clubfoot deformity are midfoot cavus, forefoot adductus, and hindfoot varus and equinus (CAVE)

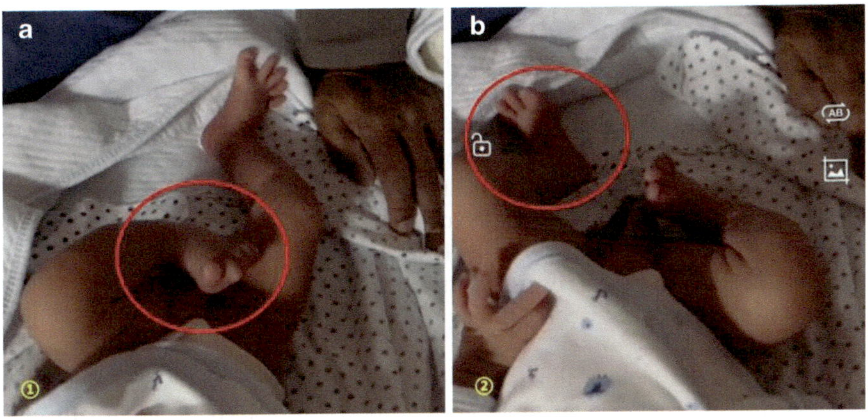

Fig. 18.2 The appearance of a foot from a still image from a video: part (**a**) and 10 s later (**b**). The images demonstrate a postural clubfoot that corrects spontaneously

radiographs and ultrasound imaging may occasionally be used in research settings [29–34]. Once a diagnosis of idiopathic clubfoot is made, parents should receive a discussion covering the prognosis, treatment options, long-term follow-up, orthotic management, and potential risks and benefits.

Treatment Timing

Early recognition and treatment of clubfoot are key to improving outcomes and reducing long-term disability [7, 10, 11, 13]. The Ponseti method, which emphasizes initiation soon after birth, depends heavily on the clinician's expertise in manipulation and casting [7]. Poorly performed manipulation and casting can lead to worsening of the deformity through ligament damage [7, 35]. Conservative treatment methods for clubfoot are now the standard of care. The French method is more complex and more expensive than the Ponseti method [12]. Therefore, the Ponseti method has become the preferred treatment method in most centers.

Misdiagnosis of clubfoot, although rare, can increase costs [11, 36, 37]. Early intervention is recommended, but has a very small risk of overtreating cases that could resolve spontaneously. In a few cases, early casting may result in slippage due to the smaller foot size [38]. Cultural practices, such as postpartum confinement practiced in China, may delay cast treatment initiation [39]. Occasionally, delayed treatment leads to gait delays [40] and early treated infants may show minimal motor delays [41, 42]. However, overall, initiating treatment for idiopathic clubfoot weeks after birth does not negatively impact outcomes [38, 43]. Lastly, the Ponseti method is also effective in older children [44] and in neglected cases in low-income nations [45].

Optimizing Resources

National and regional clubfoot programs aim to provide effective and sustainable treatment to provide high-quality care [1–3, 46, 47]. For instance, China needs an estimated 200–300 Ponseti clinics, each managing 30–50 cases annually, to provide care for 8000–10,000 new cases of clubfoot per year [47].

Clinic accessibility affects treatment outcomes, with commute time and travel distance being key factors [48]. The Ponseti method consists of two main stages: Stage I: correction, which lasts several weeks and is physician-led, and State II: maintenance, which extends over 5 years and is largely caregiver-led [9–11, 36, 37]. Stage I usually includes weekly clinic visits, although accelerated protocols have been developed [49].

Ponseti clinics include three functional areas: consultation/examination, cast removal/bathing, and manipulation/casting (Fig. 18.3). The core team usually consists of one orthopedic specialist and one to two trained assistants [50]. Families play an important role in treatment, soothing the infant, assisting with cast removal, and improving brace compliance [51]. The Pirani and Dimeglio clubfoot scoring systems can be applied before and after treatment [9–11, 43, 50] to objectively score outcomes [52–54].

How Many Casts

Families often ask about the number of casts required for clubfoot correction [52, 55]. The number of casts used depends on both intrinsic factors, such as soft tissue responsiveness, and extrinsic factors, including team expertise and family cooperation [7, 8, 50, 56]. The Ponseti manipulation method corrects all components of the

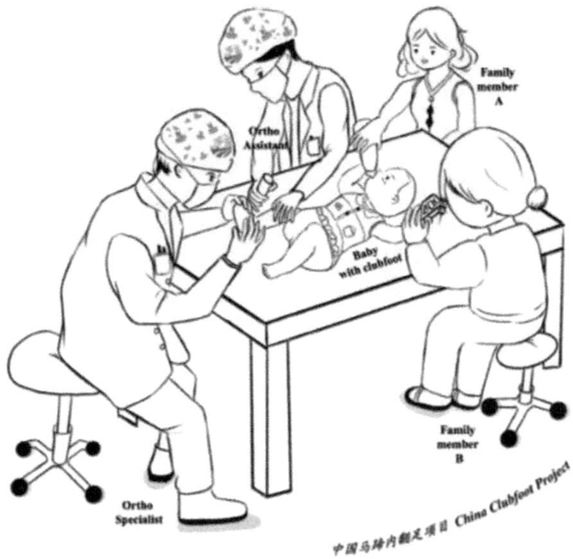

Fig. 18.3 Setting up of the treatment room

deformity simultaneously [7, 9] and avoids overstretching soft tissues [50]. The physician should provide the parents with a range for the number of casts to avoid the "anchoring effect," which can arise when clinicians rigidly adhere to a fixed number of casts [57].

Cutting the Achilles Tendon

Equinus deformity involves both calcaneal equinus and tibio-talar plantar flexion (Fig. 18.4a, b). These interrelated deformities are corrected simultaneously through dynamic midfoot–hindfoot coupling achieved by proper Ponseti manipulation [36, 58]. During manipulation to realign the navicular anteriorly with the talus, the anterior calcaneus is laterally displaced, restoring its normal relationship with the talus. This maneuver corrects both the heel varus and the calcaneal component of equinus (Fig. 18.4c–f) [7, 34].

Percutaneous Achilles tenotomy (PAT) is a small surgical procedure within the Ponseti method used to correct hindfoot deformity and achieve adequate ankle dorsiflexion. PAT is performed in approximately 90% of cases [10, 11, 44, 55]. PAT is indicated when ankle dorsiflexion remains below 15° after the casting phase [7, 9–11, 50], or to prevent midfoot breakage (rocker-bottom foot deformity) (Fig. 18.5).

The "anchoring effect" [57, 59] may influence clinical judgment in deciding about the need for PAT [52, 54]. PAT is usually reserved as the final step when hindfoot deformity persists after serial casting [9, 50]. Early PAT can occasionally be performed in select cases [59]. The procedure is often performed in the clinic

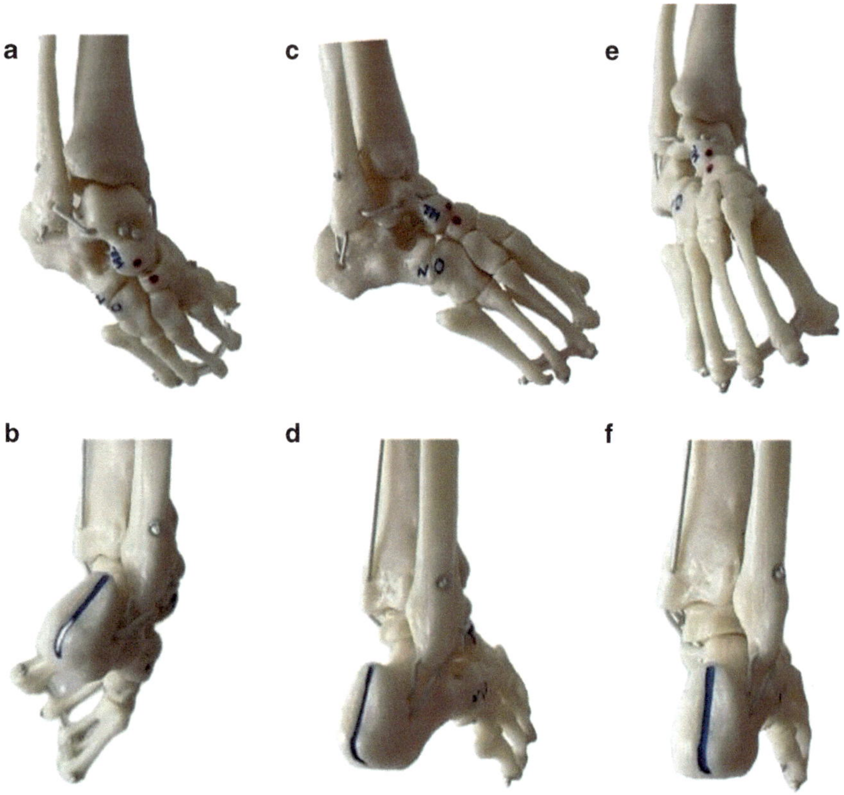

Fig. 18.4 Skeletal model of a clubfoot illustrates the relationship between the tarsal bones. Precorrected (**a**: anterior view, **b**: posterior view). Partially corrected (**c**: lateral view, **d**: posterolateral view). Fully corrected (**e**: anterior view, **f**: posterior view)

under local anesthesia [11, 60]. Confirmation of complete tendon sectioning is key [61].

Complex Clubfoot Is an Iatrogenic Condition

Complex clubfoot refers to a foot characterized by a deep transverse plantar crease from the medial to lateral side, a short first ray, toe hyperextension, severe plantar flexion of the metatarsals, and rigid equinus. Complex clubfoot often becomes apparent after unsuccessful and improper casting (Fig. 18.6) [9, 15, 62]. Although a complex clubfoot resembles an atypical clubfoot, the key distinction lies in the treatment history. Atypical clubfoot is a congenital variant with no prior intervention. Prevention of complex clubfoot relies on proper Ponseti technique. Both complex and atypical clubfoot can be effectively corrected [63]. Referral to a specialized center for further treatment may be indicated (Figs. 18.7 and 18.8) [9, 15].

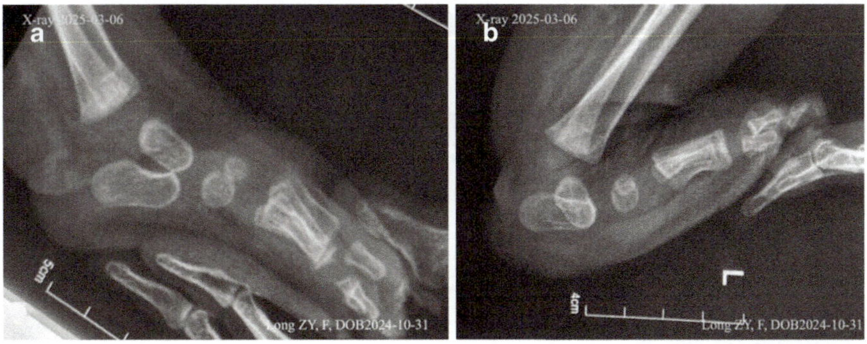

Fig. 18.5 A 14-day-old girl with clubfoot. She underwent treatment with three manipulations and castings before starting to wear the brace. At 4 months the radiograph (lateral foot in plantarflexion) shows that the talus points toward the first metatarsal. (**a**) However, the talus points away from the first metatarsal on the lateral view in dorsiflexion (rocker-bottom foot), (**b**) indicating that the midfoot is broken, due to improper manipulation and casting technique

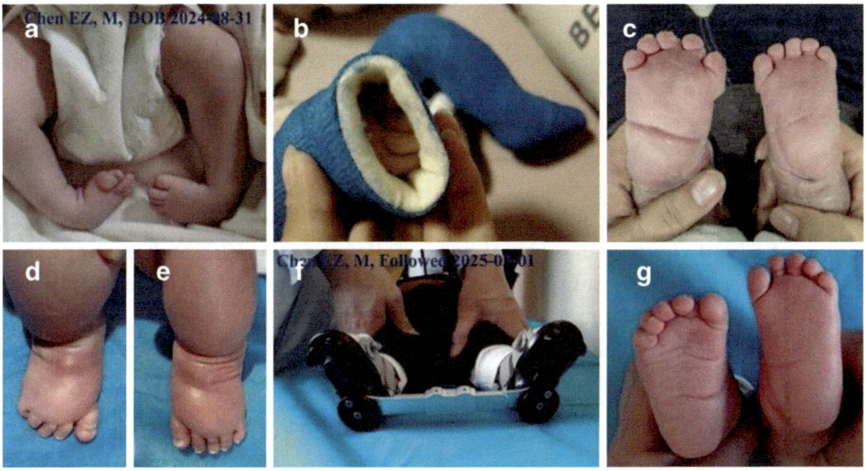

Fig. 18.6 A 3-month-old boy was born with bilateral idiopathic club feet (**a**). He underwent treatment (six manipulations castings with slippage (**b**) and PAT soon after birth elsewhere). He has bilateral swelling and shortened feet, but the right foot was even worse with the greater toe shortened and hyperextended as well as a deep, transverse plantar crease on the right side (**c**). The feet were still swollen 3 months after starting to wear a brace, following the new cycle of two manipulations and castings, without PAT (**d**, **e**). The brace was worn to maintain the feet at 30° of abduction (**f**). Over time, there was an improvement in the appearance of both feet (**g**)

Follow-Up

All patients should be closely followed during the bracing phase of management to ensure adherence to the bracing protocol and to detect signs of relapse. A well-structured follow-up protocol minimizes disruption to the patient's daily life,

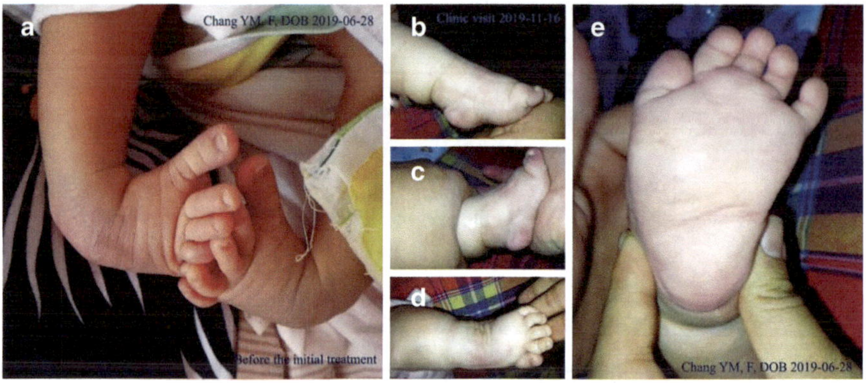

Fig. 18.7 A 5-month-old girl was born with bilateral clubfeet (**a**). She underwent 12 castings and PAT elsewhere with multiple occurrences of cast slippage. She presented with a swollen and shortened left foot in fixed plantar flexion (**b**, **c**), with the great toe shortened and hyperextended (**d**), with a transverse plantar crease (**e**). She underwent three further manipulations and castings, followed by PAT

reduces costs, supports compliance, and enables timely identification of complications [64] However, maintaining regular in-person follow-up visits during the 4–5 years of bracing can be difficult. Prioritizing patients based on relapse risk can help. The Ratio of Corrective Improvement (RCI), calculated by dividing the initial Pirani score by the number of corrective casts, identifies cases at risk for relapse. Patients with an RCI < 1 have a 27-fold higher risk of relapse compared to those with an RCI ≥ 1 [65, 66]. In our experience, follow-up at 6–12-month intervals after the initial visit, supplemented by phone communication, improves compliance monitoring and early relapse detection. Telemedicine is also clinically effective for routine follow-up [67]. Risk factors indicating more frequent follow-up include brace noncompliance and poor evertor muscle activity [68].

Bracing

Relapse risk is highest during periods of rapid growth before the age of 5–6 years [7, 69]. The Ponseti method prevents relapses through consistent bracing. The optimal bracing duration remains controversial. Noncompliance is strongly associated with recurrence [17, 36, 37]. Early recurrence predicts multiple subsequent relapses [17]. Parental education is especially critical for parents of infants <1 year [70, 71]. Hands-on demonstrations of brace application are more effective in improving compliance than verbal instructions alone [57].

The foot abduction orthosis (FAO) consists of open-toe, high-top, straight-last shoes attached to a bar set at shoulder width distance and bent 5–10°, with the convexity directed away from the child. The bar maintains approximately 60° of external rotation for the affected clubfoot and 30° for the unaffected foot [36]. Effective bracing depends on three factors: (1) proper FAO construction, (2) good shoe fit,

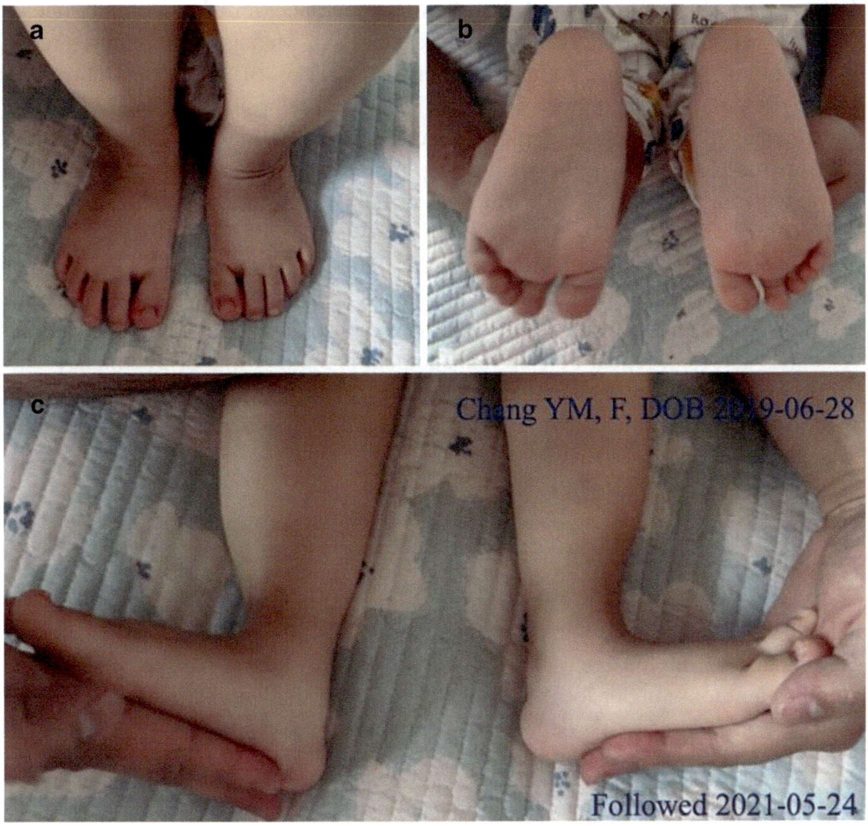

Fig. 18.8 The same girl, age 2 years. Clinical appearance after the second cycle of treatment. (**a**, **b**, **c**) The brace was worn with the feet in 30° of abduction and 15° of dorsiflexion for 3 months, 23 h/day. Thereafter, the brace was worn during sleep and naptime

and (3) adequate time wearing the FAO [36, 70]. Bracing serves two primary functions: maintaining the achieved correction and applying static tension to stretch key soft tissue structures, including the tibialis anterior, tibialis posterior, flexor digitorum longus, flexor hallucis longus, and the deltoid and spring ligaments [36].

Prevention of Relapse

Clubfoot is a developmental abnormality of the entire lower extremity. Atrophy of the postero-medial compartment is a fundamental pathological feature of idiopathic clubfoot. This atrophy is evident from the early stages of fetal development and is present at birth prior to treatment. The affected muscles exhibit reduced growth in thickness, volume, and length. As Dr. Ponseti emphasized, relapses are driven by the same underlying pathology that caused the initial deformity [7].

Relapses are characterized by the gradual reappearance of deformity components, including equinus, adductus, varus, and cavus [72]. Management requires repeat manipulation and casting, and in some cases, surgery [36]. Poor compliance with bracing is a major contributor to relapse [36]. While relapses can often be successfully managed with repeat application of the Ponseti method [73], prevention remains the best strategy. Proper bracing, including appropriate device selection, correct fit, and sufficient wear time, is critical to minimizing relapse [17, 36, 37, 58].

Progressive loss of dorsiflexion indicates a relapsing clubfoot [74]. Key risk periods for relapse include: (1) postbracing growth spurts around ages 4–5, (2) brace noncompliance, and (3) and syndromic or neuromuscular clubfoot [9, 20, 58]. When relapse is detected, repeat Ponseti management is the first line of treatment [9, 15, 36, 73, 75]. An approach that integrates early detection, targeted intervention, and parental education can potentially reduce recurrence, lower treatment costs, and increase value (Fig. 18.9).

Outcome

The Ponseti method yields excellent outcomes for idiopathic clubfoot when properly applied before the age of 1 year [10, 11, 13]. Most cases require percutaneous Achilles tenotomy under local anesthesia to correct residual equinus deformity [9, 50, 60]. Long-term success depends on parental education and adherence to bracing protocols [36, 71].

Case Example (Fig. 18.10)

A female infant was born with a right clubfoot (a) and initially underwent manipulation and casting (b, c). However, due to cast slippage, she was transferred to the author's clinic for further management. Two complete casting cycles (d–k) were performed, resulting in full correction. FAO bracing was started. At the 4-month follow-up, she demonstrated excellent foot alignment and ankle range of motion (l–o). The patient continues to wear the FAO for 16 h/day.

Summary

The current chapter presents ten practical recommendations to improve value by reducing costs while maintaining excellent outcomes when treating idiopathic clubfoot (Table 18.1).

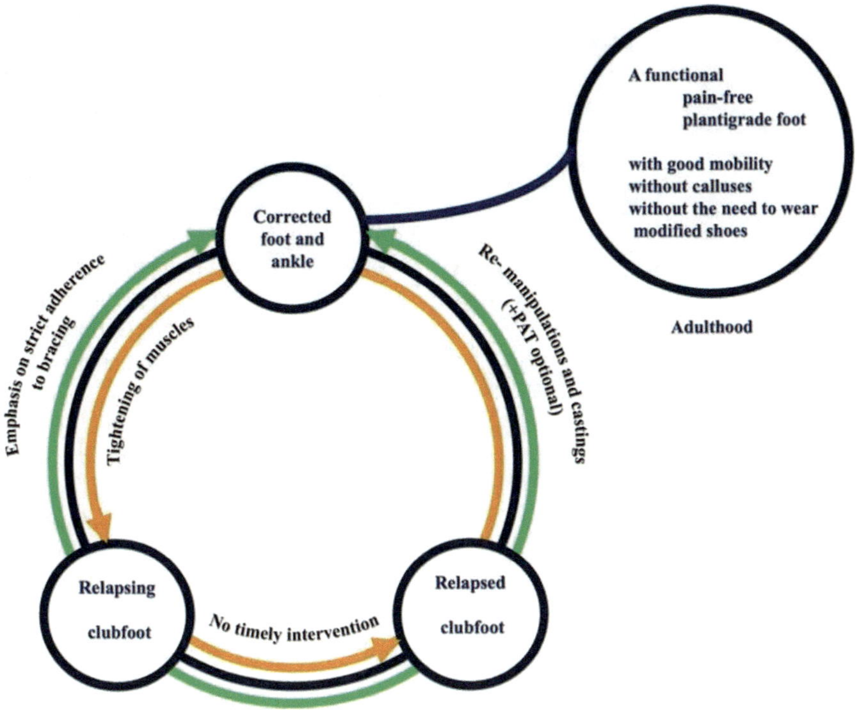

Fig. 18.9 Graph showing the relationship between the condition of corrected foot/ankle, relapsing, and relapsed clubfoot during the period of age < 1

Author Pearls

- Clubfoot treatment is not an emergency and sometimes requires early collaboration with medical specialists to rule out associated disorders.
- Establishing Ponseti clinics may improve quality of care.
- Clinic locations near transit hubs enable same-day treatment completion. Weekend clinic hours facilitate parental attendance without work conflicts.
- The technical details matter in treating the clubfoot using the Ponseti method.
- PAT in clinic using local addresses residual equinus when ankle dorsiflexion fails to reach 15°.
- Complex clubfoot is an iatrogenic condition preventable through proper Ponseti technique.
- Follow-up is important to prevent relapses. High-risk patients warrant more frequent follow-up.
- Telemedicine can be integrated into the follow-up.
- Bracing maintains correction while stretching the soft tissues.
- Parental education is key for preventing relapse.

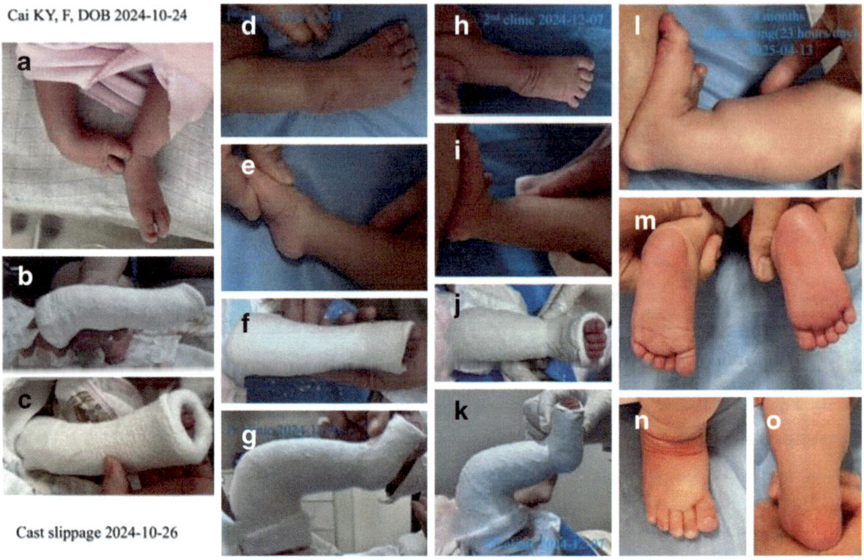

Fig. 18.10 Cast slippage

Table 18.1 Value-based practices in clubfoot treatment

Value-based practice	Value contribution
1. Prenatal counseling	Reduces parental anxiety, may improve compliance, avoids rushed decisions, and may lower treatment delays: however, may increase cost
2. Making the diagnosis	Avoid unnecessary imaging and misdiagnosis. Preventing overtreatment:
3. Timely treatment	Balance urgency with precision and cultural factors: cost neutral
4. Optimize resource use	Improve access. Reducing travel costs:
5. How many casts are needed?	Avoids rigid protocols and gives parents a range of estimated casts: cost neutral
6. Cutting the Achilles tendon?	Minimizes surgical cost by performing in-clinic tenotomy when feasible: reduces costs
7. Preventing complex clubfoot	Prevents iatrogenic harm through adherence to the Ponseti technique: reduces costs
8. Follow-up	Enables early relapse detection: reduces costs
9. Bracing	Maintains correction, prevents relapse: reduces costs
10. Prevent relapse	Prevents relapse through early detection and targeted reintervention reduces costs

Editors Comments

WLH

The Ponseti "minimal surgical approach" involving manipulation, serial casing, PAT in the clinic, and bracing is the preferred standard for clubfoot treatment and has significantly lowered costs compared to traditional surgery. Adherence to long-term bracing is essential for successful outcomes and reducing relapse. Relapses lead to higher costs and potentially more surgery. Starting treatment as soon as possible in infancy can minimize treatment duration and costs. Accelerated casting schedules, changing casts two to three times per week, are effective, reduce the duration of casting, and reduce costs. Low-cost brace options provided by NGOs such as Miraclefeet also enhance value.

RMS

The current chapter provides a detailed and actionable framework for value-based care in managing idiopathic clubfoot in infants under 1 year of age. Additional emerging strategies may further enhance value in the treatment of idiopathic clubfoot, including the use of outcomes registries, community health workers, refined clinical scoring systems, flexible follow-up options, insurance-supported brace programs, nonphysician clinicians trained to perform the Ponseti technique, and integration of patient-reported outcomes. Each of these themes will require additional research to evaluate feasibility and impact.

Acknowledgments The authors thank Jose Morcuende (Iowa, USA) and his team for their teaching and contribution to the China Clubfoot Project. We also thank Ms. Yan Zhang (Shanghai, China) for her assistance in collecting the clinical data and her preliminary editing of the current chapter.

References

1. Smythe T, Rotenberg S, Lavy C. The global birth prevalence of clubfoot: a systematic review and meta-analysis. EClinicalMedicine. 2023;63:102178.
2. China National Maternal and Child Health Monitoring and Annual Report Communication. 2022(4). http://www.mchscn.cn/ViewByStages-34/668.html. Accessed 1 June 2025.
3. Smythe T, Owen RM, Aspden A, Everhart J, Abera E, Amaraegbulam P, et al. Global clubfoot treatment in 2023: an overview of advances and outcomes. BMJ Glob Health. 2025;10(3):e017861.
4. Lu N, Zhao L, Du Q, Liu Y, Oprescu FI, Morcuende JA. From cutting to casting: impact and initial barriers to the Ponseti method of clubfoot treatment in China. Iowa Orthop J. 2010;30:1–6.
5. Hopwood S, Khan F, Kemp J, Rehm A, Ashby E. Clubfoot: an overview and the latest UK guidelines. Br J Hosp Med (Lond). 2023;84(1):1–7.
6. Li J, Li Y, Xu H, Canavese F. Clubfoot treatment in China before and after the advent of the Ponseti technique: a historical narrative review. Ann Transl Med. 2021;9(13):1107.
7. Ponseti IV. Congenital clubfoot: fundamentals of treatment. Oxford: Oxford University Press; 1996.
8. Ippolito E, De Maio F, Mancini F, Bellini D, Orefice A. Leg muscle atrophy in idiopathic congenital clubfoot: is it primitive or acquired. J Child Orthop. 2009;3(3):171–8.

9. Ponseti International Association (PIA). Clinical practice guidelines for the management of clubfoot deformity using the Ponseti method. 1 Nov 2015. http://www.ponseti.info/publications%2D%2D-resources.html. Accessed 1 June 2025.
10. Liu Y, Zhao D, Zhao L, Li H, Yang X. Congenital clubfoot: early recognition and conservative management for preventing late disabilities. Indian J Pediatr. 2016;83(11):1266–74.
11. Cady R, Hennessey TA, Schwend RM. Diagnosis and treatment of idiopathic congenital clubfoot. Pediatrics. 2022;149(2):e2021055555.
12. Elbaum R, Noel B, Degueldre V, Hallez M, Filloque E, Guerin V, et al. 20 years of functional treatment for clubfoot: advantages and limitations compared with the Ponseti method. J Pediatr Orthop B. 2022;31(4):382–90.
13. Cooper DM, Dietz FR. Treatment of idiopathic clubfoot. A thirty-year follow-up note. J Bone Joint Surg Am. 1995;77(10):1477–89.
14. Canavese F, Mansour M, Souchon L, Samba A, Dimeglio A. The "Hybrid method" for the treatment of congenital clubfoot. Ann Transl Med. 2021;9(13):1099.
15. Dragoni M, Gabrielli A, Farsetti P, Bellini D, Maglione P, Ippolito E. Complex iatrogenic clubfoot: is it a real entity? J Pediatr Orthop B. 2018;27(5):428–34.
16. Duman S, Camurcu Y, Cobden A, Ucpunar H, Karahan N, Bursali A. Clinical outcomes of iatrogenic complex clubfoot treated with modified Ponseti method. Int Orthop. 2020;44(9):1833–40.
17. Schaibley C, Torres-Izquierdo B, Hosseinzadeh P. Early clubfoot recurrence can lead to more frequent and earlier second recurrences. J Pediatr Orthop B. 2025;34(2):171–6.
18. Ruzzini L, De Salvatore S, Longo UG, Marino M, Greco A, Piergentili I, et al. Prenatal diagnosis of clubfoot: where are we now? Systematic review and meta-analysis. Diagnostics (Basel). 2021;11(12):2235.
19. Fantasia I, Dibello D, Di Carlo V, Colin G, Barbieri M, Belcaro C, et al. Prenatal diagnosis of isolated clubfoot: diagnostic accuracy and long-term postnatal outcomes. Eur J Obstet Gynecol Reprod Biol. 2021;264:60–4.
20. Shah A, Aroojis A, Mehta R. The Ponseti method of treatment for neuromuscular and syndromic (non-idiopathic) clubfeet: evaluation of a programme-based approach at a mean follow-up of 5.8 years. Int Orthop. 2021;45(1):155–63.
21. Mahan ST, Miller PE, May CJ, Kasser JR. Prospective evaluation of parental anxiety related to newborn foot disorder. J Child Orthop. 2019;13(5):500–7.
22. Radler C, Myers AK, Burghardt RD, Arrabal PP, Herzenberg JE, Grill F. Maternal attitudes towards prenatal diagnosis of idiopathic clubfoot. Ultrasound Obstet Gynecol. 2011;37(6):658–62.
23. Sun N, Yin X, Qiu L, Yang Q, Gong Y. Chinese obstetricians' attitudes, beliefs, and clinical practices related to cesarean delivery on maternal request. Women Birth. 2020;33(1):e67–71.
24. Wang K, Zou W, Lai Y, Hao C, Liu N, Ling X, et al. Accessibility, cost, and quality of an online regular follow-up visit service at an internet hospital in China: mixed methods study. J Med Internet Res. 2024;26:e54902.
25. Nizar NA, Farooki R, Mahapatra P, Halpern S, Hoogenboom T. Patient cost analysis of a community-based teledermatology service versus conventional outpatient appointments in East Kent: a retrospective study through a societal lens to reduce health inequalities. BMC Health Serv Res. 2024;24(1):1632.
26. Maheu AR, Atanda A Jr. Leveraging telehealth: utilizing digital health technology to improve patient care in orthopaedics. J Pediatr Orthop. 2022;42(Suppl 1):S8–12.
27. Bonica GM, Johns RW, Jadvar H. Telehealth and telemedicine: regulatory and medicolegal landscape. Clin Nucl Med. 2024;49(7):644–7.
28. Sirisabya A, Tooptakong T, Limpaphayom N. Common orthopedic problems in the neonate: a comparative study of 2 periods at a tertiary-care hospital. Asian Biomed. 2019;13(3):101–5.
29. Miron MC, Grimard G. Ultrasound evaluation of foot deformities in infants. Pediatr Radiol. 2016;46(2):193–209; quiz 190–2.
30. Richards BS, Faulks S, Razi O, Moualeu A, Jo CH. Nonoperatively corrected clubfoot at age 2 years: radiographs are not helpful in predicting future relapse. J Bone Joint Surg Am. 2017;99(2):155–60.

31. Lang PJ, Avoian T, Sangiorgio SN, Nazif MA, Ebramzadeh E, Zionts LE. Quantification of the ossification of the lateral cuneiform in the feet of young children with unilateral congenital talipes equinovarus. Bone Joint J. 2017;99-B(8):1109–14.
32. Sriharsha Y, Balaji G, Bharathi D, Patro DK. Do the clinical scores (Pirani and Dimeglio scores) correlate with the radiological parameters in idiopathic clubfoot in infants? A cross-sectional study. J Pediatr Orthop B. 2021;30(5):471–7.
33. Nahle IS, Miron MC, Grimard G, Abu Zeid A, Glavas PP. Ultrasound measurements in clubfoot treated with the Ponseti method and risk factors for recurrence: a retrospective study. J Child Orthop. 2022;16(1):46–54.
34. Addosooki A, Tammam H, Morsy AF, Marzouq A, Ahmed EH, Ahmed AM, et al. Correlation of radiographic parameters with clinical correction in idiopathic congenital talipes equinovarus undergoing Ponseti treatment. Int Orthop. 2022;46(8):1911.
35. Portilla-Rojas E, Jovel-Trujillo G, Ramírez L, Moreno C, Taborda JC. Factors influencing recurrence in clubfoot treatment with the Ponseti method in children under 5 years of age: a scoping review. J Pediatr Orthop B. 2025;34(2):177–84.
36. Zhao D, Liu J, Zhao L, Wu Z. Relapse of clubfoot after treatment with the Ponseti method and the function of the foot abduction orthosis. Clin Orthop Surg. 2014;6(3):245–52.
37. Alves C. Bracing in clubfoot: do we know enough? J Child Orthop. 2019;13(3):258–64.
38. Zionts LE, Sangiorgio SN, Cooper SD, Ebramzadeh E. Does clubfoot treatment need to begin as soon as possible? J Pediatr Orthop. 2016;36(6):558–64.
39. Xin J, Shian GY, Han TT, San W. Experiences of postpartum Chinese women undergoing confinement practices: a qualitative meta-synthesis. Int J Nurs Pract. 2024;30(6):e13251.
40. Bertinatto R, Forlin E, Wustro L, Tolotti JO, de Souza G. Does the presence of clubfoot delay the onset of walking? Rev Bras Ortop (Sao Paulo). 2020;55(5):637–41.
41. Hughes K, Gelfer Y, Cokljat M, Wientroub S, Yavor A, Hemo Y, et al. Does idiopathic congenital talipes equinovarus have an impact on attainment of developmental milestones? A multicentre international study. J Child Orthop. 2019;13(4):353–60.
42. Pavone V, Sapienza M, Vescio A, Caldaci A, McCracken KL, Canavese F, et al. Early developmental milestones in patients with idiopathic clubfoot treated by Ponseti method. Front Pediatr. 2022;10:869401.
43. Liu YB, Li SJ, Zhao L, Yu B, Zhao DH. Timing for Ponseti clubfoot management: does the age matter? 90 children (131 feet) with a mean follow-up of 5 years. Acta Orthop. 2018;89(6):662–7.
44. Shah A, Mehta R, Aroojis A. The Ponseti method of clubfoot treatment in walking age children: is it effective? A study of 56 children from 1 to 10 years of age. J Pediatr Orthop B. 2019;28(2):159–66.
45. Alves C, Batlle AE, Rodriguez MV. Neglected clubfoot treated by serial casting: a narrative review on how possibility takes over disability. Ann Transl Med. 2021;9(13):1103.
46. Ahmed S, Moosa S, Muhammad AA, Iftikhar S, Khan MA, Chinoy MA, et al. Eight-year review of a clubfoot treatment program in Pakistan with assessment of outcomes using the Ponseti technique: a retrospective study of 988 patients (1,458 clubfeet) aged 0 to 5 years at enrollment. J Am Acad Orthop Surg Glob Res Rev. 2022;6(4):e22.00022.
47. Zhao L, Ma ZS, Ding J. China task force takes its steady steps in "Healthy Walk"—on China Clubfoot Project during the past decade. Orthop J China. 2022;30(18):1633–6.
48. Avilucea FR, Szalay EA, Bosch PP, Sweet KR, Schwend RM. Effect of cultural factors on outcome of Ponseti treatment of clubfeet in rural America. J Bone Joint Surg Am. 2009;91(3):530–40.
49. Barik S, Nazeer M, Mani BT. Accelerated Ponseti technique: efficacy in the management of CTEV. Eur J Orthop Surg Traumatol. 2019;29(4):919–24.
50. Lohan I. Treatment of congenital clubfoot using the Ponseti method (clubfoot workshop manual), 2nd edn. www.global-help.org/publications/books/book_clubfoottreatmentmanual.html. Accessed 1 June 2025.

51. Pletch A, Morcuende J, Barriga H, Segura J, Salas A. Photovoice and clubfoot: using a participatory research method to study caregiver adherence to the Ponseti method in Perú. Iowa Orthop J. 2015;35:160–8.
52. Lampasi M, Abati CN, Bettuzzi C, Stilli S, Trisolino G. Comparison of Dimeglio and Pirani score in predicting number of casts and need for tenotomy in clubfoot correction using the Ponseti method. Int Orthop. 2018;42(10):2429–36.
53. Fan H, Liu Y, Zhao L, Chu C, An Y, Wang T, et al. The correlation of Pirani and Dimeglio scoring systems for Ponseti management at different levels of deformity severity. Sci Rep. 2017;7(1):14578.
54. Sharma A, Shukla S, Kiran B, Michail S, Agashe M. Can the Pirani score predict the number of casts and the need for tenotomy in the management of clubfoot by the Ponseti method? Malays Orthop J. 2018;12(1):26–30.
55. Ahmed H, Mohamed A, Salih M, Mohamed M, Younis A, Hussein S, et al. Assessing the influence of age, weight, and Pirani score on the number of casts during the initial phase of clubfoot treatment using the Ponseti method: a prospective study. Indian J Orthop. 2024;58(6):687–95.
56. Miller NH, Carry PM, Mark BJ, Engelman GH, Georgopoulos G, Graham S, et al. Does strict adherence to the Ponseti method improve isolated clubfoot treatment outcomes? A two-institution review. Clin Orthop Relat Res. 2016;474(1):237–43.
57. Li X, Xu H, Chu Y, Tang W, Liu X. The anchoring effect in study time allocation: labor-in-vain versus labor-and-gain. Behav Sci (Basel). 2024;14(7):567.
58. Zhao D, Li H, Zhao L, Liu J, Wu Z, Jin F. Results of clubfoot management using the Ponseti method: do the details matter? A systematic review. Clin Orthop Relat Res. 2014;472(4):1329–36.
59. Ghanem I, Ghanem D, Rassi J, Saliba I. Achilles tenotomy during Ponseti's clubfoot treatment: better early than late. J Pediatr Orthop B. 2024;33(3):251–7.
60. Rangasamy K, Baburaj V, Gopinathan NR, Sudesh P. Techniques, anaesthesia preferences, and outcomes of Achilles tenotomy during Ponseti method of idiopathic clubfoot correction: a systematic review. Foot (Edinb). 2022;52:101922.
61. Kayondo TK, El-Adwar KL, Abdullah EA, Mosa MM. Reliability of percutaneous Achilles tenotomy in the treatment of idiopathic clubfoot. J Pediatr Orthop. 2024;44(6):e566–9.
62. Patel A, Mongia AK, Sharma RK, Saini R, Chaudhary C, Singh S. Outcome of atypical & complex clubfoot managed by modified Ponseti method-a prospective study. J Foot Ankle Surg. 2022;61(5):1081–5.
63. Al-Mohrej OA, Alshaalan FN, Alhussainan TS. Is the modified Ponseti method effective in treating atypical and complex clubfoot? A systematic review. Int Orthop. 2021;45(10):2589–97.
64. Wright J, Tudor F, Luff T, Hashemi-Nejad A. Surveillance after treatment of children with developmental dysplasia of the hip: current UK practice and the proposed Stanmore protocol. J Pediatr Orthop B. 2013;22(6):509–15.
65. Kelly DM, VanderHave K, Martus JE. What's new in pediatric orthopaedics. J Bone Joint Surg Am. 2018;100(4):348–54.
66. Zhao D, Li H, Zhao L, Kuo KN, Yang X, Wu Z, et al. Prognosticating factors of relapse in clubfoot management by Ponseti method. J Pediatr Orthop. 2018;38(10):514–20.
67. Douglas C, Simmonds J, Kedroff L, Tennant S. Do live-stream telemedicine follow-up appointments for a Ponseti-treated clubfoot caseload compare favourably with a face-to-face review? Observed clinical outcomes and treatment provision during the COVID-19 pandemic. J Telemed Telecare. 2025;31(1):97–103.
68. Van Schelven H, Moerman S, Van der Steen M, Besselaar AT, Greve C. Prognostic factors for recurrent idiopathic clubfoot deformity: a systematic literature review and meta-analysis. Acta Orthop. 2022;93:11–28.
69. Sangiorgio SN, Ebramzadeh E, Morgan RD, Zionts LE. The timing and relevance of relapsed deformity in patients with idiopathic clubfoot. J Am Acad Orthop Surg. 2017;25(7):536–45.
70. Dimeo AJ Sr, Lalush DS, Grant E, Morcuende JA. Development of a surrogate biomodel for the investigation of clubfoot bracing. J Pediatr Orthop. 2012;32(7):e47–52.

71. Miller AH, Moisan A, Rhodes LN, Locke LL, Kelly DM. Caregiver impressions of bracing and its association with unsuccessful outcomes throughout the Ponseti treatment. J Pediatr Orthop. 2025;45(2):e148–55.
72. Ponseti IV. Relapsing clubfoot: causes, prevention, and treatment. Iowa Orthop J. 2002;22:55–6.
73. Liu YB, Jiang SY, Zhao L, Yu Y, Zhao DH. Can repeated Ponseti management for relapsed clubfeet produce the outcome comparable with the case without relapse? A clinical study in term of gait analysis. J Pediatr Orthop. 2020;40(1):29–35.
74. Porter ME. What is value in health care. N Engl J Med. 2010;363(26):2477–81.
75. De Mulder T, Prinsen S, Van Campenhout A. Treatment of non-idiopathic clubfeet with the Ponseti method: a systematic review. J Child Orthop. 2018;12(6):575–81.

Benign Bone Tumors and Cysts: The Value of Radiographs

19

Rikki Koehler

Introduction

Benign bone tumors are common. A longitudinal study of radiographs from 262 healthy children, conducted between 1926 and 1942, identified 35 benign tumors in 33 children, indicating a prevalence of 13% [1]. Benign bone lesions in children present with a wide range of clinical findings from incidental discoveries in asymptomatic children to low-energy fractures. Accurate diagnosis of a benign tumor or cyst is essential to guide appropriate treatment, improve care, and reduce costs.

Value-Based Themes

Proper Diagnosis Is Crucial to Increasing Value

Diagnosing the bone tumor or cyst on radiographs leads to a proper treatment plan. The surgeon must be comfortable reading the radiographs, not ordering unnecessary studies, and not performing unnecessary biopsies and resections, which would increase cost and might change the outcome.

Plain Radiograph Characteristics of Benign Bone Tumors and Cysts

The following are examples of benign bone lesions where simple evaluation and treatment provide greater value to both the patient and the hospital.

R. Koehler (✉)
Department of Orthopaedics, Children's Mercy Hospital, Kansas City, MO, USA
e-mail: rmkoehler@cmh.edu

W. L. Hennrikus, R. M. Schwend (eds.), *Value in Pediatric Orthopaedics*,
https://doi.org/10.1007/978-3-032-19570-8_19

Bone Cysts

A unicameral bone cyst (UBC) is a benign, fluid-filled cavity lined by a fibrous membrane and surrounded by thin cortical bone. UBCs most commonly occur in the proximal humerus and other metaphyseal regions of long bones in children and adolescents. The average age at presentation is 9 years old [2]. UBCs are approximately twice as common in boys as in girls. Although usually single-chambered or unicameral in most cases, the cyst can occasionally present with multiple chambers. On plain radiographs, especially in the presence of a fracture, the "fallen leaf sign" may be seen—where a fragment of cortical bone has settled dependently within the cyst (Fig. 19.1).

On plain radiographs in the case of fracture, they often present with "fallen leaf sign," where a piece of cortex falls into the cyst (Fig. 19.1).

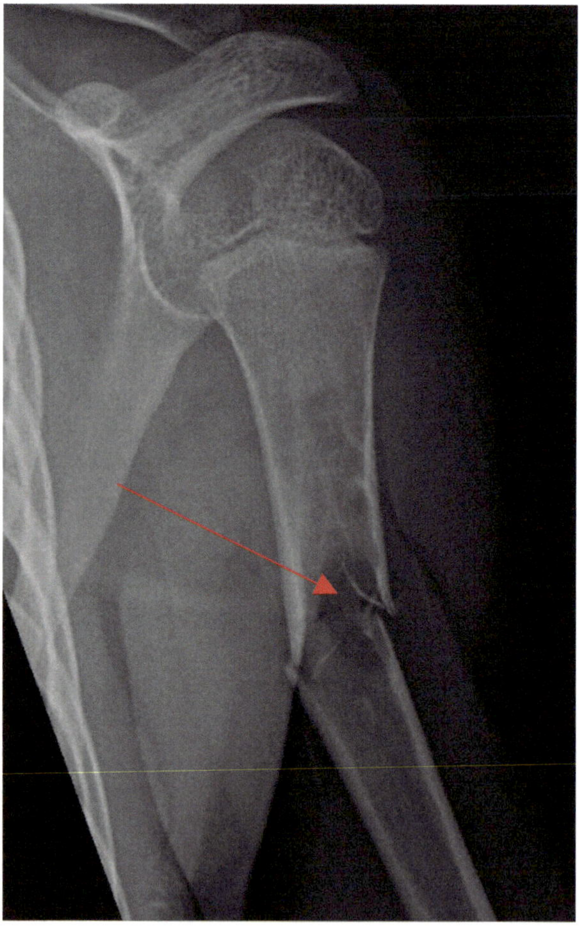

Fig. 19.1 Radiograph of 7-year-9-month-old boy depicting a "fallen leaf sign" in a unicameral bone cyst (UBC) with red arrow pointing to the "fallen leaf"

The etiology of UBCs is unknown, but they are believed to result from a disruption in normal bone development. UBCs often form in close association with the physis. In some cases, small connections between the cyst and the physis may persist. Magnetic resonance imaging (MRI) is not indicated when the cyst exhibits characteristic features on X-rays.

Unicameral bone cysts may be discovered incidentally or present with a pathological fracture. If the cyst rapidly reaccumulates following a fracture, minimally invasive treatment—such as aspiration followed by injection of a calcium sulfate or calcium phosphate matrix—can be considered. The primary goal of surgical intervention is to accelerate cyst resolution and prevent refracture. These cysts almost always resolve spontaneously after skeletal maturity, regardless of treatment. For lesions in the proximal femur, internal fixation should be strongly considered. In one series of 14 patients with pathological proximal femur fractures, due to a UBC, there was a prolonged time to union, a 64% rate of revision surgery, and a 71% overall complication rate [3]. Due to the high risk of complications associated with pathological fractures of the proximal femur, preemptive fixation is appropriate even in the absence of pain. When a cyst is located in a weight-bearing region of the pelvis, such as directly above the acetabular dome, weight-bearing restrictions, cyst aspiration, and injection should also be considered.

Aneurysmal Bone Cyst

Aneurysmal bone cysts (ABCs) are locally aggressive, blood-filled lesions that can present with pain and may lead to pathological fractures. Their etiology is unknown. On X-rays, ABCs typically exhibit cortical thinning, multiple internal septations, and, unlike UBCs, are often wider than the physis [4] (Fig. 19.2a). Diagnosis of ABC is confirmed with MRI, which characteristically shows fluid-fluid levels representing "lakes of blood" within the lesion (Fig. 19.2b). The MRI can help to rule out telangiectatic osteosarcoma, which can present with similar X-ray features as an ABC.

Treatment involves curettage and grafting with either autologous bone or a bone substitute. Various adjuvants, such as phenol or doxycycline, have been used to reduce recurrence. In fact, a recent meta-analysis evaluating doxycycline injection as a primary treatment reported a recurrence rate of only 2% [5].

Osteochondroma

Osteochondromas are benign bone tumors that project outward from the cortex and have a cartilaginous cap. They arise from the bone surface and may be either sessile or pedunculated. On radiographs, they characteristically "turn away" from the physis (Fig. 19.3). Osteochondromas are contiguous with the intramedullary canal of the host bone. Osteochondromas are associated with multiple hereditary exostoses (MHE), a genetic disorder caused by loss-of-function mutations in the *EXT1* or

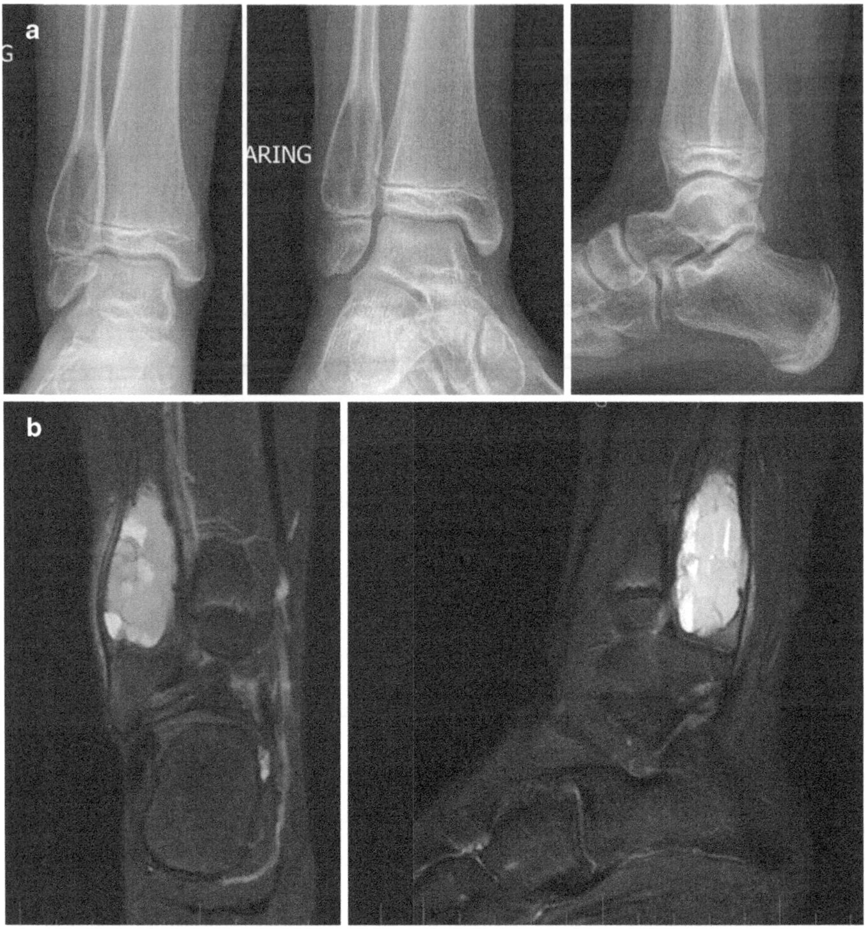

Fig. 19.2 (**a**) AP, mortise, and lateral radiographs of an 11 year + 11 month female with a right ankle aneurysmal bone cyst. (**b**) MRI demonstrating multiloculated cyst and fluid-fluid levels consistent with aneurysmal bone cyst

EXT2 genes. Patients with MHE develop multiple osteochondromas, which can lead to pain, functional impairment, and limb deformities. There is a 1–5% lifetime risk of malignant transformation to chondrosarcoma, typically occurring after skeletal maturity [6]. Routine surveillance of individual osteochondromas is not necessary, however. X-rays should be obtained for symptomatic lesions that grow or change rapidly, cause pain, produce neurologic symptoms, or result in limb malalignment. Routine X-rays of all lesions are not necessary. However, in patients old enough to undergo imaging without sedation, spinal imaging should be considered to rule out intracanal exostoses [7].

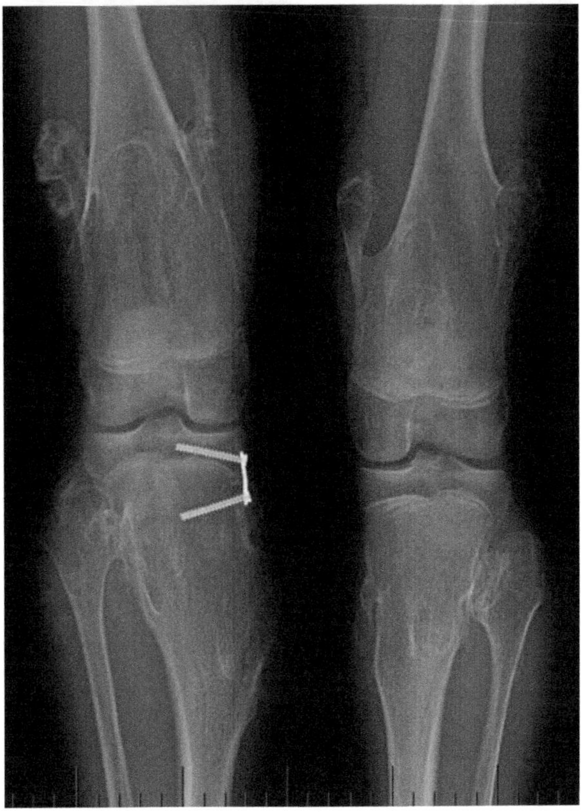

Fig. 19.3 Bilateral standing AP knee radiographs in a 15 + 9 male with multiple hereditary exostoses

Enchondroma

Enchondromas are benign cartilaginous tumors that often exhibit characteristic "popcorn" calcifications on radiographs. Multiple enchondromas can occur in the context of two conditions: Ollier disease and Maffucci syndrome. Most enchondromas are asymptomatic and can be observed. Exceptions are enchondromas located in the hand with a pathologic fracture (Fig. 19.4) or enchondromas in a weight-bearing bone. For symptomatic enchondromas, curettage and bone grafting may be considered. Malignant transformation into chondrosarcoma is rare for isolated enchondromas. However, the lifetime risk of malignant transformation is approximately 15–20% in Maffucci syndrome and 10–40% in Ollier disease [8].

Chondroblastoma

Chondroblastoma is a benign bone tumor that occurs almost exclusively in the epiphysis of teenagers (Fig. 19.5a, b). Radiographically, it appears as a lytic lesion with a sclerotic rim. Most patients present with pain. Standard treatment involves

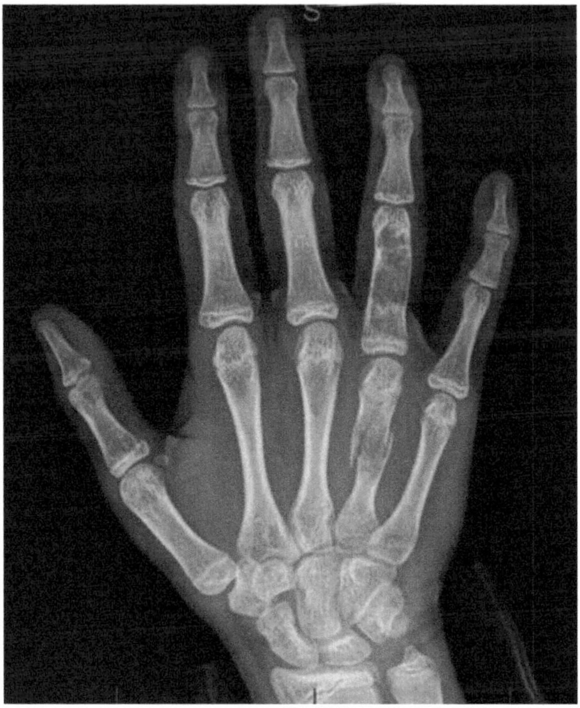

Fig. 19.4 Multiple enchondromas in the hand of a 12 + 7 female with Ollier disease. The fourth metacarpal has a pathologic fracture from the enchondroma

intralesional curettage and bone grafting, with reported recurrence rates ranging from 10% to 35% [9]. The use of adjuvants, such as cryoablation, may reduce recurrence. In one study involving ten patients treated with curettage and cryoablation, only one (10%) experienced recurrence [10].

Nonossifying Fibroma

Nonossifying fibromas are benign lesions that typically appear on radiographs as eccentric, metaphyseal defects with a characteristic "soap-bubble" appearance and a well-defined sclerotic rim (Fig. 19.6). They are usually discovered incidentally and can be observed.

Fibrous Dysplasia

Fibrous dysplasia is a condition in which normal bone is replaced by fibrous stroma. On X-rays, fibrous dysplasia appears as an expansile lesion with a characteristic ground-glass appearance and a thin, scalloped cortex (Fig. 19.7). Surgical intervention is generally reserved for lesions in major weight-bearing areas, such as the proximal femur, to reduce the risk of fracture.

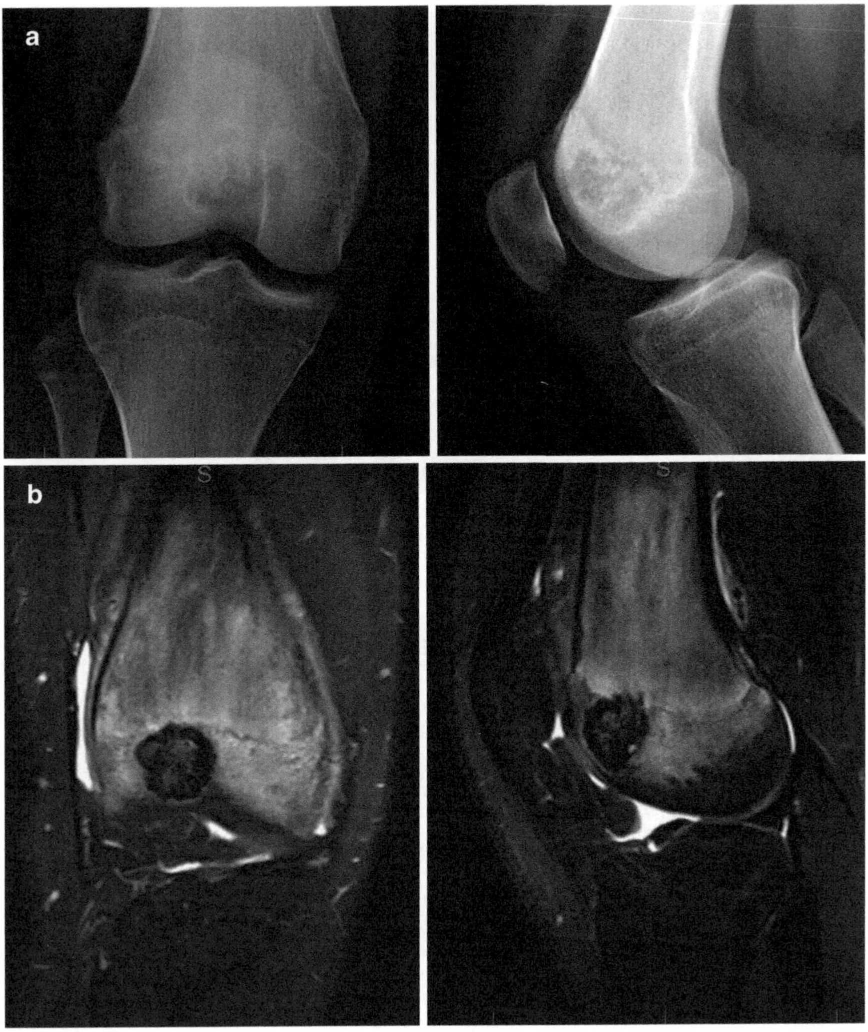

Fig. 19.5 (**a**) 15-year-old male with chondroblastoma in the right distal femur epiphysis. (**b**) MRI of the chondroblastoma demonstrating surrounding bony edema. The inflammation is associated with this painful lesion

Eosinophilic Granuloma/Langerhans Cell Histiocytosis

Langerhans cell histiocytosis (LCH) presents as a lytic, lucent bone lesion(s) (Fig. 19.8a). LCH is characterized by the proliferation of histiocytes, including immature dendritic cells and macrophages. MRI is often obtained to further evaluate the lesion, as its appearance can closely mimic infection or malignancy (Fig. 19.8b). LCH commonly affects the axial skeleton but may also occur in the diaphysis of long bones. Eosinophilic granuloma represents a less aggressive,

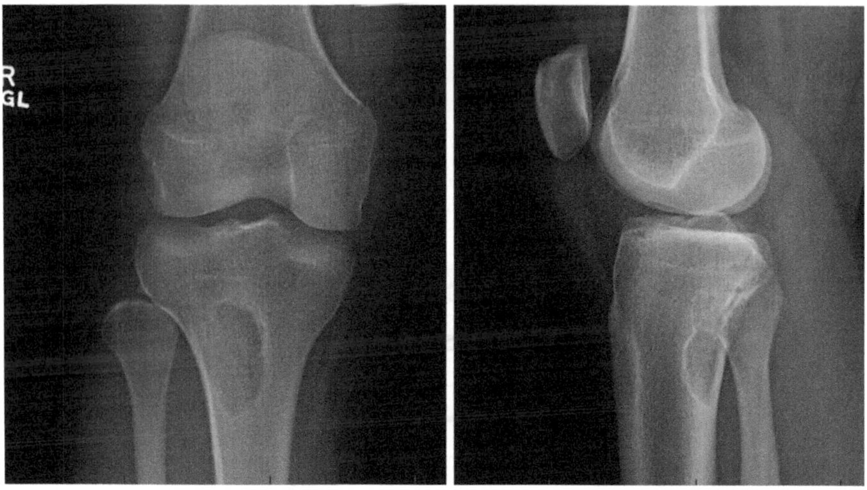

Fig. 19.6 A nonossifying fibroma was found incidentally in a 15-year-old male who had an ipsilateral fibular shaft fracture after trauma

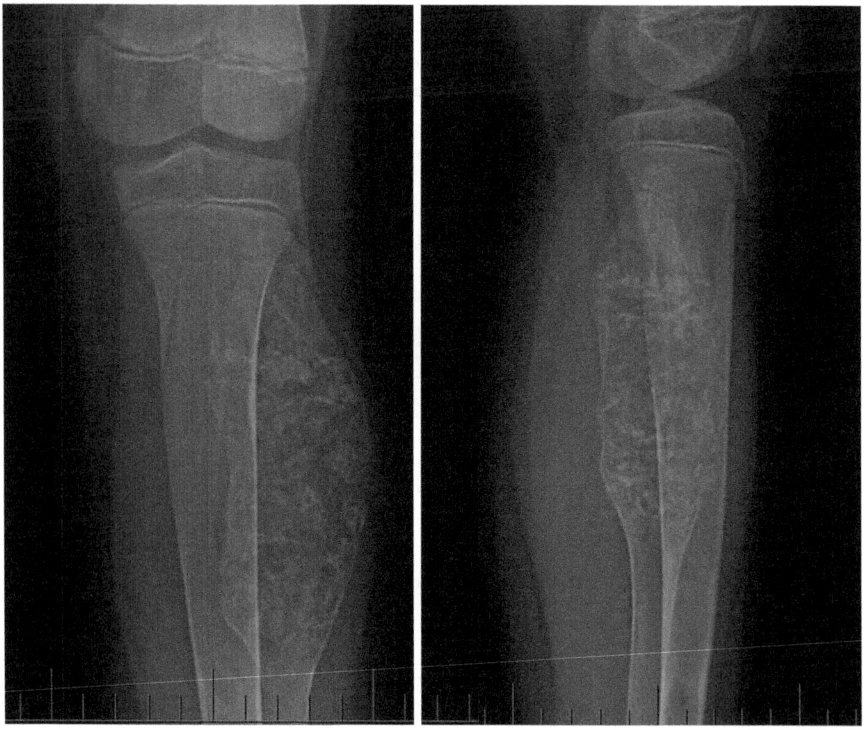

Fig. 19.7 An 8 + 2 female with fibrous dysplasia of her proximal fibula in association with McCune-Albright syndrome

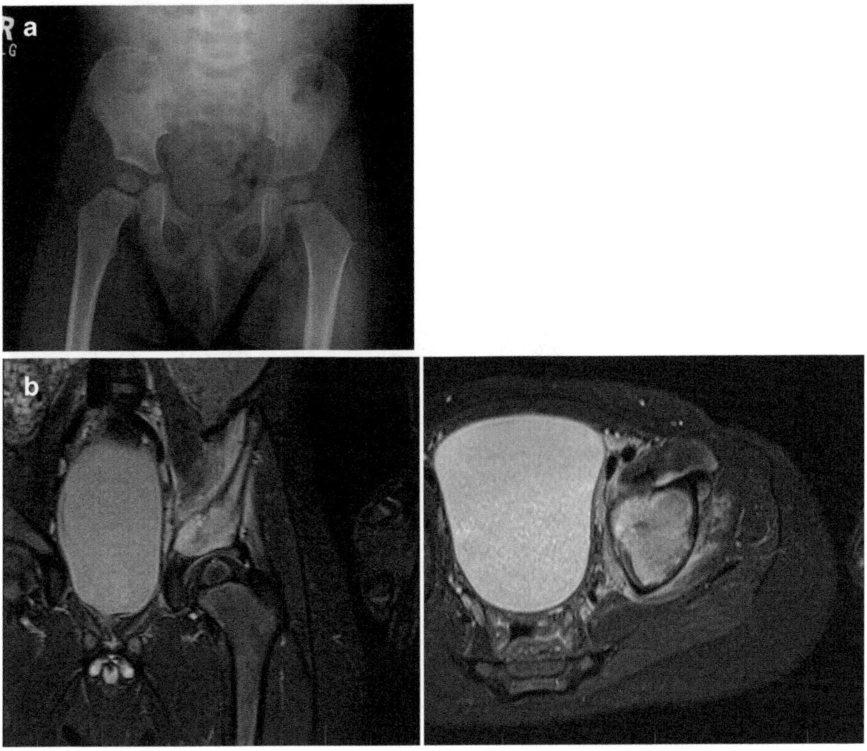

Fig. 19.8 (**a**) A 2-year + 5-month boy with LCH superior to his left acetabulum who could not bear weight. (**b**) T2 sequence, coronal and axial cuts, of the same patient with LCH

localized form of LCH. Referral to the hematology/oncology service is recommended for LCH cases to confirm diagnosis and plan treatment.

Chondromyxoid Fibroma

Chondromyxoid fibromas are rare bone tumors, accounting for approximately 0.5% of all bone lesions. They typically arise in the long bones and exhibit a mixed lytic and blastic appearance on radiographs. MRI is recommended for further evaluation. Unlike nonossifying fibromas, chondromyxoid fibromas can cause pain and swelling and may persist into skeletal maturity and adulthood. Patients often report months of localized swelling and a dull ache prior to diagnosis. Treatment involves intralesional curettage and bone grafting, with or without the use of adjuvants. The recurrence rate is relatively high, ranging from 25% to 38%. However, the overall prognosis is good [11].

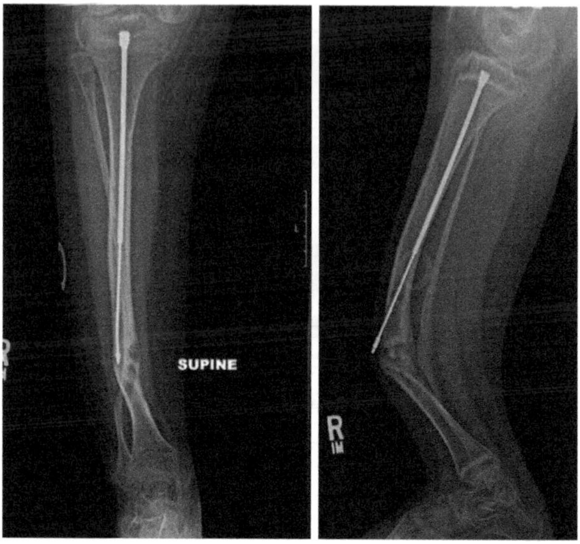

Fig. 19.9 An 13 + 3-year-old male with osteofibrous dysplasia who had had multiple acute surgical corrections starting at age 2 years old. The lesion kept *reoccurring*, which is typical in young children

Osteofibrous Dysplasia

Osteofibrous dysplasia occurs almost exclusively in the tibia and is associated with pain and apex anterior tibial bowing. On radiographs, the lesion appears bubbly and often obliterates the anterior cortex, contributing to the bowing deformity. Nonoperative management is the preferred standard in children. A clamshell orthosis may be used to help prevent fracture. Acute deformity correction is not recommended until skeletal maturity, as both the lesion and deformity tend to recur rapidly if an osteotomy is performed in young children [12] (Fig. 19.9). Anterior distal tibial guided growth is a potential option to gradually correct deformity and reduce fracture risk in cases of anterior or anterolateral bowing [13].

Osteoid Osteoma

Osteoid osteomas are small but painful bone lesions characterized by a central nidus of inflammation, typically seen on radiographs as a small, round lucency with surrounding sclerosis. The pain is often severe, worse at night, and reliably relieved by nonsteroidal anti-inflammatory drugs (NSAIDs) such as aspirin. Osteoid osteomas commonly arise within the cortex and may appear as a low-lying "sand dune" (Fig. 19.10a). While radiographs can be suggestive, computerized tomography (CT) or MRI is often better for diagnosing the lesion. However, osteoid osteoma may occasionally be missed if imaging slices are not sufficiently thin due to osteoid osteoma's small size (<1 cm) (Fig. 19.10b, c). When intervention is indicated,

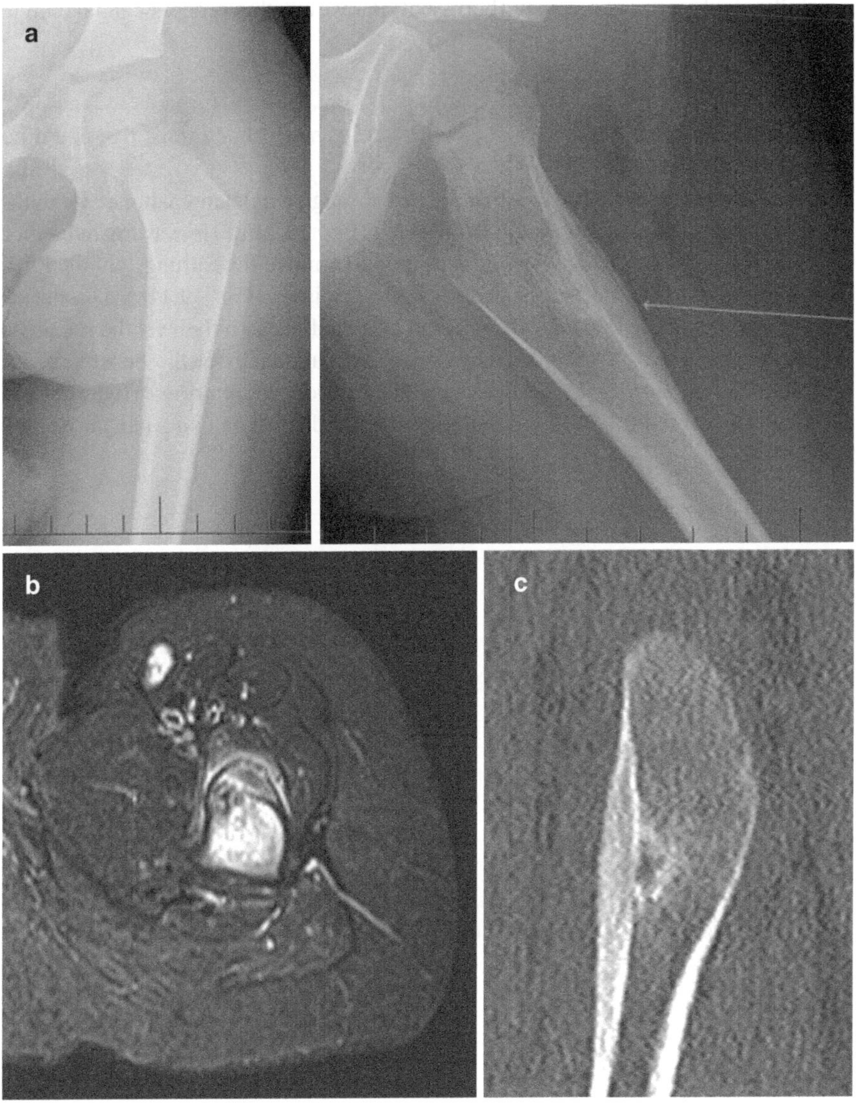

Fig. 19.10 (**a**) A 2 + 9-month female with left proximal femur osteoid osteoma. (**b**) Axial cut of the same patient above with an osteoid osteoma that demonstrates the nidus with surrounding bony edema with the adjacent raised cortical surface. (**c**) A sagittal cut of the proximal femur of the same patient showing osteoid osteoma. Notice the "sand dune"-like appearance of the adjacent cortex

radiofrequency ablation or cryoablation performed by interventional radiology (IR) can be performed unless the lesion is adjacent to critical structures such as the spinal cord, in which case surgical resection is safer [14]. If the patient and parents decide against intervention, the osteoid osteoma can be managed conservatively and typically resolves spontaneously (burns out). However, this process can take up to 33 months [15].

Case Examples

A 25-month-old boy presented with a fracture through a unicameral bone cyst in the right proximal humerus after a fall from a step (Fig. 19.11a). He was treated with a shoulder immobilizer, which he was permitted to remove for bathing.

Although the fracture had healed, the cyst persisted (Fig. 19.11b). Due to the patient's young age, the size of the residual cyst, and his activity level, he remained at risk for refracture. After a discussion with his parents about the benefits, risks, and alternatives, they elected to proceed with surgery. Aspiration, irrigation, and injection of a mixture of 75% calcium sulfate and 25% calcium phosphate was performed.

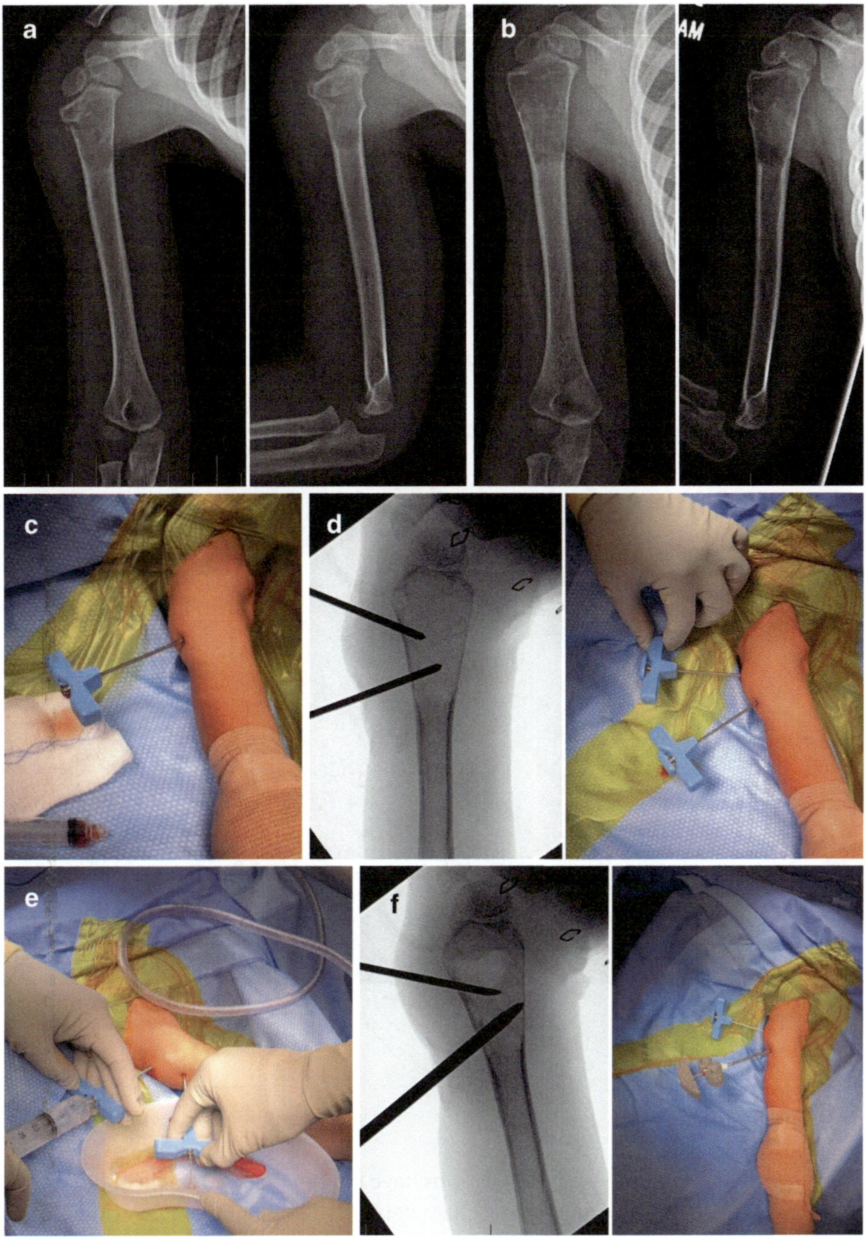

Fig. 19.11 (**a**) A 25-month-old boy with painful shoulder after he fell from a step. (**b**) Radiographs 3 months post injury. (**c**) Under fluoroscopic guidance in the operating room, a large bore bone marrow needle was placed distally into the cyst and aspirated to confirm fluid. (**d**) A second bone marrow needle was placed proximally. (**e**) 1 L of saline was irrigated between both bone marrow needles to disrupt the cyst. (**f**) A larger bore needle was then switched out distally to inject the calcium phosphate and sulfate combination (Fig. 19.12). (**g**) The calcium sulfate and phosphate combination was injected. (**h**) The calcium sulfate and phosphate combination was injected. (**i**) Radiographs performed 3 weeks later demonstrated successful cyst impregnation. The entire cyst was filled with the calcium sulfate and phosphate combination

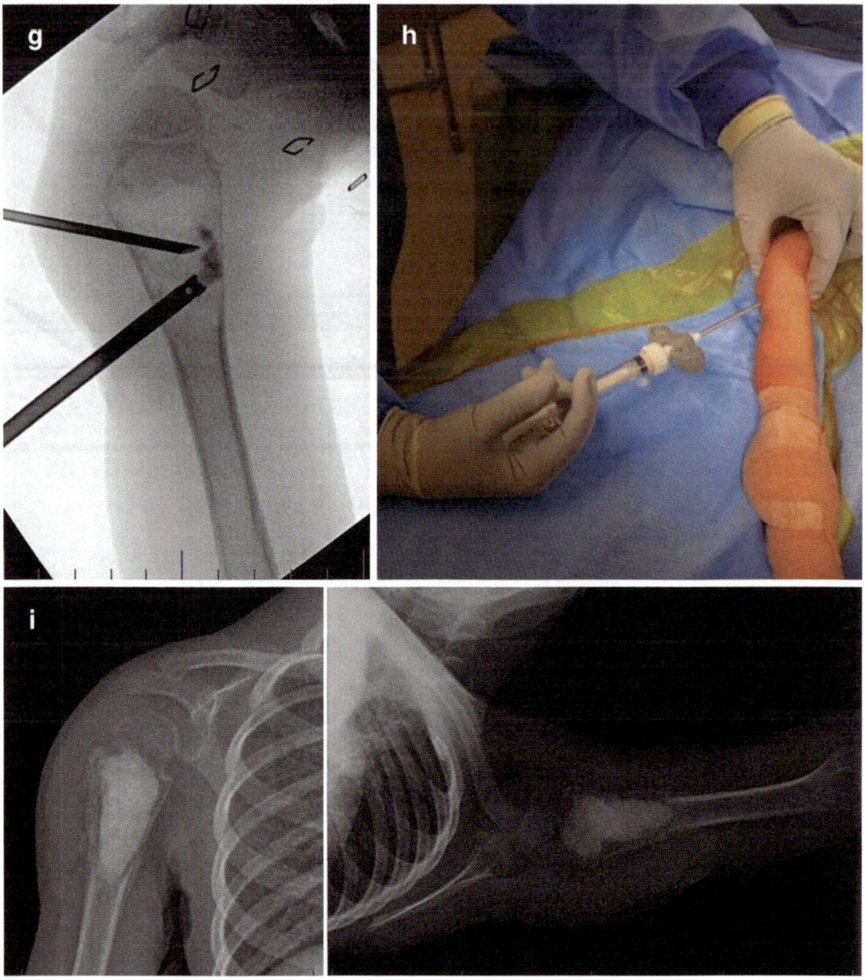

Fig. 19.11 (continued)

Summary

Recognizing which lesions on radiographs have benign radiographic features versus those with aggressive or malignant characteristics is essential in determining the need for advanced imaging and potential treatment. This approach minimizes unnecessary healthcare costs and improves value. In addition, accurate diagnosis of benign bone tumors and cysts also reduces costs by minimizing unnecessary referrals to tumor surgeons.

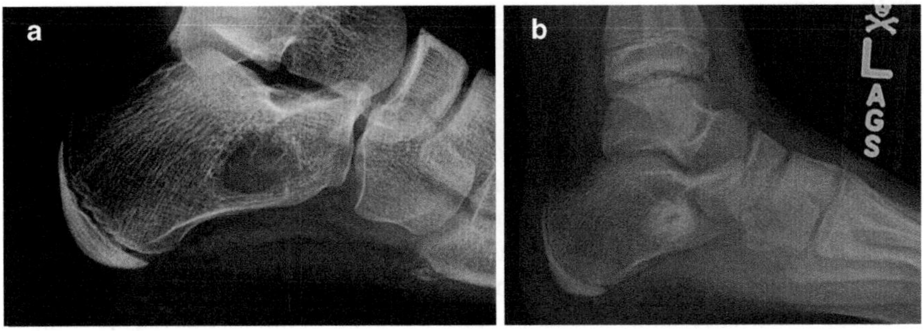

Fig. 19.12 (**a**) A second example case: Patient with heel pain. Radiograph demonstrates the calcaneal UBC prior to injection. (**b**) Resolving calcaneal cyst 7 months after calcium sulfate and phosphate injection

Author Pearls

- Most benign bone tumors in children do not require biopsy or advanced imaging when radiographic features are diagnostic.
- Some incidentally discovered lesions, such as unicameral bone cysts (UBC), nonossifying fibromas (NOF), and enchondromas, do not require follow-up.
- High-quality radiographs, combined with a careful clinical examination, often eliminate the need for advanced imaging or referral.
- Only treat ABCs aggressively when symptomatic, expanding, or located in critical areas such as the spine or proximal femur. Most cases indicated for treatment resolve with curettage, high-speed burring, and adjuvant therapy. Recurrence is common.
- Radiofrequency or cryoablation for osteoid osteoma provides lower cost, less morbidity, a quicker return to activity, and enhanced value compared to open surgery.
- Routine follow-up of lesions in patients with MHE is not needed unless symptoms arise or the lesion is located near the spine.
- Discuss the natural history and expected outcomes of benign lesions with families.
- Avoid surgery for fibrous dysplasia unless structurally necessary, such as pain or progressive deformity in weight-bearing bones.

Editors Comments

WLH

Treating benign bone tumors and cysts can be costly, but there are strategies to reduce expenses while enhancing value. As the author of the current study appropriately noted, many of these benign tumors and cysts can be safely observed without intervention. When surgery is indicated, less invasive treatment options, including radiofrequency ablation, cryoablation, sclerotherapy, or embolization, can be considered. When uncertainty exists, seeking a second opinion is advisable. Finally, explore financial assistance programs that may help patients manage expenses associated with treatment for benign bone tumors and cysts.

RMS

High-value care for benign bone tumors in children requires restraint and sometimes lies in knowing when not to intervene. Many lesions are self-limited and can be observed. Shared decision-making allows families to understand the natural history of untreated lesions and to choose observation as the treatment when appropriate. In many cases, plain radiographs are sufficient for diagnosis. Avoiding unnecessary imaging, referrals, and surgery can reduce cost and reduce family anxiety. Advanced imaging such as MRI or CT should be reserved for lesions that appear atypical or aggressive and for lesions in the proximal femur to assess fracture risk. Success should be defined by symptom resolution with minimal harm and cost. Interventions should be driven by clinical symptoms, not radiographic appearance alone. When intervention is needed, minimally invasive techniques, including image-guided ablation or percutaneous injection, can reduce morbidity, shorten hospital stays, and enhance value.

Acknowledgments I would like to thank Mark Sinclair, MD, for providing the case example.

References

1. Collier CD, Nelson GB, Conry KT, Kosmas C, Getty PJ, Liu RW. The natural history of benign bone tumors of the extremities in asymptomatic children: a longitudinal radiographic study. J Bone Joint Surg Am. 2021;103(7):575–80.
2. Porter ME. What is value in health care? N Engl J Med. 2010;363(26):2477–81.
3. Lin AJ, Siddiqui AA, Fan B, Bennett JT, Illingworth KD, Andras LM, et al. Treatments and sequelae of pediatric pathologic proximal femur fractures due to benign bone cyst. J Pediatr Orthop. 2022;42(6):e661–e6.
4. Rapp TB, Ward JP, Alaia MJ. Aneurysmal bone cyst. J Am Acad Orthop Surg. 2012;20(4):233–41.
5. Strohm JA, Strohm PC, Kühle J, Schmal H, Zwingmann J. Management of juvenile and aneurysmal bone cysts: a systematic literature review with meta-analysis. Eur J Trauma Emerg Surg. 2023;49(1):361–72.

6. Fei L, Ngoh C, Porter DE. Chondrosarcoma transformation in hereditary multiple exostoses: a systematic review and clinical and cost-effectiveness of a proposed screening model. J Bone Oncol. 2018;13:114–22.
7. Vu CL, Lindberg AW, Bompadre V, White KK, Bauer JM. Prospective spine at risk program for prevalence of intracanal spine lesions in pediatric hereditary multiple osteochondromas. Spine Deform. 2020;8(5):1069–74.
8. Lin PP, Moussallem CD, Deavers MT. Secondary chondrosarcoma. J Am Acad Orthop Surg. 2010;18(10):608–15.
9. Garin IE, Wang EH. Chondroblastoma. J Orthop Surg (Hong Kong). 2008;16(1):84–7.
10. Van Der Geest ICM, Van Noort MP, Schreuder HWB, Pruszczynski M, De Rooy JWJ, Veth RPH. The cryosurgical treatment of chondroblastoma of bone: long-term oncologic and functional results. J Surg Oncol. 2007;96(3):230–4.
11. De Mattos CB, Angsanuntsukh C, Arkader A, Dormans JP. Chondroblastoma and chondromyxoid fibroma. J Am Acad Orthop Surg. 2013;21(4):225–33.
12. Westacott D, Kannu P, Stimec J, Hopyan S, Howard A. Osteofibrous dysplasia of the tibia in children: outcome without resection. J Pediatr Orthop. 2019;39(8):e614–e21.
13. Laine JC, Novotny SA, Weber EW, Georgiadis AG, Dahl MT. Distal tibial guided growth for anterolateral bowing of the tibia: fracture may be prevented. J Bone Joint Surg Am. 2020;102(23):2077–86.
14. Le Corroller T, Vives T, Mattei J-C, Pauly V, Guenoun D, Rochwerger A, et al. Osteoid osteoma: percutaneous CT-guided cryoablation is a safe, effective, and durable treatment option in adults. Radiology. 2022;302(2):392–9.
15. Kneisl JS, Simon MA. Medical management compared with operative treatment for osteoid-osteoma. J Bone Joint Surg Am. 1992;74(2):179–85.

Part III

Sports Medicine

Adolescent Concussion: Head Bonk 101

20

Andrew Donaldson and Greg Canty

Introduction

Concussion was initially identified as a clinical entity in the tenth century [1]. However, the diagnosis and treatment of concussion continues to evolve. Concussion is best defined as a transient alteration in neurological function following direct or indirect head trauma. There is no definitive diagnostic test, and standard neuroimaging often appears normal. Treatment primarily involves relative rest, learning accommodations, graded exercise, and a graded return to activity, as outlined in the 2022 Consensus Statement on Concussion in Sport [2]. The average direct cost to evaluate and treat a high school football player who sustains a concussion is about $800 [3]. Not surprisingly, visits to the emergency department (ED) or urgent care (UC) for a concussion are more expensive. Additionally, a higher initial symptom burden was independently linked to increased costs [3]. This study offers a framework for value-based care when treating a concussion.

Concussion Evaluation

Neuroimaging in Pediatric Concussion

No definitive diagnostic test exists for concussion. As a result, concussion remains a clinical diagnosis. More severe traumatic brain injuries may need to be ruled out.

A. Donaldson
Pediatrics and Sports Medicine, Mosaic Life Care, St. Joseph, MO, USA

G. Canty (✉)
Department of Orthopedic Surgery, Children's Mercy, Kansas City, MO, USA
e-mail: gscanty@cmh.edu

W. L. Hennrikus, R. M. Schwend (eds.), *Value in Pediatric Orthopaedics*,
https://doi.org/10.1007/978-3-032-19570-8_20

Computed tomography (CT) is the most used imaging test to rule out more severe injuries due to its speed and diagnostic accuracy. A cross-sectional analysis of more than 75 million ED visits revealed a 28.1% increase in concussion-related visits over a 5-year period from 2006 to 2011 [4]. Corresponding with the rise in concussion visits, there was a 36% increase in head CT utilization among patients ultimately diagnosed with concussion [5]. One retrospective study of 151 pediatric patients referred to a multidisciplinary concussion clinic showed that 16% underwent head CT, with 79% of these scans yielding normal results [6].

While CT of the head plays a critical role in ruling out severe injuries such as brain bleeds, CT is expensive at up to $2000 per scan and exposes the child to additional radiation [4].

The American Academy of Neurology and the American Medical Society for Sports Medicine concussion management guidelines recommend obtaining neuroimaging only when evaluating for intracranial bleeding or other severe intracranial pathologies [2, 7]. The PECARN Pediatric Head Trauma Algorithm is a validated tool designed to guide ED physicians on when to obtain a head CT following pediatric head trauma. The PECARN algorithm demonstrated a negative predictive value of 99.95% and a sensitivity of 96.8% [8]. Subsequent validation studies have shown negative predictive values of 100% and sensitivities ranging from 98.8% to 100% [9, 10].

MRI is another potentially helpful imaging study. However, the utility of magnetic resonance imaging (MRI) is limited by expense, availability, and time required for completion of the exam. In the previously mentioned study of pediatric patients referred to a multidisciplinary concussion clinic, 11% underwent brain MRI, with 75% of those scans demonstrating normal results [6]. While advancements are being made in developing faster MRI protocols with greater sensitivity for detecting subtle changes to the brain following concussion, these MRI techniques have not yet been integrated into routine clinical practice [11].

Electronic Neurocognitive Testing

Computerized neurocognitive tests have been developed to assist in the diagnosis and management of concussion. These tests potentially provide increased sensitivity in detecting ongoing concussion-related pathology after symptoms have resolved and may help when making return-to-play decisions [2, 12–14]. Young athletes sometimes underreport symptoms to expedite clearance for return to sport. It is unclear whether returning to play while asymptomatic but still showing persistent neurocognitive deficits on a computerized test results in poor outcomes for the athlete.

The 2022 Consensus Statement on Concussion in Sport highlights the utility of neurocognitive testing, particularly for assessing reaction time. However, the statement emphasizes that neurocognitive testing should not be used in isolation to make clinical decisions [2]. A 2012 survey of American high schools with athletic trainers found that 40% incorporated computerized neurocognitive testing into their concussion management protocols. Athletes who underwent neurocognitive testing were significantly less likely to return to sport within 10 days and were more likely to be cleared for return by a physician rather than the athletic trainer [12].

In a study of 21 college NCAA Division-1 athletes with a concussion, 38% had persistent deficits on neurocognitive testing despite being symptom-free [13]. The authors suggest that return-to-play decisions based solely on symptoms may be inaccurate. Another study examining high school and college athletes diagnosed with concussion found that, compared to sideline concussion diagnoses, concussion symptom scales had a positive predictive value of 93% and a negative predictive value of 59%. Abnormal neurocognitive testing showed a positive predictive value of 83% and a negative predictive value of 70%. Combining symptom scales with neurocognitive testing increased diagnostic sensitivity by 19% [14]. When considering value, the potential increase in diagnostic yield from concussion testing must be weighed against the cost of cognitive testing batteries, particularly in schools and healthcare systems with limited resources. Unfortunately, there is no data on the outcomes of return-to-play decisions in asymptomatic athletes who still demonstrate abnormalities on neurocognitive testing.

Clinical Assessment Tools

The purpose of the sideline concussion evaluation is to remove an athlete with a concussion from play and prevent further injury. A potential additional benefit is identifying more severe intracranial pathology. The 2022 Consensus Statement recommends using the Concussion Recognition Tool-6 (CRT6), the Sport Concussion Assessment Tool-6 (SCAT6), and the Child Sport Concussion Assessment Tool-6 (Child SCAT6) for sideline concussion evaluation [2].

The CRT6 is designed for use by nonhealthcare personnel, such as coaches and teachers, and includes visible concussion cues, a list of concussion symptoms, and questions about awareness and red flag signs for severe pathology. The CRT6 instructs users to remove the athlete from play if a concussion is suspected and obtain a medical evaluation [15]. The CRT6 is free and accessible online. No studies to date have examined the specific value of the CRT6.

The SCAT6 and Child SCAT6 are the latest versions of the Sport Concussion Assessment Tool. The SCAT6 is designed for athletes aged 13 and older, while the Child SCAT6 is tailored for athletes aged 8–12 years [2]. These tools provide a multimodal approach to concussion assessment, with the greatest efficacy within the first 72 h after injury and decreasing validity up to 7 days post injury [16]. The SCAT6 includes an acute neurological evaluation, followed by an off-field assessment including the athlete's history, symptoms, immediate and delayed recall, concentration, coordination, and balance [17]. Child SCAT6 is similar but incorporates both child and parental symptom reporting and simplifies the assessment of cognitive functions [18]. The SCAT6 and Child SCAT6 are free and available online. The average time to administer either tool is 15 min. The SCAT6 and Child STAT6 can be used by athletic trainers or physicians on the sideline or later within 72 h after the injury. These tools help to standardize concussion assessments, improve research and quality improvement initiatives, foster communication among clinicians, and assist return-to-play decisions.

The 2022 Consensus Statement also recommends the Sport Concussion Office Assessment Tool-6 (SCOAT6) and the Child Sport Concussion Office Assessment Tool-6 (Child SCOAT6) [2]. The age distributions for these tools align with those of the SCAT6 and Child SCAT6. Designed for use in an office setting rather than on the sideline, the SCOAT6 and Child SCOAT6 serve as a baseline for reevaluation. The SCOAT6 includes an injury description, assessment of relevant medical conditions and medications that may complicate concussion diagnosis, family history of pertinent conditions, and a symptom evaluation list like the SCAT6. It also assesses immediate and delayed memory, concentration, and balance. Unlike the SCAT6, the SCOAT6 includes orthostatic vital signs, cervical spine assessment, and a general neurological examination, which features a modified Vestibular/Ocular-Motor Screening. In addition, the SCOAT6 includes screening questions for anxiety, depression, and sleep, along with a graded aerobic exercise test [19]. The Child SCOAT6 is similar but has simplified cognitive testing, includes both child and parental assessments of symptoms, and places less emphasis on screening for mental health [20].

Both the SCOAT6 and Child SCOAT6 are free and available online but are time-intensive. These tools identify athletes who may need subspecialty referrals and help to monitor recovery from the concussion [2]. They have been used for research purposes [21]. Lastly, they were developed by expert opinion consensus and have not undergone validation [2, 21].

Therapeutic Intervention

Exercise as Treatment

Strict rest until symptom resolution was once the standard approach for concussion treatment. However, recent research has highlighted the importance of early, non-contact physical activity in recovery. The 2022 Consensus Statement recommends beginning light aerobic activity 24–48 h after injury [2]. This recommendation is supported by systematic reviews and meta-analyses in both adult and pediatric concussion populations [22–24].

A 2023 meta-analysis by Chauhan et al. demonstrated that participation in physical activity improved symptom resolution and demonstrated no ill effect on quality of life [22]. Similarly, a 2023 systematic review and meta-analysis by Leddy et al. found that early introduction of light physical activity within the first 48 h post injury, followed by structured exercise therapy, reduced the risk of persistent post-concussive symptoms (PPCS). Leddy further suggested that mild symptom exacerbation is acceptable and does not slow recovery [23]. A retrospective study by Wilson et al. found that athletes who engaged in physical activity between injury and initial clinic evaluation demonstrated faster symptom resolution, fewer headaches, and better results on the Balance Error Scoring System (BESS) compared to those who remained inactive [25].

Exercise prescriptions can also treat sport-related concussion and PPCS [24]. In a multicenter clinical trial, Leddy et al. randomized athletes with concussion to either a prescribed aerobic exercise program or a stretching protocol. Athletes in the aerobic group recovered faster and demonstrated a 34% reduced risk of developing PPCS [26]. A similar randomized trial in 2019 reported comparable findings [27].

From a value-based perspective, prescribing exercise is an effective and low-cost intervention that improves concussion recovery. However, its implementation can be challenging and depends on a patient's social setting. In theory, any athlete can walk, jog, or run in their neighborhood; however, real-world limitations such as safety and climate conditions may restrict outdoor activity. Access to aerobic equipment at community facilities may also be limited due to the cost of membership. Although many young athletes have access to school-based gyms, these often have only weightlifting equipment, whose effectiveness in concussion treatment has not been established. Furthermore, some schools may restrict access to aerobic equipment until an athlete is fully symptom-free. These barriers highlight an advocacy opportunity for clinicians.

Vestibular Therapy

The 2022 Consensus Statement recommends referring patients for vestibular therapy if they continue to experience neck pain, dizziness, or headache 10 days post concussion [2]. Those with associated neck pain, after a negative C-spine radiograph, may also benefit from therapy aimed at treating cervical strain or sprain. The consensus statement also suggests the potential role of vestibular therapy in managing persistent postconcussive symptoms (PPCS) in children and adolescents. Vestibular therapy can be combined with subsymptom threshold aerobic exercise to improve concussion recovery [2, 28]. Galeno et al. demonstrated that vestibular therapy after concussion is associated with reduced dizziness, improved quality of life, and decreased gait impairment [29]. Earlier initiation of vestibular therapy has been linked to a shorter overall recovery time and a more rapid return to sport [30]. In a randomized trial of athletes with vestibular symptoms following concussion, those who received vestibular therapy were nearly four times more likely to be cleared for return to sport within 8 weeks compared to those who received general physical therapy and rested until symptom resolution [31]. Lastly, vestibular therapy has also been shown to improve gaze stability and reduce visual motion sensitivity, which are key factors for athletes preparing to return to play [32]. The utility of vestibular therapy is limited by the availability of qualified physical therapists and the cost of treatment. To date, no studies have specifically examined alternative delivery methods for vestibular therapy in the context of concussion [33]. Possibly, group vestibular therapy may be a value-enhancing intervention to improve concussion symptoms in certain clinical contexts since one therapist can treat multiple patients simultaneously [34].

Prevention

Primary prevention strategies often represent the highest-value interventions from a public health standpoint. Preventative measures can reduce the need for clinical evaluations, imaging studies, and specialist referrals, thereby lowering healthcare costs. Preventing concussion avoids postconcussive symptoms, missed time from school and sports, and potential mental health consequences. Where relevant, we have included current prices for products marketed for concussion prevention.

Rule and Policy Changes

Rule and policy changes are often the most value-enhancing strategies for concussion prevention. While there are intangible costs to rule changes, such as administrative time and effort required to implement rule changes, no direct costs are incurred, and outcomes are improved. For example, rules prohibiting body checking in youth ice hockey resulted in a 58% reduction in concussion rates [35]. In high school football, restricting the frequency and duration of full-contact practices led to a 57% decrease in concussions [36]. Lastly, following a professional baseball rule change limiting collisions between base runners and catchers, the number of concussions fell from 276 to 36 per year [37].

Helmets

Helmets were originally designed to prevent catastrophic neurological head injuries rather than concussions. While helmets play an important role in preventing catastrophic head injury, there remains insufficient evidence to support the effectiveness of helmets in preventing concussions [38]. For example, in football, helmets have not been shown to reduce the concussion rate. However, helmet fit and design influence the severity of concussion and the recovery time following concussions [35, 39]. In lacrosse, there was one study where helmet use demonstrated fewer concussions [40].

Mouthguards

A meta-analysis found that mouthguard use is associated with a 26% reduction in sport-related concussion in youth ice hockey [35]. Among youth ice hockey players, mouthguard use was associated with an odds ratio of only 0.36 for concussion, leading the study authors to recommend mandatory mouthguard use in this sport [41]. Notably, more expensive dentist-fitted mouthguards did not provide additional protection compared to inexpensive off-the-shelf options [35]. Mouth guards are a value-enhancing preventive strategy. Simply stated, the cost of an off-the-shelf mouthguard is only $20 while the cost to treat a concussion is $800 [3]. Further research is needed to evaluate the effectiveness of mouthguards in preventing concussion in other contact sports.

Jugular Vein Compression Collars

Jugular venous compression collars have been proposed as a potential method of concussion prevention by increasing intracranial blood volume, thereby reducing shear forces during head impacts [42]. Advanced neuroimaging studies in athletes after head injury have demonstrated greater disruption in white matter in athletes who did not wear a jugular vein compression collar [42, 43]. Neither study assessed the impact of jugular venous compression on concussion incidence or severity [35]. With an estimated cost of $200, jugular venous compression collars lack enough evidence to be recommended at this time.

Soft-Shell Helmet Covers

Soft-shell helmet covers have been proposed as a means of reducing concussion risk by reducing biomechanical forces during head impacts. However, no study has reported a reduction in biomechanical forces to the head with the use of these covers [44, 45]. A retrospective analysis of high school football players did not demonstrate a reduction in concussion with soft-shell helmet cover use [46]. However, one National Football League (NFL) study reported a 50% reduction in sport-related concussions among certain positions when using soft shell helmet covers [47]. The helmet covers available for public purchase differ significantly from those used in the NFL. Publicly available soft shell helmet covers cost up to $130 and currently lack enough evidence to be recommended for high school athletes.

Training Strategies

A range of exercise-based strategies has been proposed for their potential role in concussion prevention. In a nonrandomized prospective study, Morrissey et al. found that a 10-week core-strengthening program was associated with a reduction in sport-related concussion rates among high school athletes [35]. Additionally, neuromuscular training regimens, when performed as a warm-up at least three times per week, led to a 59% reduction in concussion incidence among adolescents [48] and a 60% reduction among adults [49]. Coaching education programs about equipment fit, tackling technique, and concussion awareness have reduced the incidence of concussions in youth and adolescent football [35].

Case Example

A high school football player sustained a head impact during a Friday night game and immediately reported headache and dizziness. He was evaluated on the sideline by the sports medicine physician using the SCAT6, diagnosed with a concussion, and removed from play. No neuroimaging was performed. The physician also recommended the initiation of light physical activity. One week later, the athlete followed up with his primary care doctor, who used the SCOAT6 for further assessment and provided a physical activity prescription. At the 2-week subsequent visit, most symptoms had resolved except for persistent dizziness. The athlete was referred to vestibular therapy, which successfully addressed his dizziness, and he was medically cleared to return to football. During his clearance visit, he inquired about strategies to prevent future concussions, noting that several teammates were using jugular venous compression collars. He was counseled that there is no current evidence supporting the effectiveness of jugular vein compression collars in preventing concussion. Instead, he was given a neuromuscular training program to perform as a warm-up at least three times per week. His coach applied the neuromuscular exercises to the entire team on Mondays, Tuesdays, and Thursdays. As a result, the team's concussion rate dropped to its lowest level in years.

Summary

Concussion remains a rapidly evolving topic within sports medicine. Numerous free or low-cost tools are available online to assist in the evaluation and management of concussion.

In this chapter, we highlight key aspects related to assessment, treatment, and prevention of concussion. In addition, we focus on methods to reduce costs, improve outcomes, and enhance value.

Author Pearls

1. Limit neuroimaging unless you suspect intracranial bleeding or severe intracranial pathology.
2. Encourage light, noncontact physical activity as soon as possible following concussion.
3. Consider referral to vestibular therapy early in the management of athletes with dizziness and neck pain.
4. To prevent concussions, advocate for rule changes, coaching education, less hitting in practice, and neuromuscular training programs.
5. Over-the-counter mouthguards and helmets are recommended for certain sports, such as ice hockey and lacrosse.

Editors Comments

WLH

Key pearls for concussion diagnosis include recognizing the injury promptly and identifying common symptoms such as headache, dizziness, blurred vision, confusion, memory difficulties, irritability, and sadness. Utilize the SCAT6 for standardized assessment, perform a thorough neurological examination, and obtain a CT scan only if a more serious head injury is suspected. The greatest value in concussion care lies in prevention. In your community, advocate for rule changes that reduce head contact, promote coaching education, and implement neuromuscular training programs for athletes.

RMS

Multidisciplinary concussion clinics can offer care for the athlete with prolonged symptoms, multiple concussions, or academic difficulty. Experienced physicians can guide families through complex decisions, such as when to stop playing contact sports after recurrent concussions or incomplete recovery. In addition, concussion clinics address modifiable recovery and preventive factors such as sleep hygiene, nutrition, and mental health.

References

1. McCrory PR, Berkovic SF. Concussion: the history of clinical and pathophysiological concepts and misconceptions. Neurology. 2001;57(12):2283–9. https://doi.org/10.1212/wnl.57.12.2283. PMID: 11756611.
2. Patricios JS, Schneider KJ, Dvorak J, Ahmed OH, Blauwet C, Cantu RC, Davis GA, Echemendia RJ, Makdissi M, McNamee M, Broglio S, Emery CA, Feddermann-Demont N, Fuller GW, Giza CC, Guskiewicz KM, Hainline B, Iverson GL, Kutcher JS, Leddy JJ, Maddocks D, Manley G, McCrea M, Purcell LK, Putukian M, Sato H, Tuominen MP, Turner M, Yeates KO, Herring SA, Meeuwisse W. Consensus statement on concussion in sport: the 6th international conference on concussion in sport-Amsterdam, October 2022. Br J Sports Med. 2023;57(11):695–711. https://doi.org/10.1136/bjsports-2023-106898. PMID: 37316210.
3. Yengo-Kahn AM, Kelly PD, Liles DC, McKeithan LJ, Grisham CJ, Khan MS, Lee T, Kuhn AW, Bonfield CM, Zuckerman SL. The cost of a single concussion in American high school football: a retrospective cohort study. Concussion. 2020;5(4):CNC81. https://doi.org/10.2217/cnc-2020-0012. PMID: 33204493; PMCID: PMC7653506.
4. Paul AB, Oklu R, Saini S, Prabhakar AM. How much is that head CT? Price transparency and variability in radiology. J Am Coll Radiol. 2015;12(5):453–7. https://doi.org/10.1016/j.jacr.2014.12.016. Epub 2015 Apr 1. PMID: 25841864.
5. Zonfrillo MR, Kim KH, Arbogast KB. Emergency department visits and head computed tomography utilization for concussion patients from 2006 to 2011. Acad Emerg Med. 2015;22(7):872–7. https://doi.org/10.1111/acem.12696. Epub 2015 Jun 25. PMID: 26111921; PMCID: PMC4503491.

6. Ellis MJ, Leiter J, Hall T, McDonald PJ, Sawyer S, Silver N, Bunge M, Essig M. Neuroimaging findings in pediatric sports-related concussion. J Neurosurg Pediatr. 2015;16(3):241–7. https://doi.org/10.3171/2015.1.PEDS14510. Epub 2015 Jun 2. PMID: 26031620.
7. Giza CC, Kutcher JS, Ashwal S, Barth J, Getchius TS, Gioia GA, Gronseth GS, Guskiewicz K, Mandel S, Manley G, McKeag DB, Thurman DJ, Zafonte R. Summary of evidence-based guideline update: evaluation and management of concussion in sports: report of the Guideline Development Subcommittee of the American Academy of Neurology. Neurology. 2013;80(24):2250–7. https://doi.org/10.1212/WNL.0b013e31828d57dd. Epub 2013 Mar 18. PMID: 23508730; PMCID: PMC3721093.
8. Kuppermann N, Holmes JF, Dayan PS, Hoyle JD Jr, Atabaki SM, Holubkov R, Nadel FM, Monroe D, Stanley RM, Borgialli DA, Badawy MK, Schunk JE, Quayle KS, Mahajan P, Lichenstein R, Lillis KA, Tunik MG, Jacobs ES, Callahan JM, Gorelick MH, Glass TF, Lee LK, Bachman MC, Cooper A, Powell EC, Gerardi MJ, Melville KA, Muizelaar JP, Wisner DH, Zuspan SJ, Dean JM, Wootton-Gorges SL, Pediatric Emergency Care Applied Research Network (PECARN). Identification of children at very low risk of clinically important brain injuries after head trauma: a prospective cohort study. Lancet. 2009;374(9696):1160–70. https://doi.org/10.1016/S0140-6736(09)61558-0. Epub 2009 Sept 14. Erratum in: Lancet. 2014;383(9914):308. PMID: 19758692.
9. Holmes JF, Yen K, Ugalde IT, Ishimine P, Chaudhari PP, Atigapramoj N, Badawy M, McCarten-Gibbs KA, Nielsen D, Sage AC, Tatro G, Upperman JS, Adelson PD, Tancredi DJ, Kuppermann N. PECARN prediction rules for CT imaging of children presenting to the emergency department with blunt abdominal or minor head trauma: a multicentre prospective validation study. Lancet Child Adolesc Health. 2024;8(5):339–47. https://doi.org/10.1016/S2352-4642(24)00029-4. PMID: 38609287.
10. Schonfeld D, Bressan S, Da Dalt L, Henien MN, Winnett JA, Nigrovic LE. Pediatric Emergency Care Applied Research Network head injury clinical prediction rules are reliable in practice. Arch Dis Child. 2014;99(5):427–31. https://doi.org/10.1136/archdischild-2013-305004. Epub 2014 Jan 15. PMID: 24431418.
11. Guenette JP, Shenton ME, Koerte IK. Imaging of concussion in young athletes. Neuroimaging Clin N Am. 2018;28(1):43–53. https://doi.org/10.1016/j.nic.2017.09.004. PMID: 29157852; PMCID: PMC5728158.
12. Meehan WP, d'Hemecourt P, Collins CL, Taylor AM, Dawn Comstock R. Computerized neurocognitive testing for the management of sport-related concussions. Pediatrics. 2012;129(1):38–44. https://doi.org/10.1542/peds.2011-1972.
13. Broglio SP, Macciocchi SN, Ferrara MS. Neurocognitive performance of concussed athletes when symptom free. J Athl Train. 2007;42(4):504–8. PMID: 18174938; PMCID: PMC2140076.
14. Van Kampen DA, Lovell MR, Pardini JE, Collins MW, Fu FH. The "value added" of neurocognitive testing after sports-related concussion. Am J Sports Med. 2006;34(10):1630–5. https://doi.org/10.1177/0363546506288677. Epub 2006 Jun 30. PMID: 16816151.
15. Echemendia RJ, Ahmed OH, Bailey CM, et al. The Concussion Recognition Tool 6 (CRT6). Br J Sports Med. 2023;57:692–4.
16. Echemendia RJ, Burma JS, Bruce JM, Davis GA, Giza CC, Guskiewicz KM, Naidu D, Black AM, Broglio S, Kemp S, Patricios JS, Putukian M, Zemek R, Arango-Lasprilla JC, Bailey CM, Brett BL, Didehbani N, Gioia G, Herring SA, Howell D, Master CL, Valovich McLeod TC, Meehan WP 3rd, Premji Z, Salmon D, van Ierssel J, Bhathela N, Makdissi M, Walton SR, Kissick J, Pardini J, Schneider KJ. Acute evaluation of sport-related concussion and implications for the Sport Concussion Assessment Tool (SCAT6) for adults, adolescents and children: a systematic review. Br J Sports Med. 2023;57(11):722–35. https://doi.org/10.1136/bjsports-2022-106661. PMID: 37316213.
17. Echemendia RJ, Brett BL, Broglio S, et al. Sport Concussion Assessment Tool 6 (SCAT6). Br J Sports Med. 2023;57:622–31.
18. Davis GA, Echemendia RJ, Ahmed OH, et al. Child SCAT6. Br J Sports Med. 2023;57:636–47.

19. Patricios J, Schneider GM, van Ierssel J, et al. Sport Concussion Office Assessment Tool 6 (SCOAT6). Br J Sports Med. 2023;57:651–67.
20. Davis GA, Patricios JS, Purcell LK, et al. Child SCOAT6. Br J Sports Med. 2023;57:672–88.
21. Patricios JS, Davis GA, Ahmed OH, Blauwet C, Schneider GM, Purcell LK, Echemendia RJ, Fremont P, Fuller GW, Herring SA, Harmon KG, Loosemore M, Makdissi M, O'Halloran P, Putukian M, Turner M, Webborn N, Yeates KO, van Ierssel J, Schneider KJ. Introducing the Sport Concussion Office Assessment Tool 6 (SCOAT6). Br J Sports Med. 2023;57(11):648–50. https://doi.org/10.1136/bjsports-2023-106860. Erratum in: Br J Sports Med 2023;57(21):e4. doi: 10.1136/bjsports-2023-106860corr1. PMID: 37316211.
22. Chauhan R, Cheng A, Tsow R, Sakakibara BM, Babul S, Schmidt J. Activity and recovery among youth with concussion: a meta-analysis. Pediatrics. 2023;151(5):e2022059592. https://doi.org/10.1542/peds.2022-059592.
23. Leddy JJ, Burma JS, Toomey CM, et al. Rest and exercise early after sport-related concussion: a systematic review and meta-analysis. Br J Sports Med. 2023;57:762–70.
24. Haider MN, Bezherano I, Wertheimer A, Siddiqui AH, Horn EC, Willer BS, Leddy JJ. Exercise for sport-related concussion and persistent postconcussive symptoms. Sports Health. 2021;13(2):154–60. https://doi.org/10.1177/1941738120946015. Epub 2020 Nov 4. PMID: 33147117; PMCID: PMC8167349.
25. Wilson JC, Kirkwood MW, Potter MN, Wilson PE, Provance AJ, Howell DR. Early physical activity and clinical outcomes following pediatric sport-related concussion. J Clin Transl Res. 2020;5(4):161–8. PMID: 33029564; PMCID: PMC7534529.
26. Leddy JJ, Master CL, Mannix R, Wiebe DJ, Grady MF, Meehan WP, Storey EP, Vernau BT, Brown NJ, Hunt D, Mohammed F, Mallon A, Rownd K, Arbogast KB, Cunningham A, Haider MN, Mayer AR, Willer BS. Early targeted heart rate aerobic exercise versus placebo stretching for sport-related concussion in adolescents: a randomised controlled trial. Lancet Child Adolesc Health. 2021;5(11):792–9. https://doi.org/10.1016/S2352-4642(21)00267-4. Epub 2021 Oct 1. PMID: 34600629.
27. Leddy JJ, Haider MN, Ellis MJ, et al. Early subthreshold aerobic exercise for sport-related concussion: a randomized clinical trial. JAMA Pediatr. 2019;173(4):319–25. https://doi.org/10.1001/jamapediatrics.2018.4397.
28. Schneider KJ, Critchley ML, Anderson V, et al. Targeted interventions and their effect on recovery in children, adolescents and adults who have sustained a sport-related concussion: a systematic review. Br J Sports Med. 2023;57:771–9.
29. Galeno E, Pullano E, Mourad F, Galeoto G, Frontani F. Effectiveness of vestibular rehabilitation after concussion: a systematic review of randomised controlled trial. Healthcare (Basel). 2022;11(1):90. https://doi.org/10.3390/healthcare11010090. PMID: 36611549; PMCID: PMC9819464.
30. Zargari M, Williams K, Jo J, et al. Does earlier vestibular therapy after sport-related concussion lead to faster recovery? J Neurosurg Pediatr. 2023;32(6):657–64. https://doi.org/10.3171/2023.7.PEDS23172.
31. Schneider KJ, Meeuwisse WH, Nettel-Aguirre A, et al. Cervicovestibular rehabilitation in sport-related concussion: a randomised controlled trial. Br J Sports Med. 2014;48:1294–8.
32. Broglio SP, Collins MW, Williams RM, Mucha A, Kontos AP. Current and emerging rehabilitation for concussion: a review of the evidence. Clin Sports Med. 2015;34(2):213–31. https://doi.org/10.1016/j.csm.2014.12.005. Epub 2015 Jan 24. PMID: 25818710; PMCID: PMC4387881.
33. van Vugt VA, Bosmans JE, Finch AP, van der Wouden JC, van der Horst HE, Maarsingh OR. Cost-effectiveness of internet-based vestibular rehabilitation with and without physiotherapy support for adults aged 50 and older with a chronic vestibular syndrome in general practice. BMJ Open. 2020;10(10):e035583. https://doi.org/10.1136/bmjopen-2019-035583. PMID: 33060078; PMCID: PMC7566722.
34. Han JS, Park JM, Kim Y, Seo JH, Park SY, Park SN. Group vestibular rehabilitation program: a cost-effective outpatient management option for dizzy patients. Otol Neurotol.

2022;43(9):1065–71. https://doi.org/10.1097/MAO.0000000000003675. Epub 2022 Sept 9. PMID: 36075105.

35. Eliason PH, Galarneau J, Kolstad AT, et al. Prevention strategies and modifiable risk factors for sport-related concussions and head impacts: a systematic review and meta-analysis. Br J Sports Med. 2023;57:749–61.
36. Pfaller AY, Brooks MA, Hetzel S, McGuine TA. Effect of a new rule limiting full contact practice on the incidence of sport-related concussion in high school football players. Am J Sports Med. 2019;47(10):2294–9. https://doi.org/10.1177/0363546519860120. Epub 2019 Jul 15. PMID: 31306587.
37. Green G, D'Angelo J, Coyles J, Penny I, Golfinos JG, Valadka A. Association between a rule change to reduce home plate collisions and mild traumatic brain injury and other injuries in professional baseball players. Am J Sports Med. 2019;47(11):2704–8. https://doi.org/10.1177/0363546519861525. Epub 2019 Jul 23. PMID: 31336057.
38. McGuine TA, Hetzel S, McCrea M, Brooks MA. Protective equipment and player characteristics associated with the incidence of sport-related concussion in high school football players: a multifactorial prospective study. Am J Sports Med. 2014;42(10):2470–8. https://doi.org/10.1177/0363546514541926. Epub 2014 Jul 24. PMID: 25060072; PMCID: PMC4477806.
39. Greenhill DA, Navo P, Zhao H, Torg J, Comstock RD, Boden BP. Inadequate helmet fit increases concussion severity in American high school football players. Sports Health. 2016;8(3):238–43. https://doi.org/10.1177/1941738116639027. Epub 2016 Mar 22. PMID: 27005467; PMCID: PMC4981070.
40. Comstock RD, Arakkal AT, Pierpoint LA, Fields SK. Are high school girls' lacrosse players at increased risk of concussion because they are not allowed to wear the same helmet boys' lacrosse players are required to wear? Inj Epidemiol. 2020;7(1):18. https://doi.org/10.1186/s40621-020-00242-5. PMID: 32418542; PMCID: PMC7232834.
41. Chisholm DA, Black AM, Palacios-Derflingher L, Eliason PH, Schneider KJ, Emery CA, Hagel BE. Mouthguard use in youth ice hockey and the risk of concussion: nested case-control study of 315 cases. Br J Sports Med. 2020;54(14):866–70. https://doi.org/10.1136/bjsports-2019-101011. Epub 2020 Jan 14. PMID: 31937578.
42. Myer GD, Yuan W, Barber Foss KD, Smith D, Altaye M, Reches A, Leach J, Kiefer AW, Khoury JC, Weiss M, Thomas S, Dicesare C, Adams J, Gubanich PJ, Geva A, Clark JF, Meehan WP 3rd, Mihalik JP, Krueger D. The effects of external jugular compression applied during head impact exposure on longitudinal changes in brain neuroanatomical and neurophysiological biomarkers: a preliminary investigation. Front Neurol. 2016;7:74. https://doi.org/10.3389/fneur.2016.00074. PMID: 27375546; PMCID: PMC4893920.
43. Myer GD, Yuan W, Barber Foss KD, Thomas S, Smith D, Leach J, Kiefer AW, Dicesare C, Adams J, Gubanich PJ, Kitchen K, Schneider DK, Braswell D, Krueger D, Altaye M. Analysis of head impact exposure and brain microstructure response in a season-long application of a jugular vein compression collar: a prospective, neuroimaging investigation in American football. Br J Sports Med. 2016;50(20):1276–85. https://doi.org/10.1136/bjsports-2016-096134. Epub 2016 Jun 15. PMID: 27307271; PMCID: PMC5099231.
44. Sinnott AM, Chandler MC, Van Dyke C, Mincberg DL, Pinapaka H, Lauck BJ, Mihalik JP. Efficacy of Guardian Cap soft-shell padding on head impact kinematics in American football: pilot findings. Int J Environ Res Public Health. 2023;20(21):6991. https://doi.org/10.3390/ijerph20216991. PMID: 37947549; PMCID: PMC10650906.
45. Breedlove KM, Breedlove E, Nauman E, Bowman TG, Lininger MR. The ability of an aftermarket helmet add-on device to reduce impact-force accelerations during drop tests. J Athl Train. 2017;52(9):802–8. https://doi.org/10.4085/1062-6050-52.6.01. Epub 2017 Aug 3. PMID: 28771033; PMCID: PMC5634228.
46. Hammer E, Mosiman S, Joachim MR, et al. The association between Guardian Cap use during practices and sport-related concussion risk in high school American football players. Br J Sports Med. 2025;59:257–62.

47. NFL. Guardian Cap results: "exceeded our expectations". NFL.com. 19 Sept 2022. https://www.nfl.com/playerhealthandsafety/equipment-and-innovation/engineering-technology/guardian-cap-results-exceeded-our-expectations.
48. Hislop MD, Stokes KA, Williams S, McKay CD, England ME, Kemp SPT, Trewartha G. Reducing musculoskeletal injury and concussion risk in schoolboy rugby players with a pre-activity movement control exercise programme: a cluster randomised controlled trial. Br J Sports Med. 2017;51(15):1140–6. https://doi.org/10.1136/bjsports-2016-097434. Epub 2017 May 17. PMID: 28515056; PMCID: PMC5530334.
49. Attwood MJ, Roberts SP, Trewartha G, England ME, Stokes KA. Efficacy of a movement control injury prevention programme in adult men's community rugby union: a cluster randomised controlled trial. Br J Sports Med. 2018;52(6):368–74. https://doi.org/10.1136/bjsports-2017-098005. Epub 2017 Oct 21. PMID: 29055883; PMCID: PMC5867421.

Methods to Improve Value in Pediatric/ Adolescent ACL Reconstruction

21

Josh Cummings, Kadarius Burgess, Claudius Ciecko, and Ryan Koehler

Introduction

Anterior cruciate ligament reconstruction (ACLR) surgery has become one of the most performed sports medicine surgeries in the USA, with approximately 400,000 ACLR procedures occurring each year [1]. Likewise, anterior cruciate injury (ACLI) and its treatment have also been extensively studied to advance surgical techniques and improve patient outcomes. Efforts to improve outcomes have resulted in changes in preoperative, intraoperative, and postoperative care. Much of the research has focused on improving return-to-sport rates, reducing graft failure rates, and reporting patient-reported outcomes. However, given the costs associated with ACLR, it is crucial for both patients and physicians to consider value-based decision-making throughout the entire treatment process.

Preoperative ACLR: Avoiding Delays in Treatment Through Early Diagnosis and Prehabilitation

Value-based decisions in ACLR include timely diagnosis, the use of advanced imaging, rehabilitation strategies, and the costs associated with delayed care.

J. Cummings · K. Burgess · C. Ciecko
University of Missouri Kansas City, Kansas City, MO, USA

R. Koehler (✉)
Department of Orthopaedics, Children's Mercy Hospital, Kansas City, MO, USA
e-mail: rjkoehler@cmh.edu

W. L. Hennrikus, R. M. Schwend (eds.), *Value in Pediatric Orthopaedics*,
https://doi.org/10.1007/978-3-032-19570-8_21

Using Imaging for Complete Diagnosis

Radiographic imaging has value in ACLI evaluation. Radiographs can provide important information for surgical planning, such as detecting associated fractures, assessing physeal closure in skeletally immature patients, and evaluating tibial slope. Nonspecific findings on knee X-rays in the context of ACLI may include Segond fractures, arcuate fractures, joint effusions, deep sulcus terminalis signs, or a deep lateral sulcus sign [1–3].

Magnetic resonance imaging (MRI) also adds value. MRI has a sensitivity of 95.45% and specificity of 91.67% in diagnosing ACLI [4]. Unfortunately, the average cost of a musculoskeletal MRI in the USA in 2022 was approximately $1302 [5]. While there is a lack of specific cost-effectiveness data for MRI in the context of ACLI, many considered the MRI an essential diagnostic tool particularly for identification of additional operative injuries as well as determining partial versus complete ACLI [6].

Costs of Prehabilitation Versus Quicker Return to Sport

Therapy focused on improving knee range of motion and strength before ACLR surgery is known as prehabilitation [7]. The goal of prehabilitation is to restore joint homeostasis, neuromuscular control, strength, and proprioception [8]. Patients who undergo 4–6 weeks of prehabilitation before surgery demonstrate a higher rate of return to sport, earlier return to sport, and improved postoperative range of motion and strength [9]. Patients on average returned to sports at 42.5 weeks in a no prehabilitation group compared to 34.2 weeks for the prehabilitation group. Additionally, prehabilitation patients have demonstrated a higher rate of return to sport at the preinjury level [10]. Variations in the prehabilitation protocols is common [11]. Unfortunately, prehabilitation also adds to the overall cost of care [12]. The outcomes and costs of self-guided versus therapist-guided pre-rehabilitation have not been compared. Lastly, limited data exists on how many athletes complete a prehabilitation program prior to ACLR [13].

The Heavy Cost of Delayed ACL Care

ACLI are not surgical emergencies, and most patients will have a delay before surgery of about 6 weeks to complete prehabilitation. In addition, lower income patients sometimes have additional delays. For example, higher Area Deprivation Index (ADI) percentiles and Medicaid insurance status are associated with delays in evaluation [14, 15]. Due to delays, Medicaid insurance and lower socioeconomic status (SES) are linked to an increased risk of second ACLI which is a significant increase in cost both to the athlete and the system. A 5.1% risk of a second ACLI has been calculated for every month of delay until the index surgery [14]. Furthermore, delays in treatment contribute to higher rates of meniscal tears and poorer patient-reported outcomes [16]. One study found that the cost of care increases by $8.09 for each day of diagnostic delay for operative ACLI [17]. Additionally, for every $10,000 increase in household income, the time from injury to reconstruction decreases by 19% [18]. This pattern of low family income leading to delays in care is not unique to ACLI [19].

Intraoperative ACL Care: Optimizing Outcomes Through a Value Conscious Surgical Plan

Choosing Surgery Is the First Step in Value

The decision to undergo ACLR involves upfront costs but has been shown to result in mean cost savings of $50,417 and a gain of 0.72 quality-adjusted life years (QALY) compared to rehabilitation alone [20]. Early ACLR is a more cost-effective strategy for younger, athletic patients. However, older, less active patients may benefit from a nonoperative approach or a delayed reconstruction strategy in terms of financial savings per patient and increased QALYs [21].

Selecting a Graft This Cost-Efficient and Effective

For most young athletes undergoing ACLR, autografts are preferred, because allografts have higher rates of retear and added costs [20]. Both hamstring and quadriceps autografts are good options for younger patients but can lead to weakness in the muscle groups from which the graft is harvested. In the youngest ACL patients with several years of growth remaining, an iliotibial band autograft, used in a physeal-sparing manner, or a soft tissue autograft with all epiphyseal sockets, can be performed. From a strength perspective, all autografts demonstrate higher loads to failure compared to the native ACL and are considered reasonable choices [22]. The most cost-effective graft option for pediatric and adolescent patients is controversial. Hamstring autografts have been shown to increase costs by approximately $500 compared to bone-tendon-bone autografts due to longer operative times and the higher cost of suspensory fixation compared to aperture fixation [23]. The iliotibial band autograft offers the lowest cost for pediatric patients with several years of growth remaining. This graft can be easily harvested and fixed with suture alone. However, for adolescent patients, hamstring, quadriceps tendon, and patellar bone-tendon-bone grafts all have supporting evidence. Patellar bone-tendon-bone autografts with aperture fixation, in combination with an anterolateral procedure, may be the overall most cost-effective graft.

One important consideration in graft choice is the risk of reinjury and the potential need for revision ACL reconstruction. Revision surgery increases the overall cost of ACL care. The addition of adjunct procedures to ACLR, such as lateral extra-articular tenodesis or anterolateral ligament reconstruction, reduces the risk of graft failure and is cost-effective when compared to ACLR alone [24].

Biologic Adjuncts and Navigation

The role of biologics and navigation in pediatric and adolescent ACLR remains unstudied. In the adult literature, however, platelet-rich plasma injections in ACLR have shown no beneficial effects [25]. Similarly, navigation systems hold promise, but they have not consistently led to improved outcomes when compared to traditional surgical techniques [26].

Choosing the Right Surgery Setting

Most pediatric and adolescent ACL patients are generally healthy, with few or no comorbidities, making them suitable candidates for surgery at an ambulatory surgery center (ASC). ASCs have lower overall costs by $6789 due to increased efficiency and reduced operating expenses compared to a hospital outpatient facility. However, patient costs may not differ between the two settings and can depend on insurance type, in-network status, and co-pay requirements [27, 28]. For patients with flexibility in location for the surgery, selecting the site for surgery based on network status and costs can improve value.

Local Anesthesia and Regional Block Location

The use of regional anesthesia as part of a multimodal pain management strategy for ACL reconstruction is common and has been shown in one study to be cost-effective [29]. However, another study reported no difference in postoperative pain levels or outcomes between regional blocks and surgeon-administered local anesthesia [30]. Furthermore, when regional blocks are performed in the operating room, the block increases operating room time and incurs a separate billable procedure for the anesthesia doctor, increasing the overall cost of care. Using local anesthetics more judiciously or performing regional blocks in dedicated spaces outside the operating room are potential strategies to decrease the cost of ACLR.

Postoperative ACL Care: Choosing Effective and Cost Friendly Protection Measures for Safe Return

Increasing Strength and Motion Without Increasing Cost

Postoperative rehabilitation is an important component of ACLR recovery. Most rehabilitation protocols focus on strengthening, range of motion, agility, neuromuscular control, and functional testing to ensure a safe return to sport. Early motion is generally employed to reduce postoperative knee stiffness [31]. The use of continuous passive motion (CPM) machines has not been shown to improve pain, range of motion, or swelling [32]. Optimizing a patient's time in therapy and supplementing in-person sessions with an effective home exercise program can reduce the number of visits required, lowering overall costs. Additionally, home adjuncts like neuromuscular electrical stimulation can improve muscle recovery in the muscle groups affected by autograft harvest.

Mixed Results of Bracing for an Increase in Cost

Bracing protocols after ACLR vary between surgeons and can increase overall costs. Some surgeons prescribe a post-op hinged knee brace to protect the graft and limit range-of-motion. However, one study showed no difference in outcomes between patients who are braced versus those who are unbraced during the postoperative period [33]. The use of functional ACL sports bracing for activities involving cutting, pivoting, and twisting has shown mixed results. One study concluded that functional bracing did not improve clinical outcomes related to knee stability or function [34], while another found that bracing did not reduce the rate of reinjury [35]. However, Perrone et al. found that for patients under 18 years old, functional bracing reduced the risk of graft tear [36]. Functional braces are expensive and increase the overall cost of care but potentially limit risk of costly re-injury to the knee.

Functional Testing to Safely Return to Sport

The timeline for returning to sport after ACLR varies depending on either time-specific criteria or functional testing. Dowd et al. recently reported using a series of functional tests [37]. These tests typically measure ability to perform rehab activities such as single-leg hop, single-leg triple hop, single-leg triple crossover hop, box-drop vertical jump, single-leg 4-rep max incline leg press, and a modified agility *T*-test to attempt to replicate movement patterns in sports. Passing these functional tests reduced the risk of ACL retear by 36% and reduced the risk of contralateral ACLI by 19% with younger patients were likely to fail the tests and experience a contralateral ACLI. Similarly, another study reported that passing a functional test battery including repeat sprint ability, dynamic valgus, pro agility, unilateral countermovement jump, isokinetic testing, triple hop test, and functional movement screen resulted in zero graft retears at an average follow-up of 27 months [38].

Minimizing Postoperative Imaging

Postoperative X-rays following ACLR are often used to assess tunnel placement, graft incorporation, or complications [39]. Radiographs are typically obtained at various intervals, which increases the cost and radiation exposure to the patient [40, 41]. Most post-op radiographs rarely alter clinical management and are therefore generally not cost-effective [41]. One exception is in young, growing patients, where postoperative X-rays help monitor for growth arrest. In general, post-op X-rays should be performed on a case-by-case basis based on symptoms and young age.

Conclusion

Several key themes emerge when evaluating methods to improve value for patients with ACL injury. Early diagnosis and delayed surgical treatment for prehabilitation improve outcomes and reduce overall costs. Home exercises and minimizing physical therapy visits can help reduce costs. Graft selection remains a complex decision. However, autografts and simple, inexpensive fixation methods are the most cost-effective. The addition of an anterolateral adjunct procedure for high-risk patients is also a cost-effective way to reduce the risk of graft retear. Minimizing post-op and functional bracing reduces costs. Post-op rehabilitation and functional testing before returning to high-risk sports decrease the risk of graft retear and the need for revision surgery.

Author Pearls

1. Timely diagnosis and access to MRI reduce downstream costs from instability and secondary meniscal injury.
2. Prehabilitation improves outcomes but should be tailored; structured home programs can reduce therapy costs.
3. Autografts are generally the most cost-effective graft choice for adolescents; avoid allografts due to higher retear rates and added expense.
4. Ambulatory surgery centers are safe and often less costly than hospital-based outpatient facilities.
5. Avoid routine postoperative radiographs except in skeletally immature patients at risk for growth arrest.
6. Continuous passive motion machines and routine postoperative bracing do not improve outcomes and add unnecessary cost.
7. Functional testing before return to sport reduces reinjury and prevents costly revisions.
8. Return-to-sport discussions should include not just readiness but also the long-term value of modifying activity to preserve knee health.
9. Equity matters: delays in diagnosis and surgery disproportionately affect poor patients and increase overall costs.

Case Example

A 15-year-old female high school soccer player sustained a noncontact valgus knee injury during a game. She was insured through Medicaid and lived in a rural county 2 h from the children's hospital, so she did not seek care and thought she had a "knee sprain." She returned to soccer after 2 weeks of rest and sustained a second noncontact knee injury with more knee swelling and mechanical locking this time. She was then evaluated by a medical sports medicine provider and diagnosed with an ACL tear with subsequent MRI showing additional displaced bucket handle lateral meniscus tear (Figs. 21.1 and 21.2). She was started in pre-op physical therapy with visits focused on restoring knee range of motion and function and

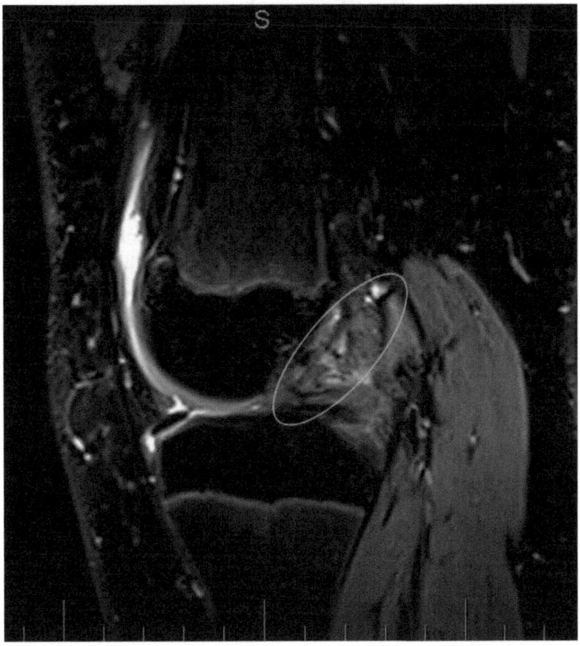

Fig. 21.1 MRI showing complete ACL tear on PD sagittal view

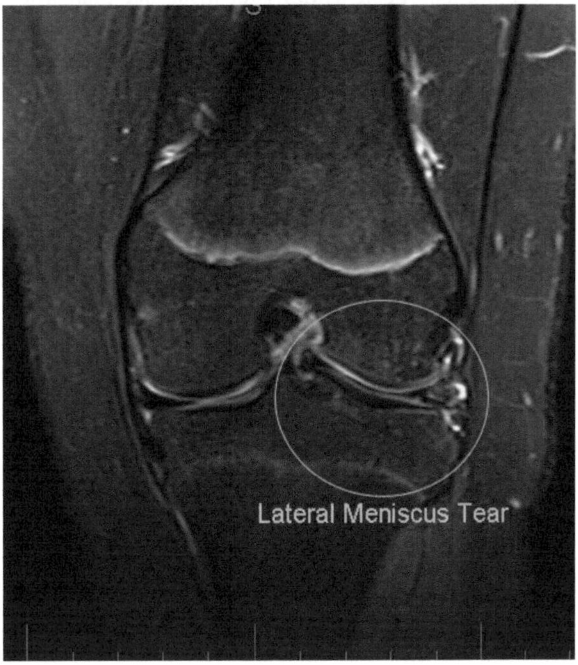

Fig. 21.2 MRI showing lateral meniscus bucket tear and T2 coronal view

completed mostly utilizing a home exercise program to minimize cost and visit utilization for after surgery. She then underwent ACL reconstruction with bone patella tendon bone autograft with aperture fixation as well as meniscus repair using an inside-out technique. Surgery was completed outpatient at an ambulatory surgery center reducing overall cost including implant and facility fees. Her follow-up visits were a combination of telehealth and in-person to reduce family cost and burden of travel. She followed an objective postoperative physical therapy protocol and passed a functional return-to-sport test battery before clearance back to soccer 12 months after surgery. At 2-year follow-up, she had no reinjury and full knee function and avoided the costs of revision surgery. This case highlights how timely diagnosis, use of home-based rehab, cost-conscious graft and facility choices, and value-based return-to-sport testing can reduce total cost while preserving long-term knee health.

Editor Comments

WLH

ACL surgery can be expensive, with estimated fees as follows: surgeon's fee $1000; anesthesia fee $2000; physical therapy fee $2000; braces, crutches, and CPM equipment fees $2000; and facility fee $15,000.

To improve value, consider the following suggestions:

- Choose a surgeon within your insurance plan who can perform the surgery at a day surgery center also in-network.
- Use your Health Savings Account (HSA) to cover out-of-pocket expenses.
- Minimize postoperative X-rays.
- Advocate for a home-based physical therapy program whenever possible.
- Limit the use of braces, as they may not be necessary.
- Continuous passive motion (CPM) devices are generally not required.
- Wait at least 9 months before returning to contact sports after ACL reconstruction.
- Negotiate with the surgery center upfront and inquire about potential discounts.
- Use the Healthcare Bluebook to compare prices at different facilities: Healthcare Bluebook.

RMS

One important area of value in ACL care that deserves emphasis is the decision about when, or even whether, to return to high-risk sports after successful ACLR. While surgical reconstruction restores knee stability, the highest costs to patients, families, and society often arise not from the surgery itself, but from reinjury. Adolescents returning to pivoting sports before adequate physical and psychological recovery face dramatically increased risks of graft failure and contralateral ACL tears, leading to additional operations, prolonged rehabilitation, and long-term osteoarthritis. Families and surgeons should weigh not only physical readiness but also the implications of sport choice and timing of return.

Not all adolescents have the desire or determination to return to sport, especially if the sport is not that enjoyable or important to them or they have other activities they prefer to do. In these situations, a discussion of the need for primary ACLR may also be appropriate for isolated complete or partial ACL injury. Shared decision-making that includes discussions about safer sport alternatives, delayed return, or permanent activity can sometimes provide the greatest overall value by reducing reinjury risk and preserving lifelong knee health.

References

1. Evans J, Nielson J, Mabrouk A. Anterior cruciate ligament (ACL) knee injuries [Internet]. Nih.gov. StatPearls Publishing; 2023. Available from: https://www.ncbi.nlm.nih.gov/books/NBK499848/
2. Adriani E, Summa P, Paola BD. Pre-operative planning in anterior cruciate ligament reconstruction revision surgery. Joints [Internet]. 2013;1(1):25. [cited 2025 Jan 22]. Available from: https://pmc.ncbi.nlm.nih.gov/articles/PMC4295686/
3. Ng WHA. Imaging of the anterior cruciate ligament. World J Orthop [Internet]. 2011;2(8):75. Available from: https://www.ncbi.nlm.nih.gov/pmc/articles/PMC3302044/
4. Zhao M, Zhou Y, Chang J, Hu J, Liu H, Wang S, et al. The accuracy of MRI in the diagnosis of anterior cruciate ligament injury. Ann Transl Med [Internet]. 2020;8(24) Available from: https://www.ncbi.nlm.nih.gov/pmc/articles/PMC7812197/#r9
5. Kjelle E, Brandsæter IØ, Andersen ER, Hofmann BM. Cost of low-value imaging worldwide: a systematic review. Applied health economics and health policy; 2024.
6. Suarez-Almazor ME, Kaul P, Kendall CJ, Saunders LD, Johnston DW. The cost-effectiveness of magnetic resonance imaging for patients with internal derangement of the knee. Int J Technol Assess Health Care [Internet]. 1999;15(2):392–405. Available from: https://pubmed.ncbi.nlm.nih.gov/10507197/
7. Cunha J, Solomon DJ. ACL prehabilitation improves postoperative strength and motion and return to sport in athletes. Arthrosc Sports Med Rehabil. 2022;4(1):e65–9.
8. Waldron K, Brown M, Calderon A, Feldman M. Anterior cruciate ligament rehabilitation and return to sport: how fast is too fast? Arthrosc Sports Med Rehabil [Internet]. 2022;4(1):e175–9. Available from: https://www.ncbi.nlm.nih.gov/pmc/articles/PMC8811519/
9. Shaarani SR, O'Hare C, Quinn A, Moyna N, Moran R, O'Byrne JM. Effect of prehabilitation on the outcome of anterior cruciate ligament reconstruction. Am J Sports Med. 2013;41(9):2117–27.
10. Failla MJ, Logerstedt DS, Grindem H, Axe MJ, Risberg MA, Engebretsen L, et al. Does extended preoperative rehabilitation influence outcomes 2 years after ACL reconstruction? Am J Sports Med. 2016;44(10):2608–14.
11. Giesche F, Niederer D, Banzer W, Vogt L. Evidence for the effects of prehabilitation before ACL-reconstruction on return to sport-related and self-reported knee function: A systematic review. Mirkov D, editor. PLoS One. 2020;15(10):e0240192.
12. Zhang JY, Cohen JR, Yeranosian MG, Lord EL, Wang JC, Petrigliano FA, et al. Rehabilitation charges associated with anterior cruciate ligament reconstruction. Sports Health Multidiscip Approach. 2015;7(6):538–41.
13. Abel R, Niederer D, Offerhaus C, Shafizadeh S, Glowa A, Froböse I, et al. Effects of exercise prehabilitation before anterior cruciate ligament reconstruction on functional outcomes during pre- and postoperative rehabilitation – protocol for a single-blinded randomised controlled trial. Trials. 2023;24(1).
14. Cherelstein RE, Natal-Albelo EJ, Kuenze CM, Curley AJ, Bodendorfer BM, Hopkins M, et al. The effect of greater area deprivation and medicaid insurance status on timing of care

and rate of reinjury after anterior cruciate ligament reconstruction. Orthop J Sports Med [Internet]. 2024;12(6):23259671241240751. Available from: https://pubmed.ncbi.nlm.nih.gov/38863506/
15. Kind AJH, Buckingham WR. Making neighborhood-disadvantage metrics accessible – the neighborhood Atlas. N Engl J Med. 2018;378(26):2456–8. AND University of Wisconsin School of Medicine Public Health. 2015 Area Deprivation Index v2.0. Downloaded from https://www.neighborhoodatlas.medicine.wisc.edu/ Feb 01, 2025.
16. Zoller SD, Toy KA, Wang PJ, Ebramzadeh E, Bowen RA. Temporal relation of meniscal tear incidence, severity, and outcome scores in adolescents undergoing anterior cruciate ligament reconstruction. 2017;25(1):215–21.
17. Cook S, Byrnes T, Hagen M, Gee A, Kweon C, Slattery C. Increased costs and health care utilization associated with delay in diagnosis of ACL injuries. Orthop J Sports Med. 2020;8(7_suppl6):2325967120S0048.
18. Leveille LA, Ladner TV, Sidhu P, Reilly CW. Delay in diagnosis and management of adolescent anterior cruciate ligament injuries in a publicly funded healthcare system. Orthop J Sports Med [Internet]. 2020;8(4_suppl3) [cited 2025 May 8]. Available from: https://pmc.ncbi.nlm.nih.gov/articles/PMC7225814/
19. Zhuang T, Eppler SL, Shapiro LM, Roe AK, Yao J, Kamal RN. Financial distress is associated with delay in seeking care for hand conditions. HAND [Internet]. 2019;16(4):511–8. [cited 2023 May 5]. Available from: https://www.ncbi.nlm.nih.gov/pmc/articles/PMC8283103/
20. Mather RC, Koenig L, Kocher MS, Dall TM, Gallo P, Scott DJ, et al. Societal and economic impact of anterior cruciate ligament tears. J Bone Joint Surg Am Vol. 2013;95(19):1751–9.
21. Deviandri R, van der Veen HC, Lubis AMT, van den Akker-Scheek I, Postma MJ. Cost-effectiveness of ACL treatment is dependent on age and activity level: a systematic review. Knee Surg Sports Traumatol Arthrosc. 2022;31(2):530–41.
22. Cruz AI, Beck JJ, Ellington MD, Mayer SW, Pennock AT, Stinson ZS, et al. Failure rates of autograft and allograft ACL reconstruction in patients 19 years of age and younger. JBJS Open Access. 2020;5(4):e20.00106–6.
23. Buerba RA, Boden SA, Lesniak B. Graft selection in contemporary anterior cruciate ligament reconstruction. JAAOS Glob Res Rev. 2021;5(10).
24. Varady NH, Oeding JF, Inclan PM, Ranawat AS, Strickland SM, Pearle AD, Rodeo SA, Williams RJ 3rd. Adding a lateral extra-articular tenodesis is cost-effective in primary anterior cruciate ligament reconstruction: a Markov analysis. Arthroscopy. 2025:S0749-8063(25)00427-X. https://doi.org/10.1016/j.arthro.2025.06.004. PMID: 40543680.
25. Zhu T, Zhou J, Hwang J, Xu X. Effects of platelet-rich plasma on clinical outcomes after anterior cruciate ligament reconstruction: a systematic review and meta-analysis. Orthop J Sports Med [Internet]. 2022;10(1):23259671211061535. [cited 2022 Feb 15]. Available from: https://pubmed.ncbi.nlm.nih.gov/35127959/
26. Saltzman BM, Cvetanovich GL, Nwachukwu BU, Mall NA, Bush-Joseph CA, Bach BR. Economic analyses in anterior cruciate ligament reconstruction. Am J Sports Med. 2015;44(5):1329–35.
27. Huyke-Hernández FA, Siljander B, Flagstad I, Only AJ, Parikh HR, Tompkins M, et al. Cost and cost driver analysis of anterior cruciate ligament reconstruction using time-driven activity-based costing. JB JS Open Access. 2022;7:4.
28. Tiao J, Wang K, Carbone AD, Herrera M, Zubizarreta N, Gladstone JN, et al. Ambulatory surgery centers significantly decrease total health care expenditures in primary anterior cruciate ligament reconstruction. Am J Sports Med. 2022;51(1):97–106.
29. Hall-Burton DM, Hudson ME, Grudziak JS, Cunningham S, Boretsky K, Boretsky KR. Regional anesthesia is cost-effective in preventing unanticipated hospital admission in pediatric patients having anterior cruciate ligament reconstruction. Reg Anesth Pain Med. 2016;41(4):527–31.
30. Stebler K, Martin R, Kirkham KR, Lambert J, De Sede A, Albrecht E. Adductor canal block versus local infiltration analgesia for postoperative pain after anterior cruciate ligament reconstruction: a single centre randomised controlled triple-blinded trial. 2019;123(2):e343–9.

31. Noyes FR, Mangine RE, Barber S. Early knee motion after open and arthroscopic anterior cruciate ligament reconstruction. Am J Sports Med. 1987;15(2):149–60.
32. Wright RW, Preston E, Fleming BC, Amendola A, Andrish JT, Bergfeld JA, et al. A systematic review of anterior cruciate ligament reconstruction rehabilitation: Part I: Continuous passive motion, early weight bearing, postoperative bracing, and home-based rehabilitation. J Knee Surg. 2008;21(3):217–24.
33. Kruse LM, Gray B, Wright RW. Rehabilitation after anterior cruciate ligament reconstruction: a systematic review. J Bone Joint Surg Am. 2012;94(19):1737–48.
34. Yang XG, Feng JT, He X, Wang F, Hu YC. The effect of knee bracing on the knee function and stability following anterior cruciate ligament reconstruction: A systematic review and meta-analysis of randomized controlled trials. Orthop Traumatol Surg Res. 2019;105(6):1107–14.
35. Marois B, Tan XW, Pauyo T, Dodin P, Ballaz L, Nault ML. Can a knee brace prevent ACL reinjury: a systematic review. Int J Environ Res Public Health. 2021;18(14).
36. Perrone GS, Webster KE, Imbriaco C, Portilla GM, Vairagade A, Murray MM, Kiapour AM. Risk of secondary ACL injury in adolescents prescribed functional bracing after ACL reconstruction. Orthop J Sports Med. 2019;7(11):2325967119879880. https://doi.org/10.1177/2325967119879880. PMID: 31763340; PMCID: PMC6851612.
37. O'Dowd DP, Stanley J, Rosenfeldt MP, Walsh S, Twaddle B, De Ruiter L, Crua E, Monk AP, Walsh S. Reduction in re-rupture rates following implementation of return-to-sport testing after anterior cruciate ligament reconstruction in 313 patients with a mean follow-up of 50 months. J ISAKOS. 2024;9(3):264–71. https://doi.org/10.1016/j.jisako.2024.01.005. Epub 2024 Jan 11. PMID: 38218452.
38. Figueroa Poblete D, Gonzalez Duque W, Landea Caroca D, Tapia Castillo C, Erskine VD. Return-to-sport tests: do they reduce risk of re-rupture after anterior cruciate ligament reconstruction? J ISAKOS. 2025;11:100399. https://doi.org/10.1016/j.jisako.2025.100399. Epub 2025 Feb 10. PMID: 39938748.
39. Grassi A, Bailey JR, Signorelli C, Carbone G, Tchonang Wakam A, Lucidi GA, et al. Magnetic resonance imaging after anterior cruciate ligament reconstruction: a practical guide. World J Orthop. 2016;7(10):638–49.
40. Stucken C, Flato R, O'Hagan T, O'Brien D, Ruiz D, Cohen SB, et al. Postoperative radiographs after ACL reconstruction are not cost-effective. Orthopedics. 2015;38(4):e339–42.
41. Werner BC, Burrus MT, Kew ME, Dempsey IJ, Gwathmey FW, Miller MD, et al. Limited utility of routine early postoperative radiography after primary ACL reconstruction. Knee. 2016;23(2):237–40.

22 Value-Based Care for Pediatric Female Athletes

Katlyn Elliott and Teri McCambridge

Introduction

Pediatric female athletes face unique health challenges which are integrally linked to biopsychosocial factors. It is well known that participation in sport provides many physical and mental health benefits, but pediatric female athletes are disproportionately affected by a number of conditions when compared to their male counterparts. Most notably are LEA and its clinical progression to RED-S, overuse injuries, stress fractures, noncontact ACL tears, and sport related concussion. The sequelae of RED-S include hormonal dysregulation, menstrual irregularities, impaired bone density, gastrointestinal disturbances, reproductive problems, impaired immunity, and cardiac and mental health problems. Pediatric female athletes are subject to immense biopsychosocial pressure, making them susceptible to mental health disorders such as anxiety, depression, body image issues, and disordered eating. The substantial impact of these conditions can lead to subsequent impaired well-being, decreased athletic performance, cessation of sport participation, and, if left untreated, long-term, potentially irreversible and costly health conditions including but not limited to delayed growth and maturation, osteopenia, osteoporosis, functional disability, chronic pain, miscarriage, infertility, and suicide.

Emerging research emphasizes the importance of addressing issues facing pediatric female athletes through a value-based care framework, highlighting the need for prevention, early detection, and multidisciplinary intervention. By integrating cost-effective validated screening tools, high risk athletes can be identified and

K. Elliott (✉)
University of Michigan Department of Family Medicine, Ann Arbor, MI, USA
e-mail: katlynel@med.umich.edu

T. McCambridge
University of Maryland St Joseph Medical Center, Towson, MD, USA
e-mail: tmccambridge@towsonortho.com

W. L. Hennrikus, R. M. Schwend (eds.), *Value in Pediatric Orthopaedics*,
https://doi.org/10.1007/978-3-032-19570-8_22

treatment can be expedited. Proactive interventions such as awareness and education of energy availability, proper nutrition, training load/volume management, as well as psychological support can also play a role in the mitigation of long-term health consequences in pediatric female athletes. This framework prioritizes prevention and early detection, placing value on improved athlete well-being, continued sport participation, and reduction of unnecessary healthcare expenditures.

Value-Based Themes

PPE

The American Academy of Pediatrics (AAP) and the American Academy of Family Physicians (AAFP) recommend that all pediatric patients have a full preparticipation physical evaluation (PPE) which is to be completed via the PPE 5 every 2–3 years with annual exams for updates and to address areas of concern [1]. The PPE serves multiple purposes including evaluation of general physical and psychological health, screening for life-threatening conditions, and importantly providing an entry point into the healthcare system for those without a primary care physician. The PPE 5 does emphasize comprehensive cardiac history to evaluate for risk factors that may predispose people to sudden cardiac death (SCD). Other important aspects of the PPE include mental health screening and inclusion of screening for disordered eating, signs of low energy availability (LEA), and sequelae of reduced energy deficiency in sport (RED-S) [2]. A study by Weiss et. al recognizes the PPE as a strategically efficient, low-cost tool for early identification of athletes at risk for LEA, therefore reinforcing its preventive value in reducing long-term health impacts as well as related healthcare expenditures if left untreated [3]. Although widely endorsed as a means to screen for conditions that may predispose athletes to injury or illness, the literature suggests that there is limited evidence supporting its effectiveness especially in regards to detecting and preventing sudden death [1].

There is ongoing debate in the medical community as to the appropriate screening recommendations to minimize the risk of sudden cardiac death in young athletes. The guidelines form the 36th Bethesda Conference recommend screening with focused personal history, family history, and PE tailored toward detection of cardiac abnormalities but did not recommend use of 12 lead ECG [4]. Many studies have debated the inclusion of EKGs to address the more than 90 competitive young athletes who die suddenly and unexpectedly in the USA each year [4]. The cost analysis completed by Schoenbaum et al. found that the standard PPE alone is not cost-effective and that in the context of the USA, ECG-inclusive screening is more effective in identifying at-risk athletes but its adoption is also limited by cost [2]. On the contrary, a study by Wheeler et al. highlights longitudinal evidence from Italy which has suggested 89% ARR in SCD risk for competitive athletes bringing risk comparable to that of age matched nonathletes. This success led the European Society of Cardiology to adopt a common European protocol including EKG as centerpiece of cardiac screening and the IOC to recommend EKG screening for Olympic athletes [4].

In summary, while PPEs are recommended and can potentially identify serious health conditions and provide a gateway into the healthcare system for young patients, the cost-effectiveness of these evaluations alone is widely debated. The available evidence regarding PPE's effectiveness in preventing SCD remains controversial and suggests that while PPEs, including ECGs, can be beneficial, their cost-effectiveness is variable and context-dependent.

Screening for RED-S

Low energy availability (LEA) is defined as insufficient energy intake to meet demands of basic metabolic functions and demands of exercise [5, 6]. LEA can be both intentional and unintentional and is now recognized as the underlying cause of RED-S. Many studies have outlined the impacts of RED-S on a broad spectrum of physiologic systems including menstrual, bone, cardiovascular, immunologic, gastrointestinal, psychological health, and athletic performance [6–14]. LEA and RED-S can be seen in both male and female athletes, although prevalence is notably higher in pediatric female athletes especially those competing in endurance and aesthetic sports, with many studies indicating risk ranging from 40 to 60% [10–15]. Long-term consequences of unrecognized and untreated LEA include menstrual dysfunction which leads to low estrogen levels. This hypoestrogenemia has a cascade of effects contributing to reduced fertility, endocrine abnormalities, and low bone marrow density which predisposes these athletes to stress fracture and premature osteoporosis. LEA is also linked to impaired immune function, increased GI distress, increased risk of cardiovascular complications, and continued psychologic distress [7–14]. Figure 22.1 visually outlines both physiologic and performance effects of LEA and RED-S.

The pervasiveness of LEA and RED-S in pediatric female athletes and the potentially irreversible long-term consequences highlight the importance of early identification and interventions via validated tools. The Low Energy Availability in Females Questionnaire (LEAF-Q) is a widely used screen to evaluate for LEA and RED-S. Studies report 78% sensitivity and 90% specificity although it is only validated for use in female athletes [4–8, 10–17]. In 2023, the IOC released the RED-S Clinical Assessment Tool version 2 (IOC RED-S CAT2) which provides an updated framework for initial LEA and RED-S screening, guidelines for a severity/risk assessment, and recommendations regarding initial treatment [12–17]. Please see Fig. 22.2 which outlines the updated traffic light severity index as well as RED-S red flags that prompt urgent management and abrupt cessation of training. Many articles highlight the importance and cost-effectiveness of early identification with validated screening tools such as the LEAF-Q and the IOC RED-S CAT2, education, as well as early multidisciplinary management involving nutritional, psychological, and medical intervention especially in the pediatric female athlete population [5, 6, 9–12, 16, 17]. Literature also notes that early screening and intervention can

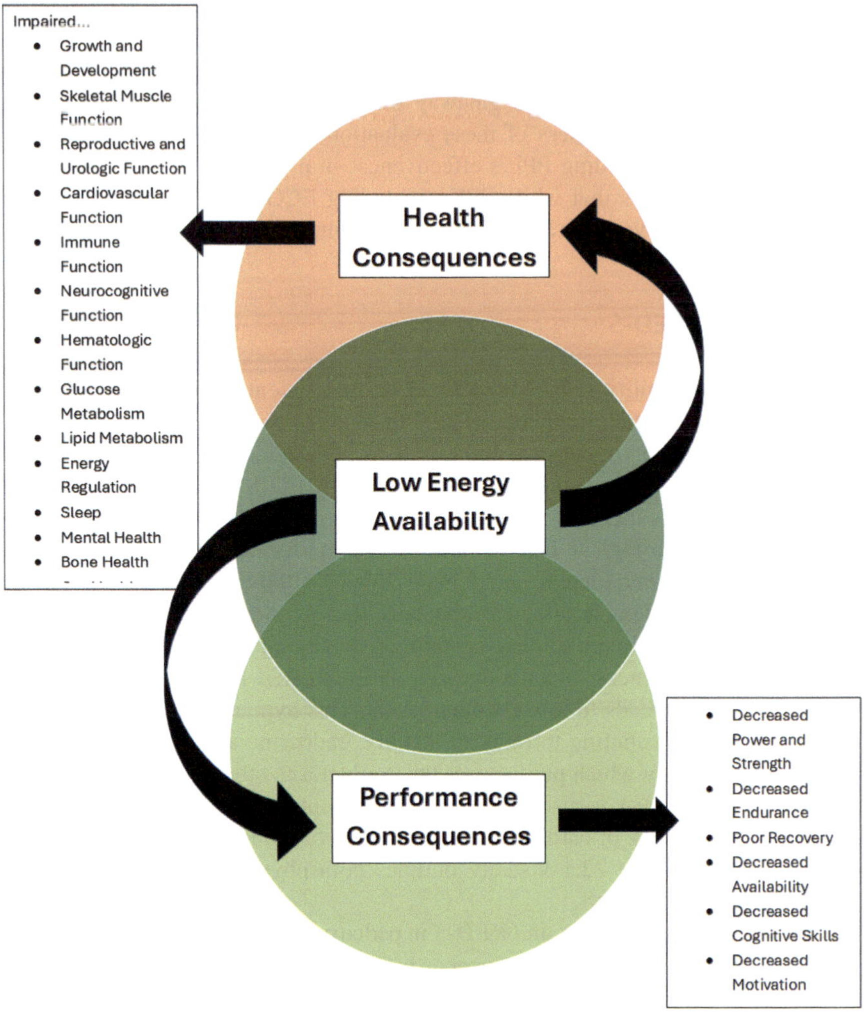

Fig. 22.1 REDs health and performance impact framework–LEA can affect many domains of health and performance in athletes. This impact can be mild and reversible in adaptable forms of LEA, although if LEA persists, these adverse outcomes are termed problematic LEA

effectively prevent progression of RED-S related sequelae and associated medical expenditure while improving pediatric overall health and mental well-being [6, 7, 10–14].

In summary, RED-S is a condition underscored by LEA and is unfortunately very common in pediatric female athletes especially those in endurance, aesthetic, and weight sensitive sports. RED-S has a broad range of physiologic and psychologic effects which should be screened for using validated tools. Although there is little true cost analysis data, the cost-effectiveness of early identification and intervention of LEA and RED-S as it has been shown to safeguard long-term athlete

Definitions		REDs diagnosis and severity index	Treatment and training/competition recommendations
REDs CAT primary indicators	Outcomes most often resulting from problematic LEA and subsequently leading to REDs signs and/or symptoms. These have the greatest measurement validity and therefore are more indicative of increased severity and risk of REDs.	**GREEN** Severity/Risk - • None to very low Clinical Criteria - • 0 primary indicators • ≤ 1 secondary indicator	• No treatment required • Full training and competition clearance
REDs CAT secondary indicators	Outcome resulting from problematic LEA leading to REDs signs and/or symptoms which have lower measured validity and demonstrate less severity and risk of REDs.	**YELLOW** Severity/Risk - • Mild Clinical Criteria – • 0 primary & ≥ 2 secondary indicators OR • 1 primary & ≤ 2 secondary indicators OR • 2 primary & ≤ 1 secondary indicator	• Treatment, monitoring and regular follow-up at appropriate intervals • Full training and competition
REDs CAT Potential indicators	Emerging outcome parameters lacking robust scientific evidence but are possibly linked to problematic LEA leading to REDs signs and symptoms. These lack validated screening tools and have poor measured validity. Given this are listed as supportive in assessment of REDs but not included in IOC REDs CAT2 severity risk assessment tool.	**ORANGE** Severity/Risk - • Moderate to High Clinical Criteria – • 1 primary & ≥ 3 secondary indicators OR • 2 primary & ≥ 2 secondary indicators OR • 3 primary & ≤ 1 secondary indicator	• Treatment, close monitoring and follow-up required Some aspects of training and/or competition may need to be modified
REDs CAT symptoms	Any REDs primary, secondary, or potential indicator that an athlete reports/ experiences	**RED** Severity/Risk - • Very High/Extreme Clinical Criteria – • 3 primary & ≥ 2 secondary indicators OR • ≥ 4 primary indicators	• Immediate treatment (hospitalization) required by frequent monitoring at daily to monthly intervals depending on severity • Significant training and competition modifications required, and in the majority of cases, removal from all training and competition is indicated
REDs CAT serious medical indicators	Serious medical indicators of REDs or eating disorders that require immediate medical attention, potential hospitalization, and immediate removal from training and competition.	**Serious Indicators** • ≤ 75% median BMI for age/sex • Electrolyte disturbance • ECG abnormalities including severe bradycardia– Adolescent: HR ≤ 45bpm • Severe hypotension ≤90/45mmHg and Orthostatics • Failure of outpatient ED treatment program • Acute complications of malnutrition • Conditions that inhibit medical treatment or monitoring while training/competing	

Fig. 22.2 Summary of IOC REDs CAT2 severity/risk stratification with sport participation guidelines and definitions. This table is adapted from the International Olympic Committee Relative Energy Deficiency in Sport clinical assessment tool 2 (IOC REDs CAT2). Overall definitions are used as a guide only, and team based approach to diagnosis and treatment decisions must consider the context of the specific athlete

health while reducing the economic burden of treating advanced RED-S complications can be inferred from evidence outlining the long-term consequences [5–14]. Given these benefits, some authors have called for policy-level integration of RED-S screening and education into youth sports and in the general pediatric population [7–9, 12–17].

Menstrual Dysfunction

A cross-sectional study by Armento et al. reported a 28% prevalence of menstrual dysfunction in high school female athletes, while Weiss et al. highlight that menstrual dysfunction is often overlooked or normalized in athletic populations [3, 18]. It is well documented in the literature that untreated menstrual dysfunction can have significant and potentially irreversible effects on bone, reproductive, endocrine, cardiovascular, and psychological health and negatively impact on performance [3, 18–23]. Long-term untreated menstrual dysfunction particularly functional hypothalamic amenorrhea (FHA) leads to chronic suppression of the hypothalamic-pituitary-ovarian axis, persistent hypoestrogenism, and anovulation potentially resulting in delayed sexual maturation, miscarriage, and infertility [20, 22, 23]. Hypoestrogenism especially during adolescence has been shown to impair bone mass acquisition leading to potentially irreversible low bone marrow density and predispose affected athletes to stress fracture and premature osteopenia/osteoporosis [20–23]. Cardiovascular complications of hypoestrogenism include altered lipid metabolism and endothelial dysfunction [20–22]. Chronic LEA is linked to endocrine dysfunction, altered thyroid and adrenal function, metabolism, as well as growth and development [21–24]. Figure 22.3 outlines the many hormonal effects of LEA. We must also consider that LEA negatively affects performance by impairing strength, recovery, and endurance while increasing injury risk. Poor performance, injury, and hormonal changes are associated with increased anxiety and depression especially in adolescent females [23, 24].

The AAP, AMSSM, and ACSM highlight that failure to identify and treat menstrual dysfunction in adolescent athletes can lead to a broad range of adverse health outcomes. These societies, as well as overwhelming literature, emphasizes the importance of early detection via screening during routine visits. A multidisciplinary approach is recommended for treatment, focusing on energy availability education and optimizing nutritional intake to prevent adverse health outcomes [3, 20, 21]. A study by Torstveit et al. also notes limited evidence supporting use of CBT to decrease circulating cortisol and improve reproductive function [14]. Studies by Ackerman et al. and Maïmoun et al. highlight that early screening and intervention for menstrual dysfunction in adolescent athletes are clinically effective, support athlete well-being, and are economically advantageous [21–23].

In summary, menstrual dysfunction in pediatric female athletes is very common, and LEA must be considered as an etiology. If left untreated, menstrual dysfunction can have a broad range of physiologic, psychologic, and performance effects. Major

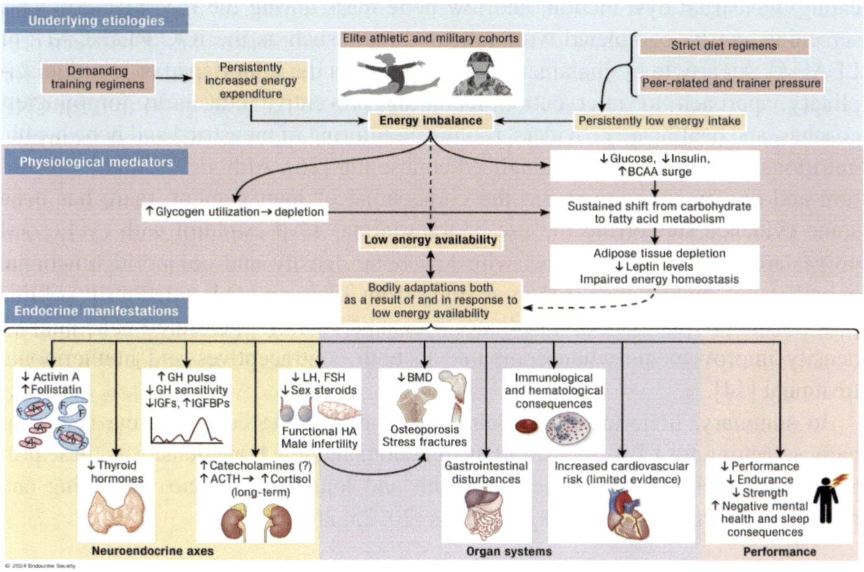

Fig. 22.3 Graphical abstract: This figure is a representation of the complex neuroendocrine manifestations and pathophysiology of RED-S [24]

societies including the AAP, AMSSM, and ACSM identify early screening and intervention as critical in preventing long-term and potentially irreversible adverse health outcomes while also being cost-effective.

Bone Health Implications

Pediatric female athletes are at risk for compromised bone health due to several factors, primarily related to low energy availability (LEA), menstrual dysfunctions (late menarche, oligomenorrhea, amenorrhea), low body weight/BMI [3, 19], and prolonged participation in endurance or aesthetic sports [20, 25, 26]. LEA either intentionally or unintentionally leads to estradiol suppression impairing calcium metabolism leading to increased bone resorption and decreased bone formation in addition to being an independent or compounding factor in menstrual dysfunction [3, 19, 25]. These conditions lead to suboptimal bone accrual during youth that may not be fully reversible and predispose female athletes to increased lifetime risk of premature osteoporosis, stress fractures, functional disability, and chronic pain, especially if left untreated [25, 26]. Given 90% of peak bone mass is acquired by age 18, low BMD in college-aged athletes often reflects missed opportunities for prevention in adolescence, suggesting the importance for earlier identification and intervention [25, 26].

Both the AAP and the American Medical Society for Sports Medicine (AMSSM) emphasize that female athletes should be screened for signs of LEA, disordered eating, menstrual dysfunction, and low bone mass during the PPE [19, 20]. This screening can be completed with validated tools such as the IOC RED CAT2 or LEAF-Q. An article by Ihalainen et al. emphasizes the importance of a multidisciplinary approach to intervention including preventive education for athletes, coaches, and healthcare providers, routine monitoring of menstrual and bone health, nutritional support, and individualized counseling [26]. Although primary prevention and nutritional support are the cornerstone of management, there has been some evidence supporting the use of transdermal 17-β estradiol with cyclic oral progesterone in female athletes with low bone density and comorbid functional hypothalamic amenorrhea (FHA). A study from Torstveit et al. noted utility of this pharmacologic treatment as an adjunct with superior DXA measured bone marrow density improvements when compared to both contraceptives and nonhormonal treatment [14].

In summary, literature overwhelmingly supports the cost-effective nature of early screening for LEA, menstrual dysfunction, and low bone density as these proactive measures safeguard skeletal health and long-term athlete well-being and reduce long-term healthcare expenditures [20, 25, 26].

Cardiovascular Implications

When discussing cardiac concerns in athletes, we must acknowledge that athletes are at nearly 2.5x higher risk of SCD than that of age matched nonathlete population [27]. It has been noted in the literature that female athletes have a significantly lower incidence of sport related SCD when compared to males; however, female athletes exhibit different forms of structural and electrical remodeling when exposed to sport [27–29]. Female athletes have a tendency toward eccentric cardiac remodeling with smaller left ventricular mass and less pronounced wall thickness as compared to males, while electrically female athletes generally have longer QT intervals, greater sinoatrial node automaticity, and enhanced atrioventricular node function as compared to male athletes [3, 28–33]. Other common cardiac complications faced by female athletes include endothelial dysfunction and lipid abnormalities that are linked to hypoestrogen states.

Low estrogen states in pediatric female athletes are often due to LEA and/or menstrual dysfunction such as amenorrhea or oligomenorrhea. Overall estrogen is cardioprotective, and studies have shown that amenorrheic athletes exhibit impaired flow-mediated dilation of the brachial artery, indicating endothelial dysfunction which is a marker for early atherosclerosis and cardiovascular disease [19, 32, 34, 35]. Additionally, amenorrheic athletes tend to have higher levels of total cholesterol, LDL, and lower HDL compared to their eumenorrheic counterparts. These lipid abnormalities further contribute to the risk of developing cardiovascular disease [14, 35]. In more severe cases of LEA, other potentially life-threatening cardiac complications such as severe bradycardia and orthostatic hypotension should be considered. These conditions may require a higher level of care and abrupt cessation of training [27–29].

In summary, there are sex specific structural, electrical, and hormonal differences in female athletes that should be acknowledged to avoid overlooking or misclassifying findings [30–32]. The AAP and AMSSM both emphasize the importance of early detection and treatment of LEA, RED-S, and menstrual dysfunction to mitigate cardiovascular risks [19, 34, 35]. This strategy is supported by research from Grosman-Rimon et al. which highlighted that energy and hormonal imbalances can be corrected through nutritional adjustments and restoration of menstrual cycles, therefore improving endothelial dysfunction and lipid profile abnormalities [35].

Immunologic Implications

Pediatric female athletes are prone to immunosuppression due to the LEA in the setting of high-intensity prolonged training, poor nutrition, and subsequent hormonal dysregulation. Several studies as well as the European College of Sport Science, ACSM, and the IOC highlight that overtraining and LEA can lead to prolonged immune depression, making athletes more prone to infections (upper respiratory and gastrointestinal infections), prolonged recovery from illness, and delayed wound healing [19, 24, 36–40]. This immunosuppression is characterized by decreased salivary IgA levels, reduced neutrophil function, altered cytokine responses, and elevated levels of cortisol, IL-6, and TNF-α—these changes indicate a pro-inflammatory state compromising both innate and adaptive immunity [24, 37–39]. Nutritional status also plays a critical role in maintaining immune function such that deficiencies in energy; macronutrients particularly carbohydrates and protein; micronutrients such as vitamins A, C, D, E, B6, and B12; omega 3 fatty acids; and minerals like iron and zinc can impair immune cell function, increase inflammation, and exacerbate training-related stress [19, 36, 40]. Additionally, hormonal changes associated with LEA can influence immune function. Menstrual dysfunction, often a result of LEA, leads to estrogen deficiencies which reduce immune protection while increasing levels of pro-inflammatory markers such as cortisol, interleukin-6 (IL-6), and tumor necrosis factor-alpha subsequently negatively impacting the athletes' immune health and overall growth [19, 24, 36, 40].

The International Society of Sports Nutrition's 2023 position emphasizes the importance of nutritional demands of pediatric female athletes, highlighting how inadequate nutrition and LEA can contribute to immune dysfunction [40]. Appropriate nutritional support and use of supplements as needed are essential in addressing LEA. Evidence supports the use of vitamin D supplementation to reduce infection incidence and duration [36, 39]. The International Society of Sports Nutrition also recommends creatine and iron supplementation for female athletes due to their efficacy in supporting muscle function and overall health [36–40]. This position statement, as well as several supporting studies, promotes the value of early, cost-effective screening via validated tools as a method for primary prevention and way to mitigate the adverse health effects of LEA and overtraining, improve immunity, and subsequently improve long-term health and performance outcomes for young female athletes [19, 24, 40].

In summary, immunological concerns, such as increased susceptibility to infections and impaired recovery, highlight the need for early screening, proper nutritional interventions, and tailored support of pediatric female athletes from a multidisciplinary team as recommended by AMSSM [19]. Maintaining immune health through proper nutrition in pediatric female athletes is economically efficient as it reduces healthcare utilization and can enhance performance and ensure participation.

GI Implications

Gastrointestinal concerns in pediatric female athletes are multifaceted. It is important to determine the true cause of the gastrointestinal complaints and rule out conditions such as inflammatory bowel syndrome, inflammatory bowel disease, and celiac disease that are all more prevalent in females [14, 41, 42]. Female athletes often report higher rates of gastrointestinal dysfunction, which can be exacerbated by both regular and irregular menstrual cycles as well as psychological stress associated with body image and performance pressures [11, 42]. Cross- sectional studies have demonstrated a higher prevalence of GI issues in female athletes with LEA compared with those with adequate energy availability [14]. The stress of high-intensity or prolonged training and LEA sequelae including nutritional deficiencies, electrolyte imbalances, and hormonal dysregulation are believed to lead to a cascade of physiological disruptions resulting in compromised gastrointestinal function that can manifest as dysbiosis, delayed gastric emptying, reduced gut motility, altered gut hormone secretion, and impaired nutritional absorption [10, 11, 19, 24, 41–43]. Moreover, the stress of prolonged or intense exercise, combined with LEA, can lead to ischemia and damage to the gut mucosa, contributing to gastrointestinal distress during exercise which we now refer to as exercise-associated gastrointestinal symptoms (Ex-GIS) and exercise-induced gastrointestinal syndrome (EIGS) [10, 11, 19, 24, 41, 42]. Additionally, chronic LEA can lead to hormonal imbalances, including reduced levels of gastrointestinal hormones like ghrelin and peptide YY, which further disrupt normal gastrointestinal function ultimately compounding the effects of LEA potentially affecting growth, hormonal balance, and bone health [10, 11, 24].

The American Medical Society for Sports Medicine highlights that LEA and its sequelae can contribute to many gastrointestinal problems in female athletes, and a systematic review and meta-analysis by Gallant et al. found that the prevalence of gastrointestinal symptoms is notably higher and more severe in females with LEA and RED-S when compared to males with similar disease [10, 11, 14, 24]. Early identification of LEA via validated screening tools as well as early intervention via nutritional support is crucial to prevent long-term adverse health consequences and the associated healthcare expenditure. Adequate nutrition and hydration is the primary management. Once this is achieved, gut training and feeding tolerance adjustments can help manage exercise-induced gastrointestinal symptoms. Dietary adjustments such as adopting a low FODMAP (fermentable oligo-, di-, monosaccharides and polyols) diet reduce symptoms like flatulence, diarrhea, and abdominal pain [41, 43].

In summary, GI distress is common among pediatric female athletes and even more prevalent in those exposed to LEA and its related nutritional and hormonal dysregulation. GI symptoms may serve as both a consequence and an indicator of low energy availability; therefore, early identification via proactive screening and early intervention is a cost-effective strategy to improve overall growth, health, and performance of pediatric female athletes as well as mitigate unnecessary associated healthcare expenditure.

Nutritional Counseling

Nutritional concerns in pediatric female athletes are multifaceted but center around adequate energy availability (EA) to meet the demands of growth, development, and athletic performance [3, 44]. In general, recommendations for macronutrient intake for athletes include 1.2–1.7 g/kg/day of carbohydrates to support blood glucose levels during exercise and replenishing muscle glycogen stores, 1.0–1.2 g per kilogram of body weight per day of protein to support muscle repair and growth, and 25–35% of total daily calories in healthy fats which are essential for hormonal regulation and overall health [44–46]. Unfortunately pediatric female athletes are often at risk for deficiencies in iron, calcium, and vitamin D, which can impair cognitive performance and exercise capacity and compromise bone health leading to increased risk of stress fractures and impaired immune function, respectively [14, 19, 24, 40, 45–47]. Monitoring of these micronutrients can be considered depending on the athlete's clinical presentation, but supplementation should only be considered when a deficiency is identified through screening or when dietary intake cannot meet an athlete's nutritional needs [40, 45–47]. Nutrition education regarding the importance of hydration before, during, and after exercise optimizes performance, reduces injury risk, and supports recovery in pediatric female athletes [40, 45, 48].

The ACSM, Academy of Nutrition and Dietetics, and Dietitians of Canada emphasize the need for comprehensive nutritional screening for pediatric female athletes and individualized nutrition plans with consideration of the unique needs of female athletes [45]. This consensus statement as well as endorsement from AMSSM and the AAP emphasizes the critical nature of early identification and intervention to mitigate these risks of LEA [3, 19, 48]. Screening for LEA via validated screening tools that focus on energy availability (LEAF-Q– Low Energy Availability in Females Questionnaire, IOC RED-S Clinical Assessment Tool 2), hydration status, dietary assessment (FFQ–Food Frequency Questionnaire), potential for disordered eating (EDSA–Eating Disorder Screen for Athletes, EDE-Q–Eating Disorder Examination Questionnaire or EAT-26–Eating Attitudes Test), menstrual dysfunction, growth and development (height, weight, and body composition) as well as regular follow up with a multidisciplinary team after initiation of appropriate intervention [3, 19, 40, 45, 47, 48].

In summary, nutritional counseling that focuses on adequate energy availability, balanced nutrition, hydration, and necessary supplementation is critical. Physicians should be aware of the signs and sequelae of LEA. Early identification and appropriate nutritional intervention are critical in the prevention of long-term complications, improved athletic performance, and provide cost-effective care for pediatric female athletes.

Mental Health Counseling

A total of 13–20% of children living in the USA experience a mental disorder annually, with rates only increasing [49, 50]. Mental health counseling is crucial for pediatric female athletes due to the unique stressors they face. These stressors can significantly impact their mental health and well-being. Pediatric female athletes are at increased risk for a range of psychological issues, including anxiety (general and performance related), depression, disordered eating, overtraining, burnout, injury related stress, vulnerability to abuse and harassment, and body image issues as well as potentially conflicting societal expectations surrounding femininity, beauty, and strength which can be further compounded if competing in aesthetic or weight sensitive sports [19, 24, 51–55].

Both the 2017 ACSM Team Physician Consensus statement and the 2020 AMSSM position statement on mental health emphasize the critical importance of mental health screening in female pediatric athletes. They emphasize that mental health is as vital as physical health in athletes [19, 52, 54]. The AAP guidelines suggest that anxiety screening should begin after the age of 8, while depression and suicide risk screening should start after the age of 12 years [50, 56]. In addition to screening for these internalizing disorders, there should be routine comprehensive surveillance of the abovementioned stressors affecting pediatric female athletes via validated tools. Further management of mental health disorders should be multidisciplinary, involving physicians, mental health professionals, dietitians, coaches, and athletic trainers working collaboratively to educate and create a supportive environment to address the physical and psychological manifestations of mental health disorders [19, 51, 54]. Evidence does suggest that mental health counseling and CBT can directly enhance athletic performance by improving focus, resilience, and confidence, facilitating injury recovery, helping manage both performance related anxiety and disordered eating, and contributing to athlete safety [19, 51–55]. Despite literature supporting early identification and continued screening for mental health concerns in pediatric female athletes, symptoms tend to be underreported secondary to the fear of stigma and lack of appropriate mental health resources [52, 53].

In summary, mental health concerns are common among athletes, and female athletes face unique biopsychosocial challenges. Research and governing bodies such as ACSM, AMSSM, and AAP all emphasize the importance of early, regular mental health screening, using validated tools as well as a multidisciplinary care model to identify and manage these concerns effectively [19, 52–56]. Mental health support, especially if provided early, is essential for athlete safety, performance, and long-term athlete well-being. Given this, it can be inferred that early mental health screening is cost-effective.

Prevention of Overuse Injuries

Overuse injuries such as gymnast's wrist, lower extremity stress injury, Osgood Schlatter, Jumper's knee, and patellofemoral syndrome are extremely common and unfortunately on the rise. Brenner et al. note that overuse injuries in pediatric athletes account for nearly half sport related injuries in children and adolescents [57]. In children, growing bone apophyses and epiphyses especially of the lower extremity are particularly vulnerable and susceptible to injury with cumulative repetitive stress and inadequate rest [57, 58]. The 2014 AMSSM position statement by DiFiori et al. highlight the rising prevalence of overuse injuries and burnout in youth sports, attributed largely to early sports specialization, high training volumes, and lack of adequate rest [58]. Other risk factors include being female, participation in endurance sports, and prior overuse injury [57, 58].

Although there is limited actual cost analysis to support the cost-effectiveness of prevention strategies, guidance from AMSSM, AOSSM, and AAP stresses that implementation of low-cost preventive measures such as delayed specialization, appropriate training limits, mandatory structured rest periods, and education of coaches and parents can substantially decrease injury rates as well as subsequent healthcare expenditure [57–59]. General AAP and AMSSM recomendations for training load include avoiding trainging volume greater than their age in hours per week as well as increasing training intensity, duration or frequency no more than 10% from week to week [57–59]. These governing bodies also recommend one to two off days per week as well as scheduled breaks throughout the year, with the AAP endorsing breaks of 2–3 months from each sport annually [57–59]. There has been some evidence supporting the utility of proactive injury prevention programs in youth sport. Watson, Soomro, and Rossler et al. noted decreased injury burden and economic benefits of implementing proactive injury prevention programs in youth soccer and team sport programs, respectively [59–61].

In summary, overuse injuries are plaguing youth athletes particularly pediatric female athletes. Governing bodies including the AAP, AOSSM, and AMSSM recognize that implementing preventive strategies such as delayed specialization, appropriate training limits, mandatory structured rest periods, and education for coaches and parents can substantially decrease injury rates and keep children active while subsequently limiting healthcare expenditure. Despite lack of true cost analysis studies, it can be inferred that prioritizing prevention promotes sustained athletic participation, healthier youth, and lower healthcare expenditures.

Healthy Lifestyle

Proper sleep, stress modification, and appropriate nutrition (discussed earlier) are essential for recovery, injury prevention, and optimal performance in pediatric female athletes and are overall large contributors to leading a healthy life.

Sleep

Sleep in the pediatric population plays a critical role in growth and recovery and positively influences both physical and mental well-being [62–64]. However, a study by Gooderick et al. notes that more than 70% of athletes are regularly operating in a sleep debt [2]. Evidence highlights that inadequate sleep is linked to increased injury risk, impaired recovery, weakened immune function, hormonal dysregulation, mood disturbances, as well as reduced cognitive and physical performance [52, 63, 64]. Given these adverse effects and the prevalence of inadequate sleep in pediatric athletes, simple, noninvasive, low-cost strategies such as sleep hygiene education, decreased screen time before bed, and prioritization of sleep as a pillar of youth athlete health and performance can contribute to healthy pediatric female athletes [19, 52, 62–64]. It is also clear that further research into targeted sleep interventions specific to athletic populations is needed.

Stress

In pediatric female athletes, significant psychosocial stressors and physical stressors such as overtraining, burnout, and LEA directly impact recovery and overall well-being. Female athletes are subject to unique societal pressures including inaccurate female norms and sport inequity as well as psychosocial pressures including body image concerns, overtraining, and pressure to balance academic and athletic commitments [19, 57, 65]. These stressors are intricately linked and exacerbate mental health disorders. The AMSSM and AAP recognize that female athletes are at increased risk for mental health disorders including depression, anxiety, and disordered eating [57, 65]. Overtraining, burnout, and low energy available are all discussed in above sections but also contribute to significant physical and mental stressors in pediatric female athletes [3, 19, 57]. The effects of the above stressors are multifaceted and can be severe, we must highlight some stress reduction strategies. CBT and mental health counselling which are both endorsed as gold standard for stress and mental health disorders by the AMSSM [54, 66]. There has also been initiative in the sports community to provide education and promotion of open communication of stress and mental health issues, and this has been shown to reduce stigma and encourage athletes to seek help [57]. Other notable strategies endorsed by athletes to reduce stress include mindfulness, resilience training, and engaging social support networks [54, 66–68]. CBT does have evidence to support its cost-effectiveness as it has been shown to enhance focus, resilience, and confidence and facilitate injury recovery [54, 66]. The other strategies noted here have limited cost analysis data. The cost-effectiveness of stress reduction in pediatric female athletes can be inferred as it would allow for improved athlete well-being and mental and physical health.

Increased Injury Risk

Three quarters of US households have children who play sports, and female participation in sports is on the rise. Increased athletic participation has resulted in more injuries; >3.5 million sports injuries are reported annually [69]. Three of the most common injuries in pediatric female athletes include noncontact ACL tears, stress fractures, and concussions. In this section, we will be analyzing potential injury prevention strategies and their cost-effectiveness.

Prevention of Noncontact ACL Injuries

One of the most common injuries plaguing pediatric female athletes is noncontact ACL tears. Epidemiological studies have shown that the prevalence of ACL injuries is four to six times higher in females than males, and this has been attributed to a combination of sex specific anatomic, hormonal, and biomechanical factors [69, 70]. Overall, the medical literature including a consensus statement from the American Academy of Pediatrics Council on Sports Medicine and Fitness highlights the effectiveness of multicomponent neuromuscular and strength "prehab" programs in reducing ACL injuries among female athletes, with reductions ranging from 56% to 88%, while also noting the practical scalability of these programs [59, 69–76]. A cost-effectiveness analysis published in the *Journal of Bone and Joint Surgery* noted that implementation of universal neuromuscular training for all athletes was more cost-effective as compared to screening and implementing these prehab programs in only high risk athletes [69]. Given the cost of surgical intervention ranging from 5000 to 17000 dollars and comprehensive rehab needed to return female athletes to sport reaching up to 38,000 dollars [71, 72], it can be inferred that implementing universal preventative multicomponent neuromuscular training programs among young female athletes is both a clinically and economically advantageous approach to reducing ACL injuries.

Concussion Prevention

In a 2018 AAP and 2019 AMSSM report on sport related concussion, it was noted that female athletes in sports such as soccer and basketball have higher rates of concussion and often report more severe symptoms with longer recovery times as compared to males [77–79]. Applying this policy to rule changes such as delaying the introduction of heading in soccer as well as implementation of education programs such as the CDC's HEADS UP program with coaches and parents has been shown to promote safe behavior and reduce concussion incidence [78, 79]. The adoption of equipment such as helmets and mouthguards can prevent severe head and dental injuries, but their role in concussion prevention is less clear [79]. Direct cost analysis data specific to pediatric female athletes and concussions is limited, but it can be inferred that implementation of rule changes, use of protective equipment, and educational programs likely have some benefit in reducing severity of concussions and likely lowering long-term healthcare costs.

Prevention of Stress Fractures

Research demonstrates that pediatric female athletes at the high school and collegiate level are at increased risk for stress injury and fractures as compared to males. NCAA female athletes are almost two times more likely to sustain a stress fracture especially if participating in high risk sports such as endurance athletics, gymnastics, and dance [25, 80]. Evidence emphasizes risk factors for stress fracture in pediatric female athletes include low BMI, menstrual dysfunction (amenorrhea, oligomenorrhea, or delayed menarche), low bone marrow density, disordered eating, high training volume, and previous stress fracture [25, 58]. Many of these risk factors contribute to and or are sequelae of LEA and its progressions to RED-S. Given this, the AMSSM emphasizes the importance of screening for the LEA/RED-S in female athletes in an effort to prevent stress fractures [58]. There is limited cost analysis data in this population on stress fracture prevention, but it can be inferred that early screening for LEA and optimizing nutritional deficits especially deficiencies of calcium and vitamin D are cost-effective strategies in the prevention of stress fracture in pediatric female athlete as they allow for continued sport participation, improve athlete well-being, and limit unnecessary healthcare expenditure.

Case Example

A 17-year-old female high school track athlete with past medical history of previously diagnosed female athlete triad (2023), previously diagnosed left tibial stress fracture (2023), right proximal tibial stress fracture (2024), and depression presents to clinic on May 29, 2025, complaining of swelling and sharp pain in her left leg that started on May 13, 2025, immediately following PR-ing in her final 2 mile race of her track season. Pt was taken to the Emergency Department where she was advised to continue with Tylenol, Motrin, and ace bandage. Since then, she and her mother reported being unable to go back to school because of her pain and difficulty with bearing weight.

In regards to her previous diagnoses, she was advised to see a nutritionist and supplement calcium—unfortunately, this was never completed. Other lab workup in 2023 was unremarkable. Pt does not eat calcium or like taking oral pills, but otherwise has no reported dietary restrictions. Pt reports that she has a well-balanced diet and has attempted to increase her protein intake. Pt weights per chart review have been stable, with slight increase over 3 years from 115 lbs to 118 lbs. In August 2023, during initial diagnosis of female athlete triad, she did have menstrual dysfunction which she reports has resolved, and her current menstrual cycles are regular. Currently pt does not take any medications or supplements but did previously take sertraline for depression. Pt training volume is reported to not have changed and runs almost daily, and she has incorporated strength training as part of her routine this season.

On the physical exam, pt was limping and had some obvious poor dentition. On inspection is a soft tissue edema from the distal third of her left tibia with a visible ecchymotic area just superior to the medial malleolus. Pt had point tenderness of the distal one-third of her left anterior medial tibia and positive bump test and unfortunately is unable to complete the hop test in the setting of pain. Pt was otherwise neurovascularly intact. Pt did have two view weight-bearing left tib-fib X-ray completed on office noting obvious distal third of tibia stress fracture with soft tissue swelling surrounding fracture line.

Given the above history, physical exam, and imaging, pt was diagnosed with her third tibial stress fracture since 2023 (two on left, one on right) likely due to RED-S or female athlete triad syndromes. For patient's stress fracture, she was placed in a long walking boot and crutches if needed with complete activity restriction until 4-week follow-up in which a 45-min appointment has been scheduled to complete full RED-S screening questionnaire and to go over DEXA scan and lab workup (CBC, CMP, TSH, free T4, iron panel, vitamin D, vitamin B12) which was ordered today.

Summary

Pediatric female athletes face unique health challenges which are influenced by biopsychosocial pressures. LEA and its progression to RED-S have broad physiologic and psychologic consequences that must be recognized early. For the many of the challenges facing pediatric female athletes investigated in this chapter, early screening and multidisciplinary intervention improved athlete health and well-being while decreasing long-term healthcare expenditure.

Author Pearls

- It is our charge to continue to advocate for research involving pediatric female athlete populations.
- Evidence suggests that the PPE is not cost-effective in identifying or preventing SCD in young athletes although it is an opportunity to complete other appropriate screening as well as serve as an entry point into the healthcare system for those without a primary care physician.
- All physicians caring for pediatric female athletes should be familiar with signs of LEA and multisystem sequelae of RED-S including menstrual dysfunction, hormonal imbalance, impaired bone health, GI distress, cardiovascular complications, impaired immunity, psychological distress, increased injury risk, and poor performance.
- Early identification via screening with validated tools such as the LEAF-Q and IOC RED-S CAT2 combined with early intervention by a multidisciplinary team is imperative in the successful management of LEA and RED-S. This strategy of primary prevention is likely cost-effective given the large downstream costs of chronic management of RED-S sequelae.

- Menstrual dysfunction in pediatric female athletes is very common, and LEA must be considered as an etiology. If left untreated, menstrual dysfunction can have a broad range of physiologic, psychologic, and literature supports early and continued screening in pediatric females.
- Pediatric female athletes are at risk for compromised bone health due to LEA, menstrual dysfunctions, low body weight/BMI, and prolonged participation in endurance or aesthetic sports. Literature overwhelmingly supports the cost-effective nature of early screening for LEA, menstrual dysfunction, and low bone density as these proactive measures safeguard skeletal health in pediatric female athletes.
- There are structural, electrical, and hormonal differences in female athletes that impact their cardiac health. With early identification, energy and hormonal imbalances can be corrected, mitigating the risk and improving endothelial dysfunction and lipid profile abnormalities.
- Immunological concerns related to LEA include increased susceptibility to infections and impaired recovery.
- GI distress is common among pediatric female athletes, and GI symptoms may serve as both a consequence and an indicator of low energy availability.
- Individualized nutrition plans emphasizing appropriate energy availability for training load accompanied by adequate hydration, balanced nutrition with intake of macro- and micronutrients, and as needed supplementation are critical. Physicians should be aware of the signs and sequelae of LEA, as early identification and appropriate nutritional intervention are crucial in the prevention of long-term complications, improved athletic performance, and provide cost-effective care for pediatric female athletes.
- Pediatric female athletes face unique biopsychosocial challenges which contribute to a variety of mental health issues. Early and regular mental health screening with validated tools and a multidisciplinary care model are essential for athlete safety, performance, and long-term well-being. Given this, it can be inferred that early mental health screening is cost-effective.
- Implementing preventive strategies such as delayed specialization, appropriate training limits, mandatory structured rest periods, and education for coaches and parents can substantially decrease rates of overuse injuries and keep children active while subsequently limiting healthcare expenditure.
- Proper sleep, stress modification, and appropriate nutrition (discussed earlier) are essential for recovery, injury prevention, and optimal performance in pediatric female athletes and are overall large contributors to leading a healthy life.

Editor Comments

WLH

This comprehensive and practical treatise by Drs. Elliott and McCambridge offers a thorough review of strategies to enhance value in the care of pediatric female athletes. These athletes often present with complex medical and surgical concerns that are best addressed through a collaborative, multidisciplinary approach ideally led by a pediatric sports medicine physician.

RMS

Future efforts should prioritize the development of prospective registries to track outcomes of RED-S and related interventions. Evaluating the cost-effectiveness of screening tools across diverse athletic populations and advocating for standardized education and policy reforms in youth sports are also critical next steps. Additional research is needed to explore long-term recovery and treatment adherence among athletes with RED-S in order to define high-value care pathways.

References

1. MacDonald J, Schaefer M, Stumph J. The preparticipation physical evaluation. Am Fam Physician. 2021;103(9):539–46. PMID: 33929170.
2. Schoenbaum M, Denchev P, Vitiello B, Kaltman JR. Economic evaluation of strategies to reduce sudden cardiac death in young athletes. Pediatrics. 2012;130(2):e380–9.
3. Weiss Kelly AK, Hecht S. The female athlete triad. Pediatrics. 2016;138(2):e20160922.
4. Wheeler MT, Heidenreich PA, Froelicher VF, Hlatky MA, Ashley EA. Cost-effectiveness of preparticipation screening for prevention of sudden cardiac death in young athletes. Ann Intern Med. 2010;152(5):276–86. https://doi.org/10.7326/0003-4819-152-5-201003020-00005. PMID: 20194233; PMCID: PMC2873148.
5. Mountjoy M, Sundgot-Borgen J, Meyer NL, Burke LM. The International Olympic Committee (IOC) consensus statement on relative energy deficiency in sport (RED-S). Br J Sports Med. 2014;48(7):491–7. https://doi.org/10.1136/bjsports-2014-093502.
6. Mountjoy M, Sundgot-Borgen J, Burke LM, et al. Relative energy deficiency in sport (RED-S): a position statement from the International Olympic Committee. Int J Sport Nutr Exercise Metab. 2018;28(4):365–75. https://doi.org/10.1123/ijsnem.2018-0127.
7. Stellingwerff T, Mountjoy M, McCluskey WT, et al. Review of the scientific rationale, development and validation of the International Olympic Committee Relative Energy Deficiency in Sport Clinical Assessment Tool: V.2 (IOC REDs CAT2) – by a subgroup of the IOC consensus on REDs. Br J Sports Med. 2023;57:1109–21.
8. Łuszczki E, Jagielski P, Bartosiewicz A, Kuchciak M, Dereń K, Stolarczyk A, Pakosz P, Oleksy L. The LEAF questionnaire is a good screening tool for the identification of the Female Athlete Triad/Relative Energy Deficiency in Sport among young football players. PeerJ. 2021;9:e12118. https://doi.org/10.7717/peerj.12118. PMID: 34557358; PMCID: PMC8420870.
9. Wasserfurth P, Halioua R, Toepffer D, Lautz Z, Engel H, Melin AK, Torstveit MK, Claussen MC, Koehler K. Screening for relative energy deficiency in sport: detection of clinical indicators in female endurance athletes. Med Sci Sports Exerc. 2025; https://doi.org/10.1249/MSS.0000000000003644. Epub ahead of print. PMID: 39780352.
10. Gallant TL, Ong LF, Wong L, Sparks M, Wilson E, Puglisi JL, Gerriets VA. Low energy availability and relative energy deficiency in sport: a systematic review and meta-analysis. Sports Med. 2025;55(2):325–39. https://doi.org/10.1007/s40279-024-02130-0. Epub 2024 Nov 1. PMID: 39485653.

11. Logue DM, Madigan SM, Melin A, Delahunt E, Heinen M, Donnell SM, Corish CA. Low energy availability in athletes 2020: an updated narrative review of prevalence, risk, within-day energy balance, knowledge, and impact on sports performance. Nutrients. 2020;12(3):835. https://doi.org/10.3390/nu12030835. PMID: 32245088; PMCID: PMC7146210.
12. International olympic committee relative energy deficiency in sport clinical assessment tool 2 (IOC REDs CAT2). Br J Sports Med. 2023;57:1068–9.
13. Carl RL, Johnson MD, Martin TJ, Council on Sports Medicine and Fitness. Promotion of healthy weight-control practices in young athletes. Pediatrics. 2017;140(3):e20171871. https://doi.org/10.1542/peds.2017-1871. Epub 2017 Aug 21. PMID: 28827381.
14. Torstveit MK, Ackerman KE, Constantini N, et al. Primary, secondary and tertiary prevention of Relative Energy Deficiency in Sport (REDs): a narrative review by a subgroup of the IOC consensus on REDs. Br J Sports Med. 2023;57:1119–28.
15. Melin A, Tornberg AB, Skouby S, Faber J, Ritz C, Sjödin A, Sundgot-Borgen J. The LEAF questionnaire: a screening tool for the identification of female athletes at risk for the female athlete triad. Br J Sports Med. 2014;48(7):540–5. https://doi.org/10.1136/bjsports-2013-093240. PMID: 24563388.
16. Witkoś J, Błażejewski G, Gierach M. The Low Energy Availability in Females Questionnaire (LEAF-Q) as a useful tool to identify female triathletes at risk for menstrual disorders related to low energy availability. Nutrients. 2023;15(3):650. https://doi.org/10.3390/nu15030650. PMID: 36771357; PMCID: PMC9920150.
17. Sundgot-Borgen J, Torstveit MK. Prevalence of eating disorders in elite female athletes. Int J Sport Nutr Exerc Metab. 2013;23(5):435–47. https://doi.org/10.1123/ijsnem.23.5.435.
18. Armento A, VanBaak K, Seehusen CN, Sweeney EA, Wilson JC, Howell DR. Presence and perceptions of menstrual dysfunction and associated quality of life measures among high school female athletes. J Athl Train. 2021;56(10):1094–9. https://doi.org/10.4085/624-20. PMID: 33626156; PMCID: PMC8530419.
19. Female Athlete Issues for the Team Physician. A consensus statement – 2017 update. Med Sci Sports Exerc. 2018;50(5):1113–22. https://doi.org/10.1249/MSS.0000000000001603. PMID: 29652732.
20. Maïmoun L, Georgopoulos NA, Sultan C. Endocrine disorders in adolescent and young female athletes: impact on growth, menstrual cycles, and bone mass acquisition. J Clin Endocrinol Metab. 2014;99(11):4037–50. https://doi.org/10.1210/jc.2013-3030. Epub 2014 Mar 6. PMID: 24601725.
21. Ackerman KE, Misra M. Amenorrhoea in adolescent female athletes. Lancet Child Adolesc Health. 2018;2(9):677–88. https://doi.org/10.1016/S2352-4642(18)30145-7. Epub 2018 Jul 6. PMID: 30119761.
22. Nattiv A, Loucks AB, Manore MM, Sanborn CF, Sundgot-Borgen J, Warren MP. American College of Sports Medicine. American College of Sports Medicine position stand. The female athlete triad. Med Sci Sports Exerc. 2007;39(10):1867–82. https://doi.org/10.1249/mss.0b013e318149f111. PMID: 17909417.
23. Huhmann K. Menses requires energy: a review of how disordered eating, excessive exercise, and high stress lead to menstrual irregularities. Clin Ther. 2020;42(3):401–7. https://doi.org/10.1016/j.clinthera.2020.01.016. Epub 2020 Mar 2. PMID: 32139174.
24. Angelidi AM, Stefanakis K, Chou SH, Valenzuela-Vallejo L, Dipla K, Boutari C, Ntoskas K, Tokmakidis P, Kokkinos A, Goulis DG, Papadaki HA, Mantzoros CS. Relative Energy Deficiency in Sport (REDs): endocrine manifestations, pathophysiology and treatments. Endocr Rev. 2024;45(5):676–708. https://doi.org/10.1210/endrev/bnae011. PMID: 38488566.
25. Tenforde AS, Carlson JL, Sainani KL, Chang AO, Kim JH, Golden NH, Fredericson M. Sport and triad risk factors influence bone mineral density in collegiate athletes. Med Sci Sports Exerc. 2018;50(12):2536–43. https://doi.org/10.1249/MSS.0000000000001711. PMID: 29975299.
26. Ihalainen JK, Mikkonen RS, Ackerman KE, Heikura IA, Mjøsund K, Valtonen M, Hackney AC. Beyond menstrual dysfunction: does altered endocrine function caused by problematic low energy availability impair health and sports performance in female athletes? Sports

Med. 2024;54(9):2267–89. https://doi.org/10.1007/s40279-024-02065-6. PMID: 38995599; PMCID: PMC11393114.
27. Donovan DJ, Nelson JE, Monaco MA. The cardiac preparticipation sports evaluation. Curr Opin Pediatr. 2023;35(5):546–52. https://doi.org/10.1097/MOP.0000000000001284. PMID: 37555798.
28. Rajan D, Garcia R, Svane J, Tfelt-Hansen J. Risk of sports-related sudden cardiac death in women. Eur Heart J. 2022;43(12):1198–206. https://doi.org/10.1093/eurheartj/ehab833. PMID: 34894223.
29. Afaghi S, Rahimi FS, Soltani P, Kiani A, Abedini A. Sex-specific differences in cardiovascular adaptations and risks in elite athletes: bridging the gap in sports cardiology. Clin Cardiol. 2024;47(9):e70006. https://doi.org/10.1002/clc.70006. PMID: 39228309; PMCID: PMC11372237.
30. D'Ascenzi F, Cavigli L, Marchese A, Taddeucci S, Cappelli E, Roselli A, et al. Electrical and structural remodelling in female athlete's heart: a comparative study in women vs men athletes and controls. Int J Cardiol. 2024;400:131808. https://doi.org/10.1016/j.ijcard.2024.131808. PMID: 38262482.
31. Hoch AZ, Lal S, Jurva JW, Gutterman DD. The female athlete triad and cardiovascular dysfunction. Phys Med Rehabil Clin N Am. 2007;18(3):385–400, vii–viii. https://doi.org/10.1016/j.pmr.2007.05.001. PMID: 17678758.
32. Rao SJ, Shah AB. Exercise and the female heart. Clin Ther. 2022;44(1):41–9. https://doi.org/10.1016/j.clinthera.2021.11.018. PMID: 34930659.
33. Li L, Le Douairon LS, Ding S, Schnell F. Sex differences in the incidence of sudden cardiac arrest/death in competitive athletes: a systematic review and meta-analysis. Sports Med. 2025;55(3):697–712. https://doi.org/10.1007/s40279-024-02163-5. PMID: 39752044; PMCID: PMC11985649.
34. Rickenlund A, Eriksson MJ, Schenck-Gustafsson K, Hirschberg AL. Amenorrhea in female athletes is associated with endothelial dysfunction and unfavorable lipid profile. J Clin Endocrinol Metab. 2005;90(3):1354–9. https://doi.org/10.1210/jc.2004-1286. PMID: 15572426.
35. Grosman-Rimon L, Wright E, Freedman D, Kachel E, Hui S, Epstein I, et al. Can improvement in hormonal and energy balance reverse cardiovascular risk factors in athletes with amenorrhea? Am J Physiol Heart Circ Physiol. 2019;317(3):H487–95. https://doi.org/10.1152/ajpheart.00242.2019. PMID: 31322425.
36. Gleeson M. Immunological aspects of sport nutrition. Immunol Cell Biol. 2016;94(2):117–23. https://doi.org/10.1038/icb.2015.109. PMID: 26634839.
37. Meeusen R, Duclos M, Foster C, Fry A, Gleeson M, Nieman D, et al. Prevention, diagnosis, and treatment of the overtraining syndrome: joint consensus statement of the European College of Sport Science and the American College of Sports Medicine. Med Sci Sports Exerc. 2013;45(1):186–205. https://doi.org/10.1249/MSS.0b013e318279a10a. PMID: 23247672.
38. Tringali C, Scala L, Silvestri I, Vitale J, Scurati R, Michielon G, et al. Protective role of 17-β-estradiol towards IL-6 leukocyte expression induced by intense training in young female athletes. J Sports Sci. 2014;32(5):452–61. https://doi.org/10.1080/02640414.2013.830190. PMID: 24016202.
39. Walsh NP. Nutrition and athlete immune health: new perspectives on an old paradigm. Sports Med. 2019;49(Suppl 2):153–68. https://doi.org/10.1007/s40279-019-01160-3. PMID: 31691927; PMCID: PMC6901425.
40. Sims ST, Kerksick CM, Smith-Ryan AE, Janse de Jonge XAK, Hirsch KR, Arent SM, et al. International society of sports nutrition position stand: nutritional concerns of the female athlete. J Int Soc Sports Nutr. 2023;20(1):2204066. https://doi.org/10.1080/15502783.2023.2204066. PMID: 37221858; PMCID: PMC10210857.
41. Costa RJS, Gaskell SK, Henningsen K, Jeacocke NA, Martinez IG, Mika A, et al. Sports Dietitians Australia and Ultra Sports Science Foundation Joint Position Statement: a practitioner guide to the prevention and management of exercise-associated gastrointestinal perturba-

tions and symptoms. Sports Med. 2025; https://doi.org/10.1007/s40279-025-02186-6. Epub ahead of print. PMID: 40195264.
42. Diduch BK. Gastrointestinal conditions in the female athlete. Clin Sports Med. 2017;36(4):655–69. https://doi.org/10.1016/j.csm.2017.06.001. PMID: 28886820.
43. Lis DM. Exit gluten-free and enter low FODMAPs: a novel dietary strategy to reduce gastrointestinal symptoms in athletes. Sports Med. 2019;49(Suppl 1):87–97. https://doi.org/10.1007/s40279-018-01034-0. PMID: 30671907; PMCID: PMC6445805.
44. Grabia M, Perkowski J, Socha K, Markiewicz-Żukowska R. Female Athlete Triad and Relative Energy Deficiency in Sport (REDs): nutritional management. Nutrients. 2024;16(3):359. https://doi.org/10.3390/nu16030359. PMID: 38337644; PMCID: PMC10857508.
45. American Dietetic Association; Dietitians of Canada; American College of Sports Medicine, Rodriguez NR, Di Marco NM, Langley S. American College of Sports Medicine position stand. Nutrition and athletic performance. Med Sci Sports Exerc. 2009;41(3):709–31. https://doi.org/10.1249/MSS.0b013e31890eb86. PMID: 19225360.
46. McClung JP, Gaffney-Stomberg E, Lee JJ. Female athletes: a population at risk of vitamin and mineral deficiencies affecting health and performance. J Trace Elem Med Biol. 2014;28(4):388–92. https://doi.org/10.1016/j.jtemb.2014.06.022. Epub 2014 Jul 5. PMID: 25060302.
47. Desbrow B, McCormack J, Burke LM, Cox GR, Fallon K, Hislop M, Logan R, Marino N, Sawyer SM, Shaw G, Star A, Vidgen H, Leveritt M. Sports Dietitians Australia position statement: sports nutrition for the adolescent athlete. Int J Sport Nutr Exerc Metab. 2014;24(5):570–84. https://doi.org/10.1123/ijsnem.2014-0031. Epub 2014 Mar 25. PMID: 24668620.
48. Javed A, Tebben PJ, Fischer PR, Lteif AN. Female athlete triad and its components: toward improved screening and management. Mayo Clin Proc. 2013;88(9):996–1009. https://doi.org/10.1016/j.mayocp.2013.07.001. PMID: 24001492.
49. Perou R, Bitsko RH, Blumberg SJ, Pastor P, Ghandour RM, Gfroerer JC, Hedden SL, Crosby AE, Visser SN, Schieve LA, Parks SE, Hall JE, Brody D, Simile CM, Thompson WW, Baio J, Avenevoli S, Kogan MD, Huang LN. Centers for Disease Control and Prevention (CDC). Mental health surveillance among children – United States, 2005–2011. MMWR Suppl. 2013;62(2):1–35. PMID: 23677130.
50. Beers LS, Godoy L, John T, Long M, Biel MG, Anthony B, Mlynarski L, Moon R, Weissman M. Mental health screening quality improvement learning collaborative in pediatric primary care. Pediatrics. 2017;140(6):e20162966. https://doi.org/10.1542/peds.2016-2966. Epub 2017 Nov 7. PMID: 29114061.
51. Jasser J, Patel DR, Beenen KT. The role of psychologists in sport medicine practice. Pediatr Clin North Am. 2022;69(5):975–88. https://doi.org/10.1016/j.pcl.2022.05.010. PMID: 36207107.
52. Chang CJ, Putukian M, Aerni G, Diamond AB, Hong ES, Ingram YM, Reardon CL, Wolanin AT. American Medical Society for Sports Medicine position statement: mental health issues and psychological factors in athletes: detection, management, effect on performance, and prevention-executive summary. Clin J Sport Med. 2020;30(2):91–5. https://doi.org/10.1097/JSM.0000000000000799. PMID: 32000168.
53. Pascoe M, Pankowiak A, Woessner M, Brockett CL, Hanlon C, Spaaij R, Robertson S, McLachlan F, Parker A. Gender-specific psychosocial stressors influencing mental health among women elite and semielite athletes: a narrative review. Br J Sports Med. 2022;56(23):1381–7. https://doi.org/10.1136/bjsports-2022-105540. Epub 2022 Oct 11. PMID: 36220199.
54. Psychological issues related to illness and injury in athletes and the team physician: a consensus statement-2016 update. Med Sci Sports Exerc. 2017;49(5):1043–54. https://doi.org/10.1249/MSS.0000000000001247. PMID: 28410329.
55. Edwards CD, Weatherbee P, Aron CM. Unique considerations for female athletes: a psychiatric perspective. Psychiatric Annals. 2024;54(11):e295–300. https://doi.org/10.3928/00485713-20241107-01.

56. Le LK, Esturas AC, Mihalopoulos C, Chiotelis O, Bucholc J, Chatterton ML, Engel L. Cost-effectiveness evidence of mental health prevention and promotion interventions: a systematic review of economic evaluations. PLoS Med. 2021;18(5):e1003606. https://doi.org/10.1371/journal.pmed.1003606. PMID: 33974641; PMCID: PMC8148329.
57. Brenner JS, Watson A, Council on Sports Medicine and Fitness. Overuse injuries, overtraining, and burnout in young athletes. Pediatrics. 2024;153(2):e2023065129. https://doi.org/10.1542/peds.2023-065129. PMID: 38247370.
58. DiFiori JP, Benjamin HJ, Brenner J, Gregory A, Jayanthi N, Landry GL, Luke A. Overuse injuries and burnout in youth sports: a position statement from the American Medical Society for Sports Medicine. Clin J Sport Med. 2014;24(1):3–20. https://doi.org/10.1097/JSM.0000000000000060. PMID: 24366013.
59. Watson A, Mjaanes JM, Council on Sports Medicine and Fitness. Soccer injuries in children and adolescents. Pediatrics. 2019;144(5):e20192759. https://doi.org/10.1542/peds.2019-2759. PMID: 31659001.
60. Soomro N, Sanders R, Hackett D, Hubka T, Ebrahimi S, Freeston J, Cobley S. The efficacy of injury prevention programs in adolescent team sports: a meta-analysis. Am J Sports Med. 2016;44(9):2415–24. https://doi.org/10.1177/0363546515618372. Epub 2015 Dec 16. PMID: 26673035.
61. Rössler R, Donath L, Verhagen E, Junge A, Schweizer T, Faude O. Exercise-based injury prevention in child and adolescent sport: a systematic review and meta-analysis. Sports Med. 2014;44(12):1733–48. https://doi.org/10.1007/s40279-014-0234-2. PMID: 25129698.
62. Mason L, Connolly J, Devenney LE, Lacey K, O'Donovan J, Doherty R. Sleep, nutrition, and injury risk in adolescent athletes: a narrative review. Nutrients. 2023;15(24):5101. https://doi.org/10.3390/nu15245101. PMID: 38140360; PMCID: PMC10745648.
63. Gooderick J, Clash R, Fisher H, Maxwell N, Hayes M. The use of individualised, media-based sleep hygiene education for professional female footballers. Eur J Sport Sci. 2025;25(2):e12247. https://doi.org/10.1002/ejsc.12247. PMID: 39776218; PMCID: PMC11706236.
64. Fox JL, Scanlan AT, Stanton R, Sargent C. Insufficient sleep in young athletes? Causes, consequences, and potential treatments. Sports Med. 2020;50(3):461–70. https://doi.org/10.1007/s40279-019-01220-8. PMID: 31679145.
65. Beisecker L, Harrison P, Josephson M, DeFreese JD. Depression, anxiety and stress among female student-athletes: a systematic review and meta-analysis. Br J Sports Med. 2024;58(5):278–85. https://doi.org/10.1136/bjsports-2023-107328. PMID: 38233087.
66. McManama O'Brien KH, Rowan M, Willoughby K, Griffith K, Christino MA. Psychological resilience in young female athletes. Int J Environ Res Public Health. 2021;18(16):8668. https://doi.org/10.3390/ijerph18168668. PMID: 34444426; PMCID: PMC8392459.
67. Zisopoulou T, Varvogli L. Stress management methods in children and adolescents: past, present, and future. Horm Res Paediatr. 2023;96(1):97–107. https://doi.org/10.1159/000526946. Epub 2022 Sep 12. PMID: 36096110.
68. Lundqvist C, Schary DP, Eklöf E, Zand S, Jacobsson J. Elite lean athletes at sports high schools face multiple risks for mental health concerns and are in need of psychosocial support. PLoS One. 2023;18(4):e0284725. https://doi.org/10.1371/journal.pone.0284725. PMID: 37083747; PMCID: PMC10121048.
69. Swart E, Redler L, Fabricant PD, Mandelbaum BR, Ahmad CS, Wang YC. Prevention and screening programs for anterior cruciate ligament injuries in young athletes: a cost-effectiveness analysis. J Bone Joint Surg Am. 2014;96(9):705–11. https://doi.org/10.2106/JBJS.M.00560. PMID: 24806006; PMCID: PMC4001460.
70. Webster KE, Hewett TE. Meta-analysis of meta-analyses of anterior cruciate ligament injury reduction training programs. J Orthop Res. 2018;36(10):2696–708. https://doi.org/10.1002/jor.24043. Epub 2018 Jun 13. PMID: 29737024.
71. Padua DA, DiStefano LJ, Hewett TE, Garrett WE, Marshall SW, Golden GM, Shultz SJ, Sigward SM. National athletic trainers' association position statement: prevention of anterior cruciate ligament injury. J Athl Train. 2018;53(1):5–19. https://doi.org/10.4085/1062-6050-99-16. Epub 2018 Jan 9. PMID: 29314903; PMCID: PMC5800728.

72. Stricker PR, Faigenbaum AD, McCambridge TM, Council on Sports Medicine and Fitness. Resistance training for children and adolescents. Pediatrics. 2020;145(6):e20201011. https://doi.org/10.1542/peds.2020-1011. PMID: 32457216.
73. Huang YL, Jung J, Mulligan CMS, Oh J, Norcross MF. A majority of anterior cruciate ligament injuries can be prevented by injury prevention programs: a systematic review of randomized controlled trials and cluster-randomized controlled trials with meta-analysis. Am J Sports Med. 2020;48(6):1505–15. https://doi.org/10.1177/0363546519870175. Epub 2019 Aug 30. PMID: 31469584.
74. Moksnes H, Grindem H. Prevention and rehabilitation of paediatric anterior cruciate ligament injuries. Knee Surg Sports Traumatol Arthrosc. 2016;24(3):730–6. https://doi.org/10.1007/s00167-015-3856-5. Epub 2015 Nov 14. PMID: 26572630.
75. Arundale AJH, Bizzini M, Giordano A, Hewett TE, Logerstedt DS, Mandelbaum B, Scalzitti DA, Silvers-Granelli H, Snyder-Mackler L. Exercise-based knee and anterior cruciate ligament injury prevention. J Orthop Sports Phys Ther. 2018;48(9):A1–A42. https://doi.org/10.2519/jospt.2018.0303. PMID: 30170521.
76. Noyes FR, Barber Westin SD. Anterior cruciate ligament injury prevention training in female athletes: a systematic review of injury reduction and results of athletic performance tests. Sports Health. 2012;4(1):36–46. https://doi.org/10.1177/1941738111430203. PMID: 23016067; PMCID: PMC3435901.
77. Halstead ME, Walter KD, Moffatt K, Council on Sports Medicine and Fitness. Sport-related concussion in children and adolescents. Pediatrics. 2018;142(6):e20183074. https://doi.org/10.1542/peds.2018-3074. Epub 2018 Nov 12. PMID: 30420472.
78. Feiss R, Lutz M, Reiche E, Moody J, Pangelinan M. A systematic review of the effectiveness of concussion education programs for coaches and parents of youth athletes. Int J Environ Res Public Health. 2020;17(8):2665. https://doi.org/10.3390/ijerph17082665. PMID: 32294972; PMCID: PMC7216205.
79. Harmon KG, Clugston JR, Dec K, Hainline B, Herring SA, Kane S, Kontos AP, Leddy JJ, McCrea MA, Poddar SK, Putukian M, Wilson JC, Roberts WO. American medical society for sports medicine position statement on concussion in sport. Clin J Sport Med. 2019;29(2):87–100. https://doi.org/10.1097/JSM.0000000000000720. Erratum in: Clin J Sport Med. 2019;29(3):256. doi:10.1097/JSM.0000000000000764. PMID: 30730386.
80. Bishop ME, Ahlmen A, Rosendorf J, Erickson BJ, Cohen S. Bone stress injuries in female athletes. Ann Joint. 2021;6:37. https://doi.org/10.21037/aoj.2020.04.04.

Value-Based Care for First-Time Pediatric Patellofemoral Dislocations

23

David M. Kell, Brendon C. Mitchell, Akbar N. Syed, and Theodore J. Ganley

Introduction

Lateral patellar dislocations are among the most common knee injuries in children and adolescents, with an estimated incidence ranging from 2 to 77 per 100,000 individuals [1–8]. After a first-time dislocation, recurrence rates range from 15% to 60%, increasing the risk of cumulative chondral damage and the eventual development of osteoarthritis [2, 9]. Physicians must weigh the risk of recurrence and arthritis complications against the importance of minimizing time away from physical activity for the youth athlete.

Management of first-time patellar dislocations is controversial. Historically, patients without an associated osteochondral fracture were treated nonoperatively with a brief period of immobilization followed by physical therapy to gradually restore function and return the patient to pre-injury activity levels [3, 10–12]. However, recent literature has supported surgical intervention after first-time dislocations as a strategy to reduce recurrence and protect against further chondral injury [13, 14].

Ultimately, the treatment decision should be individualized, taking into account the patient's anatomical risk factors, activity goals, and preferences [7]. Management strategies must balance the potential benefits of surgical intervention and the

D. M. Kell · B. C. Mitchell · A. N. Syed
Orthopedics Center, The Children's Hospital of Philadelphia, Philadelphia, PA, USA
e-mail: kelld1@chop.edu; mitchellb4@chop.edu; syeda@chop.edu

T. J. Ganley (✉)
Orthopedics Center, The Children's Hospital of Philadelphia, Philadelphia, PA, USA

Perelman School of Medicine at the University of Pennsylvania, Philadelphia, PA, USA
e-mail: ganley@chop.edu

W. L. Hennrikus, R. M. Schwend (eds.), *Value in Pediatric Orthopaedics*,
https://doi.org/10.1007/978-3-032-19570-8_23

arthritis risks of conservative treatment while also considering the financial implications of each approach. The main goal should be to preserve long-term joint health and optimize functional outcomes while minimizing unnecessary procedures, complications, and costs.

Value-Based Themes

Preoperative Decision-Making

Emergency Department Costs

Patients who experience a patellar dislocation should be evaluated in the emergency department (ED) if they are unable to reduce the dislocation, report severe pain or significant swelling, cannot bear weight, or show signs of neurovascular compromise, such as numbness, tingling, or absent distal pulses. However, Li et al. found that while 87.6% of first-time dislocators sought initial care in the ED, fewer than one-third with recurrent instability did so, suggesting that improved patient education may help reduce unnecessary ED visits [15]. Emergency department visits were associated with an average of $1994 more in charges compared to initial treatment in outpatient settings [15]. Enhancing patient awareness about appropriate care pathways represents one key opportunity to improve the value of care.

Magnetic Resonance Imaging

One indication for surgery after a first-time patellar dislocation is the presence of an osteochondral fracture or loose body, which occurs in 35–76% of cases [11, 16, 17]. MRI is considered the gold standard for identifying a loose body. While plain radiographs are less expensive, they are less sensitive than MRI and can miss up to 33% of loose bodies [18, 19]. In resource-limited settings, it may not always be possible to obtain an MRI [20]. However, without MRI, there is a greater risk that a loose body could go undetected, leading to an increased risk of post-traumatic osteoarthritis [21, 22].

In cases where MRI is not accessible, certain patient characteristics can help guide clinical decision-making. For example, children who have ligamentous laxity (e.g., those with a high Beighton score and an easily dislocatable patella), present without a joint effusion, and have experienced an atraumatic injury are at lower risk for an osteochondral fracture and can forgo MRI [23]. Additionally, female patients, skeletally immature patients, and those with patella alta on radiographs have a reduced risk of an osteochondral fracture following dislocation [23]. On the other hand, a laterally positioned tibial tubercle is a risk factor for osteochondral fracture [16, 23, 24].

Nonoperative Treatment: Bracing

There is no consensus on the effectiveness of a patellar stabilizing brace following a first-time dislocation [3, 25, 26]. In most cases, initial treatment with a brief period of immobilization, followed by physical therapy, is recommended [14]. Although there is variation in the type of immobilization prescribed, two randomized controlled trials have shown that a neoprene, non-hinged knee brace, or taping resulted in better functional outcomes and reduced quadriceps muscle atrophy compared to knee motion-restricting braces or casting [14, 27, 28]. While further research is needed, taping and neoprene sleeves are both effective and inexpensive [27].

Surgical Treatment Considerations

Surgical treatment of first-time patellar dislocations has traditionally been based on the presence of a loose body. Depending on the patient's anatomical risk factors (e.g., elevated tibial tubercle-trochlear groove distance [TT-TG], Caton-Deschamps Index [CDI], or trochlear dysplasia), surgeons may also perform medial patellofemoral ligament (MPFL) reconstruction along with loose body removal. One study has shown that only 26% of patients who received conservative treatment for a first-time patellar dislocation returned to unrestricted activity 3 years later [29]. Additionally, Gurusamy et al. reported that patients who underwent both loose body removal and MPFL reconstruction had five times lower recurrence rates compared to those who did not [30].

A multicenter prospective study on patellar dislocations recently reported that, at 5 years post-intervention, initial surgical treatment was more cost-effective [24]. While surgical intervention has been shown to reduce the risk of recurrent dislocations and further chondral damage, the potential for complications (e.g., infection, stiffness, arthrofibrosis, or neurovascular injury) must also be considered [31–34]. Nwachukwu et al. found that while nonoperative treatment was the least expensive initial option, it was also the least cost-effective in the long run. In contrast, both immediate and delayed surgical interventions (following an initial period of nonoperative treatment) offered greater quality-adjusted life years per dollar spent [35].

Both surgical approaches were deemed cost-effective, depending on the probability of recurrent instability, which is influenced by anatomical factors (e.g., patella alta, trochlear dysplasia) and patient activity goals (e.g., high-level sports participation, frequent cutting or pivoting) [7, 35]. These findings underscore the importance of considering patient functional outcomes and goals, particularly since most dislocations occur during athletic activity. While preliminary evidence suggests that immediate surgical intervention may be more cost-effective for patients at high risk for recurrent instability, more long-term studies are needed. Recently, pediatric orthopedic surgeons reached a 99% consensus recommending nonoperative treatment for patients with a first-time dislocation without osteochondral fractures [14].

Intraoperative Decision-Making

Medial patellofemoral ligament (MPFL) reconstruction is a commonly performed procedure for patellar stabilization and often utilizes various patellar-sided fixation techniques. Many of these methods involve bony fixation. Some require creating tunnels in the patella. The choice of approach ultimately depends on surgeon preference, with an emphasis on minimizing complications and the risk for reinjury, while optimizing recovery [3, 36–43].

Patellar Fixation Implants

Patellar graft fixation can be performed with implant-based or implant-less techniques. Each technique has varying implications for cost, safety, and outcomes. Implant options include interference screws, endo-buttons, and suture anchors. Short-term studies comparing patellar bone socket fixation to cortical surface fixation have found similar patient-reported outcomes [44, 45]. However, both endobuttons and interference screws risk patellar fracture [46]. In contrast, suture anchors mitigate the risk of fracture, potentially improve long-term functional outcomes, and reduce implant costs. Suture anchors are a viable option in value-based care [46–48]. In addition, if bony tunnel fixation is selected, double tunnel techniques are more effective at reducing failure rates and reoperation compared to single tunnel techniques [49, 50].

Alternatively, fixation techniques not using implants such as converging tunnels or the basketweave approach eliminate the cost of implants [51]. Both the basketweave and quadriceps tendon turndown are soft-tissue fixation methods that avoid injuring the physis (Fig. 23.1) [52–54]. In contrast, bony fixation strategies use implants that increase the cost of surgery compared to soft-tissue techniques [55]. A recent multicenter study found no significant differences in short- or long-term complications with or without implants [56]. Overall, soft-tissue fixation techniques offer a more cost-effective option compared to the more expensive fixation strategies using implants.

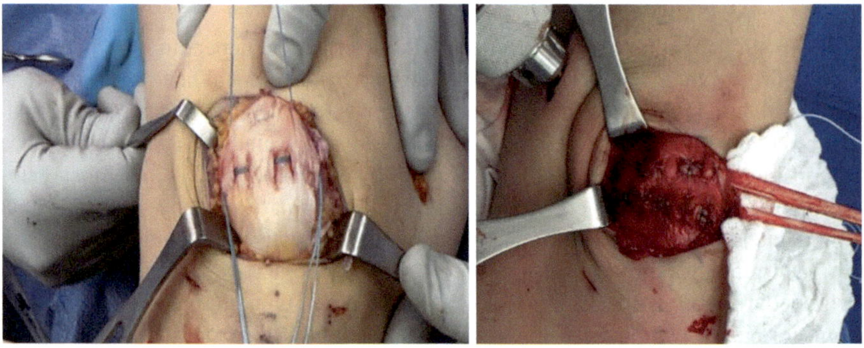

Fig. 23.1 Basketweave preparation with passing sutures and whipstitched MPFL/MQTFL allograft limb with pretzel stitching at weave transition points. Whipstitched limbs were passed subfascially through lateral patellar retinaculum and tied to provide secondary pullout fixation. (Williams et al. [51], requesting permission)

Soft-Tissue Graft Selection

Both autografts and allografts are viable graft options for MPFL reconstruction. Allografts provide equivalent clinical outcomes with the added benefits of lower cost and reduced reoperation rates [57, 58]. A matched-cohort analysis found no significant differences in failure rates, complications, or patient-reported outcomes between the two graft types [57]. Notably, Hendawi et al. found that autografts were approximately $1058 less expensive than allografts. However, the time required for autograft harvesting increased OR costs by $445. In addition, autografts resulted in a 29% higher reoperation rate which added $34,740 in costs to the payor and $4500 in costs to the hospital [58]. Conversely, allografts offer shorter operative time and improved graft survivorship and are therefore the more cost-effective option.

Femoral Fixation

An anatomical MPFL reconstruction is recommended to preserve physiological patellofemoral kinematics [3, 52, 59–62]. Graft fixation at Schottle's point is considered the anatomic origin of the MPFL. Nonanatomic constructs are typically fixed to the medial collateral ligament (MCL) or adductor magnus tendon origin [62, 63]. Malpositioning of the femoral fixation, such as placing it too proximally, can increase patellofemoral loads during knee flexion [61, 64]. However, malpositioning can be avoided by using intraoperative fluoroscopy to optimize graft positioning [65].

When evaluating the most cost-effective implant for fixation, a prospective RCT and a systematic review found no significant differences in clinical outcomes, complications, or re-dislocation rates comparing suture anchors and interference screws [66, 67]. However, a cadaveric study showed that suspensory fixation (e.g., cortical button, TightRope) demonstrated the highest load to failure with the lowest number of graft failures [68]. Suspensory fixation implants, such as a cortical button, are priced similarly to interference screws and suture anchors and are therefore cost-effective.

Other Considerations

Although MPFL reconstruction remains the primary procedure for patients undergoing surgery after a first-time dislocation, a thorough assessment of all patient risk factors is crucial to avoid treatment failure and unnecessary costs. For instance, overall alignment should be evaluated and corrected when needed such as performing hemi-epiphysiodesis for excessive genu valgum [69]. A tibial tubercle osteotomy may be considered for patients with an elevated tibial tubercle-trochlear groove distance or patellar alta [70]. Similarly, a trochleoplasty may be indicated for patients with trochlear dysplasia [71].

Postoperative Decision-Making

Postoperative care following MPFL reconstruction has not been standardized but often includes initial partial weight-bearing with gradual increases in range of motion and quadriceps strengthening [72]. Cost-effective care combines rehabilitation to minimize the risk of arthrofibrosis with limiting the time spent in physical therapy. Studies indicate that early weight-bearing and range of motion are safe and effective and reduce the risk of arthrofibrosis [73]. A hinged knee brace may also be used [74]. However, no significant differences in recurrent instability rates or return-to-sport timelines are reported between patients who were braced or not braced [75]. In addition, excessive knee immobilization can lead to increased quadriceps muscle atrophy and longer rehabilitation time [27].

Case Example

A 16-year-old male sustained his first patellar dislocation after twisting and falling while playing soccer. The patella was reduced in the emergency department, and plain radiographs were obtained demonstrating a small knee effusion but no acute osseous abnormalities. The patient was placed in a knee immobilizer and referred to our pediatric sports medicine clinic for follow-up.

Two weeks later, he was seen in clinic by our nonoperative sports medicine colleague. An MRI was obtained which revealed a small 4 mm intra-articular loose body and a joint effusion with fluid-fluid levels, consistent with hemarthrosis (Fig. 23.2). Additionally, he had a Caton-Deschamps Index (CDI) of 1.18, a tibial tubercle-trochlear groove (TT-TG) distance of 26.1 mm, and a sulcus angle of 140 degrees.

He was then referred to the senior author and pediatric sports medicine surgeon. On examination, he was unable to perform a straight leg raise. He exhibited bilateral ligamentous laxity, including significant knee hyperextension and three to four quadrants of lateral patellar translation. The knee was aspirated in the office, removing 70 ccs of bloody fluid. After discussing treatment options, the patient and his family consented to operative intervention, which included loose body removal and MPFL reconstruction.

Intraoperatively, there was Outerbridge grade 3 chondromalacia on the distal lateral trochlea. A chondroplasty was performed to address the loose, frayed chondral tissue in this area. Additionally, the patella was observed to be laterally

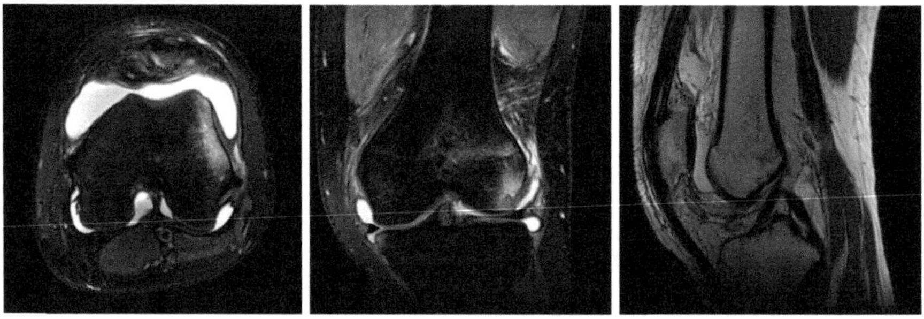

Fig. 23.2 MRI of the injured knee 2 weeks after initial injury

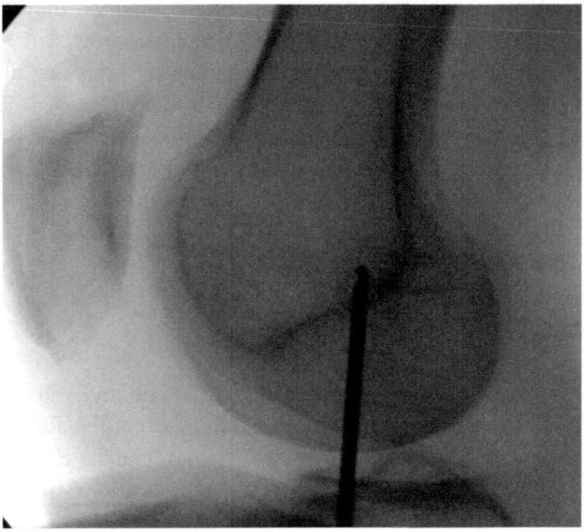

Fig. 23.3 Fluoroscopic images to identify Schottle's point

translated in extension, with engagement within the trochlea occurring only at deeper ranges of flexion.

An MPFL reconstruction was performed using a posterior tibial tendon allograft. The graft was whipstitched at both ends and looped over a suture button construct. The basketweave technique, employing high-strength non-resorbable sutures, was used to fix the two limbs of the graft to the patella and quadriceps tendon. Intraoperative fluoroscopy was used to identify Schottle's point and ensure anatomic reconstruction (Fig. 23.3). A tunnel was drilled in the femur at this location, and the graft was tensioned using the suture button construct. He was fitted with a hinged knee brace, locked in extension, and referred to physical therapy. He remained toe-touch weight-bearing for 2 weeks and gradually increased his weight-bearing and range of motion, progressing from 25 degrees to 135 degrees over a 6-week period.

Summary

This chapter aims to highlight both nonoperative and operative strategies that optimize patient outcomes, reduce costs, and enhance value when treating first-time patellar dislocations.

Author Pearls

- Understand the ABCs of treating patellar dislocations: activity modifications, bracing, and conservative treatment.
- Prevent early arthritic changes by fixing avulsed fractures as indicated.

- Make your first surgery your last surgery—the most cost-effective treatment involves minimizing the need for reoperations.
- Evaluate lower extremity alignment—correcting alignment via guided growth early or osteotomy late.
- Council patients on the risk for reinjury—educate patients about the risks for re-dislocation after nonoperative and operative treatment.

Comments from the Editors

WLH

First-time pediatric patella dislocation—oh my! What a challenging topic to tackle; but, the authors nicely did just that and more! Value enhancing pearls include the following: see the patent in clinic rather than the ED if possible; use a patella sleeve or taping in cases without surgical indications; if surgery is indicated to fix or remove an osteochondral fragment, strongly consider an MPFL reconstruction using an allograft and suture anchors at the same setting; begin weight-bearing immediately postoperatively. For patients with excessive valgus, consider adding guided growth.

RMS

In the management of first-time patellar dislocations in pediatric patients, high-value care begins with identifying those children who do not require surgical intervention. Patients without osteochondral fractures or high-risk anatomic features are better managed nonoperatively. Evidence supports the use of early activity modification, quadriceps strengthening, and cost-effective bracing options such as neoprene sleeves or taping, which offer functional benefits, while minimizing quadriceps atrophy and rehabilitation time. These strategies reduce unnecessary imaging, emergency department utilization, and operative costs. Reserving surgery for patients with intra-articular loose bodies or significant instability risk factors ensures optimal outcomes while aligning with value-based care principles.

References

1. Hsiao M, Owens BD, Burks R, Sturdivant RX, Cameron KL. Incidence of acute traumatic patellar dislocation among active-duty United States military service members. Am J Sports Med. 2010;38(10):1997–2004.
2. Fithian DC, Paxton EW, Stone ML, et al. Epidemiology and natural history of acute patellar dislocation. Am J Sports Med. 2004;32(5):1114–21.
3. Hennrikus W, Pylawka T. Patello-femoral instability in immature athletes. J Bone Joint Surg. 2013;95A:176–83.

4. Sillanpää P, Mattila VM, Iivonen T, Visuri T, Pihlajamäki H. Incidence and risk factors of acute traumatic primary patellar dislocation. Med Sci Sports Exerc. 2008;40(4):606–11.
5. Sanders TL, Pareek A, Hewett TE, Stuart MJ, Dahm DL, Krych AJ. Incidence of first-time lateral patellar dislocation: a 21-year population-based study. Sports Health. 2018;10(2):146–51.
6. Gravesen KS, Kallemose T, Blønd L, Troelsen A, Barfod KW. High incidence of acute and recurrent patellar dislocations: a retrospective nationwide epidemiological study involving 24.154 primary dislocations. Knee Surg Sports Traumatol Arthrosc. 2018;26(4):1204–9.
7. Waterman BR, Belmont PJ Jr, Owens BD. Patellar dislocation in the United States: role of sex, age, race, and athletic participation. J Knee Surg. 2012;25(1):51–7.
8. Nietosvaara Y, Aalto K, Kallio PE. Acute patellar dislocation in children: incidence and associated osteochondral fractures. J Pediatr Orthop. 1994;14(4):513–5.
9. Sanders TL, Pareek A, Johnson NR, Stuart MJ, Dahm DL, Krych AJ. Patellofemoral arthritis after lateral patellar dislocation: a matched population-based analysis. Am J Sports Med. 2017;45(5):1012–7.
10. Cash JD, Hughston JC. Treatment of acute patellar dislocation. Am J Sports Med. 1988;16(3):244–9.
11. Wolfe S, Varacallo M, Thomas JD, Carroll JJ, Kahwaji CI. Patellar instability. In: StatPearls. StatPearls Publishing; 2023.
12. Dixit S, Deu RS. Nonoperative treatment of patellar instability. Sports Med Arthrosc. 2017;25(2):72–7.
13. Balcarek P, Blønd L, Beaufils P, et al. Management of first-time patellar dislocation: the ESSKA 2024 formal consensus-Part 2. Knee Surg Sports Traumatol Arthrosc. 2025; https://doi.org/10.1002/ksa.12637.
14. Parikh SN, Schlechter JA, Veerkamp MW, et al. Consensus-based guidelines for management of first-time patellar dislocation in adolescents. J Pediatr Orthop. 2024;44(4):e369–74.
15. Li LT, Bokshan SL, Lemme NJ, Testa EJ, Owens BD, Cruz AI Jr. Predictors of surgery and cost of care associated with patellar instability in the pediatric and young adult population. Arthrosc Sports Med Rehabil. 2021;3(5):e1279–86.
16. İğrek S, Şahbat Y, Koç E, Çeliksöz AH, Topkar OM. Patellar lateralization, absence of joint hypermobility, and the mechanism of injury are associated with osteochondral fracture after first-time acute lateral patellar dislocation in adolescents: an MRI-based evaluation. J Pediatr Orthop. 2024; https://doi.org/10.1097/BPO.0000000000002629.
17. Khan SA, Baghdadi S, Carey JL, Moores TS, Sheth NP, Ganley T. Osteochondral fractures after patellar dislocation: current concepts. J Am Acad Orthop Surg Glob Res Rev. 2021;5(12). https://doi.org/10.5435/JAAOSGlobal-D-21-00155.
18. Missed Transient Patellar Dislocation in Younger Patients With Traumatic Knee Injuries.
19. Stanitski CL, Paletta GA Jr. Articular cartilage injury with acute patellar dislocation in adolescents. Arthroscopic and radiographic correlation. Am J Sports Med. 1998;26(1):52–5.
20. Hilabi BS, Alghamdi SA, Almanaa M. Impact of magnetic resonance imaging on healthcare in low- and middle-income countries. Cureus. 2023;15(4):e37698.
21. Showery JE, Kusnezov NA, Dunn JC, Bader JO, Belmont PJ Jr, Waterman BR. The rising incidence of degenerative and posttraumatic osteoarthritis of the knee in the United States military. J Arthroplasty. 2016;31(10):2108–14.
22. Gomoll AH, Madry H, Knutsen G, et al. The subchondral bone in articular cartilage repair: current problems in the surgical management. Knee Surg Sports Traumatol Arthrosc. 2010;18(4):434–47.
23. Yi Z, Zhang X, Wu M, Jiang J, Xia Y. Factors associated with an increased risk of osteochondral injuries after patellar dislocations: a systematic review. J Orthop Surg Res. 2023;18(1):822.
24. McGinley JJ, Ellis HB, Propp B, et al. Radiological risk factors for osteochondral fractures in patients with first-time and recurrent patellar instability: data from the JUPITER cohort. Am J Sports Med. 2025;53(4):839–47.
25. van Gemert JP, de Vree LM, Hessels RAPA, Gaakeer MI. Patellar dislocation: cylinder cast, splint or brace? An evidence-based review of the literature. Int J Emerg Med. 2012;5(1):45.

26. Vermeulen D, van der Valk MR, Kaas L. Plaster, splint, brace, tape or functional mobilization after first-time patellar dislocation: what's the evidence? EFORT Open Rev. 2019;4(3):110–4.
27. Honkonen EE, Sillanpää PJ, Reito A, Mäenpää H, Mattila VM. A randomized controlled trial comparing a patella-stabilizing, motion-restricting knee brace versus a neoprene non-hinged knee brace after a first-time traumatic patellar dislocation. Am J Sports Med. 2022;50(7):1867–75.
28. Rood A, Boons H, Ploegmakers J, van der Stappen W, Koëter S. Tape versus cast for non-operative treatment of primary patellar dislocation: a randomized controlled trial. Arch Orthop Trauma Surg. 2012;132(8):1199–203.
29. Magnussen RA, Verlage M, Stock E, et al. Primary patellar dislocations without surgical stabilization or recurrence: how well are these patients really doing? Knee Surg Sports Traumatol Arthrosc. 2017;25(8):2352–6.
30. Gurusamy P, Pedowitz JM, Carroll AN, et al. Medial patellofemoral ligament reconstruction for adolescents with acute first-time patellar dislocation with an associated loose body. Am J Sports Med. 2021;49(8):2159–64.
31. Lewallen L, McIntosh A, Dahm D. First-time patellofemoral dislocation: risk factors for recurrent instability. J Knee Surg. 2015;28(4):303–9.
32. Nwachukwu BU, So C, Schairer WW, Green DW, Dodwell ER. Surgical versus conservative management of acute patellar dislocation in children and adolescents: a systematic review. Knee Surg Sports Traumatol Arthrosc. 2016;24(3):760–7.
33. Bitar AC, Demange MK, D'Elia CO, Camanho GL. Traumatic patellar dislocation: nonoperative treatment compared with MPFL reconstruction using patellar tendon. Am J Sports Med. 2012;40(1):114–22.
34. Gao B, Dwivedi S, Fabricant PD, Cruz AI Jr. Patterns in outcomes reporting of operatively managed pediatric patellofemoral instability: a systematic review and meta-analysis. Am J Sports Med. 2019;47(6):1516–24.
35. Nwachukwu BU, So C, Schairer WW, et al. Economic decision model for first-time traumatic patellar dislocations in adolescents. Am J Sports Med. 2017;45(10):2267–75.
36. Ahmad R, Jayasekera N, Schranz P, Mandalia V. Medial patellofemoral ligament reconstruction: a technique with a "v"-shaped patellar tunnel. Arthrosc Tech. 2014;3(5):e589–92.
37. Russ SD, Tompkins M, Nuckley D, Macalena J. Biomechanical comparison of patellar fixation techniques in medial patellofemoral ligament reconstruction. Am J Sports Med. 2015;43(1):195–9.
38. Ahmad CS, Brown GD, Stein BS. The docking technique for medial patellofemoral ligament reconstruction. Am J Sports Med. 2009;37(10):2021–7.
39. Kang H, Cao J, Yu D, Zheng Z, Wang F. Comparison of 2 different techniques for anatomic reconstruction of the medial patellofemoral ligament. Am J Sports Med. 2013;41(5):1013–21.
40. Kim TS, Kim HJ, Ra IH, Kyung HS. Medial patellofemoral ligament reconstruction for recurrent patellar instability using a gracilis autograft without bone tunnel. Clin Orthop Surg. 2015;7(4):457.
41. Nakagawa S, Arai Y, Kan H, et al. Medial patellofemoral ligament reconstruction procedure using a suspensory femoral fixation system. Arthrosc Tech. 2013;2(4):e491–5.
42. Lorbach O, Haupert A, Efe T, et al. Biomechanical evaluation of MPFL reconstructions: differences in dynamic contact pressure between gracilis and fascia lata graft. Knee Surg Sports Traumatol Arthrosc. 2017;25(8):2502–10.
43. Haupert A, Lorbach O. Anatomic reconstruction of the medial patellofemoral ligament using the fascia Lata as an autograft. Arthrosc Tech. 2015;4(1):e57–63.
44. Desai VS, Tagliero AJ, Parkes CW, et al. Systematic review of medial patellofemoral ligament reconstruction techniques: comparison of patellar bone socket and cortical surface fixation techniques. Arthroscopy. 2019;35(5):1618–28.
45. Migliorini F, Driessen A, Quack V, Schenker H, Tingart M, Eschweiler J. Patellar fixation graft via suture anchors versus tunnel techniques during isolated MPFL reconstruction for recurrent patellofemoral instability: a systematic review of the literature. Arch Orthop Trauma Surg. 2020;140(9):1201–10.

46. Jackson GR, Tuthill T, Gopinatth V, et al. Complication rates after medial patellofemoral ligament reconstruction range from 0% to 32% with 0% to 11% recurrent instability: a systematic review. Arthroscopy. 2023;39(5):1345–56.
47. Mountney J, Senavongse W, Amis AA, Thomas NP. Tensile strength of the medial patellofemoral ligament before and after repair or reconstruction. J Bone Joint Surg Br. 2005;87(1):36–40.
48. Astur DC, Gouveia GB, de Borges SJH, et al. Medial patellofemoral ligament reconstruction: a longitudinal study comparison of 2 techniques with 2 and 5-years follow-up. Open Orthop J. 2015;9(1):198–203.
49. Mohammed R, Hunt N, Gibbon AJ. Patellar complications in single versus double tunnel medial patellofemoral ligament reconstruction. J Orthop Surg (Hong Kong). 2017;25(1):2309499017691007.
50. Wang CH, Ma LF, Zhou JW, et al. Double-bundle anatomical versus single-bundle isometric medial patellofemoral ligament reconstruction for patellar dislocation. Int Orthop. 2013;37(4):617–24.
51. Williams BA, Logterman S, Weltsch D, Lawrence JT. Patellar stabilization using modified basket-weave allograft MPFL/MQTFL reconstruction. Univ Pennsylvania Orthop J. 2021;31:141–4.
52. Nelitz M, Dreyhaupt J, Reichel H, Woelfle J, Lippacher S. Anatomic reconstruction of the medial patellofemoral ligament in children and adolescents with open growth plates: surgical technique and clinical outcome. Am J Sports Med. 2013;41(1):58–63.
53. Fink C, Veselko M, Herbort M, Hoser C. Minimally invasive reconstruction of the medial patellofemoral ligament using quadriceps tendon. Arthrosc Tech. 2014;3(3):e325–9.
54. Kodkani PS. Basket-weave technique for medial patellofemoral ligament reconstruction. Arthrosc Tech. 2015;4(3):e279–86.
55. Tanaka MJ. All-soft-tissue medial patellofemoral complex reconstruction for revisions and skeletally immature knees. Arthrosc Tech. 2024;13(12):103125.
56. O2101: isolated medial patellofemoral ligament reconstruction with and without bony patellar fixation in young patients – a multicenter comparison of three operative techniques.
57. Henstenburg J, Pezzulo JD, Farronato DM, et al. Comparison of clinical outcomes after medial patellofemoral ligament reconstruction with allograft versus autograft: a matched-cohort analysis. Orthop J Sports Med. 2024;12(7):23259671241256983.
58. Hendawi T, Godshaw B, Flowers C, Stephens I, Haber L, Waldron S. Autograft vs allograft comparison in pediatric medial patellofemoral ligament reconstruction. Ochsner J. 2019;19(2):96–101.
59. Bicos J, Fulkerson JP, Amis A. Current concepts review: the medial patellofemoral ligament. Am J Sports Med. 2007;35(3):484–92.
60. Schöttle P, Schmeling A, Romero J, Weiler A. Anatomical reconstruction of the medial patellofemoral ligament using a free gracilis autograft. Arch Orthop Trauma Surg. 2009;129(3):305–9.
61. Elias JJ, Cosgarea AJ. Technical errors during medial patellofemoral ligament reconstruction could overload medial patellofemoral cartilage: a computational analysis. Am J Sports Med. 2006;34(9):1478–85.
62. Schöttle PB, Schmeling A, Rosenstiel N, Weiler A. Radiographic landmarks for femoral tunnel placement in medial patellofemoral ligament reconstruction. Am J Sports Med. 2007;35(5):801–4.
63. Kalinterakis G, Vlastos I, Gianzina E, et al. MPFL reconstruction in skeletally immature patients: comparison between anatomic and non-anatomic femoral fixation-systematic review. Children (Basel). 2024;11(11). https://doi.org/10.3390/children11111275.
64. Amis AA, Firer P, Mountney J, Senavongse W, Thomas NP. Anatomy and biomechanics of the medial patellofemoral ligament. Knee. 2003;10(3):215–20.
65. Parikh SN, Nathan ST, Wall EJ, Eismann EA. Complications of medial patellofemoral ligament reconstruction in young patients. Am J Sports Med. 2013;41(5):1030–8.
66. Migliorini F, Baroncini A, Eschweiler J, Tingart M, Maffulli N. Interference screws vs. suture anchors for isolated medial patellofemoral ligament femoral fixation: a systematic review. J Sport Health Sci. 2022;11(1):123–9.

67. Lind M, Nielsen T, Miller L, Sørensen OG, Mygind-Klavsen B, Faunø P. RCT assessing two femoral fixation strategies. The bone femoral fixation technique used an interference screw in the femur, while the soft- tissue fixation technique looped the graft around the adductor magnus tendon. Arthrosc J Arthrosc Relat Surg. 2019;35:1130–7.
68. Vezolc L, Gunst S, Gras LL, et al. What is the best fixation method in medial patellofemoral ligament reconstruction? A biomechanical comparison of common methods for femoral graft attachment. SICOT J. 2024;10:7.
69. Parikh SN, Redman C, Gopinathan NR. Simultaneous treatment for patellar instability and genu valgum in skeletally immature patients: a preliminary study. J Pediatr Orthop B. 2019;28(2):132–8.
70. Niu EL, Williams BA, Stinson Z, et al. Tibial tubercle osteotomy in the adolescent patient. J Pediatr Orthop Soc N Am. 2023;5(4):750.
71. Nelitz M. Trochleoplasty in children and adolescents. In: Patellofemoral pain, instability, and arthritis. Springer: Berlin/Heidelberg; 2020. p. 545–9.
72. Greenberg E, Hannon J, Chaclas N, et al. Variable guidelines for pediatric medial patellofemoral ligament reconstruction rehabilitation exists across PRiSM member organizations. HSS J. 2024;20(3):365–70.
73. Rahnel T, Weitz FK, Launonen AP, Sillanpää PJ, Hyvärinen AV. Evaluation of an active rehabilitation program with early weightbearing and no immobilization after tibial tubercle distalization. Orthop J Sports Med. 2024;12(11):23259671241287169.
74. DeFrancesco CJ, Storey EP, Shea KG, Kocher MS, Ganley TJ. Challenges in the management of anterior cruciate ligament ruptures in skeletally immature patients. Instr Course Lect. 2018;67:391–402.
75. Schaver AL, Tranovich MA, O'Reilly OC, et al. Postoperative bracing after medial patellofemoral ligament reconstruction. J Knee Surg. 2024;37(9):631–7.

24 Methods to Improve Value During the Preparticipation Sports Evaluation

Rebecca Carl and Cameron Hayes

PPE Overview

Goals

The primary goal of the preparticipation physical evaluation PPE is to promote the safety of athletes. This is achieved through preseason screening aimed at identifying conditions that may be life-threatening or disabling. The PPE also assesses personal and family history to uncover potential underlying health concerns. The PPE determines whether the athlete can safely participate in their desired sport or if modifications, additional testing, and treatment are warranted. However, no evidence exists demonstrating PPE effectiveness. Instead, consensus expert opinion is used to support the PPE as a practical strategy to achieve athlete safety [1].

Ideally, the PPE is conducted by the athlete's primary care doctor, who is familiar with their medical history. Unfortunately, some athletes do not have a primary care doctor. Therefore, a second goal of the PPE is to serve as an entry point into the healthcare system for athletes lacking a primary care physician. For these athletes, the PPE is an opportunity to document medical history, current medications, prior injuries, and any hereditary or chronic conditions and potentially find a medical home that will provide continuity of care.

A third potential goal of the PPE is to provide a setting for athletes to ask questions about health and lifestyle topics such as risky behaviors, substance use, sexuality, and mental health themes. This goal underscores the benefit of conducting the PPE in a private primary care office setting rather than in an open gymnasium. A related fourth goal of the PPE is to give the physician an opportunity to educate the

R. Carl (✉) · C. Hayes
Lurie Children's Hospital, Chicago, IL, USA
e-mail: rcarl@luriechildrens.org; chayes@luriechildrens.org

W. L. Hennrikus, R. M. Schwend (eds.), *Value in Pediatric Orthopaedics*,
https://doi.org/10.1007/978-3-032-19570-8_24

athlete on topics such as nutrition, hydration, supplements, overtraining, and other healthy life habits.

Ethical Considerations

Ethical considerations arise when performing a PPE such as athlete privacy, the legal implications of restricting participation, and maintaining the confidentiality of sensitive information disclosed during the evaluation. Coaches, school administrators, or athletic organizations sometimes request access to medical information, creating a conflict between protecting the athlete's privacy and ensuring team safety. The regulations defined by the Health Insurance Portability and Accountability Act (HIPAA) must be followed. The American Academy of Pediatrics (AAP), in collaboration with six other medical societies, has developed PPE guidelines and intake forms for pediatric athletes. These guidelines state that only the minimum necessary protected health information (PHI) required for determining medical clearance and ensuring safe sport participation should be shared with schools and athletic organizations.

Another ethical concern involves decisions to deny or limit an athlete's participation based on medical findings. These complex decisions carry personal, social, and financial consequences, particularly for those high school athletes pursuing athletic scholarships. If the athlete or their parents perceive the restriction as unjust, inconsistent, or discriminatory, a legal challenge could occur. Lastly, concerns may also arise regarding the consistency of the PPE across different settings such as open gymnasiums vs. private practice offices. Such inconsistencies pose legal risks if an athlete is deemed eligible to play but later suffers harm from an undetected condition.

General Screening Considerations

Ideally, the PPE should be integrated into annual preventive care visits conducted by the athlete's primary care physician in the office. Incorporating standardized PPE questions and physical examination components into routine health supervision improves efficiency and reduces the risk of omitting critical elements [2]. Additionally, embedding the standardized PPE form into the electronic health record improves data collection and future potential research [3].

Medical history is a key component of the PPE. In evaluations of high school and collegiate athletes, history alone has been shown to identify approximately 88% of general medical conditions and up to 75% of musculoskeletal conditions [4]. To improve accuracy, the history forms should ideally be completed in advance of the PPE, with input from both the athlete and a parent. History should include questions about symptoms such as chest pain, syncope, or shortness of breath during exercise, as well as any family history of SCD or known cardiovascular conditions in relatives under age 50 years. Physicians should review these forms in private with the athlete during the PPE to verify the information about musculoskeletal, cardiovascular, concussion, and mental health history.

The physical examination should begin with measurement of vital signs and visual acuity. Elevated blood pressure and visual impairment are among the most common abnormalities identified during the PPE [5]. Reviewing growth curve data can help detect atypical weight changes that may indicate disordered eating or underlying endocrine disorders. The physical examination should be guided by concerns raised during the medical history. Unfortunately, no screening protocol has been shown to reliably predict all injury risk in athletes [6]. Instead, broadly implemented injury prevention programs that emphasize biomechanical training and neuromuscular control can be implemented to reduce the risk of some athletic injuries [7].

The most important component of the PPE is determining the athlete's medical clearance to play. In general, athletes will fall into one of three categories: cleared for full participation, restricted from participation pending further evaluation, or restricted from some or all athletic activities without the need for additional assessment. Eligibility decisions should be guided by clinical guidelines, such as those from the American Academy of Pediatrics (AAP) or the American Heart Association (AHA). Restrictions may depend on the physical demands and risk profiles of the sport, as well as the athlete's medical condition. Overall, about 14% of athletes will require additional evaluation before a final eligibility decision can be made, and 98% will ultimately be cleared to play in their chosen sport [8]. Physicians should engage in shared decision-making, discussing the risks and benefits of participation and considering accommodation, including assistive devices, to allow sport involvement when appropriate. In addition, eligibility determinations should be revisited periodically, as an athlete's medical status and associated risks may change over time.

Special Populations

While the PPE is designed to screen for general medical, musculoskeletal, and cardiovascular conditions applicable to all athletes, additional considerations are necessary for specific groups of athletes including female athletes, athletes with disabilities, and transgender athletes. These populations may have additional health concerns that warrant further evaluation.

Female athletes may face unique challenges related to the female athlete triad or its broader conceptualization—the Relative Energy Deficiency in Sport (RED-S)—which focuses on menstrual health, adequate caloric intake, and bone density. Questions about menstrual history and eating habits should be addressed early as prompt identification of RED-S can prevent long-term consequences like stress fractures and osteoporosis. Obtaining an accurate dietary history may be difficult in athletes with disordered eating due to the athlete's concerns about restricted athletic participation because of this eating behavior. Female athletes are also at higher risk for noncontact ACL injuries, patellofemoral pain, and adolescent idiopathic scoliosis [9]. In addition, female athletes have higher rates of sport-related concussion and longer recovery times after experiencing a concussion [10].

Athletes with disabilities require an individualized approach to the PPE, tailored to their physical or cognitive disability. The primary goal of the PPE for disabled athletes is to promote safe participation in sports whenever possible. The PPE for these athletes should also address disability-specific factors such as assistive device use, skin integrity in those who use wheelchairs or prosthetics, and potential overuse injuries resulting from compensatory movement patterns. Many conditions identified through history and physical examination will not preclude participation but may warrant further evaluation or rehabilitation before playing sports. Effective communication with the athlete, parents, and any involved healthcare team members is essential to understand how their disability may affect sport participation. Lastly, PPE facilities should be accessible to accommodate all athletes.

Transgender athletes present another cohort of athletes for whom physicians must balance medical, ethical, and regulatory considerations. The PPE should focus on current health status and any medical or hormonal treatments the athlete may be receiving. Physicians should maintain a respectful, nonjudgmental environment. The policies of athletic governing bodies regarding transgender athlete participation and hormone use are variable. At the high school level, the National Federation of State High School Associations (NFHS) states that policies regarding transgender athlete participation be handled by individual states and local communities. On the other hand, the International Olympic Committee (IOC) has its own policies regarding athlete participation as it relates to gender identity and testosterone levels. These policies will likely continue to evolve.

Value-Based Themes

General Principles

The value of the PPE remains low. A major problem is the lack of high-quality research demonstrating any effectiveness of the PPE in reducing athlete morbidity and mortality [11]. Limited evidence supports cardiovascular and musculoskeletal screening [2]. Another key limitation is the lack of standardization across states and clinical settings. Although the National Federation of State High School Associations (NFHS) recommends a PPE for all student-athletes prior to sport participation, NFHS lacks the authority to mandate or enforce a uniform approach, leading to variation in how the evaluation is conducted in each state. On the other hand, the PPE remains a key opportunity to engage a broader segment of the youth population that plays sports [12].

The optimal strategy for cardiovascular screening during the PPE remains controversial. The EKG provides improved sensitivity over history and physical examination alone in detecting previously undiagnosed cardiac disorders [13]. However, the American Heart Association (AHA) and American College of Cardiology (ACC) recommend against the universal screening with EKG and echocardiography. The American Medical Society for Sports Medicine (AMSSM) advocates for a selective, case-based approach, to ECG screening [14].

Cardiovascular Screening

Sudden cardiac death (SCD) in young athletes during physical exertion/sports is rare [15]. SCD occurs in approximately 1 in 80,000 high school athletes and 1 in 50,000 collegiate athletes [16]. Identifying athletes at risk for SCD is challenging as these athletes often appear healthy and asymptomatic despite harboring a potentially life-threatening cardiovascular condition [17]. Early and accurate detection is critical; however, there is no consensus on the most effective strategy for cardiovascular screening.

History and physical examination have been the traditional approach for cardiovascular preparticipation screening [18]. However, the sensitivity of history alone for detecting cardiovascular disorders is about 20% [19]. Despite the low sensitivity, screening history questions may prompt further evaluation and, in some cases, prevent morbidity or mortality. One study estimated that history and physical examination alone resulted in a gain of 0.56 life-years per 1000 athletes screened, compared to no screening at all [20]. The cost-effectiveness of this traditional screening model was calculated at $199,000 per life-year saved [20].

While screening with history and physical examination offers some benefits, it also has notable limitations. One major concern is that up to 80% of athletes who experience SCD are asymptomatic at the time of the PPE, making it difficult to identify them using history and physical examination [17]. Additionally, PPE questionnaires depend on the athlete's understanding and honesty. When concerning symptoms are reported, they may be misinterpreted by the physician as normal responses to vigorous exercise. Physical examination presents further challenges, particularly in the realm of cardiac auscultation. Distinguishing between physiological and pathologic heart murmurs can be difficult even for experienced clinicians [21], especially when the examination is performed in an open gymnasium.

The addition of a screening EKG to the standard PPE increases the detection of potentially lethal cardiac disorders in athletes [22]. EKG is five times more sensitive than history and ten times more sensitive than physical examination for the screening of cardiovascular disease in athletes [19]. Up to 60% of disorders associated with SCD in young athletes have detectable EKG changes [23]. In studies at academic centers with considerable experience with EKG screening, the addition of EKG to the PPE increases the sensitivity of detecting previously undiagnosed cardiac disorders [24]. One study found that screening with EKG and cardiovascular-focused history and physical examination saved an average of 2.6 life-years per 1000 athletes screened compared to those who received no screening [20]. The addition of EKG to the PPE results in an average additional cost of $89 per athlete and yields a cost-effectiveness ratio of $42,900 per life-year saved when compared to PPE alone [20].

Other studies have demonstrated that adding an EKG to PPE is not cost-effective. Schoenbaum et al. used decision analysis modeling to evaluate various cardiovascular screening strategies, considering overall costs, quality-adjusted life years (QALYs), and premature deaths prevented [25]. They reported that including an

EKG resulted in an incremental cost-effectiveness of $68,800 per QALY and prevented 131 additional cases of SCD at a cost of $900,000 per case. Most of these added costs were due to false-positive EKG results, which triggered further evaluation and unnecessary and expensive use of healthcare resources. Given that the commonly accepted societal willingness to pay is approximately $50,000 per QALY [26], the authors concluded that adding an EKG to preparticipation screening is not cost-effective.

One of the limitations of EKG screening is its low specificity due to challenges in accurate interpretation. Although standardized interpretation criteria have improved consistency to some extent, these standards remain imperfect. Even among experienced physicians, there is considerable interobserver variability when reading an EKG, leading to both false-positive and false-negative results [27]. False-positive rates of EKG screening are cited in the range of 2.5–6.6% when conducted by a physician with experience with EKG interpretation in athletes [22]. In cases of false positives, athletes may undergo unnecessary additional testing, increasing healthcare costs and potentially causing psychological stress. With millions of high school athletes participating in sports each year, false-positive EKG readings can create a substantial financial burden. Beyond interpretation challenges, EKG is also limited by its dependence on the presence of detectable electrical abnormalities, which may not be present in all at-risk athletes. Overall, while EKG may play a role in select populations, technical and economic barriers limit its feasibility as a universal tool for the PPE.

Conclusions

Unfortunately, the value of the PPE remains low. A major problem is the lack of high-quality research demonstrating any effectiveness of the PPE in reducing athlete morbidity and mortality.

Another key limitation is the lack of standardization across states and clinical settings.

In the context of cardiovascular screening, a focused history and physical examination can detect some conditions at minimal cost. In resource-rich settings, the addition of an EKG to the standard PPE may improve sensitivity for identifying cardiovascular disorders that could result in SCD. However, the optimal strategy for cardiovascular screening and value enhancement during the PPE remains unknown.

Case Example

A 15-year-old high school sophomore presented to his primary care doctor for a PPE before the upcoming high school football season. He reported experiencing palpitations and lightheadedness during some workouts over the summer. He also described a syncopal episode during an especially intense session, which he

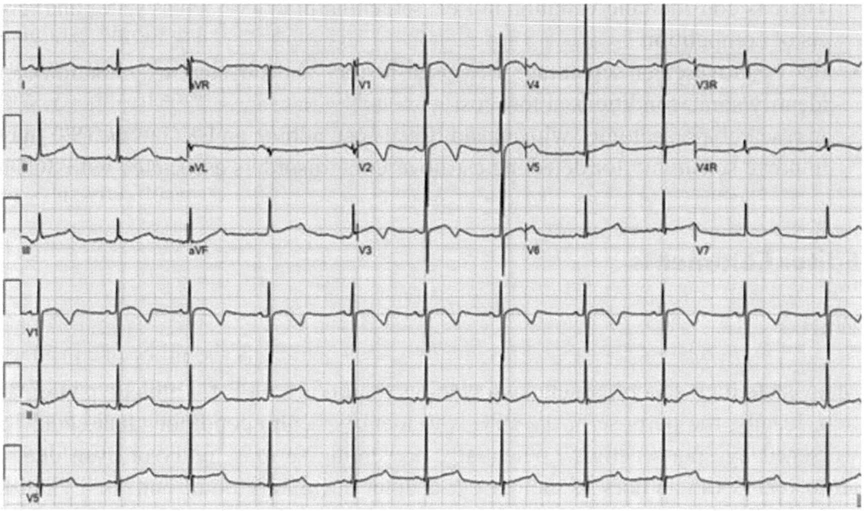

Fig. 24.1 EKG with stress testing showing prolonged QT interval

attributed to inadequate hydration. Notably, he had a family history of SCD in his maternal uncle at the age of 28 years. On examination, his vital signs were age-appropriate, and no heart murmurs were appreciated. However, given the concerning history, his primary care physician ordered an EKG and referred him to a pediatric cardiologist for further evaluation.

His resting EKG did not reveal ventricular arrhythmias but was notable for a prolonged QT interval, with a corrected QT (QTc) of 520 milliseconds. The cardiologist expressed concern for congenital long QT syndrome and recommended further evaluation, including an exercise stress test and genetic testing. The stress test (Fig. 24.1) showed a QTc of 560 milliseconds 3 min into the recovery phase. Genetic testing identified a mutation in the *KCNH1* gene, confirming the diagnosis of congenital long QT syndrome. He was initiated on beta-blocker therapy and monitored for symptom recurrence. At his 3-month follow-up, he remained asymptomatic, with no further episodes of palpitations or lightheadedness. After a shared decision-making discussion with his cardiologist and parents, he was cleared to return to sports, provided he would participate in a supervised setting with access to an automated external defibrillator (AED).

Author Pearls

- The PPE is an important opportunity to screen for health conditions and support safe participation in sports.
- The PPE serves as an entry point into the healthcare system for patients who do not have a primary care physician.
- High-quality evidence supporting the effectiveness of the PPE is lacking.

- There is considerable variation in PPE screening practices across states and levels of competition.
- For cardiovascular screening, a focused history and physical examination can identify some conditions at low cost.
- In research rich settings, with an additional cost, adding an EKG to the PPE may improve sensitivity for detecting cardiovascular disorders associated with SCD.

Editor Comments

WLH

Many state high school athletic associations require the PPE for athletic participation. Ideally, the purpose of the PPE is to identify health conditions that could be worsened by sports activity, potentially preventing serious injury or even death. However, as the authors of the current chapter accurately point out, the PPE has limited effectiveness in detecting conditions that predispose athletes to injury or sudden cardiac events. Additionally, several challenges hinder the utility of the PPE, including cost, timing, time constraints, inconvenience, lack of standardization, risk of disqualification for minor findings, and the potential for false positives. Lastly, what about medical evaluations for students who do not participate in high school sports? The PPE is currently only required for student-athletes, leaving a gap in preventive care for the broader student population.

RMS

The PPE, when performed in the physician's office, offers a possible opportunity to address sensitive adolescent health concerns—including mental health, substance use, disordered eating, sexuality, gender identity, pregnancy, and contraception. Clinicians should respond with empathy, professionalism, and a clear understanding of state-specific confidentiality laws. Most states allow minors to consent to certain services—such as contraception, STI care, mental health, and substance use treatment—while parental consent is still required for other types of care. Respect for adolescent autonomy, confidentiality, and the therapeutic relationship should guide PPE encounters. Physicians must also be aware of mandated reporting requirements, including for suicidal ideation and suspected abuse. A thoughtful, legally informed approach can help make the PPE a meaningful point of engagement in adolescent healthcare—not just a clearance formality.

References

1. Wingfield K, Matheson GO, Meeuwisse WH. Preparticipation evaluation: an evidence-based review. Clin J Sport Med. 2004;14(3):109–22.
2. LaBotz M, Bernhardt DT. Preparticipation physical examination: is it time to stop doing the sports physical? Br J Sports Med. 2017;51(3):151–2.

3. Kriz PK, Clyne AILIS, Ford SR. Preparticipation physical exams: the Rhode Island perspective, a call for standardization. RI Med J. 2016;99:18–22.
4. Koester MC, Amundson CL. Preparticipation screening of high school athletes: are recommendations enough? Phys Sports Med. 2003;31(8):35–8.
5. Dixit S, DiFiori J. Prevalence of hypertension and prehypertension in collegiate student athletes. Clin J Sport Med. 2006;16(5):440.
6. Bahr R. Why screening tests to predict injury do not work – and probably never will…: a critical review. Br J Sports Med. 2016;50(13):776–80.
7. Hewett TE, Myer GD, Ford KR, Heidt RS Jr, Colosimo AJ, McLean SG, Succop P. Biomechanical measures of neuromuscular control and valgus loading of the knee predict anterior cruciate ligament injury risk in female athletes: a prospective study. Am J Sports Med. 2005;33(4):492–501.
8. Smith J, Laskowski ER. The preparticipation physical examination: Mayo Clinic experience with 2,739 examinations. In: Mayo Clinic proceedings, vol. 73, No. 5. Elsevier; 1998. p. 419–29.
9. Loud KJ, Micheli LJ. Common athletic injuries in adolescent girls. Curr Opin Pediatr. 2001;13(4):317–22.
10. Schallmo MS, Weiner JA, Hsu WK. Sport and sex-specific reporting trends in the epidemiology of concussions sustained by high school athletes. JBJS. 2017;99(15):1314–20.
11. Best TM. The preparticipation evaluation: an opportunity for change and consensus. Clin J Sport Med. 2004;14(3):107–8.
12. Park MJ, Brindis CD, Vaughn B, Barry M, Guzman L, Berger A. Adolescent health highlight: health care services. Child Trends; 2013.
13. Baggish AL, Hutter AM Jr, Wang F, Yared K, Weiner RB, Kupperman E, Wood MJ. Cardiovascular screening in college athletes with and without electrocardiography: a cross-sectional study. Ann Intern Med. 2010;152(5):269–75.
14. Drezner JA, O'Connor FG, Harmon KG, Fields KB, Asplund CA, Asif IM, Roberts WO. AMSSM position statement on cardiovascular preparticipation screening in athletes: current evidence, knowledge gaps, recommendations and future directions. Br J Sports Med. 2017;51(3):153–67.
15. Maron BJ, Carney KP, Lever HM, Lewis JF, Barac I, Casey SA, Sherrid MV. Relationship of race to sudden cardiac death in competitive athletes with hypertrophic cardiomyopathy. J Am Coll Cardiol. 2003;41(6):974–80.
16. Harmon KG, Drezner JA, Wilson MG, Sharma S. Incidence of sudden cardiac death in athletes: a state-of-the-art review. Heart. 2014;100(16):1227–34.
17. Maron BJ, Shirani J, Poliac LC, Mathenge R, Roberts WC, Mueller FO. Sudden death in young competitive athletes: clinical, demographic, and pathological profiles. JAMA. 1996;276(3):199–204.
18. Maron BJ, Thompson PD, Ackerman MJ, Balady G, Berger S, Cohen D, Puffer JC. Recommendations and considerations related to preparticipation screening for cardiovascular abnormalities in competitive athletes: 2007 update: a scientific statement from the American Heart Association Council on Nutrition, Physical Activity, and Metabolism: endorsed by the American College of Cardiology Foundation. Circulation. 2007;115(12):1643–55.
19. Harmon KG, Zigman M, Drezner JA. The effectiveness of screening history, physical exam, and ECG to detect potentially lethal cardiac disorders in athletes: a systematic review/meta-analysis. J Electrocardiol. 2015;48(3):329–38.
20. Wheeler MT, Heidenreich PA, Froelicher VF, Hlatky MA, Ashley EA. Cost-effectiveness of preparticipation screening for prevention of sudden cardiac death in young athletes. Ann Intern Med. 2010;152(5):276–86.
21. O'Connor FG, Johnson JD, Chapin M, Oriscello RG, Taylor DC. A pilot study of clinical agreement in cardiovascular preparticipation examinations: how good is the standard of care? Clin J Sport Med. 2005;15(3):177–9.
22. Fudge J, Harmon KG, Owens DS, Prutkin JM, Salerno JC, Asif IM, Drezner JA. Cardiovascular screening in adolescents and young adults: a prospective study comparing the Pre-participation Physical Evaluation Monograph 4th Edition and ECG. Br J Sports Med. 2014;48(15):1172–8.

23. Maron BJ, Haas TS, Murphy CJ, Ahluwalia A, Rutten-Ramos S. Incidence and causes of sudden death in US college athletes. J Am Coll Cardiol. 2014;63(16):1636–43.
24. Wilson MG, Basavarajaiah S, Whyte GP, Cox S, Loosemore M, Sharma S. Efficacy of personal symptom and family history questionnaires when screening for inherited cardiac pathologies: the role of electrocardiography. Br J Sports Med. 2008;42(3):207–11.
25. Schoenbaum M, Denchev P, Vitiello B, Kaltman JR. Economic evaluation of strategies to reduce sudden cardiac death in young athletes. Pediatrics. 2012;130(2):e380–9.
26. Kouakou CR, Poder TG. Willingness to pay for a quality-adjusted life year: a systematic review with meta-regression. Eur J Health Econ. 2022;23(2):277–99.
27. Brosnan M, La Gerche A, Kumar S, Lo W, Kalman J, Prior D. Modest agreement in ECG interpretation limits the application of ECG screening in young athletes. Heart Rhythm. 2015;12(1):130–6.

Part IV

Practice Management

Value-Based Care in Pediatric Orthopedic Urgent Care Centers

25

C. J. Froemming and Kevin Latz

Introduction

Musculoskeletal injuries account for nearly one in five pediatric emergency department visits [1]. However, many of these injuries do not require the high-acuity, high-cost resources of an emergency department. While orthopedic urgent care centers have grown in popularity, few are specifically designed for pediatric patients. Adult-centered care models often overlook the unique physiological and developmental needs of children and adolescents [2, 3].

POUCCs provide efficient, cost-effective care by providing timely evaluation, imaging, and treatment in children for isolated musculoskeletal injuries including fractures, dislocations, strains, sprains, and sports-related injuries. POUCC effectiveness can be maximized through strategies such as optimized scheduling, the use of physician extenders, integration of telemedicine, and streamlined surgery and referrals. These approaches may help to reduce wait times and potentially improve patient satisfaction. The POUCC model aligns with the Institute for Healthcare Improvement's Triple Aim framework: improving population health, enhancing the patient experience, and reducing healthcare costs [4].

C. J. Froemming
Saint Louis University School of Medicine, St. Louis, MO, USA
e-mail: carrie.froemming@health.slu.edu

K. Latz (✉)
Children's Mercy Hospital, Kansas City, MO, USA
e-mail: klatz@cmh.edu

W. L. Hennrikus, R. M. Schwend (eds.), *Value in Pediatric Orthopaedics*,
https://doi.org/10.1007/978-3-032-19570-8_25

Right Patient, Right Setting, Right Time

One of the most critical factors in determining value in pediatric orthopedic urgent care is appropriate patient selection. About 20% of emergency department (ED) visits are due to musculoskeletal complaints, many of which can be managed in an urgent care setting [5]. Children with isolated fractures, sprains, minor dislocations, or soft tissue injuries are appropriate for urgent care. In contrast, polytrauma, open fractures, suspected non-accidental trauma, or injuries requiring surgery should be directed to the ED. Protocols must be established that include clear exclusion criteria and decision support tools to guide proper care location.

Triage protocols help reduce inappropriate ED or POUCC utilization, lower costs, and improve patient satisfaction [6]. Orthopedic urgent care centers and walk-in clinics have reduced the number of orthopedic cases seen in the ED and reduced ED-generated orthopedic referrals [5, 7]. This shift theoretically improves access to hospital services for patients with non-orthopedic conditions [5, 7].

Minimize Cost

Urgent care centers can provide the same care at less cost compared to EDs. Patients with the same diagnoses are often charged up to ten times more at hospital-based EDs than at urgent care centers [8]. In some urgent care settings, professional fees are lower when the patient is seen by a nurse practitioner or by a physician assistant rather than by a physician. Facility fees may also be lower at an urgent care center compared to an ED. One study reported that treating a cohort of patients with low-acuity orthopedic injuries in an urgent care setting, rather than in the ED, resulted in about $62,000 in savings over 6 months [9]. In New York, the average charge for an orthopedic urgent care visit was $670, compared to $1800 for a similar ED visit. This cost difference also benefits patients with high-deductible insurance plans [9]. Overall, national estimates suggest that redirecting up to 27% of ED visits to urgent care centers could result in about $4.4 billion in savings annually [6].

Working at the Highest Scope of Practice

POUCCs often utilize flexible staffing models that enhance cost-efficiency without theoretically reducing the quality of care. For example, physician assistants (PAs) and nurse practitioners (NPs) can manage many common orthopedic injuries with high diagnostic and treatment accuracy [10]. In some states, staffing POUCC with PAs and NPs rather than physicians allows the physician extenders to theoretically work independently at the full extent of their licensure [11]. To maintain safe, high-quality care, the PAs and NPs must undergo supervision from orthopedic surgeons, outcome monitoring, and continuous training. This staffing approach reduces labor costs and maintains access to specialized orthopedic care when needed [12]. Depending on state laws about physician extender oversight, physician leadership philosophies, and potential liability concerns, some POUCC may choose to always have a pediatric orthopedic surgeon on-site when PAs and NPs are seeing patients.

Definitive Fracture Management

POUCC can handle a high volume of fractures. For example, one facility in Los Angeles treated an average of 9619 fractures annually between 2019 and 2023 [13]. To deliver effective care, a fully equipped urgent care center must provide on-site radiography and the ability to manage displaced fractures, including closed reduction and casting/splinting. These services enable definitive treatment at the point of care, which reduces costs and improves patient satisfaction [14].

Coordination with Other Medical Professionals

POUCCs are best integrated into a larger orthopedic care network with efficient referral pathways to surgical and sports medicine specialists. About 75% of cases presenting to orthopedic urgent care can be definitively treated on-site; about 5% of cases are indicated for surgery [15, 16]. Timely referral for surgical treatment remains crucial. For example, a displaced forearm fracture may initially be managed at the POUCC with splinting and pain control, with surgery scheduled at a same-day surgery center in the next few days. This approach ensures continuity of care, avoids unnecessary hospital admissions, and reduces costs [17]. Lastly, healthcare systems must ensure capacity for advanced imaging, referrals to surgeons and subspecialists, operating room time, and follow-up visits to accommodate internal referrals generated by an urgent care clinic.

Same Day/Walk-In Appointments and Expedited Care

Timeliness for appointments is a key component of success for a POUCC. For example, same-day access, walk-in availability, and open appointment slots enable POUCC to efficiently manage acute musculoskeletal injuries. Clinics that prioritize chronic cases over acute cases risk losing their ability to treat urgent patients effectively. Maintaining acute availability every day is key. Rapid access for an appointment in the POUCC reduces unnecessary ED visits and improves patient satisfactions [18]. In addition, one study reported that patients treated at an urgent care center experienced significantly shorter initial wait times (17 min vs. 46 min), reduced visit durations (43 min vs. 156 min), and faster follow-up to orthopedic subspecialists (1.2 days vs. 3.4 days) [5].

Integration with Telehealth

For some cases, telehealth enables POUCC to conduct virtual triage visits and offer follow-up care virtually. Children with routine, nonsurgical musculoskeletal injuries are often unnecessarily transferred from community hospitals or pediatric clinics to tertiary institutions, leading to increased transportation costs, delayed treatment, and additional stress and cost for families [19]. Integrating telehealth into POUCC enhances access to care, particularly for rural or underserved populations. One pediatric orthopedic program demonstrated that implementing telehealth e-consultations prevented unnecessary hospital transfers and reduced average care costs by thousands of dollars per patient [20]. In addition, clinician-to-clinician telemedicine e-consultations are more cost-effective than reflexive ambulance transfers in nearly all scenarios of pediatric musculoskeletal trauma [21]. By incorporating telehealth, POUCC can improve access and convenience while reducing costs.

Case Example

A 12-year-old boy was playing recreational soccer when he collided with another player and fell onto his outstretched hand, resulting in wrist pain and visible swelling. His mom took him to a general ED that lacked pediatric orthopedic expertise. Radiographs revealed an isolated, displaced distal radius fracture. The ED team applied an unmolded short-arm fiberglass cast (Fig. 25.1). This led to further displacement. The patient was ultimately indicated for surgical intervention once seen a pediatric hospital (Fig. 25.2). The costs of the general ED visit and subsequent surgery, along with the time and travel burden on the family, may have been avoided if the patient had initially received initial care at a POUCC.

Summary

Pediatric orthopedic urgent care centers enhance value comparted to emergency departments for managing musculoskeletal injuries in children. The success of POUCC hinges on proper patient selection, skilled PAs and NPs working under orthopedic supervision, access to imaging, and the capacity for coordinated

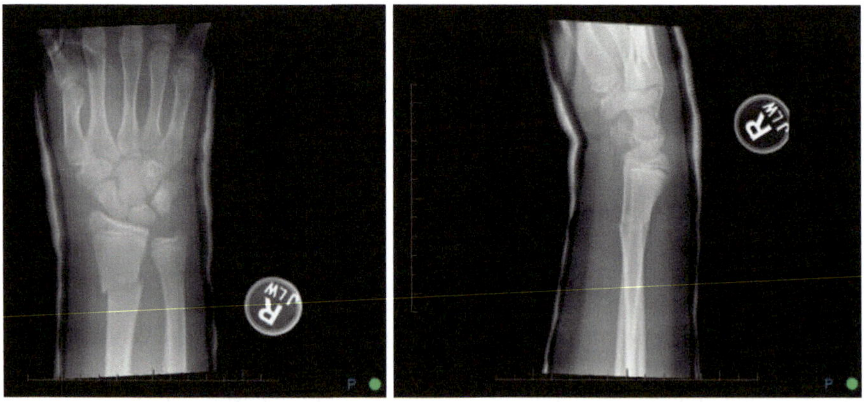

Fig. 25.1 PA and lateral radiographs after the patient received an unmolded short-arm cast

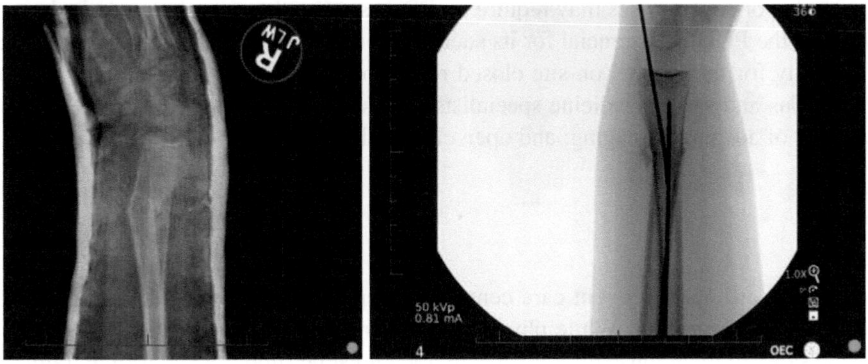

Fig. 25.2 Lateral radiograph showing loss of reduction and subsequent surgical treatment

definitive treatment and follow-up. Overall, POUCCs enhance value by improving access, reducing costs, maintaining excellent outcomes, and increasing patient satisfaction.

Author Pearls

- Up to 30% of pediatric ED visits are for orthopedic injuries, many of which can be managed at an urgent care center.
- Physician assistants and nurse practitioners can provide safe, cost-effective musculoskeletal care and are key members of the POUCC team.
- Facility fees and professional fees can be lower in urgent care settings compared to EDs.
- Providing definitive care at the point of service (e.g., splinting, reduction, and immobilization) enhances value.
- Telehealth e-consultations can prevent unnecessary patient transfers to tertiary centers.
- Healthcare systems must ensure capacity for follow-up visits, advanced imaging, and referrals to surgeons and subspecialists to accommodate internal referrals generated by an urgent care clinic.

Comments by the Editors

WLH

POUCCs offer specialized care for bone, muscle, and joint injuries, potentially enhancing value by providing faster, more convenient, and less expensive treatment than a general ED. However, POUCCs may not be suitable for all injuries, and more complex or severe cases may require an ED. As the authors emphasized, the back-end of the POUCC is crucial for its success. For example, the hospital must ensure capacity for immediate, on-site closed reductions and castings; urgent referrals to surgeons and sports medicine specialists: access to operating rooms; timely availability of advanced imaging; and open clinic follow-up slots.

RMS

Pediatric orthopedic urgent care centers deliver value when integrated into a collaborative care model. While physician assistants and nurse practitioners can provide safe, efficient musculoskeletal care, they must be supported by formal training and close supervision by orthopedic surgeons. Review of PA and NP notes, oversight agreements, and accessible specialty support are crucial for ensuring safety, accountability, and quality care. The true value of this model lies in the teamwork it fosters providing timely expert care without compromising outcomes or patient trust.

References

1. de Inocencio J, Carro M, Flores M, Carpio C, Mesa S, Marín M. Epidemiology of musculoskeletal pain in a pediatric emergency department. Rheumatol Int. 2016;36(1):83–9.
2. Gladden PB, Wilson CH, Suk M. Pediatric orthopedic trauma: principles of management. Semin Pediatr Surg. 2004;13(2):119–25.
3. Musgrave DS, Mendelson SA. Pediatric orthopedic trauma: principles in management. Crit Care Med. 2002;30(11 Suppl):S431–43.
4. Berwick DM, Nolan TW, Whittington J. The triple aim: care, health, and cost. Health Aff. 2008;27(3):759–69.
5. Anderson TJ, Althausen PL. The role of dedicated musculoskeletal urgent care centers in reducing cost and improving access to orthopaedic care. J Orthop Trauma. 2016;30(Suppl 5):S3–s6.
6. Weinick RM, Burns RM, Mehrotra A. Many emergency department visits could be managed at urgent care centers and retail clinics. Health Aff (Millwood). 2010;29(9):1630–6.
7. MacKechnie MC, Nadeau M, Deering E, Thaller J, MacKechnie MA. Orthopaedic walk-in clinics: a model to lessen the burden on emergency departments during the COVID-19 pandemic. J Orthop. 2020;20:293–6.
8. Ho V, Metcalfe L, Dark C, Vu L, Weber E, Shelton G Jr, et al. Comparing utilization and costs of care in freestanding emergency departments, hospital emergency departments, and urgent care centers. Ann Emerg Med. 2017;70(6):846–57.e3.
9. Pean CA, Bird ML, Buchalter DB, Yang SS, Egol KA. Orthopaedic urgent care versus the emergency department: cost implications for low-energy fracture care. J Am Acad Orthop Surg. 2022;30(3):e371–e4.
10. Boman E, Duvaland E, Gaarde K, Leary A, Rauhala A, Fagerström L. Implementation of advanced practice nursing for minor orthopedic injuries in the emergency care context: a non-inferiority study. Int J Nurs Stud. 2021;118:103910.
11. Enslin S. Optimizing the Role of Advanced Providers (APPs): involving APPs in practice operations: ASGE; Available from: https://www.asge.org/home/resources/publications/practical-solutions/practical-solutions-april-optimizing-the-role-of-advanced-practice-providers

12. Spence BG, Ricci J, McCuaig F. Nurse practitioners in orthopaedic surgical settings: a review of the literature. Orthop Nurs. 2019;38(1):17–24.
13. Abbott A, Swertfager K, Bloom S, Jackson NJ, Goldman J. Pediatric fracture epidemiology in an orthopaedic urgent care setting. J Pediatr Orthop Soc N Am. 2025:100216.
14. Krause P. Pediatric orthopedic urgent care: efficient care for minor musculoskeletal injuries. J Pediatr Orthop. 2021;41(6):e438–e44.
15. Badia A, Irizarry J, Rylander E, Cela T. Orthopedic Immediate Care. J Orthop Experience Innov. 2020;1(1).
16. Henry TW, Lutsky K, Beredjiklian P, Matzon J. The five-year growth of an orthopedic urgent care center: identifying patient and center trends. Cureus. 2022;14(12).
17. Schmale GAML. Telemedicine in pediatric orthopaedics: value and cost-effectiveness. J Am Acad Orthop Surg. 2020;28(11):e486–e93.
18. Orthopedics M. [cited 2025]. Available from: https://midamericaortho.com/blog/275-orthopaedic-immediate-care-vs-the-emergency-room
19. Mowrer G, Pilla N, Sorenson S, Armstron D, Hennrikus W. Emergency pediatric orthopaedic transfer criteria: a pilot study. J Surg Orthop Adv. 2023;32:182–6.
20. Study AC. Nemours Children's Health: Telemedicine and Pediatric Orthopaedic Triage; Available from: https://www.aha.org/role-hospitals-nemours-childrens-health-how-telemedicine-can-cut-costs-and-speeds-care-pediatric-orthopedic-injuries
21. Maheu AR, Shih YC, LeBrun DG, Fabricant PD, Atanda AW Jr. A telemedicine solution to minimize unnecessary emergency department transfers for low-acuity pediatric orthopaedic patients: a model for cost minimization. J Am Acad Orthop Surg. 2024;32(9):e443–e51.

The Value of Reusing Orthopedic-Related Equipment

26

Michaela Booker, Ellen Tsay, and Sanjeev Sabharwal

Introduction

Compared to other countries, the USA has one of the highest per capita healthcare costs estimated to be 2.5 times higher than the global average [1]. These elevated costs can limit access to care and contribute to health inequities [2, 33]. In addition, hospitals, especially operating rooms, generate substantial medical waste which can negatively impact the environment [4–6]. The combined effects of high healthcare costs and environmental harm from disposed waste can also contribute to poor health outcomes [6, 7]. In response to these challenges, some countries have implemented systems for reusing orthopedic-related equipment such as external fixator components [8, 11]. In contrast, reuse of medical equipment remains uncommon in the USA. However, adopting safe and effective reuse strategies for orthopedic equipment could enhance value by reducing medical waste and healthcare costs. The current chapter explores the value of reusing surgical and orthopedic-related equipment, the associated costs, and potential pathways for broader implementation.

Definitions

In Table 26.1, we define several terms used in this chapter. We will focus on the reuse and refurbishing of commonly used orthopedic-related equipment.

This table defines key terms related to the life cycle management of orthopedic-related equipment. It includes definitions for "repurpose," "reuse," and "refurbish,"

M. Booker · E. Tsay · S. Sabharwal (✉)
University of California, San Francisco, Department of Orthopaedic Surgery, San Francisco, CA, USA
e-mail: Michaela.booker@ucsf.edu; ellen.tsay@ucsf.edu; sanjeev.sabharwal@ucsf.ed

W. L. Hennrikus, R. M. Schwend (eds.), *Value in Pediatric Orthopaedics*, https://doi.org/10.1007/978-3-032-19570-8_26

Table 26.1 Reuse and refurbishing of orthopaedic-related equipment

Repurpose	To use a device for the purpose other than originally intended
Reuse	To use an equipment or device for more than one deployment of its intended function
Refurbish	To process a previously used device for reuse after confirming appropriate fitness to use based on specific standards [1]

each describing different methods of extending or altering the use of medical devices.

1. *The Value of Reusing Orthopedic-Related Equipment*

Reusing orthopedic-related equipment adds value in three key areas: ethical, environmental, and economic.

(a) *Enhanced Delivery of Ethically Grounded Surgical Care*

Reusing orthopedic equipment supports two core principles of medical ethics: justice and beneficence. By facilitating broader access to care, reuse of orthopedic equipment helps ensure that more patients such as patients in low- and middle-income countries (LMICs) receive the treatment they need. In these environments, patients sometimes face barriers to accessing timely and appropriate care due to limited availability of surgical resources such as implants and instruments [13]. Instead of discarding certain items after a single use, some orthopedic equipment can be safely sterilized or refurbished and redistributed to meet the needs of underserved populations, both locally and globally [13, 14].

High-income countries (HICs) have greater resources but are not immune to health disparities [15]. Millions of Americans are either uninsured or enrolled in public insurance programs for low-income individuals, veterans, or military members. These populations can experience poorer health outcomes [16–26]. Uninsured patients may delay recommended tests and treatments due to financial concerns [3]. Reinvesting cost savings from the reuse of orthopedic equipment could help improve access and health inequities for these vulnerable populations.

(b) *Minimizing the Negative Impact of Surgical Waste on the Environment*

According to the 2009 *Lancet* Climate Change Commission, climate change is the biggest global health threat of the twenty-first century [5, 27, 28]. The USA is among the top 3 global contributors to greenhouse gas emissions [29, 30]. The USA generates over four billion pounds of medical waste annually [31–33]. The health consequences of climate change are evident. For example, in the late 1990s, smoke from the uncontrolled burning of tropical forests following an El Niño weather event led to respiratory illness in Indonesia and Brazil [34]. In 1998, Hurricane Mitch caused extensive deforestation and flooding across Central America, creating stagnant water that resulted in outbreaks of cholera, malaria, and dengue fever [4].

Climate change can exacerbate global health risks and be potentially influenced by the environmental impact of medical waste.

The operating room (OR) accounts for 50–70% of total medical waste [29]. As such, the OR represents a key target for interventions aimed at reducing medical waste [16, 31, 35–38]. A large portion of this waste is attributed to single-use devices (SUDs), making the replacement of single-use devices with reusable alternatives a promising strategy. For example, reusing a disposable laryngeal masks up to 40 times reduced environmental impact by 50% by limiting the production and polymerization of polyvinyl chloride (PVC) [30]. Similarly, reusing surgical gowns and drapes consumes 50–66% less energy and generates 86% less waste compared to disposable counterparts [39]. Furthermore, reusing rigid sterilization containers (RSCs) rather than using single-use polypropylene packaging for surgical instruments lowers carbon emissions and eco-costs by 85% [40].

Given the potential global health consequences of climate change, developing systems to reduce surgical waste can potentially enhance health outcomes worldwide.

(c) *Reduction of the Economic Burden of Surgical Care*

High healthcare costs often limit access to care in low- and middle-income countries (LMICs) [13]. However, patients in high-income countries (HICs) also face barriers because of substantial price markups for medical services and devices, leading to poor cost-effectiveness [40, 41]. For example, a ventriculoperitoneal shunt system costs $650 in the USA but only $35 in India [41]. According to a PBS report, the USA spends roughly $900 per person annually on healthcare administrative costs, compared to $300 in France [42]. Similarly, the average hospital stay costs $18,000 in the USA, versus $6200 in other countries [42]. Nearly half of American adults now report being unable to afford healthcare resulting in delayed or lack of medical treatment [3, 17].

Reusing medical equipment can lead to cost savings. For example, two studies have shown that reusing external fixator components reduces expenses [8, 13]. Dirschl et al. reported a 34% reduction in mean hospital charges from $1864 to $1238 over a 15-month period following the implementation of a reuse program for external fixator parts [9]. Similarly, at one US trauma center, reusing refurbished external fixator components, saved $65,452 over 30 months [10]. A systematic review found that reusing laparoscopic equipment resulted in annual cost savings of $17,500 [43]. Another study reported that switching to reusable instrument sets for dermatologic procedures saved approximately £7 per procedure compared to disposable alternatives.

2. *The Costs of Reusing Orthopedic-Related Equipment*

While reusing orthopedic equipment can enhance value, reuse also entails challenges and costs that limit widespread implementation.

(a) *Sterility and Safety*

A primary concern when considering the reuse of orthopedic equipment is safety, specifically whether reuse increases the risk of infection or mechanical failure. The following section examines several commonly reused orthopedic devices, focusing on safety considerations, sterilization protocols, and the associated costs of instrument reprocessing.

(i) *Sterility Concerns*

The evidence on the sterility of reused orthopedic equipment is mixed and varies depending on the type of device. For example, tourniquets are frequently contaminated but can be effectively sterilized for reuse. Mufarrih et al. demonstrated that a weekly disinfection protocol using a 30-min sodium hypochlorite soak eliminated all detectable organisms on tourniquets [44]. Disposable gowns and drapes, introduced in the 1980s, have not been shown to conclusively reduce surgical site infections compared to reusable alternatives [45]. However existing data is limited [38, 45–50].

External fixator components have been more thoroughly studied. Research shows no differences in pin site infection rates, fixation loss, or loosening when reused [4, 11, 52]. While these findings are reassuring, the risk of infection is not zero. Although direct studies on protein contamination in reused external fixators are limited, evidence from other surgical instruments raises some concerns. For example, Baxter et al. found that reprocessed instruments from five national hospitals in England and Wales retained median residual protein levels ranging from 163 to 756 micrograms per instrument, despite standard cleaning and sterilization protocols [53]. This suggests that some devices, including external fixation components, may retain proteinaceous material even after reprocessing.

(ii) *Mechanical Integrity Concerns*

In addition to sterility, mechanical integrity is a critical consideration when reusing surgical instruments after reprocessing. As with sterility data, evidence on mechanical durability varies by device type. For example, Darvish et al. compared new vs. reprocessed drill bits and found that reprocessed bits exhibited shortened chisel edges that reduced drilling efficiency and compromised mechanical performance [55]. In contrast, studies on arthroscopic shaver blades have shown minimal visible wear after a single use [56, 57]. For external fixation systems, components such as bolts and wires require particular scrutiny. Wosar et al. found that cannulated and slotted bolts failed to maintain 70% of the initial wire tension after seven and four uses, respectively [58]. These findings underscore that mechanical degradation is highly device-specific and dependent on the number of reuses. As such, the safe reuse of surgical instruments demands equipment-specific guidelines and testing.

(iii) *Upholding Sterility and Mechanical Integrity*

Preventing the adverse effects of improper re-sterilization and mechanical wear comes at a cost. In some cases, this cost can exceed the savings from reusing equipment. In one study, single-use devices in lumbar spine surgery demonstrated a cost savings of $181 compared to reused instruments due to the cost of reprocessing and re-sterilization [59]. Similarly, a separate study comparing disposable and reusable instrument kits in lumbar fusions showed a cost advantage for disposable kits due to the high cost of sterilizing reusable components [60].

Lastly, when evaluating infection prevention methods for reused equipment, a major challenge is the lack of safety data and the absence of standardized policies for reporting adverse outcomes. These gaps hinder the development of evidence-based recommendations. Additionally, many existing safety studies are supported by industry funding [61, 62] which may introduce biases and affect the reliability of conclusions. Independent research and comprehensive reporting are needed about infection prevention.

(b) *The Hidden Cost of Reusing*

In addition to the expected costs of infection prevention when reusing orthopedic instruments, there are also hidden costs to consider, such as tool repair, replacement, and ongoing maintenance. A cost analysis by Schaer et al. compared laparoscopic SUDs with reusable instruments, incorporating both expected and hidden costs [63]. For reusable instruments, hidden costs included depreciation, repair, replacement, cleaning, sterilization, and associated labor [63]. The study found that the annual cost of SUDs was seven times higher than that of reusable instruments; however, the hidden costs accounted for 56% of the total expense for reusable options [63]. Maintenance and repair remain essential considerations. Using a life cycle assessment, Rizan et al. analyzed the cost of repairing surgical scissors, including purchase, decontamination, repair, and waste disposal. They found that repairing scissors was more cost-effective than purchasing new ones [64]. However, the frequency and feasibility of repairs were uncertain and unpredictable. In some cases, the cumulative cost of upkeep may exceed that of replacement.

(c) *Risk of Liability*

In 2007, a survey of 287 Canadian acute-care hospitals revealed that 75% did not reuse SUDs, primarily due to concerns about potential litigation [65, 66]. In the USA, the federal government regulates the reuse of reprocessed SUDs through two pieces of legislation passed in 2000 and 2002. This legislation established regulatory requirements that allowed the reuse of certain FDA Class I and II medical devices [67–69]. The majority of reusable SUDs (about 75%) fall into the Class II category [36] (Table 26.2).

This table outlines the three FDA medical device classes, categorized according to the level of risk associated with their use.

Table 26.2 Description of FDA medical device classes [69]

Class	Risk level	Description	Examples
Class I	Low risk	Subject to general controls (e.g., labeling, registration). Most are exempt from premarket notification	Bandages, tongue depressors, manual instruments
Class II	Moderate risk	Subject to general and special controls. Often requires 510(k) premarket notification	Surgical drapes, orthopedic implants, infusion pumps
Class III	High risk	Requires premarket approval (PMA). Supports or sustains life or presents high risk	Pacemakers, heart valves, implantable defibrillators

Following these policy changes, reporting violations have occurred primarily involving the reuse of devices labeled by the FDA as single use. These violations have resulted in prison sentences and fines for both hospitals and individual physicians [70–73]. While these cases are extreme, they underscore the importance of adhering to regulations on equipment reuse and validate the concerns regarding liability and potential litigation.

W Erosion of Public Trust

The reuse of surgical equipment is sometimes viewed negatively by the public. For example, in one study examining public perceptions of SUDs, 45% of participants expressed doubts about the safety of reprocessing and reusing the surgical equipment [74]. Similarly, when nursing students were surveyed about their attitudes toward reprocessed SUDs, they identified public concern over safety as the most significant perceived barrier [75]. Reused equipment is often seen as inferior, due in part to its lower cost [11, 51, 54]. Building public trust in reprocessed equipment involves addressing misconceptions and conducting rigorous safety research.

(d) *The Need for Infrastructure Development*

The lack of infrastructure, knowledge, and training is a barrier to implementing sustainable, environmentally friendly practices in orthopedics [38]. Currently, there are no protocols for assessing the suitability of reusing orthopedic equipment, nor is there a workforce trained to reprocess such equipment [8, 65, 66, 76–80]. These gaps contribute to concerns about safety and litigation and discourage hospitals and surgeons from adopting reuse practices [65, 66].

3. *Potential Solutions*

Having reviewed the value and cost of reusing SUDs, the next section explores potential solutions to overcome barriers to the reuse of orthopedic equipment.

(a) *Reverse Innovation*

These are examples where HICs can further study and adopt successful reuse protocols that have been studied and reported as successful and safe in resource-limited environments.

Reverse innovation is a well-established concept in the business world that refers to the flow of ideas from lower- to higher-income settings [81]. This approach is effective because resource-limited environments are often more motivated to innovate and implement new systems and technologies. With fewer regulatory and cultural barriers, these innovations can be adopted more rapidly in low-income countries [81]. For example, to reduce costs for the UK's National Health Service (NHS), the Institute of Global Health Innovation (IGHI) implemented the Arbutus Drill Cover System, originally developed in Kampala, Uganda. This system employs a sterilizable, reusable cover for surgical drills, with the potential to reduce costs by about 94% [82]. Similarly, in 2021, during COVID-19 pandemic, two physicians in India developed and published safety guidelines for face shield reuse [83]. These two examples demonstrate how high-income countries can learn from and potentially adopt safe, evidence-based reuse protocols developed in low-income countries.

(b) *Establishing Standards*

There is a lack of research on the safety of reusing orthopedic-related surgical equipment. For example, the number of times certain instruments can be safely and effectively reused remains unclear. A potential solution involves establishing universal standards and protocols for reusing orthopedic equipment. Doing so could alleviate safety concerns and reduce the fear of litigation.

Medical and legal teams must be well-informed about regulatory guidelines and should work collaboratively to advise surgeons and hospitals on issues of safety, efficacy, and liability. Professional associations and regulatory bodies play a key role by developing clear guidelines that include criteria for equipment selection, screening, evaluation, and preparation for reuse with patient safety as a top priority [54, 77, 82]. In addition, workflows should incorporate recordkeeping systems that track reused equipment, including data on the recommended lifespan and number of prior uses. In addition, adverse event reporting systems and specific reuse protocols should be developed. These frameworks would serve as a foundation for guidelines on the safe reuse of orthopedic surgical equipment [77].

Conclusion

As one of the highest per capita healthcare spenders globally, the USA would potentially benefit from developing models that reduce overall healthcare delivery costs and expand patient access. The operating room is a major source of medical waste, contributing to climate change and adverse health outcomes. Implementing strategies to reduce surgical waste could help mitigate these effects and improve population health. Reusing surgical and orthopedic-related equipment enhances value by delivering care that is safe, cost-effective, locally relevant, and environmentally sustainable. Lastly, further research is needed to better understand the financial and environmental implications of reusing orthopedic equipment before such practices can be adopted on a larger scale.

Chapter Pearls

- Reusing pediatric orthopedic equipment can reduce environmental impact and lower healthcare costs.
- Barriers to widespread adoption include concerns about patient safety, liability risks, negative public perceptions, and logistical challenges such as limited infrastructure and quality control measures.
- Some low- and middle-income countries already have established models of equipment reuse that could be adapted by high-income countries like the USA.
- Further research is needed to evaluate the safety and efficacy of reusing various orthopedic devices and to develop standardized reuse guideline.

Disclaimer

This chapter was adapted from the original JBJS Review article [12] written by Dr. Ellen Tsay and Dr. Sanjeev Sabharwal with permission from JBJS.

Editor Comments

WLH

Reusing orthopedic equipment presents a promising opportunity to enhance value in pediatric orthopedics and is already a common practice in many low- and middle-income countries. However, widespread adoption in the USA is hindered by several challenges, including concerns about patient safety, liability risks, negative public perception, and inadequate quality control infrastructure. Further research is needed to explore the safety, efficacy, and broader implications of this cost-saving and environmentally sustainable approach.

RMS

A common question is how to send supplies, instruments, implants, and equipment to low- and middle-income countries (LMICs). The following is a list of organizations that accept and process these donations.

Organization	Website	Unique feature	Approx. dollar value
Doc to Dock	https://www.doctodock.org	Ships containers (~$500 K value) from surplus US hospital supplies by request	$500 K/container
Primis Medical	https://primismedical.com	Salt Lake City-based; manages $100 M+ in medical assets under CEO Doug Beck; uses TAP platform	$100 M+
MedShare	https://www.medshare.org	Dual distribution centers; offers recipient-customized online inventory	$100 M+
Project C.U.R.E.	https://www.projectcure.org	Ships ~2 customized 40-ft containers per week worldwide; largest US distributor	$40–45 M/year
SIGN Fracture Care International	https://www.signfracturecare.org	Orthopedic-specific; manufactures implants and trains surgeons in LMICs	$8.7 M/year
Afya Foundation	https://www.afyafoundation.org	Web-based item selection for LMIC partners; focus on Africa and the Caribbean	Tens of millions (estimated)

References

1. Egol KA, Capriccioso CE, Konda SR, et al. Cost-effective trauma implant selection: AAOS exhibit selection. J Bone Jt Surg. 2014;96(22):e189. https://doi.org/10.2106/JBJS.N.00514.
2. Tzenios N. The determinants of access to healthcare: a review of individual, structural, and systemic factors. J Humanit Appl Sci Res. 2019;2(1):1–14.
3. Montero A, Kearney A, Hamel L, Brodie M. Americans' challenges with health care costs. Kaiser Family Foundation. 2022;14. Accessed 3 Aug 2023. https://www.kff.org/health-costs/issue-brief/americans-challenges-with-health-care-costs/.
4. Epstein PR. Climate and health. Science. 1999;285(5426):347–8. https://doi.org/10.1126/science.285.5426.347.
5. Bekkar B, Pacheco S, Basu R, DeNicola N. Association of air pollution and heat exposure with preterm birth, low birth weight, and stillbirth in the US: a systematic review. JAMA Netw Open. 2020;3(6):e208243. https://doi.org/10.1001/jamanetworkopen.2020.8243.
6. Eckelman MJ, Sherman J. Environmental impacts of the U.S. health care system and effects on public health. PLoS One. 2016;11(6):e0157014. https://doi.org/10.1371/journal.pone.0157014.
7. Chen KJ, Rascoe A, Su CA, et al. Value challenge: a bottoms-up approach to minimizing cost and waste in orthopaedic surgery. JBJS Open Access. 2023;8(2). https://doi.org/10.2106/JBJS.OA.22.00129.
8. Cinthuja P, Wijesinghe PCI, Silva P. Use of external fixators in developing countries: a short socioeconomic analysis. Cost Eff Resour Alloc. 2022;20(1):14. https://doi.org/10.1186/s12962-022-00353-4.
9. Dirschl DR, Smith IJ. Reuse of external skeletal fixator components: effects on costs and complications. J Trauma Acute Care Surg. 1998;44(5):855.
10. Sung JK, Levin R, Siegel J, Einhorn TA, Creevy WR, Tornetta PI. Reuse of external fixation components: a randomized trial. J Orthop Trauma. Accessed 12 May 2025. https://journals.lww.com/jorthotrauma/fulltext/2008/02000/Reuse_of_External_Fixation_Components__A.9.aspx.

11. Mahapatra S, Rengarajan N. Use of recycled external fixators in management of compound injuries. Expert Rev Med Devices. 2017;14(1):83–5. https://doi.org/10.1080/17434440.2017.1265886.
12. Tsay EL, Sabharwal S. Reuse of orthopaedic equipment: barriers and opportunities. JBJS Rev. 2024;12(3):e23.00117. https://doi.org/10.2106/JBJS.RVW.23.00117.
13. Pulate A, Olivier LC, Agashe S, Rallan R, Kamal V, Nast-Kolb D. Adaptation of Ilizarov ring fixator to the economic situation of developing countries. Arch Orthop Trauma Surg. 2001;121(1–2):79–82. https://doi.org/10.1007/s004020000159.
14. Cuncannon A, Dosani A, Fast O. Sterile processing in low- and middle-income countries: an integrative review. J Infect Prev. 2021;22(1):28–38. https://doi.org/10.1177/1757177420947468.
15. National Academies of Sciences, Engineering, and Medicine; Health and Medicine Division; Board on Population Health and Public Health Practice; Committee on Community Based Solutions to Promote Health Equity in the United States. https://www.ncbi.nlm.nih.gov/books/NBK425848/.
16. Rizan C, Steinbach I, Nicholson R, Lillywhite R, Reed M, Bhutta MF. The carbon footprint of surgical operations: a systematic review. Ann Surg. 2020;272(6):986–95. https://doi.org/10.1097/SLA.0000000000003951.
17. Gunja MZ, Gumas ED, Williams II RD. U.S. health care from a global perspective, 2022: accelerating spending, worsening outcomes. Published online 31 Jan 2023. Accessed 2 Aug 2023. https://www.commonwealthfund.org/publications/issue-briefs/2023/jan/us-health-care-global-perspective-2022#:~:text=In%202021%2C%20the%20U.S.%20spent,higher%20than%20in%20South%20Korea.
18. Resad Ferati S, Parisien RL, Joslin P, Knapp B, Li X, Curry EJ. Socioeconomic status impacts access to orthopaedic specialty care. JBJS Rev. 2022;10(2):e21. https://doi.org/10.2106/JBJS.RVW.21.00139.
19. Hanchate AD, Zhang Y, Felson DT, Ash AS. Exploring the determinants of racial and ethnic disparities in total knee arthroplasty: health insurance, income, and assets. Med Care. 2008;46(5):481–8. https://doi.org/10.1097/MLR.0b013e3181621e9c.
20. Almaguer AM, Hsu AR, Pearson JM, et al. Do geographic region, medicaid status, and academic affiliation affect access to care among medicaid and privately insured Total hip arthroplasty patients? J Arthroplast. 2019;34(12):2866–71. https://doi.org/10.1016/j.arth.2019.07.030.
21. Wiznia DH, Nwachuku E, Roth A, et al. The influence of medical insurance on patient access to orthopaedic surgery sports medicine appointments under the affordable care act. Orthop J Sports Med. 2017;5(7):2325967117714140. https://doi.org/10.1177/2325967117714140.
22. Baraga MG, Smith MK, Tanner JP, Kaplan LD, Lesniak BP. Anterior cruciate ligament injury and access to care in South Florida: does insurance status play a role? J Bone Joint Surg Am. 2012;94(24):e183. https://doi.org/10.2106/JBJS.K.00852.
23. Sabharwal S, Zhao C, McClemens E, Kaufmann A. Pediatric orthopaedic patients presenting to a university emergency department after visiting another emergency department: demographics and health insurance status. J Pediatr Orthop. 2007;27(6):690–4. https://doi.org/10.1097/BPO.0b013e3181425653.
24. Kim CY, Wiznia DH, Wang Y, et al. The effect of insurance type on patient access to carpal tunnel release under the affordable care act. J Hand Surg. 2016;41(4):503–509.e1. https://doi.org/10.1016/j.jhsa.2016.01.007.
25. Pierce TR, Mehlman CT, Tamai J, Skaggs DL. Access to care for the adolescent anterior cruciate ligament patient with Medicaid versus private insurance. J Pediatr Orthop. 2012;32(3):245–8. https://doi.org/10.1097/BPO.0b013e31824abf20.
26. Fletcher ND, Sirmon BJ, Mansour AS, Carpenter WE, Ward LA. Impact of insurance status on ability to return for outpatient management of pediatric supracondylar humerus fractures. J Child Orthop. 2016;10(5):421–7. https://doi.org/10.1007/s11832-016-0769-x.
27. Intergovernmental Panel on Climate Change (IPCC). The ocean and cryosphere in a changing climate: special report of the intergovernmental panel on climate change. 1st ed. Cambridge University Press; 2022. https://doi.org/10.1017/9781009157964.

28. Costello A, Abbas M, Allen A, et al. Managing the health effects of climate change: Lancet and University College London Institute for Global Health Commission. Lancet Lond Engl. 2009;373(9676):1693–733. https://doi.org/10.1016/S0140-6736(09)60935-1.
29. Popovich N, Plumer B. Who has the most historical responsibility for climate change? The New York Times https://www.nytimes.com/interactive/2021/11/12/climate/cop26-emissions-compensation.html. 12 Nov 2021. Accessed 2 Apr 2023.
30. Eckelman M, Mosher M, Gonzalez A, Sherman J. Comparative life cycle assessment of disposable and reusable laryngeal mask airways. Anesth Analg. 2012;114(5):1067–72. https://doi.org/10.1213/ANE.0b013e31824f6959.
31. Kwakye G, Brat GA, Makary MA. Green surgical practices for health care. Arch Surg Chic Ill 1960. 2011;146(2):131–6. https://doi.org/10.1001/archsurg.2010.343.
32. American Hospital Association. Fast Facts on U.S. Hospitals, 2022. Published online 2022. Accessed 6 June 2023. https://www.aha.org/statistics/fast-facts-us-hospitals.
33. Singh N, Ogunseitan OA, Tang Y. Medical waste: current challenges and future opportunities for sustainable management. Crit Rev Environ Sci Technol. 2022;52(11):2000–22. https://doi.org/10.1080/10643389.2021.1885325.
34. Epstein PR. Extreme weather events: the health and economic consequences of the 1997/98 El Niño and La Niña. Center for Health and the Global Environment; 1999.
35. Axelrod D, Bell C, Feldman J. Greening the operating room and perioperative arena: environmental sustainability for anesthesia practice. Published online October 2014. Accessed 2 Apr 2023. https://www.asahq.org/about-asa/governance-and-committees/asa-committees/environmental-sustainability/greening-the-operating-room#15.
36. The Business Case for Greening the OR. Published online 2011. Accessed 2 Apr 2023. https://practicegreenhealth.org/sites/default/files/upload-files/gor_fullset_webmaterials.pdf.
37. van Straten B, van der Heiden DR, Robertson D, et al. Surgical waste reprocessing: injection molding using recycled blue wrapping paper from the operating room. J Clean Prod. 2021;322:129121. https://doi.org/10.1016/j.jclepro.2021.129121.
38. Phoon KM, Afzal I, Sochart DH, Asopa V, Gikas P, Kader D. Environmental sustainability in orthopaedic surgery. Bone Jt Open. 2022;3(8):628–40.
39. Overcash M. A comparison of reusable and disposable perioperative textiles: sustainability state-of-the-art 2012. Anesth Analg. 2012;114(5):1055–66.
40. Friedericy HJ, van Egmond CW, Vogtländer JG, van der Eijk AC, Jansen FW. Reducing the environmental impact of sterilization packaging for surgical instruments in the operating room: a comparative life cycle assessment of disposable versus reusable systems. Sustainability. 2022;14(1):430. https://doi.org/10.3390/su14010430.
41. Cotton M, Henry J, Hasek L. Value innovation: an important aspect of global surgical care. Glob Health. 2014;10(1):1. https://doi.org/10.1186/1744-8603-10-1.
42. Health costs: how the U.S. compares with other countries | The Rundown | PBS NewsHour.
43. Hailey D, Jacobs PD, Ries NM, Polisena J. Reuse of single use medical devices in Canada: clinical and economic outcomes, legal and ethical issues, and current hospital practice. Int J Technol Assess Health Care. 2008;24(4):430–6. https://doi.org/10.1017/S0266462308080562.
44. Mufarrih SH, Qureshi NQ, Rashid RH, et al. Microbial colonization of pneumatic tourniquets in the orthopedic operating room. Cureus. Published online 2 Aug 2019. https://doi.org/10.7759/cureus.5308.
45. Sharplin P, Hooper G. Is the repair of reusable surgical drapes safe? A pilot study. Orthop Surg. 2019;2:1121.
46. Overcash M. A comparison of reusable and disposable perioperative textiles: sustainability state-of-the-art 2012. Anesth Analg. 2012;114(5):1055–66. https://doi.org/10.1213/ANE.0b013e31824d9cc3.
47. Kieser DC, Wyatt MC, Beswick A, Kunutsor S, Hooper GJ. Does the type of surgical drape (disposable versus non-disposable) affect the risk of subsequent surgical site infection? J Orthop. 2018;15(2):566–70. https://doi.org/10.1016/j.jor.2018.05.015.
48. Rutala WA, Weber DJ. A review of single-use and reusable gowns and drapes in health care. Infect Control Hosp Epidemiol. 2001;22(4):248–57. https://doi.org/10.1086/501895.

49. Bellchambers J. A prospective study of wound infection in coronary artery surgery. Eur J Cardiothorac Surg. 1999;15(1):45–50. https://doi.org/10.1016/S1010-7940(98)00255-3.
50. Showalter BM, Crantford JC, Russell GB, et al. The effect of reusable versus disposable draping material on infection rates in implant-based breast reconstruction: a prospective randomized trial. Ann Plast Surg. 2014;72(6):S165–9. https://doi.org/10.1097/SAP.0000000000000086.
51. Sung JK, Levin R, Siegel J, Einhorn TA, Creevy WR, Tornetta P. Reuse of external fixation components: a randomized trial. J Orthop Trauma. 2008;22(2):126–30. https://doi.org/10.1097/BOT.0b013e318162e55c.
52. Dirschl DR, Smith IJ. Reuse of external skeletal fixator components: effects on costs and complications. J Trauma. 1998;44(5):855–8. https://doi.org/10.1097/00005373-199805000-00018.
53. Baxter RL, Baxter HC, Campbell GA, et al. Quantitative analysis of residual protein contamination on reprocessed surgical instruments. J Hosp Infect. 2006;63(4):439–44. https://doi.org/10.1016/j.jhin.2006.03.011.
54. Friedman LGM, Suk M. The ethical implications of reusing external fixation systems: a used car or a plastic water bottle? J Orthop Exp Innov. 2021;2(2). https://doi.org/10.60118/001c.25910.
55. Darvish K, Shafieian M, Rehman S. The effect of tip geometry on the mechanical performance of unused and reprocessed orthopaedic drill bits. Proc Inst Mech Eng Part H. 2009;223(5):625–35. https://doi.org/10.1243/09544119JEIM555.
56. Kobayashi M, Nakagawa Y, Okamoto Y, Nakamura S, Nakamura T. Structural damage and chemical contaminants on reprocessed arthroscopic shaver blades. Am J Sports Med. 2009;37(2):266–73. https://doi.org/10.1177/0363546508325668.
57. King JS, Pink MM, Jobe CM. Assessment of reprocessed arthroscopic shaver blades. Arthrosc J Arthrosc Relat Surg. 2006;22(10):1046–52. https://doi.org/10.1016/j.arthro.2006.07.021.
58. Wosar MA, Marcellin-Little DJ, Roe SC. Influence of bolt tightening torque, wire size, and component reuse on wire fixation in circular external fixation. Vet Surg. 2002;31(6):571–6. https://doi.org/10.1053/jvet.2002.34672.
59. Bouthors C, Nguyen J, Durand L, Dubory A, Raspaud S, Court C. Single-use versus reusable medical devices in spinal fusion surgery: a hospital micro-costing analysis. Eur J Orthop Surg Traumatol. 2019;29(8):1631–7. https://doi.org/10.1007/s00590-019-02517-0.
60. Ottardi C, Damonti A, Porazzi E, et al. A comparative analysis of a disposable and a reusable pedicle screw instrument kit for lumbar arthrodesis: integrating HTA and MCDA. Health Econ Rev. 2017;7(1):1–10. https://doi.org/10.1186/s13561-017-0153-7.
61. Mansur J. In: Soule BM, editor. Reuse of single-use devices: understanding risks and strategies for decision-making for health care organizations. Joint Commission International. Published online 2017. Accessed 2 Aug 2023. https://www.jointcommissioninternational.org/-/media/jci/jci-documents/offerings/other-resources/white-papers/jci_white_paper_reuse_of_single_use_devices.pdf.
62. Southworth PM. Infections and exposures: reported incidents associated with unsuccessful decontamination of reusable surgical instruments. J Hosp Infect. 2014;88(3):127–31. https://doi.org/10.1016/j.jhin.2014.08.007.
63. Schaer GN, Koechli OR, Haller U. Single-use versus reusable laparoscopic surgical instruments: a comparative cost analysis. Am J Obstet Gynecol. 1995;173(6):1812–5. https://doi.org/10.1016/0002-9378(95)90432-8.
64. Rizan C, Brophy T, Lillywhite R, Reed M, Bhutta MF. Life cycle assessment and life cycle cost of repairing surgical scissors. Int J Life Cycle Assess. 2022;27(6):780–95. https://doi.org/10.1007/s11367-022-02064-7.
65. Polisena J, Hailey D, Moulton K, et al. Reprocessing and reuse of single-use medical devices: a National Survey of Canadian Acute-Care Hospitals. Infect Control Hosp Epidemiol. 2008;29(5):437–9. https://doi.org/10.1086/587648.
66. Thamyongkit S, Bachabi M, Thompson JM, Shafiq B, Hasenboehler EA. Use of reprocessed external fixators in orthopaedic surgery: a survey of 243 orthopaedic trauma surgeons. Patient Saf Surg. 2018;12(1):10. https://doi.org/10.1186/s13037-018-0156-2.

67. Dept of Health and Human Services. Code of Federal Regulations Title 21, Chapter I, Subchapter H, Parts 807 and 814 2023;1(4). Accessed 4 June 2023. https://www.ecfr.gov/current/title-21/chapter-I/subchapter-H.
68. Food and Drug Administration, Health and Human Services. Guidance for industry on enforcement priorities for single-use devices reprocessed by third parties and hospitals; availability. Fed Regist. 2000;65(157):49583–5.
69. Classify Your Medical Device: Device Classification Panels. U.S. Food & Drug Administration. 31 Aug 2018. Accessed 2 Aug 2023. https://www.fda.gov/medical-devices/classify-your-medical-device/device-classification-panels.
70. United States v. The Prometheus Group., et al. (W.D. Michigan). https://www.justice.gov/usao-wdmi/pr/2025_0326_Prometheus_Settlement.
71. West Michigan Urogynecologist Sentenced to Prison for Healthcare Fraud and Adulteration of Medical Devices. United States Attorney's Office. 29 Oct 2020. Accessed 5 Aug 2023. https://www.justice.gov/usao-wdmi/pr/2020_1029_Beyer_Wright.
72. United States Attorney's Office, District of Nevada. Las Vegas Urologist sentenced to four years in prison for re-using needle guides during prostate procedures. Published online 5 May 2015. Accessed 2 Aug 2023. https://www.justice.gov/usao-nv/pr/las-vegas-urologist-sentenced-four-years-prison-re-using-needle-guides-during-prostate.
73. Khatun R. Reusing medical devices: Maharashtra Govt files cases against top hospitals. Business Medical Dialogues. https://businessmedicaldialoguesin/reusing-medical-devices-maharashtra-govt-files-cases-against-top-hospitals. 28 Mar 2018. Accessed 2 Aug 2023.
74. Wang D, Wu J. Reprocessing and reuse of single-use medical devices in China: a pilot survey. BMC Public Health. 2019;19(1):1–10. https://doi.org/10.1186/s12889-019-6835-9.
75. Maben-Tenney L. Nursing attitudes toward the use of reprocessed single-use medical devices. HIM 1990-2015. Published online 1 Aug 2012. https://stars.library.ucf.edu/honorstheses1990-2015/1337.
76. Costa D d M, Lopes LK d O, Vickery K, et al. Reprocessing safety issues associated with complex-design orthopaedic loaned surgical instruments and implants. Injury. 2018;49(11):2005–12. https://doi.org/10.1016/j.injury.2018.09.006.
77. Magetsari R, van der Houwen EB, Bakker MTJ, et al. Biomechanical and surface physicochemical analyses of used osteosynthesis plates and screws—potential for reuse in developing countries? J Biomed Mater Res B Appl Biomater. 2006;79B(2):236–44. https://doi.org/10.1002/jbm.b.30534.
78. Panta G, Richardson AK, Shaw IC, Coope PA. Compliance of primary and secondary care public hospitals with standard practices for reprocessing and steam sterilization of reusable medical devices in Nepal: findings from nation-wide multicenter clustered audits. BMC Health Serv Res. 2020;20(1):923. https://doi.org/10.1186/s12913-020-05788-0.
79. Stephens A, Assang A. What do you mean you can't sterilize it? The reusable medical device matrix. Can Oper Room Nurs J. 2010;28(4):6–11. 20–24.
80. Fast O, Fast C, Fast D, Veltjens S, Salami Z, White MC. Limited sterile processing capabilities for safe surgery in low-income and middle-income countries: experience in the Republic of Congo, Madagascar and Benin. BMJ Glob Health. 2017;2(Suppl 4):e000428. https://doi.org/10.1136/bmjgh-2017-000428.
81. DePasse JW, Lee PT. A model for 'reverse innovation' in health care. Glob Health. 2013;9(1):40. https://doi.org/10.1186/1744-8603-9-40.
82. Prime M, Attaelmanan I, Imbuldeniya A, Harris M, Darzi A, Bhatti Y. From Malawi to Middlesex: the case of the Arbutus Drill Cover System as an example of the cost-saving potential of frugal innovations for the UK NHS. BMJ Innov. Published online 30 Mar 2018:bmjinnov. https://doi.org/10.1136/bmjinnov-2017-000233.
83. Khan MM, Parab SR. Safety guidelines for sterility of face shields during COVID 19 pandemic. Indian J Otolaryngol Head Neck Surg. 2021;73(1):85–6. https://doi.org/10.1007/s12070-020-01865-2.

27 Operating Room Efficiency: At Home and Abroad

Brian A. Shaw and Richard M. Schwend

Introduction

Enhancing value in the operating room is essential. The OR is among the most resource-intensive areas in any hospital, contributing significantly to healthcare expenditures, solid waste generation, and greenhouse gas emissions [1, 2]. Factors such as excessive use of disposable supplies, redundant instrumentation, expensive implants, inefficient scheduling, last-minute cancellations, unnecessary procedures, and inexperienced surgical teams all drive costs up. Globally, quality improvement programs in the OR have demonstrated success in reducing both costs and environmental impact [3]. Supporting staff well-being is also an important component of the value equation [4]. In order to retain and advance your staff, treat them as if you are recruiting them; otherwise, you may end up needing to recruit new staff at significant cost.

At home in your domestic practice or while on international surgical mission trips, value-based care focuses on achieving the best patient outcomes at the lowest cost. In the OR, simple, targeted strategies can enhance value by increasing efficiency, improving clinical outcomes, and promoting environmental sustainability [5]. Methods to enhance value include the following:

- Optimize patient selection and preoperative planning.
- Standardize surgical procedures and implants (Fig. 27.1).
- Eliminate unnecessary imaging.

B. A. Shaw (✉)
University of Colorado Medical School, Children's Hospital of Colorado-Colorado Springs, Colorado Springs, CO, USA

R. M. Schwend
Children's Mercy Hospital, Kansas City, MO, USA
e-mail: rmschwend@cmh.edu

W. L. Hennrikus, R. M. Schwend (eds.), *Value in Pediatric Orthopaedics*,
https://doi.org/10.1007/978-3-032-19570-8_27

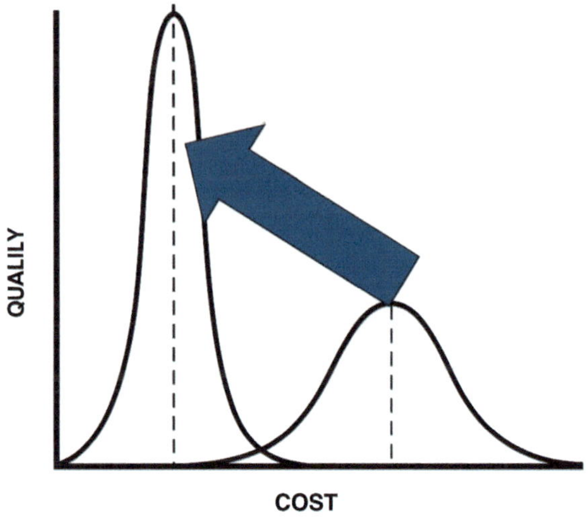

Fig. 27.1 The goal of improving the value of surgical care in the OR is to reduce variability, lower costs, and enhance quality. However, defining quality can be challenging, as it varies depending on the perspective of the patient, family, surgeon, or hospital

- Eliminate redundant instrument trays.
- Minimize use of disposable items.
- Use cost-effective supplies and techniques.
- Engage key stakeholders to identify inefficiencies and eliminate waste [6].
- Improve working conditions and mentor, recognize, and retain talented staff.

Value-Based Themes

Optimizing Preoperative Planning

Preoperative planning is essential. Careful case selection, including the avoidance of high-risk revisions when the risk-benefit ratio is unfavorable, can help reduce complications and total OR time. In low-income nations while on international surgical mission trips, preoperative imaging should be optimized to minimize reliance on intraoperative fluoroscopy. Fluoroscopy may be unavailable, unreliable, or of poor quality. In many overseas locations, surgeons should be prepared to perform surgery without fluoroscopy. Schedule procedures to do that you could perform confidently and routinely at home. Avoid pressure from local host surgeons to undertake high-risk cases based on unrealistic expectations from the family or team.

Case Example Before international surgical mission trips, our pediatric orthopedic team conducts a Zoom-based preoperative conference with the local host physician to improve case selection and ensure that the necessary equipment and implants are available upon arrival.

Enhancing Communication

Effective communication among surgeons, anesthesiologists, and OR staff is essential for improving efficiency and outcomes. In international settings, teams have used WhatsApp or email to coordinating cases prior to arrival and follow-up after departure. Once on site, holding a weekly preoperative, multidisciplinary indications case conference can be valuable for planning strategies related to patient positioning, airway management (e.g., intubation vs. mask ventilation), anesthesia type (including spinal or peripheral nerve blocks), special equipment considerations, and perioperative medications.

Case Example A pediatric orthopedic team conducting a 1-week international outreach trip used WhatsApp to communicate with local host surgeons prior to arrival and during 6-week postoperative follow-up appointments. At the end of the week trip, a comprehensive case conference was presented reviewing the surgical cases performed that week. Education for the local surgeons and trainees and a detailed sign-out were emphasized. Follow-up care by the local surgeons was scheduled.

Database for Postoperative Follow-Up, Research, and Funding

Long-term patient follow-up is essential. Utilizing databases enables teams to track outcomes, ensure continuity of care, and report outcomes research. In the context of international surgical mission trips, maintaining clinical data also strengthens the ability to secure funding, as many foundations request measurable results. Two foundations that support international orthopedic surgical care include the Oracle Health Foundation (Oracle Health Foundation Grant Request) and Shriners Children's (Shriners Children's).

Case Example Our pediatric orthopedic surgical international team uses a REDCap database to document patient demographics, surgical procedures, complications, outcomes, and follow-up care. This database has helped local physicians monitor patients postoperatively and has supported collaborative research (https://projectredcap.org/?action=login).

Dedicated Orthopedic Trauma Operating Room

Domestically, implementing a daily add-on trauma room reduces the number of late-night surgical cases, potentially improves outcomes and reduces complications, and improves overall morale of the surgical team. Sankar et al. demonstrated that after-hours cases decreased by 48% with the introduction of a next-day trauma room [7]. In addition, fewer complications were reported for surgically treated supracondylar fractures.

Case Example All Type II supracondylar humerus fractures and some Type III fractures can be stabilized with a splint and managed surgically the next day during daylight hours in an add-on trauma room. However, supracondylar fractures with associated vascular compromise, risk of compartment syndrome, or skin compromise should be treated urgently without delay at the time of presentation.

Incorporating Donated Supplies for International Surgical Mission Trips

Some medical supply companies provide donated implants and surgical instruments for international mission trips. Giving your local representative ample lead time of several month increases the likelihood of securing needed items. Additionally, check that your surgical power tools and implant systems are compatible to avoid intraoperative issues while volunteering in a low-income nation.

Case Example One pediatric orthopedic team reduces costs by utilizing donated bone graft materials from LifeNet Health for orthopedic procedures performed at the low-income country hospital. Another team borrowed instrument sets from a manufacturer, reimburses the company only for the implants used, and gave the sets to the local in-country representative at the conclusion of the mission trip. This approach avoided the logistical challenges of transporting surgical sets back to the USA on commercial flights.

Reducing Disposable Waste

Domestically, only the food industry generates more annual waste than the healthcare industry [8]. Healthcare facilities in the USA produce over four billion pounds of waste and nearly 10% of total greenhouse gas emissions each year [1, 9, 10]. Operating rooms are responsible for up to 70% of hospital medical waste, much of which is avoidable [1, 11, 12]. About 20% of overall supply costs are attributed to wasted supplies [13]. Institutional, behavioral, and business barriers often hinder change, highlighting the need for a possible broader culture shift [14].

Environmentally conscious decisions in the OR can potentially reduce both waste and costs [6, 15]. For example, awareness of disposable item costs can influence behavior [13]. Simple measures such as using reusable sharps containers and minimizing the use of disposable drapes and instruments can reduce waste and costs. Eliminating frequently unused items from surgical packs could prevent over 6000 tons of waste annually, improve supply chain efficiency, and reduce costs [16]. Separating hazardous from nonhazardous waste can also reduce disposal costs [12].

Sustainability in the OR is guided by the "5 Rs": refuse, reduce, reuse, repurpose, and recycle [3]. "Lean and green" is a guiding principle [8]. One author reported that using a scorecard program with financial incentives to encourage surgeons to reduce waste led to a 10% reduction in waste and surgical costs [17]. At one international surgical mission site, surgeons reduce costs by using single gloves, with no appreciable increase in the infection rates [18].

Case Example One hospital reported $968 in waste per neurosurgical case, with $653 (67%) attributed to unused supplies. Interventions such as price transparency, education of surgeons and nurses about waste, simplifying preference cards, and clear guidelines on which supplies should be opened versus kept on standby helped to reduce this waste [19]. Prepackaged surgical packs may contribute to waste and increased costs. The two authors of the current study combined have organized international surgical mission trips for over 50 years without using prepackaged surgical packs.

Improving Anesthesia Workflow Efficiency

Anesthesia plays a key role in operating room efficiency at home or overseas. Delays in induction and emergence can prolong OR time. The use of drugs to reverse neuromuscular blockade shortens OR time and expedites room turnover [20]. In appropriate cases, the use of tranexamic acid improves patient safety while reducing transfusion costs [5]. Lastly, portable ultrasound machines enable accurate placement of peripheral nerve blocks.

Case Example In international surgical mission trips where anesthesia resources may be limited, careful planning of anesthesia techniques can reduce operative time. When possible, at the home institution or when practicing on an international mission trip, local infiltration with bupivacaine can be performed to help reduce pain. For instance, during reduction and pinning of supracondylar humerus fractures, injecting bupivacaine directly into the fracture site is safe and quick and provides effective analgesia that often eliminates the need for postoperative narcotics [21]. Caudal block anesthesia is effective for hip procedures in young children; however, local wound infiltration may be a safer and equally effective alternative [22].

Reducing Surgical Time

Surgical time is defined as the interval from incision to dressing application [23]. With the average cost of OR time estimated at as high as $120 per minute, small reductions in surgical time can lead to cost savings.

In adolescent idiopathic scoliosis (AIS) surgery, propensity-matched studies have shown that shorter surgical times are associated with less blood loss, fewer transfusions, shorter lengths of stay, and fewer intraoperative neuromonitoring (IOM) alerts compared to longer procedures [24].

One strategy to reduce surgical time is to utilize a consistent and dedicated OR team and have two experienced surgeons scrub together on complex procedures [25]. In addition, hip and knee arthroplasty surgeons have reduced costs by sharing unblinded clinical and financial data, including surgical times [26].

Case Example One author of the current chapter utilizes a consistent OR team and two experienced surgeons to consistently complete two AIS cases in 1 day [25] (Fig. 27.2). At other institution, the second author of the current study uses a single surgeon working with an experienced physician assistant and a consistent OR team to also complete two AIS cases per day.

Simplifying Surgical Instrument Trays

Typically, only about 20% of the instruments in a surgical tray are used during a case, making tray simplification one of the most practical strategies to improve OR efficiency [27]. Reducing the number of instruments can decrease setup time, sterilization costs, and waste. Dyas et al. found that streamlining instrument trays reduced costs, reduced preparation time, minimized decontamination time, and decreased physical strain on staff [28].

Case Example After visiting the OR of an international colleague, who only used the most essential instruments for surgery, all fitting on a single Mayo stand (Fig. 27.3a), we returned home and reduced the number of surgical trays for spine cases from 22 to 6. This reduction reduced the total instrument weight from 440 pounds to 220 pounds (Fig. 27.3b, c). The decreased mass of instruments reduced the workload on our sterile processing staff, reduced setup time, reduced costs, improved team morale, and simplified training for new staff. We estimated a cost savings of about $2400 per case due to reduced processing and operating room time.

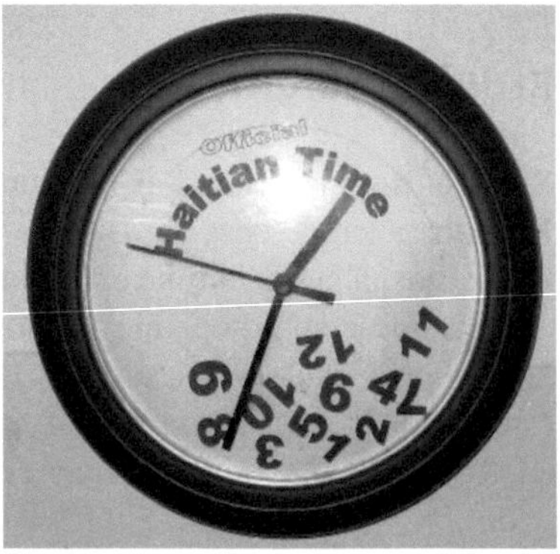

Fig. 27.2 *Pay attention to the clock.* As part of the time-out, we recommend discussing the anticipated duration of the surgery with the OR staff to promote efficient use of OR time, help the anesthesiologist to plan appropriately, and alert the recovery room to plan for an estimated time of patient arrival

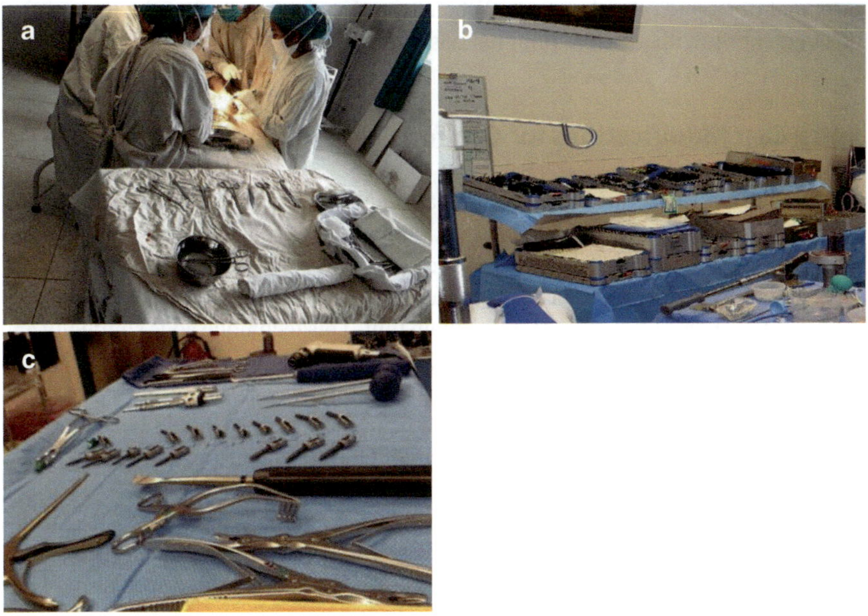

Fig. 27.3 (**a**) Example of simple instrument setup on a Mayo stand (**b**) A typical spine case previously used 22 trays, weighed 440 lbs., and required a two-level back table (**c**) After consolidating to six trays on the back table, the most frequently used instruments were placed on the Mayo stand. Pedicle screws were premeasured using preoperative imaging, and only the anticipated screws were processed for the case

Using Cost-Effective Implants and Techniques

Implant selection plays an important role in cost reduction. Surgeon education about implant pricing and implant waste is essential to achieving meaningful savings [29]. Using nonproprietary implants can also reduce costs. The implementation of shared-savings programs for surgical supplies can decrease inventory costs [30]. One innovative shared-savings program attempted to align surgeon and hospital incentives by returning 50% of implant savings to the surgical division [30]. Through single-source contracting, one center reduced annual spine implant costs by half, from $four million to $two million. Implant waste was mitigated through targeted surgeon education and waste reduction initiatives which also reduced costs [31]. The use of K-wire fixation saves time and reduces implant costs [18]. In addition, augmenting K-wire fixation with casting, rather than solely using more expensive implants, also improves value.

Case Example Osteotomies can be fixed using inexpensive K-wires instead of more expensive blade plates. A bolt cutter can be purchased from a local hardware store if an appropriate K-wire cutting tool is unavailable. Bone staples are another inexpensive and versatile option for stabilizing osteotomies around the foot, ankle, proximal tibia, and other locations. When using K-wires or staples, the fixation can be augmenting with a cast at minimal cost.

Spica Cast Modifications for Comfort, Ease of Care, and Transport

Traditional spica casts with connecting bars can sometimes be difficult to transport and manage postoperatively. A modified spica design that uses posterior splints instead of a bar between the lower limbs can be more practical for patient handling. Longitudinally applied posterior fiberglass splints add strength to the cast while allowing the sides of the spica cast to remain thin. This technique adds simplicity and safety when bivalving or removing the spica. In addition, overall, the cast is thinner and lighter with less fiberglass making it easier for parents to lift and carry. In countries without air-conditioning, plaster hip spica or spine casts should be avoided, as they tend to deteriorate quickly once the child returns home from the hospital.

Case Example In low-income countries, access to specialized spica casting tables may be limited. In addition, for patients with early-onset scoliosis, tables such as Risser, Cotrel, or Mehta are often prohibitively expensive. To address these specialized table deficiencies, we have successfully used a simple, low-cost alternative: an aluminum bar placed between two standard tables. The child is supported on the bar while fiberglass is applied to create the hip or spine cast. The bar is pre-lubricated with petroleum jelly, and once casting is complete, the bar can be easily slid out and removed (Fig. 27.4).

Preparing for Resource-Limited Operating Room Environments

Surgeons volunteering on international mission trips must adapt to limited resources, including lack of fluoroscopy, limited surgical tools and implants, and variability in anesthesia techniques. Pre-trip preparation, including packing K-wires of known quality and diameter and bone staples, can facilitate surgical success.

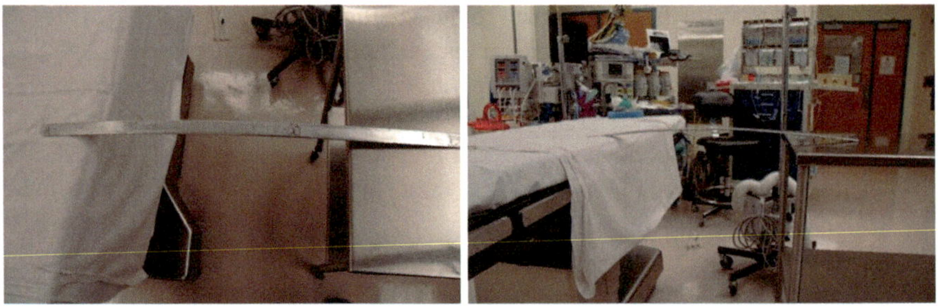

Fig. 27.4 An aluminum bar suspended between two standard tables serves as a simple and inexpensive substitute for a spica or spine casting table. This is our preferred device for applying casts in young children when specialized casting tables are not available

Summary

In both domestic and international settings, improving value in the operating room involves a multifaceted approach that reduces costs, enhances efficiency, and maintains high-quality patient care. Key elements include effective preoperative planning, clear communication, and the use of databases for follow-up and research. Practical strategies including establishing a dedicated, daily trauma OR room, streamlining surgical trays, optimizing implant selection, minimizing disposable waste, improving anesthesia efficiency, reducing surgical times, using an innovative spica/spine casting table, and incorporating donated supplies can all enhance value.

Author Pearls

- The following list of pearl applies primarily to international surgical mission trips.
- Invite experienced surgeons who are adaptable, practical, ethical, and committed to teaching the host team.
- Prioritize simplicity. Avoid unnecessary implants and use K-wires whenever possible. Smooth, non-buried K-wires are easier for host surgeons to remove.
- In young children, we prefer the Pemberton pelvic osteotomy and suture the bone graft rather than using K-wires that need to be subsequently removed.
- Supplement K-wire fixation with fiberglass casting. In warm international climates, fiberglass holds up better than plaster. A thin fiberglass cast can be reinforced with well-placed longitudinal splints.
- Bring essential tools—but not excessive equipment—to avoid logistical issues.
- Be flexible with imaging. In low-income nations, intraoperative fluoroscopy may be unavailable. For some cases, we often proceed without a C-arm and obtain a flat-plate radiograph at the end of the procedure.
- Improve communication by using platforms like WhatsApp and Zoom for pre-trip case reviews to help with surgical planning and logistics.
- Reduce waste by minimizing the use of disposable supplies.
- Minimize the number of instruments and trays to increase efficiency.
- Include the host surgeon in every procedure.
- Emphasize long-term follow-up.
- Use local medical students as translators if possible. The students also gain educational and patient care experience.
- Avoid placing Vicryl sutures near or at the skin. Vicryl can cause inflammatory reactions and extrusion, which may be confused for infection by local staff after you are gone.

References

1. Lee RJ, Mears SC. Greening of orthopedic surgery. Orthopedics. 2012;35(6):e940–4.
2. Eckelman MJ, Huang K, Lagasse R, Senay E, Dubrow R, Sherman JD. Health care pollution and public health damage in the United States: an update. Health Aff (Millwood). 2020;39(12):2071–9.

3. Sullivan GA, Petit HJ, Reiter AJ, Westrick JC, Hu A, Dunn JB, et al. Environmental impact and cost savings of operating room quality improvement initiatives: a scoping review. J Am Coll Surg. 2023;236(2):411–23.
4. Schouten AM, Flipse SM, van Nieuwenhuizen KE, Jansen FW, van der Eijk AC, van den Dobbelsteen JJ. Operating room performance optimization metrics: a systematic review. J Med Syst. 2023;47(1):19.
5. Gurnea TP, Frye WP, Althausen PL. Operating room supply costs in orthopaedic trauma: cost containment opportunities. J Orthop Trauma. 2016;30(Suppl 5):S21–S6.
6. Petit HJ, Sullivan GA, Hughes IM, Pittman KL, Myers JA, Cocoma SM, et al. Exploring barriers and facilitators to reducing the environmental impact of the operating room. J Surg Res. 2023;292:197–205.
7. Brusalis CM, Shah AS, Luan X, Lutts MK, Sankar WN. A dedicated orthopaedic trauma operating room improves efficiency at a pediatric center. J Bone Joint Surg Am. 2017;99(1):42–7.
8. Van Demark RE Jr, Smith VJS, Fiegen A. Lean and green hand surgery. J Hand Surg Am. 2018;43(2):179–81.
9. Wormer BA, Augenstein VA, Carpenter CL, Burton PV, Yokeley WT, Prabhu AS, et al. The green operating room: simple changes to reduce cost and our carbon footprint. Am Surg. 2013;79(7):666–71.
10. Yates EF, Bowder AN, Roa L, Velin L, Goodman AS, Nguyen LL, et al. Empowering surgeons, anesthesiologists, and obstetricians to incorporate environmental sustainability in the operating room. Ann Surg. 2021;273(6):1108–14.
11. Bravo D, Gaston RG, Melamed E. Environmentally responsible hand surgery: past, present, and future. J Hand Surg Am. 2020;45(5):444–8.
12. Talbot S, Moore D. Waste management in the operating theatre. Surgeon. 2024;22(4):248–52.
13. Chasseigne V, Leguelinel-Blache G, Nguyen TL, de Tayrac R, Prudhomme M, Kinowski JM, et al. Assessing the costs of disposable and reusable supplies wasted during surgeries. Int J Surg. 2018;53:18–23.
14. Pillay L, Winkel KD, Kariotis T. Developing the green operating room: exploring barriers and opportunities to reducing operating room waste. Med J Aust. 2024;221(5):279–84.
15. Brown C, Meals C. Four ways plastic surgeons can fight climate change. Plast Reconstr Surg Glob Open. 2020;8(7):e2961.
16. Cunningham AJ, Krakauer K, Schofield C, Kenron D, Krishnaswami S. Reducing disposable surgical items: decreasing environmental impact and costs at a children's hospital, a pilot study. J Surg Res. 2023;288:309–14.
17. Zygourakis CC, Valencia V, Moriates C, Boscardin CK, Catschegn S, Rajkomar A, et al. Association between surgeon scorecard use and operating room costs. JAMA Surg. 2017;152(3):284–91.
18. Taylor ZR, Hamblin RW, Shaw BA, Navas-Solares JC, Shaw LF. Special report: the Moore pediatric surgery center: an evolving model for pediatric orthopaedic surgical care in a limited resource environment. J Pediatr Orthop. 2023;43(3):181–6.
19. Zygourakis CC, Yoon S, Valencia V, Boscardin C, Moriates C, Gonzales R, et al. Operating room waste: disposable supply utilization in neurosurgical procedures. J Neurosurg. 2017;126(2):620–5.
20. Zhang B, Hepner DL, Tran MH, Friedman M, Korn JR, Menzin J. Neuromuscular blockade, reversal agent use, and operating room time: retrospective analysis of US inpatient surgeries. Curr Med Res Opin. 2009;25(4):943–50.
21. Kim K, Armstrong D, Hennrikus W. Methods to reduce opioid use druing treatment of pediatric supracondylar fractures. Injury. 2021;52:1331–5.
22. Zundel S, Conz F, Fuchs J, Blumenstock G, Guerrero-Rodrigues A, Grasshoff C, et al. Caudal block versus wound infiltration for inguinal procedures in young children: a randomized clinical study. Eur J Pediatr Surg. 2023;33(5):354–9.
23. Wagala NN, Marasigan JAM, Mian HM, Schwend RM. Operative time in adolescent idiopathic scoliosis surgery: a need for a standard definition. J Pediatr Orthop B. 2021;30(3):205–10.

24. Noe MC, Hagaman D, Sipp B, Qureshi F, Warren JR, Kaji E, et al. The effect of surgical time on perioperative complications in adolescent idiopathic scoliosis cases. A propensity score analysis. Spine Deform. 2024;12(4):1053–60.
25. Warren JR, Link RC, Bonanni S, Noe MC, Anderson JT, Schwend RM. Two AIS cases, 2 surgeons, 1 operating room, 1 day: faster and safer than 1 case in a day. J Pediatr Orthop. 2024;44(8):502–7.
26. Winegar AL, Jackson LW, Sambare TD, Liu TC, Banks SR, Erlinger TP, et al. A surgeon scorecard is associated with improved value in elective primary hip and knee arthroplasty. J Bone Joint Surg Am. 2019;101(2):152–9.
27. Yalamanchi P, Miller JE, Prout S, Matthews E, Spagnol C, Harrington S, et al. Association of operating room costs with head and neck surgical instrumentation optimization: a surgeon-led quality improvement initiative. JAMA Otolaryngol Head Neck Surg. 2022;148(5):402–7.
28. Dyas AR, Lovell KM, Balentine CJ, Wang TN, Porterfield JR Jr, Chen H, et al. Reducing cost and improving operating room efficiency: examination of surgical instrument processing. J Surg Res. 2018;229:15–9.
29. Soroceanu A, Canacari E, Brown E, Robinson A, McGuire KJ. Intraoperative waste in spine surgery: incidence, cost, and effectiveness of an educational program. Spine (Phila Pa 1976). 2011;36(19):E1270–3.
30. Eiferman D, Bhakta A, Khan S. Implementation of a shared-savings program for surgical supplies decreases inventory cost. Surgery. 2015;158(4):996–1000. discussion -2.
31. Payne A, Slover J, Inneh I, Hutzler L, Iorio R, Bosco JA 3rd. Orthopedic implant waste: analysis and quantification. Am J Orthop (Belle Mead NJ). 2015;44(12):554–60.

Magnetic Resonance Imaging: The Value Proposition

28

Charles T. Mehlman

Introduction

Canada currently has 432 MRI units for a population of about 40 million. This figure can be compared to the 438 MRI units in the Dallas-Fort Worth metropolitan area or the 465 scanners in Chicago [3, 4]. One may ask, do certain regions have an overabundance of MRI units or do other regions have too few? However, concerns have been raised regarding the overuse of diagnostic imaging [5]. In addition, MRI remains a costly medical resource, particularly when performed in a hospital setting (Table 28.1). In recent years, there has been a marked increase in the use of advanced imaging, including MRI, in pediatric emergency departments [6]. The cost of these MRIs is further amplified when anesthesia is required for pediatric patients. Nearly 15% of all pediatric MRI examinations performed during emergency department visits necessitate general anesthesia [7].

Some argue that "defensive imaging" contributes to the increase in MRI utilization [8]. In certain markets, MRI accounts for nearly 20% of orthopedic studies [9]. Among orthopedic trauma surgeons in the USA, the rate of defensively ordered MRIs is about 30% [10]. Health policy researchers also note that reduced imaging rates are linked to states that have implemented tort reform [11]. The frequency of reflexively ordered MRIs, MRIs ordered out of simple habit, or MRIs ordered due to family demands remains speculative. The current chapter focuses on a select list of pediatric orthopedic scenarios for which MRI has been commonly used and studied, framing these situations within value-based themes.

C. T. Mehlman (✉)
Dayton Children's Hospital, Dayton, OH, USA
e-mail: Charles.mehlman@cchmc.org

W. L. Hennrikus, R. M. Schwend (eds.), *Value in Pediatric Orthopaedics*,
https://doi.org/10.1007/978-3-032-19570-8_28

Table 28.1 Publicly available Cincinnati Children's Hospital MRI charges

	Hospital fee	Radiologist fee	Total
Knee joint	$3937	$319	$4256
Pelvis	$5398	$514	$5912
Upper spine	$3833	$347	$4180
Middle spine	$4006	$347	$4353
Lower spine	$4019	$349	$4368

Charges may be different than other US pediatric hospitals. Reimbursed costs may be lower

Table 28.2 Rates of coexisting osteomyelitis in setting of septic arthritis

Joint	Rate (%)	Source
Shoulder	78	Ernat et al. 2017 J Ped Orthop [15]
Knee	65	Monsalve et al. 2015 AJR [16]
Elbow	58	Nduaguba et al. 2016 J Ped Orthop [17]
Hip	48	Nguyen et al. 2017 J Ped Orthop [18]
Ankle	31	Montgomery et al. 2013 J Ped Orthop [19]

Value-Based Themes

Acute Musculoskeletal Infection in Children

Pediatric musculoskeletal infections pose a significant burden at many children's hospitals, with approximately 3000 infection-related consultations reported annually at some hospitals [12]. The diagnosis of septic arthritis is relatively straightforward, typically requiring a detailed history, physical examination, basic laboratory tests, and joint aspiration. However, determining whether acute hematogenous osteomyelitis and/or a subperiosteal abscess are present can be more challenging [13]. Available literature indicates that different joints exhibit varying rates of these associated conditions (Table 28.2). A common limitation in these studies is that the diagnosis of osteomyelitis is based on MRI findings rather than culture confirmation, which can make it difficult to distinguish between reactive marrow changes and true disease [14].

Classic teaching suggests that joints with an intra-articular metaphysis are at higher risk for simultaneous septic arthritis and acute hematogenous osteomyelitis. Traditionally, the joints on this list include the hip, shoulder, elbow, and ankle. For reasons that remain unclear to this author, the knee—despite having an intra-articular portion of the distal metaphyseal femur—has not typically been included in this group (Fig. 28.1).

In addition, two separate studies, both heavily focused on septic hips and knees, identified symptom duration as a key predictor of associated osteomyelitis, with a 4-day symptom duration emerging as the critical threshold [20, 21].

There is a "chicken and egg" aspect of this discussion. Because septic arthritis is more commonly encountered than osteomyelitis, the current focus tends to be on the child who presents primarily with septic arthritis, rather than the opposite

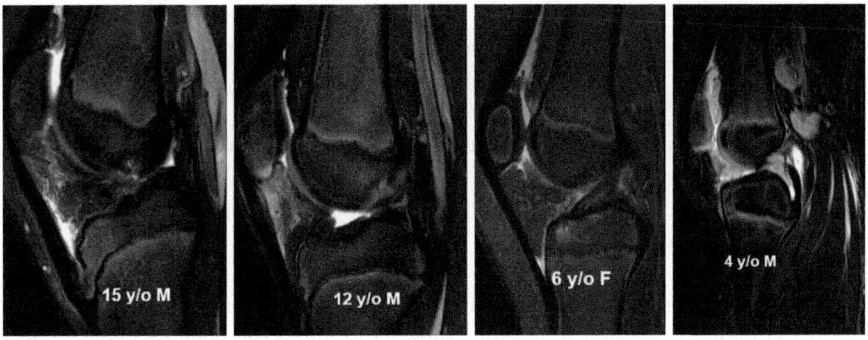

Fig. 28.1 Substantial portions of the distal metaphyseal femur are intra-articular

scenario where acute hematogenous osteomyelitis is the initial concern. The advent of MRI has greatly enhanced our ability to identify bone-related findings associated with septic arthritis. As a result, a new wave of MRI protocols designed to aid in the diagnosis of musculoskeletal infections has emerged in recent years [22].

On the other hand, the limitations of infection-related MRI must be mentioned, particularly in the context of repeat imaging. For example, in a study of children with acute hematogenous osteomyelitis, researchers at the Children's Hospital of Philadelphia found that only 11% of more than 100 repeat MRIs led to a change in treatment, highlighting the minimal impact of repeat imaging [23]. Similarly, the same group reported that 50% of MRIs performed at their hospital would have been deemed unnecessary if the indications for imaging developed in Houston had been applied [24]. These findings underscore the importance of regional variation in the management of musculoskeletal infections.

Outcomes One way to assess the influence of MRI on clinical outcomes is to consider what would likely occur if MRI were unavailable in clinical care. For cases of septic arthritis of the hip and knee, the absence of MRI could theoretically lead to missed adjacent pericapsular abscesses or acute osteomyelitis and potentially a greater likelihood of repeat surgical interventions. However, this assumption is not supported by existing literature.

Several pediatric septic arthritis studies have reported outcomes in settings where MRI was not used or used infrequently. For example, in a 1986 study from St. Christopher's Hospital, Philadelphia, involving 95 patients, predominantly with septic knees, who were treated with a combination of multiple aspirations and some open surgical debridement without MRI, no relapses were reported [101]. A Taiwanese study of septic arthritis in 58 children managed without MRI also reported no relapses [102]. A sentinel study from Seattle Children's Hospital, in which MRI was not utilized, analyzed predictors of repeat surgery for septic arthritis involving hips and knees. In that study, elevated CRP levels and positive blood cultures were identified as statistically significant predictors of repeat surgery in a multivariable analysis [103] (Table 28.3). These three studies demonstrate that MRI

Table 28.3 Septic arthritis of the hip and knee

	Single surgery (n = 84)	Multiple surgeries (n = 21)
CRP (mg/dl)	7.91 (±7.14)	17.64 (±9.85)
Blood culture	23% (19/84)	67% (14/21)

Elevated CRP and positive blood cultures are significant predictors of needing repeat surgery

may be used more selectively, potentially reserved for patients with predictors of more severe disease or for patients who do not respond to standard first-line management.

A multicenter study conducted in Georgia, South Carolina, and Tennessee analyzed 138 pediatric patients with septic hips and found no association between preoperative MRI and the need for a second surgery [104]. Identified risk factors for return to the operating room included an elevated initial ESR (>40 mm/h), CRP (>10 mg/dL), MRSA infection, and the presence of concomitant osteomyelitis [104].

Proponents of aggressive MRI utilization also claim MRI decreases the length of hospital stay and overall cost of care [105, 106]. However, a multicenter study from four hospitals in Michigan, New York, Ontario, and Texas evaluated 104 patients with osteomyelitis and septic arthritis involving hips and knees [107]. When comparing patients who did and did not undergo preoperative MRI, the study found no significant differences in length of stay, number of surgeries required, or readmission rates. Notably, patients who received MRI were significantly less likely to undergo surgery on the day of admission, raising concerns about potential delays in treatment due to the time it takes to obtain MRI imaging [107].

MRI Screening in the Setting of Scoliosis

Due to concerns about spinal cord abnormalities including syringomyelia and tethered cord, and their potential impact on scoliosis management, MRI has been utilized as a screening tool in some scoliosis contexts [25]. Studies from the 1990s and early 2000s investigated the use of spinal MRI in patients with adolescent idiopathic scoliosis (AIS). One study focused on atypical curve patterns, such as left thoracic curves, and reported a 7% incidence of neurologic abnormalities, none of which required neurosurgical intervention [26]. Another study reported that clinical features such as severe unexplained headache, neck pain or stiffness, abnormal spinal movement patterns, and neurologic signs like cavus foot deformity provide a practical basis for ordering spinal MRI in scoliosis patients [27].

Multiple studies have emphasized the limited utility of MRI screening in asymptomatic patients with adolescent idiopathic scoliosis (AIS). Bob Winter and colleagues prospectively evaluated 140 neurologically normal AIS patients and identified four neurologic abnormalities, none of which were indicated for neurosurgical intervention [28]. Similarly, Twee Do and coauthors conducted a prospective study involving 327 neurologically normal AIS patients and found seven neurologic abnormalities, again with no cases needing neurosurgical treatment [29]. In addition, MRI scans have also been reported to be normal in patients with very large idiopathic curves (greater than 70 degrees) [30]. AIS of the thoracic spine is typically associated with hypokyphosis. Richards and colleagues, on the other hand, noted that patients with accentuated thoracic kyphosis are at increased risk for neural axis abnormalities [31]. This finding was further validated by a large multicenter study, which identified thoracic hyperkyphosis and juvenile onset as significant predictors of an abnormal spinal MRI. In contrast, factors such as left-sided curves, male sex, Risser sign <1, large curve magnitude, triple major curves, and obesity were not predictive [32].

Outcomes Today, MRI screening in AIS patients is approaching the status of accepted science. However, routine screening MRI in AIS has not demonstrated clinical value. On the other hand, MRI evaluation of the neural axis is warranted when specific neurologic warning signs are present. In addition, patients with other forms of scoliosis such as congenital scoliosis, Marfan-associated scoliosis, or scoliosis related to neurofibromatosis may derive benefit from MRI.

Pediatric Knee Imaging

An increasing reliance on knee MRI has contributed to a decline in emphasis on the physical examination of the knee [33–35]. In fact, documented physical examinations are present in only about half of knee MRI orders placed by primary care physicians [36], and even within the specialty of orthopedics, the importance of a careful knee examination has been called into question. Over time, this trend has led to a dependence on MRI over clinical assessment, to address ligamentous and meniscal concerns.

This shift away from the physical examination has financial consequences, as the cost of a knee MRI is substantial. For example, among 35 children's hospitals, the negotiated price for a single knee MRI ranged from $458 to $2619 [37]. For young children, typically under 7 years old, the cost of MRI can increase by another $5000 when general anesthesia is needed to complete the study.

The menisci are among the most frequently injured structures in the knees in children [38]. However, the accuracy of knee MRI in pediatric patients aged 4–14 years is significantly lower than in adolescents aged 15–17 years [39]. This reduced diagnostic accuracy is due to the increased vascularity of the meniscus in younger children [40]. Notably, neonatal menisci, including the central region, are six times more vascular compared to adult menisci [41]. In addition, the utility of MRI in evaluating meniscal healing after repair surgery has been questioned. Clinical examination has superior reliability in assessing postoperative meniscal healing [42].

Luhmann prospectively studied nearly 100 pediatric knee patients and reported that the orthopedic surgeon's preoperative diagnosis was significantly more accurate ($p < 0.05$) than the radiologist's MRI interpretation [43]. For pediatric anterior cruciate ligament (ACL) injuries, the longstanding clinical question is whether an associated meniscal tear is present. Dawkins and colleagues published findings that cast doubt on MRI's reliability in this setting, demonstrating only moderate accuracy in detecting such tears [44] (Table 28.4). Notably, MRI missed up to 76% of lateral meniscus root tears in children [45].

In recent years, there has been an explosion in clinical research focused on another pediatric knee condition: patellofemoral instability [46–49]. MRI studies have shown that osteochondral fractures and loose bodies occur in about 43% of children with a first-time patella dislocation and in 35% of those with recurrent dislocation [50]. These findings have led some orthopedic surgeons to routinely obtain a post-dislocation MRI scan. In the absence of mechanical symptoms, other orthopedic surgeons may adopt a watchful waiting approach and not proceed to an MRI. Normative values for tibial tubercle-trochlear groove (TTTG) distance have been established in children [51]. These values contribute to our understanding of both normal and pathological anatomy [52–55]. However, questions remain regarding the reliability of MRI in guiding surgical decision-making for patellofemoral instability [56]. This skepticism is reinforced by studies demonstrating a lack of correlation between imaging measurements of adolescent patellar instability and patient-reported outcome [57].

Another important pediatric knee condition is juvenile osteochondritis dissecans (OCD). MRI has been promoted as the standard of care for the diagnosis and classification of OCD [58]. Beyond identifying the precise anatomic location of the lesion, MRI is often used to assess lesion stability, a critical factor influencing treatment decisions. However, concerns have been raised regarding the clinical utility of MRI in juvenile OCD [59]. For example, when arthroscopic evaluation is used as the gold standard, MRI accurately predicts lesion stability in only 40–60% of cases [60–63].

The limited ability of MRI to accurately predict lesion stability in juvenile OCD is particularly concerning given the costs associated with obtaining these studies. Compounding this concern is the fact that effective treatments exist for both stable and unstable lesions [64–67]. Since these treatments almost universally involve arthroscopic surgery, there is a strong argument for broadening the indications for arthroscopy to serve both diagnostic and therapeutic purposes. The Research on Osteochondritis Dissecans of the Knee (ROCK) group has advanced our understanding of OCD [68].

Outcomes MRI does not reliably identify meniscal injuries or assess the stability of OCD lesions. Reducing the use of MRI in the evaluation of pediatric knee patients would lead to a renewed emphasis on physical examination of the knee. The knee is the largest and most accessible joint in the human body for physical examination

Table 28.4 Diagnostic performance of MRI to detect meniscal injury in pediatric ACL patients (406 patients; mean age, 15.4 years; range: 10–18 years; Dawkins et al. [44])

	Sensitivity (%)	Specificity (%)	PPV (%)	NPV (%)
Lateral meniscal tear	51.0	86.5	78.3	65.0
Medial meniscal tear	83.2	80.6	62.3	92.5
Any meniscal tear	75.0	72.1	81.5	63.8

PPV positive predictive value, *NPV* negative predictive value assessment. Minimizing MRI use would also result in an increase in diagnostic arthroscopy. However, arthroscopy has its own risk benefit balance and cost considerations. With recent advances in arthroscopic technology, such as office-based needle arthroscopy, this shift could add value, particularly for older pediatric patients.

Pediatric Hip Imaging

The classic "big three" pediatric hip disorders include developmental dysplasia of the hip (DDH), Legg-Calvé-Perthes (LCP) disease, and slipped capital femoral epiphysis (SCFE). More recently, femoro-acetabular impingement (FAI) has emerged as a fourth addition to this list. Each of these conditions can result in substantial musculoskeletal impairment in the pediatric population. MRI has been widely utilized across all four disorders. MRI's overall track record in evaluating these hip disorders is, at best, mixed. In addition, the need for general anesthesia in young children to perform the MRI adds cost and some risk.

For infants with DDH, MRI has value in assessing the quality of reduction following closed or open reduction and spica casting [69–72]. MRI does not reliably predict the future development of postoperative avascular necrosis and has no added prognostic value [73]. In symptomatic adolescents and young adults with DDH evaluated for periacetabular osteotomy, MRI is utilized for staging osteoarthrosis [74, 75]. MRI has proven useful in some research settings [76, 77].

Over time, the management of LCP disease has shifted back and forth from non-operative treatment to surgical intervention [78, 79]. MRI has emerged as a helpful tool in identifying which patients are more likely to benefit from surgery. In particular, the severity of femoral head avascularity is a critical factor in LCP, and perfusion MRI has demonstrated reliability in both quantifying vascular compromise and predicting future femoral head deformity [80, 81]. However, some authors have expressed caution, noting that increased use of MRI in LCP has been associated with higher rates of surgery without evidence of improved long-term clinical outcomes [82].

Several challenging issues remain in the management of SCFE. These include improving outcomes after unstable slips, addressing residual deformities in stable slips, and determining when the so-called "pre-slipped" contralateral hip warrants prophylactic screw stabilization. In cases of unstable SCFE, the main concern is femoral head vascularity. Both bone scan and MRI continue to have proponents for predicting avascular necrosis (AVN) [83–87]. Surprisingly, even intraoperative monitoring using a pressure probe in the femoral head has been shown to be unreliable in predicting AVN [88]. While advocates of corrective osteotomy emphasize potential long-term benefits, reported iatrogenic AVN rates remain high at up to 20% [89–91]. As for the contralateral hip, studies both supporting and opposing the utility of MRI for detecting pre-slip changes have been published [92, 93].

The abnormal biomechanics of FAI place the articular cartilage and acetabular labrum at risk for damage. FAI is most commonly idiopathic; however, a combination of activity-related stress and presumed genetic predispositions underlies the development of FAI [94, 95]. Accurate diagnosis of FAI and associated labral pathology requires careful integration of hip symptoms, physical examination, and imaging findings. On the other hand, multiple studies have reported a high prevalence of FAI positive hip MRI findings in asymptomatic individuals. For example, in an adult population aged 27–43 years, Schmitz et al. reported a 26% prevalence of asymptomatic paralabral cysts and an 86% prevalence of asymptomatic labral tears on MRI [96]. Similarly, Dutch researchers studying a comparable young adult population concluded that MRI arthrography provided no additional value beyond the clinical diagnosis of labral pathology [97]. In a prospective study of 67 asymptomatic male collegiate football players with a mean age of 21 years, 95% of hips demonstrated at least one imaging sign of FAI, and 77% exhibited more than one [98]. Despite the high prevalence of imaging abnormalities, nonoperative management protocols are effective for many cases of FAI [99]. Researchers at Duke University have emphasized that clinical history, physical examination, plain radiographs, and diagnostic injections should be prioritized over routine use of MRI for FAI [100].

Outcomes In young patients with DDH, the absence of MRI would lead to renewed reliance on intraoperative arthrography and on CT or ultrasound for postreduction and casting assessment. In adolescents and young adults with DDH undergoing evaluation for periacetabular osteotomy, less use of MRI would result in increased use of hip arthroscopy for osteoarthritis staging. The role of perfusion MRI in guiding surgical decision-making for LCP disease remains uncertain. In cases of suspected contralateral pre-slip in SCFE, MRI would not be missed, since well-established plain radiographic and clinical criteria are sufficient for decision-making. The most contentious use of MRI in hip pathology relates to FAI. If MRI were eliminated in this setting, there would be increased use of ultrasound-guided intra-articular anesthetic injections for diagnostic and symptom clarification purposes, as well as a lowered threshold for proceeding to hip arthroscopy in appropriate patients.

Case Examples

Case 1 An 8-year-old boy presented with a 5-day history of left knee pain and limping. Fever and vomiting occurred during the week before the onset of knee symptoms. His oral temperature was 37.8 °C. A left knee effusion was present. Plain X-rays of the left knee were read as normal by the radiologist (Fig. 28.2). Laboratory evaluation revealed a peripheral white blood cell count of 9310/μL, C-reactive protein (CRP) of 9.40 mg/dL, and erythrocyte sedimentation rate (ESR) of 91 mm/h.

Arthrocentesis of the left knee was performed in the emergency department, yielding 14,850 white blood cells/μL with a differential of 76% segmented neutrophils, 17% lymphocytes, and 7% monocytes. Synovial fluid was sent for aerobic and anaerobic cultures, and a peripheral blood culture was also obtained. Based on his history, physical examination, and initial laboratory findings, most pediatric

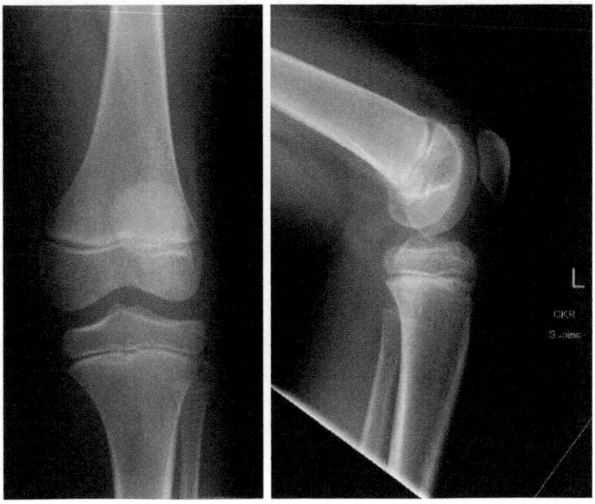

Fig. 28.2 AP and lateral radiograph of the left knee at presentation

orthopedic surgeons would proceed with irrigation and debridement, most likely via arthroscopy. Most pediatric orthopedic surgeons would also likely aspirate the distal femur metaphysis and drill the bone at the same setting to rule out associated osteomyelitis. However, a preoperative MRI of the left knee was obtained and revealed an additional posterior subperiosteal abscess (Fig. 28.3). This case highlights the added value of MRI in guiding appropriate surgical management.

The MRI findings potentially altered the surgical plan if the surgeon had not also aspirated and drilled the distal femur metaphysis. In addition to arthroscopic irrigation, debridement, and drain placement, a distal lateral approach to the femur was performed to evacuate the subperiosteal abscess and place iodoform gauze packing. Both blood and knee joint cultures grew methicillin-sensitive *Staphylococcus aureus* (MSSA) within 24 h. The knee joint drain and distal femur packing were removed on postoperative day 3. The child subsequently recovered uneventfully.

Case 2 A 13-year-old boy presented with scoliosis and associated non-radiating, sports-related low back pain. There was no family history of scoliosis. Physical examination revealed a mild leg length discrepancy, a cavus deformity of the right foot, and multiple myoclonus beats in the right foot. Radiographic imaging confirmed that he was not hyperkyphotic, the triradiate cartilage was open, and he was graded as Risser 1 (Fig. 28.4a).

An MRI obtained due to his cavus foot and myoclonus beats revealed a Chiari I cranio-cervical malformation and a large spinal cord syrinx (Fig. 28.4b). The patient subsequently underwent suboccipital decompression performed by pediatric neurosurgery. Despite surgical decompression and scoliosis bracing, his spinal curvature gradually progressed, and he underwent posterior spinal fusion with instrumentation 3 years later (Fig. 28.5).

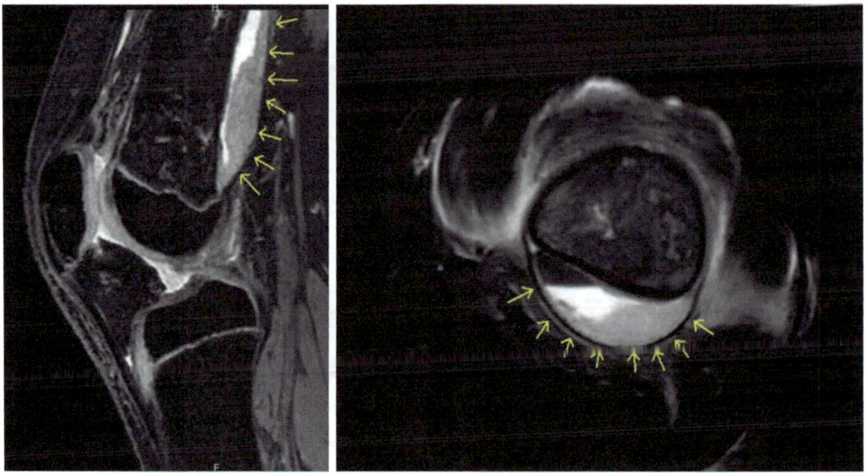

Fig. 28.3 Sagittal and transverse magnetic resonance images revealed large layered subperiosteal fluid collection

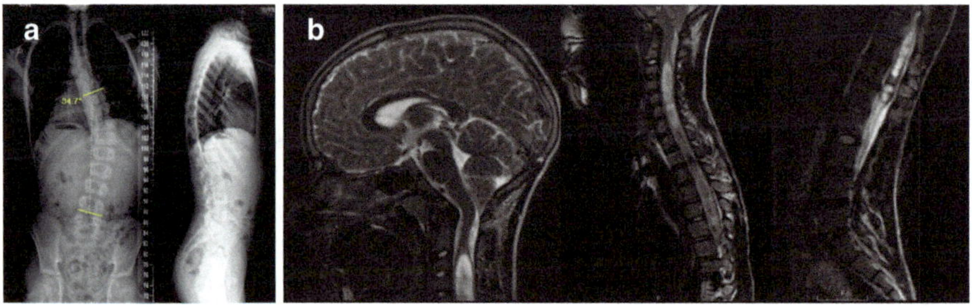

Fig. 28.4 (**a**) PA and lateral scoliosis X-rays demonstrate mild leg length difference, nearly 35-degree apex right thoracolumbar curve, and normal sagittal alignment. (**b**) MRI revealed Chiari I and extensive spinal cord syrinx

Case 3 A 12-year-old boy experienced right knee pain, particularly during crouching while playing catcher for his travel baseball team. He did not have mechanical symptoms. Plain radiographs revealed an osteochondritis dissecans (OCD) lesion located in the posteromedial aspect of the medial femoral condyle (Fig. 28.6).

A right knee MRI was obtained, which demonstrated intact articular cartilage over the OCD lesion, with associated adjacent bone marrow edema. No loose bodies were identified, and no additional abnormalities were noted (Fig. 28.7).

The patient was treated with two 6-week courses of cast immobilization, separated by a 1-week "honeymoon" period without casting. This was followed by physical therapy and the use of a hinged knee brace designed to unload the medial compartment. Follow-up radiographs obtained 1 year and 3 months later demonstrated healing of the lesion (Fig. 28.8). He was asymptomatic and returned to playing baseball at his same position.

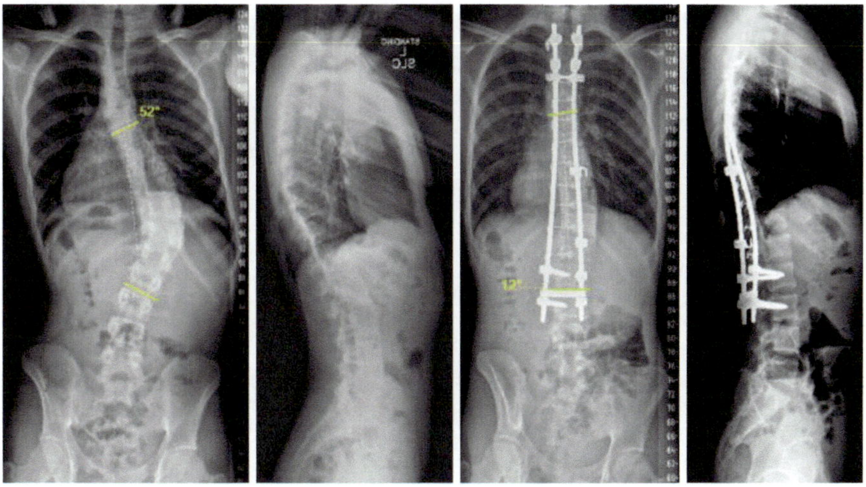

Fig. 28.5 Immediate pre-op PA and lateral and early post-op PA and lateral radiograph

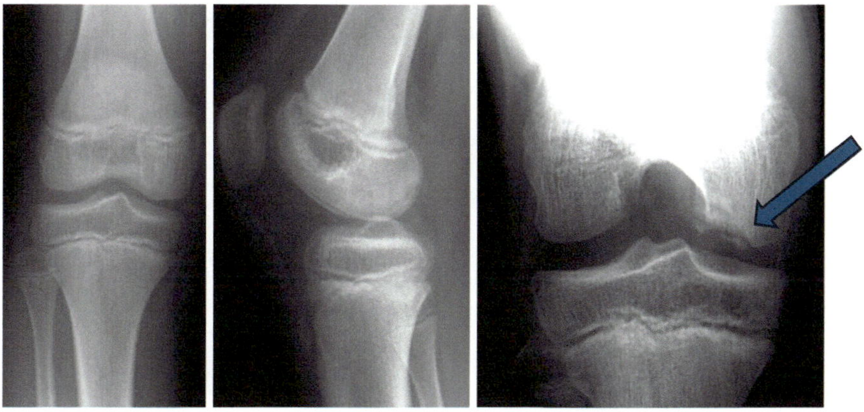

Fig. 28.6 AP, lateral, and notch views of the right knee. (Notch view; arrow shows the lesion)

Case 4 A 4-year-old male presented with a painless limp and radiographic findings consistent with Legg-Calvé-Perthes disease of the left hip (Fig. 28.9a). A gadolinium-enhanced MRI revealed diminished perfusion to the left capital femoral epiphysis, with approximately 80% of the epiphysis being non-perfused (Fig. 28.9b, c). Initial management was nonoperative; however, 8 months later, progressive femoral head deformity and restricted abduction prompted surgical intervention. He underwent a medial soft tissue release (adductor longus and medial hip capsule) followed by Petrie casting (Fig. 28.9d). Six weeks later, he underwent containment surgery via shelf arthroplasty. At 8 months postoperatively, imaging showed satisfactory periacetabular bone healing, progressive femoral head re-ossification, and restoration of full range of motion (Fig. 28.9e, f). At 8-year follow-up, radiographs were

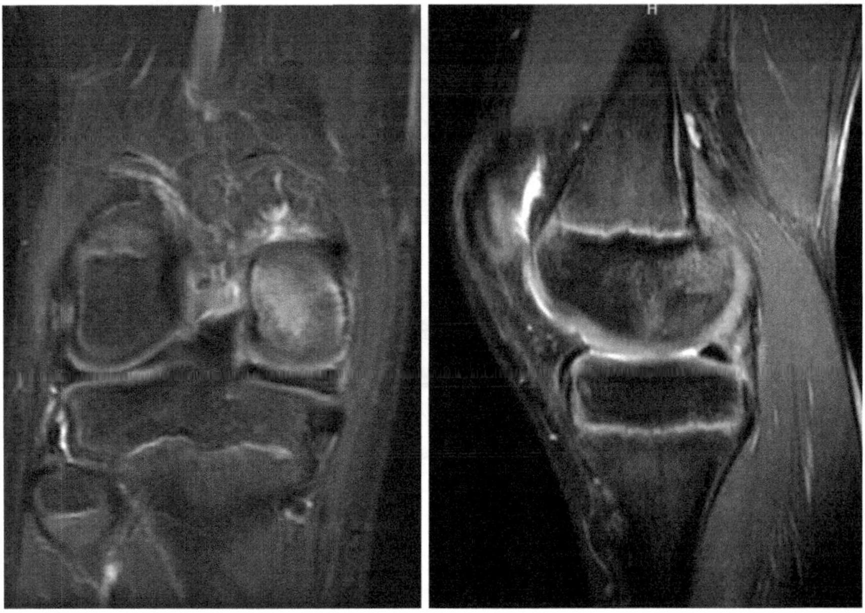

Fig. 28.7 Coronal and sagittal MRI views of the right knee

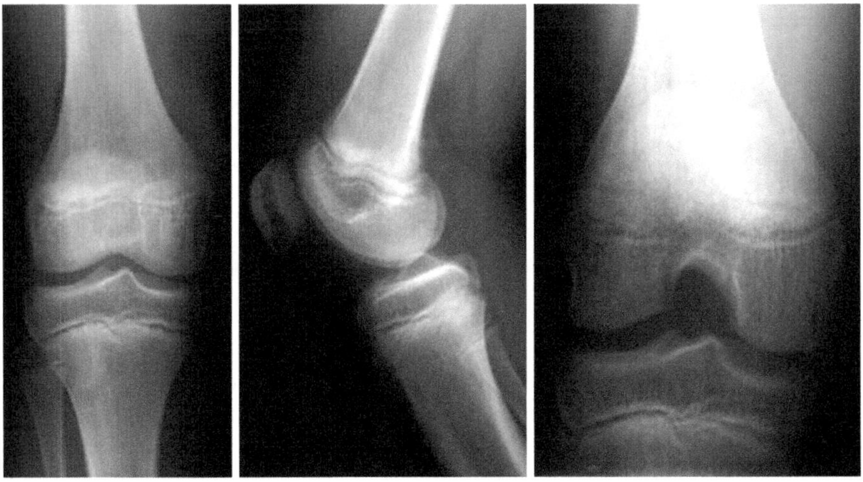

Fig. 28.8 One-year, 3-month follow-up AP, lateral, and notch views of the right knee

consistent with a Stulberg I classification, indicating favorable long-term hip morphology (Fig. 28.9g, h). The perfusion MRI did not influence the clinical decision-making process in a timely manner.

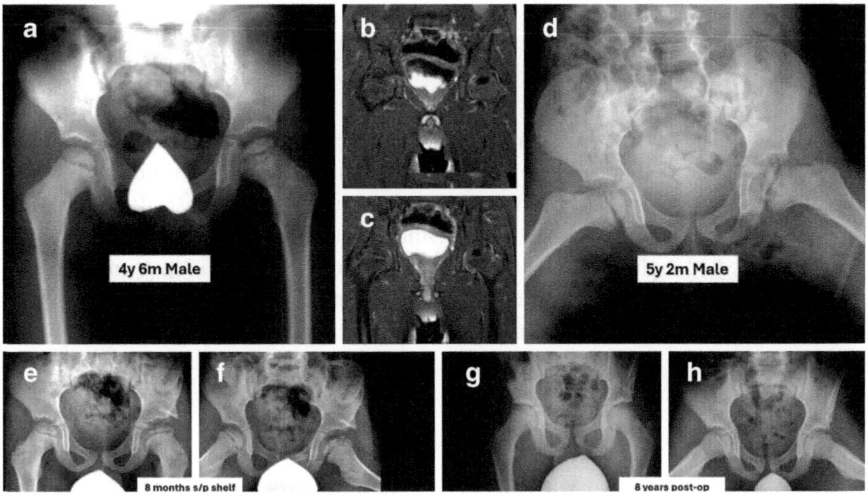

Fig. 28.9 Four-year-old boy with left hip Legg-Calvé-Perthes disease

Summary

Questions remain regarding the appropriate role of MRI across a wide range of pediatric orthopedic clinical cases. Among the examples presented in this chapter, there are instances where MRI clearly adds value. However, there are also cases in which MRI shows no value or has negative value by just increasing time and cost. Routine (what might be termed reflexive) MRI ordering should be critically evaluated, particularly for cases where imaging would also require general anesthesia. Value is enhanced with selective MRI use.

Author Pearls

1. *Infection*: Selective use of MRI when the clinical prodrome exceeds 4 days adds value to the management of pediatric septic arthritis.
2. *Scoliosis*: A small subset of patients with presumed AIS who exhibit neurologic abnormalities benefit from MRI of the neural axis.
3. *Knee*: Despite the common perception of its near infallibility, MRI of the pediatric knee sometimes yields unreliable and inaccurate information.
4. *Hip*: The value of MRI in pediatric hip conditions varies depending on the patient's age and specific diagnosis.

Editor Comments

WLH

Dr. Mehlman has written a "classic" chapter focusing on value and the use and abuse of MRI in pediatric orthopedics. MRI was first applied to musculoskeletal diagnoses in about 1985. Unfortunately, and surprisingly, the cost of MRI has not gone down in the intervening 40 years. Other strategies for saving money when an MRI is indicated include having the MRI performed at a freestanding imaging center over a hospital, negotiating cash prices or self-pay discounts, and verifying your insurance coverage to ensure in-network facilities and prices.

RMS

MRI has transformed pediatric orthopedics, but its value lies in mindful and selective use. Emerging abbreviated MRI protocols may lower cost, reduce anesthesia, and improve efficiency, potentially changing the value equation in the future. At the same time, alternatives such as ultrasound and office-based needle arthroscopy are gaining popularity. Ultimately, imaging should complement, not replace, the physical examination and thoughtful clinical judgment.

References

1. Anzai Y, Minoshima S, Lee VS. Enhancing value of MRI: a call for action. J Magn Reson Imaging. 2019;49:e40–8.
2. Smith-Bindman R, Kwan ML, Marlow EC, Theis MK, Balch W, et al. Trends in use of medical imaging in the US health care systems and in Ontario, Canada 2000–2016. JAMA. 2019;322:843–56.
3. Canadian Medical Imaging Inventory 2022–2023:MRI. Canadian Agency for Drugs and Technologies in Health. 2024 August. Report no. HC0024-06.
4. Definitive Healthcare. How many imaging centers are in the US? Published 17 Jan 2025. Accessed 8 Apr 2025 https://www.definitivehc.com/resources/healthcare-insights/imaging-centers-us.
5. Cohen E, Rodean J, Diong C, Hall M, et al. Low-value diagnostic imaging use in pediatric emergency department in the United States and Canada. JAMA Pediatr. 2019;173:e191439.
6. Marin JR, Rodean J, Hall M, Alpern ER, Aronson PL, et al. Trends in use of advanced imaging in pediatric emergency departments 2009–2018. JAMA Pediatr. 2020;174:e202209.
7. Hayatghaibi SE, Kandil AI, Zhang B, Alves VV, Ayyala RS, Dillman JR, Trout AT. Trends in anesthesia/sedation for computed tomography and magnetic resonance imaging encounters in pediatric emergency departments 2012–2022. JAMA Pediatr. 2023;177:1105–7.
8. Studdert DM, Mello MM, Sage WM, DesRoches CM, Peugh J, Zapert K, Brennan TA. Defensive medicine among high-risk specialist physicians in a volatile malpractice environment. JAMA. 2005;293:2609–17.
9. Miller RA, Sampson NF, Flynn JM. The prevalence of defensive orthopaedic imaging: a prospective practice audit in Pennsylvania. J Bone Joint Surg-Am. 2012;94:e18. (1–6).

10. Sathiyakumar V, Jahangir AA, Mir HR, Obremskey WT, Lee YM, Apfeld JC, Sethi MK. The prevalence of and costs of defensive medicine among orthopaedic trauma surgeons: a national survey study. J Orthop Trauma. 2013;27:592–8.
11. Li S, Dor A, Deyo D, Hughes DR. The impact of state tort reforms on imaging utilization. J Am Coll Radiol. 2017;14:149–56.
12. Schoenecker JG, et al. (CORTICES Group). Defining the volume of consultations for musculoskeletal infection encountered by pediatric orthopaedic services in the United States. PLoS One. 2020;15:e0234055.
13. Hartman NR, Gerard JM, Puryear A, Sethi A, Flood RG. Clinical characteristics of acute hematogenous osteomyelitis with and without subperiosteal abscesses in the acute care setting. Pediatr Emerg Care. 2022;38:e1224–8.
14. Mehlman CT, Rosenfeld S, et al. Predicting the presence of adjacent infection in septic arthritis in children. J Pediatr Orthop. 2016;36:e64.
15. Ernat J, Riccio AI, Fitzpatrick K, Jo CH, Wimberly RL. Osteomyelitis is commonly associated with septic arthritis of the shoulder in children. J Pediatr Orthop. 2017;37:547–52.
16. Monsalve J, Kan JH, Bisset GS, Zhang W, Rosenfeld SB. Septic arthritis in children: frequency of coexisting unsuspected osteomyelitis and implications on imaging work-up and management. AJR. 2015;204:1289–95.
17. Nduaguba AM, Flynn JM, Sankar WN. Septic arthritis of the elbow in children: clinical presentation and microbiological profile. J Pediatr Orthop. 2016;36:75–9.
18. Nguyen A, Kan JH, Bisset G, Rosenfeld S. Kocher criteria revisited in the era of MRI: how often does Kocher criteria identify underlying osteomyelitis? J Pediatr Orthop. 2017;37:e114–9.
19. Montgomery CO, Siegel E, Blasier RD, Suva LJ. Concurrent septic arthritis and osteomyelitis in children. J Pediatr Orthop. 2013;33:464–7.
20. Rosenfeld S, Bernstein DT, Daran S, et al. Predicting the presence of adjacent infections in septic arthritis in children. J Pediatr Orthop. 2016;36:70–4.
21. Siddiqui AA, Andras LM, Illingsworth KD, Skaggs DL. Pain for greater than 4 days is highly predictive of concomitant osteomyelitis in children with septic arthritis. J Pediatr Orthop. 2021;41:255–9.
22. Chan KS, McBride D, Wild J, Kwon S, Samet J, Gibly RF. A rapid MRI protocol for the evaluation of acute pediatric musculoskeletal infections: eliminating contrast and decreasing anesthesia scan time and hospital length of stay and charges. J Bone Joint Surg Am. 2024;106:700–7.
23. Courtney PM, Flynn JM, Jaramillo D, Horn BD, Calabro K, Spiegel DA. Clinical indications for repeat MRI in children with acute hematogenous osteomyelitis. J Pediatr Orthop. 2010;30:883–7.
24. Refakis CA, Arkader A, Baldwin KD, Spiegel DA, Sankar WN. Predicting periarticular infection in children with septic arthritis of the hip: regionally derived criteria may not apply to all populations. J Pediatr Orthop. 2019;39:268–74.
25. Lee H, Janjua F, Ragab A, Moran J, Haims A, et al. Total spine MRI for the preoperative evaluation of adolescent idiopathic scoliosis: part 1. Curr Probl Diagn Radiol. 2024;53:405–14.
26. Mejia EA, Hennrikus WL, Schwend RM, Means JB. A prospective evaluation of idiopathic left thoracic scoliosis with magnetic resonance imaging. J Pediatr Orthop. 1996;16:354–8.
27. Schwend RM, Hennrikus W, Hall JE, Means B. Childhood scoliosis: clinical indications for magnetic resonance imaging. J Bone Joint Surg Am. 1995;77:46–53.
28. Winter RB, Lonstein JE, Heithoff KB, Kirkham JA. Magnetic resonance imaging evaluation of the adolescent patient with idiopathic scoliosis before spinal instrumentation and fusion: a prospective double-blind study of 140 patients. Spine. 1997;22:855–8. jei O.
29. Do T, Fras C, Burke S, Widmann RF, Rawlins B, Boachie-Adjei O. Clinical value of routine magnetic resonance imaging in idiopathic scoliosis: a prospective study of three hundred and twenty-seven patients. J Bone Joint Surg Am. 2001;83:577–9.
30. Obrien MF, Lenke LG, Bridwell KH, Blanke K, Baldus C. Preoperative spinal canal investigation in adolescent idiopathic scoliosis curves > or = 70 degrees. Spine. 1994;19:1606–10.

31. Richards BS, Sucato DJ, Johnston CE, Diab M, Sarwark JF, Lenke LG, Parent S. Right thoracic curves in presumed adolescent idiopathic scoliosis: which clinical and radiographic findings correlate with a preoperative abnormal magnetic resonance image? Spine. 2010;35:1855–60.
32. Diab M, Landman Z, Lubicky J, Dormans J, Erickson M, Richards BS. Use and outcome of MRI in the surgical treatment of adolescent idiopathic scoliosis. Spine. 2011;36:667–71.
33. Stanitski CI. Correlation of arthroscopic and clinical examinations with magnetic resonance imaging findings of injured knees in children and adolescents. Am J Sports Med. 1998;26:2–6.
34. Kocher MS, DiCanzio J, Zurakowski D, Micheli LJ. Diagnostic performance of clinical examination and selective magnetic resonance imaging in the evaluation of intraarticular knee disorders in children and adolescents. Am J Sports Med. 2001;29:292–6.
35. Hofmann B, Havik V, Andersen ER, et al. Low-value MRI of the knee in Norway: a register-based study to identify the proportion of potentially low-value MRIs and estimate related costs. BMJ Open. 2023;14:e081860.
36. Wylie JD, Crim JR, Working ZM, Schmidt RL, Burks RT. Physician provider type influences utilization and diagnostic utility of magnetic resonance imaging of the knee. J Bone Joint Surg Am. 2015;97:56–62.
37. Hayatghaibi SE, Alves VV, Ayyala RS, Dillman JR, Trout AT. Transparency and variability in pricing for pediatric outpatient imaging in US hospitals. JAMA Netw Open. 2022;5:e220736.
38. Cabral J, Sinikumpu J. Clinical considerations of anatomy and magnetic resonance imaging in pediatric meniscal tear with imaging-based treatment options. J Child Orthop. 2023;17:63–9.
39. McDermott MJ, Bathgate B, Gillingham BL, Hennrikus WL. Correlation of MRI and arthroscopic diagnosis of knee pathology in children and adolescents. J Pediatr Orthop. 1998;18:675–8.
40. Takeda Y, Ikata T, Yoshida S, et al. MRI high-signal intensity in the menisci of asymptomatic children. J Bone Joint Surg Am. 1998;80:463–7.
41. Lin KM, Gadinsky NE, Klinger CE, Dyke JP, Rodeo SA, Green DW, Fabricant PD, Helfet DL, Shea KG, Lazaro LE. Increased vascularity in the neonatal versus adult meniscus: evaluation with magnetic resonance imaging. Cartilage. 2021;13:1562S–9S.
42. Schoenecker JH, Tollefsen LV, Solaiman RH, et al. A lack of joint line tenderness is consistent with a healed meniscus but positive clinical examination findings and MRI scans are inconsistent in identifying failure after meniscal repair: a systematic review and subgroup meta-analysis. Am J Sports Med. 2025;53:1750–60.
43. Luhmann SJ, Schootman M, Gordon JE, Wright RW. Magnetic resonance imaging of the knee in children and adolescents: its role in clinical decision-making. J Bone Joint Surg Am. 2005;87:497–502.
44. Dawkins BJ, Kolin DA, Park J, Fabricant PD, Gilmore A, Seeley M, Mistovich RJ. Sensitivity and specificity of MRI in diagnosing concomitant meniscal injuries in pediatric and adolescent ACL tears. Ortho J Sports Med. 2022;10:23259671221079338. https://doi.org/10.1177/23259671221079338. eCollection.
45. Schlechter J, Pak T, Gornick B, McDonald E. Magnetic resonance imaging of lateral meniscus root tears in the pediatric and adolescent knee. Orthop J Sports Med. 2022;10:23259671221114629. https://doi.org/10.1177/23259671221114629.
46. Kamalapathy P, Rush J, Montgomery SR, et al. A national perspective of patellar instability in children and adolescents in the United State: MPFL reconstruction is three times higher than the incidence of isolated lateral release. Arthroscopy. 2022;38:466–73.
47. Parikh SN, Wall EJ. Patellar fracture after medial patellofemoral ligament surgery: a report of five cases. J Bone Joint Surg Am. 2011;93:e97. (1–8).
48. Parikh SN, Schlechter JA, Veerkamp MW, et al. Consensus-based guidelines for management of first-time patellar dislocation in adolescents. J Pediatr Orthop. 2024;44:e369–74.
49. Masquijo J, Parkih SN, Kothari A. Evaluation of the optimal femoral fixation site for medial patellofemoral ligament reconstruction in the skeletally immature patient. Orthopedics. 2023;46:108–13.

50. Qiu RY, Fitzpatrick DWD, Cohen D, et al. MRI as the optimal imaging modality for assessment and management of osteochondral fractures and loose bodies following traumatic patellar dislocation: a systematic review. Knee Surg Sports Traumatol Arthrosc. 2023;31:1744–52.
51. Park SJ, Won SH, Park MS, Sung KH. Normative values of tibial tubercle-trochlear groove distance and tibial tubercle-posterior cruciate ligament distance in children. Am J Sports Med. 2023;51:1785–91.
52. Hemke R, van den Berg JM, Nusman CM, et al. Contrast-enhanced MRI findings of the knee in healthy children: establishing normal values. Eur Radiol. 2018;28:1167–74.
53. Cheng J, Shah AA, Wang JW, et al. Anterior attachment of the medial patellofemoral ligament: morphological characteristics. J Bone Joint Surg Am. 2025;107:741–8.
54. Kemmeren LAM, Oei EHG, van Middlekoop M, et al. Prevalence of abnormalities and normal variants in the adolescent knee on MRI in a population -based cohort of 3800 knees. Am J Sports Med. 2024;52:3039–45.
55. Kinsella SD, Rider SM, Fury MS, Tepolt FA, Eckland K, Kocher MS. Concomitant posterolateral corner injuries in skeletally immature patients with acute anterior cruciate ligament injuries. J Pediatr Orthop. 2020;40:271–6.
56. Fabricant PD, Heath MR, Mintz DN, Emery K, Veerkamp M, Gruber S, Green DW, Strickland SM, Wall EJ, JUPITER study group, Shubin-Stein BE, Parikh SN. Many radiographic and magnetic resonance imaging assessments for surgical decision making in pediatric patellofemoral instability patients demonstrate poor interrater reliability. Arthroscopy. 2022;38:2702–13.
57. Eysturoy NH, Husum HC, Ingelsrud LH, Blond L, Barfod KW. Correlation between radiological measurements for patellar instability and patient-reported outcome measurements in adolescents: a study from the Faroese knee cohort. Am J Sports Med. 2025;53:172–80.
58. Chau MM, Klimstra MA, Wise KL, et al. Current concepts: osteochondritis dissecans. J Bone Joint Surg Am. 2021;103:1132–51.
59. Hu H, Zhang C, Chen J, et al. Clinical value of MRI in assessing the stability of osteochondritis dissecans lesions: a systematic review and meta-analysis. Am J Roentgenol. 2019;213:147–54.
60. Heywood CS, Benke MT, Brindle K, Fine KM. Correlation of magnetic resonance imaging to arthroscopic findings of stability in juvenile osteochondritis dissecans. Arthroscopy. 2011;27:194–9.
61. Samora WP, Chevillet J, Adler B, Young GS, Klingele KE. Juvenile osteochondritis dissecans of the knee: predictors of lesion stability. J Pediatr Orthop. 2012;32:1–4.
62. Ellermann JM, Donald B, Rohr S, et al. Magnetic resonance imaging of osteochondritis dissecans: validation study for the ICRS classification system. Acad Radiol. 2016;23:724–9.
63. Robbach BP, Paulus AC, Niethammer TR, et al. Discrepancy between morphological findings in juvenile osteochondritis dissecans (OCD): a comparison of magnetic resonance imaging (MRI) and arthroscopy. Knee Surg Sports Traumatol Arthrosc. 2016;24:1259–64.
64. Wall EJ, Vourazeris J, Myer GD, Emery KH, et al. The healing potential of stable juvenile osteochondritis dissecans knee lesions. J Bone Joint Surg Am. 2008;90:2655–64.
65. Heyworth BE, Ganley TJ, Liotta ES, et al. Transarticular versus retroarticular drilling of stable osteochondritis dissecans of the knee: a prospective multicenter randomized controlled trial by the ROCK group. Am J Sports Med. 2023;51:1392–402.
66. Husen M, Vanderweiden GS, Custers RJH, et al. Internal fixation of unstable osteochondritis dissecans of the knee: long-term outcomes in skeletally immature and mature patients. Am J Sports Med. 2023;51:1403–13.
67. Johnstone T, Espiritu J, Tompkins M, et al. Which osteochondritis dissecans lesions will heal nonoperatively? An application of machine learning to the ROCK prospective cohort. Orthop J Sports Med. 2024;12:1–9.
68. Edmonds EW, Polousky J. A review of knowledge in osteochondritis dissecans 123 years of minimal evolution from König to the ROCK group. Clin Orthop Rel Res. 2013;471:1118–26.

69. Laor T, Roy DR, Mehlman CT. Limited magnetic resonance imaging examination after surgical reduction of developmental dysplasia of the hip. J Pediatr Orthop. 2000;20:572–4.
70. Struder K, Williams N, Struder P, Baker M, Glynn A, Foster BK, Cundy PJ. Obstacles to reduction in infantile developmental dysplasia of the hip. J Child Orthop. 2017;11:358–66.
71. Dibello D, Odoni L, Pederiva F, DiCarlo V. MRI in postreduction evaluation of developmental dysplasia of the hip: our experience. J Pediatr Orthop. 2019;39:449–52.
72. Jia H, Wang L, Chang Y, et al. Assessment of irreducible aspects in developmental hip dysplasia by magnetic resonance imaging. PMC Pediatrics. 2020;20:550. (1–7).
73. Nguyen JC, Back SJ, Barrera CA, Patel M, Nguyen MK, Hong S, Sankar WN. Developmental dysplasia of the hip: can contrast-enhanced MRI predict the development of avascular necrosis following surgery? Skeletal Radiol. 2021;50:389–97.
74. Schmitz MR, Murtha AS, Clohisy JC, Anchor Study Group. Developmental dysplasia of the hip in adolescents and young adults. J Am Acad Orthop Surg. 2020;28:91–101.
75. Selberg CM, Chidsey B, Skelton A, Mayer S. Pelvic osteotomies in the child and young adult hip: indications and surgical technique. J Am Acad Orthop Surg. 2020;28:e230–7.
76. Nakamura T, Yamaguchi R, Wada A, et al. A longitudinal study for the prediction of the mature acetabular morphology using childhood magnetic resonance imaging. J Orthop Sci. 2021;26:644–9.
77. Xu C, Pan X, Song B, Zhang G, Zhang D. A modified non-contrast MRI in the preoperative examination of periacetabular osteotomy at 3.0T. J Orthop Surg Res. 2025;20:121. (1–8).
78. Nguyen NT, Klein G, Dogbey G, McCourt JB, Mehlman CT. Operative versus nonoperative treatments for Legg-Calve-Perthes disease: a meta-analysis. J Pediatr Orthop. 2012;32:697–705.
79. Saran N, Varghese R, Mulpuri K. Do femoral or salter innominate osteotomies improve femoral head sphericity in Legg-Clave-Perthes disease? A meta-analysis. Clin Orthop Relat Res. 2012;470:2383–93.
80. Chong DY, Schrader T, Laine JC, Yang S, Gilbert SR, Kim HKW. Reliability and validity of visual estimation of femoral head hypoperfusion on perfusion MRI in Legg-Calve-Perthes disease. J Pediatr Orthop. 2021;41:e780–6.
81. Kang MS, Zimmerhanzel D, Haider S, Kim HKW. Eary-stage femoral head hypoperfusion correlates with femoral head deformity at intermediate follow-up in Legg-Calve-Perthes disease. J Bone Joint Surg Am. 2025;107:36–45.
82. Kalenderer O, Erkus S, Sarikaya IA, Turgut A, Inan M. The MRI effect in clinical decision process in Perthes disease: more complex imaging more complicated surgeries. Acta Chir Orthop Traumatol Cechoslov. 2022;89:134–8.
83. Edouard C, Raphael V, Hubert D. Is the femoral head dead or alive before surgery of slipped capital femoral epiphysis? Interest of perfusion magnetic resonance imaging. J Clin Orthop Trauma. 2014;5:18–26.
84. Gelfand MJ, Strife JL, Graham EJ, Crawford AH. Bone scintigraphy in slipped capital femoral epiphysis. Clin Nucl Med. 1983;8:613–5.
85. Gelfand MJ, Ball WS, Oestreich AE, Crawford AH, Jolson R, Perlman A. Transient loss of femoral head Tc-99m diphosphonate uptake with prolonged maintenance of femoral head architecture. Clin Nucl Med. 1983;8:347–54.
86. Napora JK, Gilmore A, Son-Hing JP, Grimberg DC, Thompson GH, Liu RW. Early MRI detection and closed bone graft epiphysiodesis may alter the course of avascular necrosis following unstable slipped capital femoral epiphysis. J Pediatr Orthop. 2018;38:202–7.
87. Parikh AK, Washington ER, Bobbey AJ, Spottswood SE. Evaluation of femoral head viability via bone scintigraphy in the postoperative pediatric patient. Pediatr Radiol. 2018;48:350–8.
88. Ellsworth BK, Lee JY, Batley MG, Sankar WN. Intraoperative epiphyseal perfusion monitoring does not reliably predict osteonecrosis following treatment of unstable SCFE. J Pediatr Orthop. 2024;44:e400–5.

89. Cullen MC, Crawford AH. The management of severe avascular necrosis following slipped capital femoral epiphysis by transtrochanteric rotational osteotomy: results of successful treatment in two cases with long-term follow-up. Iowa Orthop J. 1995;15:209–16.
90. Crawford AH. Role of osteotomy in the treatment of slipped capital femoral epiphysis. J Pediatr Orthop B. 1996;5:102–9.
91. Winson DMG, Cundy WJ, Roser MJN, et al. Subcapital realignment osteotomy for the treatment of moderate and severe slipped upper femoral epiphysis: a retrospective study of 123 hips in a tertiary center. J Child Orthop. 2024;18:379–85.
92. Samora JB, Adler B, Druhan S, Brown SA, Erickson J, Samora WP, Klingele KE. MRI in idiopathic stable slipped capital femoral epiphysis: evaluation of contralateral pre-slip. J Child Orthop. 2018;12:454–60.
93. Wensaas A, Wiig O, Hellund JC, et al. Magnetic resonance imaging at primary diagnosis cannot predict contralateral slip in slipped capital femoral epiphysis. Skeletal Radiol. 2017;46:1687–94.
94. Bedi A, Kelly BT. Current concepts review: femoroacetabular impingement. J Bone Joint Surg Am. 2013;95-A:82–92.
95. Skendzel JG, Weber AE, Ross JR, Larson CL, Leunig M, Kelly RT, Bedi A. The approach to the evaluation and surgical treatment of mechanical hip pain in the young patient. J Bone Joint Surg-Am. 2013;95-A:e133. (1–16).
96. Schmitz MR, Campbell SE, Fajardo RS, Kadrmas WR. Identification of acetabular labral pathology in asymptomatic volunteers using optimized noncontrast 1.5 -T magnetic resonance imaging. Am J Sports Med. 2012;40:1337–41.
97. Reurink G, Jansen SPL, Bisselink JM, et al. Reliability and validity of diagnosing acetabular labral lesions with magnetic resonance arthrography. J Bone Joint Surg Am. 2012;94:1643–8.
98. Kapron AL, Anderson AE, Aoki SK, et al. Radiographic prevalence of femoroacetabular impingement in collegiate football players. J Bone Joint Surg Am. 2011;93:e111. (1–10).
99. Zogby AM, Boman JD, Johnson KP, Upasani VV, Pennock AT. Nonoperative management of femoroacetabular impingement in adolescents: clinical outcomes at a mean of 5 years a prospective study. Am J Sports Med. 2021;49:2960–7.
100. Cunningham DJ, Paranjape CS, Harris JD, et al. Advanced imaging adds little value in the diagnosis of femoroacetabular impingement syndrome. J Bone Joint Surg Am. 2017;99:e133. (1–9).
101. Welkon CJ, Long SS, Fisher MC, Alburger PD. Pyogenic arthritis in infants and children: a review of 95 cases. Pediatr Infect Dis. 1986;5:669–76.
102. Wang CL, Wang SM, Yang YJ, et al. Septic arthritis in children: relationship of causative pathogens complications and outcome. J Microbiol Immunol Infect. 2003;36:41–6.
103. Telleria JJM, Cotter RA, Bompadre V, Steinman SE. Laboratory predictors for risk of revision surgery in pediatric septic arthritis. J Child Orthop. 2016;10:247–54.
104. Murphy RF, Plumblee L, Barfield WB, Murphy JS, Fuerstenau N, Spence DD, Kelly DM, Dow MA, Mooney JF III. Septic arthritis of the hip - risk factors associated with secondary surgery. J Am Acad Orthop Surg. 2019;27:321–6.
105. Hamilton EC, Villani MC, Klosterman MM, Jo C, Liu J, Copley LAB. Children with primary septic arthritis have a markedly lower risk of adverse outcomes than those with contiguous osteomyelitis. J Bone Joint Surg Am. 2021;103:1229–37.
106. Robinette ED, Brower L, Schaffzin JK, Whitlock P, Shah SS, Connelly B. Use of a clinical care algorithm to improve care for children with hematogenous osteomyelitis. Pediatrics. 2019;143:e20180387.
107. Englert EG, Braithwaite CL, Aguirre-Flores ME, et al. Pediatric patients with osteomyelitis and/or septic joint undergoing surgical debridement have equivalent short-term outcomes with or without preoperative MRI. Children. 2024;11:300. https://doi.org/10.3390/children11030300.

Mini-C-Arm in Pediatric Orthopaedic Surgery: Small But Mighty

29

Lisa Bonsignore-Opp, Katherine Bach, Ashraf N. El Naga, and David Gendelberg

Introduction

Pediatric orthopedic surgery addresses a wide range of musculoskeletal conditions. The diversity of patients and pathologies presents unique challenges for surgical teams, particularly in balancing outcomes and cost. Procedural techniques are often difficult to standardize. Intraoperative imaging plays a critical role in the accurate diagnosis and management of pediatric orthopedic conditions by providing real-time visualization and guidance during surgery enabling precise decision-making. In the emergency department, effective use of imaging can reduce hospital resource utilization and enhance value.

A variety of radiographic technologies are available to assess bony architecture, including the full-size C-arm, flat-panel radiographs, and computed tomography (CT) scans. These imaging modalities differ in terms of physical absorbed dose (measured in Grays, Gy) and effective dose or dose equivalent that includes biologic effect (measured in Sieverts, Sv). CT serves as a proxy for the biological impact of radiation exposure. Compared to other radiologic equipment, the mini-C-arm offers a low-cost, low-dose alternative, albeit with trade-offs such as reduced field of view and limited soft tissue penetration. However, when used appropriately, the mini-C-arm supports value-based care by enhancing outcomes while lowering costs.

L. Bonsignore-Opp · K. Bach · A. N. El Naga · D. Gendelberg (✉)
Department of Orthopaedics, University of California, San Francisco, San Francisco, CA, USA
e-mail: lisa.bonsignore-opp@ucsf.edu; kelly.bach@ucsf.edu; ashraf.elnaga@ucsf.edu; david.gendelberg@ucsf.edu

W. L. Hennrikus, R. M. Schwend (eds.), *Value in Pediatric Orthopaedics*, https://doi.org/10.1007/978-3-032-19570-8_29

Value-Based Themes

Reducing Radiation Exposure

(a) *To the Patient*

Radiation exposure is a particular concern in children, as skeletally immature patients are more susceptible to the long-term effects of ionizing radiation, including the accumulation of genetic mutations that may lead to illness later in life. Studies have shown that exposure to 50 mGy (milligray) during childhood triples the risk of developing leukemia [4]. While this level of radiation is rarely reached during one orthopedic procedure, patients with complex conditions requiring multiple surgeries or CT scans face increased cumulative risk. For example, a recent study published in *The Journal of the American Medical Association* projected that the 93 million CT scans performed in the U.S. in 2023 could result in more than 100,000 future cancer diagnoses [5].

For the same fluoroscopy time and distance, the mini-C-arm emits significantly less radiation to the patient compared to the traditional full-size C-arm and reduces scatter exposure (Fig. 29.1) [1–3].

For reference, an adult size person (surface area 1.5 m^2) at sea level receives an annual background radiation dose area product (DAP) of 3 $mGy \cdot m^2$ per year. For upper extremity surgeries, the mini-C-arm typically results in radiation exposure to the operative field ranging from 0.001 to 0.017 $mGy \cdot m^2$ (the units used in radiologic imaging, also termed DAP or dose area product), though values can vary depending on the specific device and institution [1, 6]. This dose would be the equivalent of 3 h to 2 days of background radiation at sea level. For lower extremity procedures, exposure generally ranges from 0.008 to 0.024 $mGy \cdot m^2$ when using the mini-C-arm [1, 7, 8]. These values remain well below the established safety thresholds for pediatric radiation exposure.

Percutaneous techniques are common in pediatric orthopedics and often rely on imaging to assess fracture reduction and hardware placement. The use of a mini-C-arm during percutaneous procedures results in lower radiation exposure compared to open surgery performed with a full-size C-arm [9]. For instance, in pediatric supracondylar humerus fracture fixation, the mini-C arm resulted in lower overall patient radiation exposure compared to the full-size C-arm, thus improving value [10].

(b) *To the Surgeon*

The harmful effects of radiation exposure are well documented, and there is an increasing focus on improving safety for healthcare workers who face occupational radiation exposure. Orthopedic surgeons are at elevated risk for cancer due to cumulative radiation, with breast cancer incidence reported to be nearly four times higher than in the general US population [11, 12]. To mitigate this risk, the US Centers for Disease Control and the Nuclear Regulatory Commission advocate for the ALARA

Feature	Mini -C-arm	Full-Size C-Arm
Size	- **Smaller** arc and footprint - More compact	- **Larger** arcand footprint
Maneuverability	- Higher, better workplace access	- Lower, requires more space
Portability	- Highly portable	- Less portable
Operator	- **Surgeon-operated** in many cases	- Typically requires an **x-ray tech**
Cost (Initial)	- Generally **lower** purchase price	- Generally **higher** purchase price
Cost (Operational)	- **Potentially lower due to no need for a tech in some cases** - **Lower electrical utilization**	- Potentially higher due to tech costs - Higher electrical utilization
Radiation Exposure	- Generally lower for extremities, but depends on usage and training	- Generally higher, but depends on usage and training
Field of View	- Limited to **extremities and smaller body parts**	- Larger, suitable for **pelvis and spine**
Imaging Quality	- Excellent for extremities, may be lower for larger or denser anatomy	- **Generally higher for a wider range of body parts**
Power of X-ray Generator	- Lower power	- Higher power
Accuracy	- High accuracy for extremity procedures	- High accuracy for a broader range of procedures
Applications	- **Primarily extremity surgery, some limited shoulder scans**	- **Both extremity and axial surgery**

Fig. 29.1 Comparison of mini-C-arm versus full-size traditional C-arm

(as low as reasonably achievable) principle, which emphasizes minimizing exposure time, maximizing distance from the source, and using appropriate shielding [13, 14].

A 2013 study found that most surveyed surgeons reported using lead aprons while operating with a mini-C-arm [15]. However, the same study revealed that many did not regularly wear dosimeter badges, making it difficult to accurately assess their cumulative radiation exposure.

Scatter radiation from the mini-C-arm remains below occupational safety thresholds for the body, thyroid, hands, and eyes [3, 16, 17, 24]. Additionally, physician exposure is generally lower than with the full-size C-arm [2, 18, 19]. However, in certain procedures, the mini-C-arm may increase radiation exposure to the surgeon's hands due to the proximity of the X-ray beam to their hands [20, 21]. However, the exposure remains well below the recommended occupational dose limits for the hands [22, 24]. One study estimated that a surgeon would need to perform over 18,000 mini-C-arm-assisted cases annually to exceed the recommended hand dose [25].

Several commercially available options can further reduce hand exposure, including lead-free metal oxide gloves, leaded gloves, and radiation-attenuating cream. Each of these products has been demonstrated to reduce radiation to the hands during mini-C-arm use [23, 26].

Radiation-induced damage to the lens of the eye typically results from scattering. The use of metal instrumentation can increase scatter by reflecting radiation, thereby placing the lens at greater risk [27]. Therefore, lead eyewear is recommended for both the surgeon and first assistant during fluoroscopic procedures [23, 27].

Although radiation exposure from the mini-C-arm is relatively low, proper training is essential to ensure safe use and minimize potential harm. An elegant 2020 study by Gendelberg et al. demonstrated that formal radiation safety training significantly reduced radiation exposure to patients as well as residents performing pediatric both-bone forearm or distal radius fracture reductions in the emergency department [28]. A follow-up study confirmed that these reductions in radiation exposure were sustained nearly 1 year after the initial training [29]. Additionally, residents with greater experience in a specific reduction technique were shown to use less radiation [30], underscoring the importance of radiation safety education to improve value.

The literature on mini-C-arm use supports several best practice guidelines that can enhance value (Fig. 29.2). In general, vertical beam orientation (i.e., perpendicular to the floor) is safer than horizontal orientation, as vertical orientation avoids directing radiation toward the patient or surgeon [31]. The optimal configuration to minimize scatter is with the X-ray tube positioned beneath the extremity and the image receiver above [31]. In the operating room, the X-ray tube should be placed below the table rather than resting on it [32]. Radiation exposure can also be reduced by limiting magnification, using collimation, and positioning the limb appropriately when obtaining orthogonal views [28]. Unlike the full-size C-arm, the mini-C-arm should be directly controlled by the surgeon to reduce unnecessary imaging caused by potential communication errors. When available, laser guidance (e.g., C-arm crosshairs) can improve targeting accuracy and further decrease the number of images required [33].

Most of the current safety data on mini-C-arm use is derived from upper extremity and hand surgery. One study evaluating mini-C-arm use in foot and ankle procedures demonstrated radiation exposure levels well below the recommended safety

Fig. 29.2 Summary of best practice guidelines

Practice
All team members wear lead aprons during fluoroscopy with any size C-arm
All team members utilize radiation dosimeters
Practice ALARA (as low as reasonably achievable) techniques to reduce radiation to lowest acceptable level
Remove physician' shands from x-ray beam as able
Surgeon and first assistant wear lead glasses
Use laser guidance when localizing images
Wear hand-shielding products when available

thresholds [34]. However, additional research is needed to better understand the safety profile of mini-C-arm use in lower extremity surgery.

(c) *To the Surgical Team*

Radiation exposure decreases exponentially with increased distance from the source. Doubling the distance results in a fourfold reduction in exposure. Given that the mini-C-arm produces less radiation per image and generates less scatter than a full-size unit, exposure to other surgical team members positioned farther from the source is greatly reduced. At 40 cm from the image source, radiation dose approaches 0 μGy [35]. In simulated surgical environments, mini-C-arm use has been associated with low radiation exposure for all operating room staff and would require over 20 h of exposure without protective lead shielding to reach a cumulative dose of 1 mSv [4].

Earlier guidelines suggested that individuals located more than 1 meter from the image source did not require protective equipment; however, these recommendations were based on first-generation machines with lower radiation output [36]. Current standards advise that all operating room personnel wear lead aprons and thyroid shields during use of both full-size and mini-C-arm devices [37].

Additional recommended best practices to improve value include mandatory radiation safety training for staff, provision of dosimeter badges, routine equipment servicing and maintenance, and regular audits of usage and radiation exposure [38].

Alleviating Strain on Hospital Resources

(a) *In the Emergency Department*

The mini-C-arm is frequently used in the emergency department (ED) to assist with pediatric fracture reductions. In this setting, the mini-C-arm enhances value by improving fracture reduction quality, reducing radiation exposure, reducing the need for repeat reductions, and shortening the duration of orthopedic consultations [39].

In addition to aiding fracture reduction, the mini-C-arm images can serve as definitive postreduction images. No significant difference in re-manipulation rates or surgical intervention rates occurred when comparing mini-C-arm to traditional flat-panel imaging [40, 41]. At one institution, implementing this approach reduced ED time by an average of 33 min per patient [40, 42]. However, adult fracture reductions in the ED derived less benefit from fluoroscopic-assisted distal radius reductions [43, 44].

(b) *In the Operating Room*

Unlike the full-size C-arm, which requires a radiographic technician, the mini-C-arm offers the advantage of being surgeon-operated. At a single center in the UK, use of the full-size C-arm accounted for 11% of operating room delays waiting for an available technician [45]. The introduction of the mini-C-arm eliminated these delays and reduced radiographic technician workload by 15% [45]. Enhancing operating room efficiency reduces costs and improves value. In fact, the time and money saved through mini-C-arm use offset the total cost of the mini-C-arm within 5 years [46]. In addition to reducing technician demand and operative delays, the mini-C-arm has substantially lower capital and maintenance costs than full-size units. Its lower complexity reduces servicing needs and operating overhead, further contributing to its value in high-volume pediatric orthopedic practices. Furthermore, the mini-C-arm has significantly lower initial and ongoing costs compared to the full-size C-arm. For example, in Australia, it was reported to cost AU$100,000 less to purchase a mini-C-arm and AU$35,000 less per year to operate compared to a full-size C-arm [47].

(c) *In the Clinic*

Like its use in the emergency department, the mini-C-arm can also be effectively utilized in the clinic setting as an alternative to traditional flat-panel imaging. Its use for postoperative radiographic evaluation has been successfully implemented for monitoring femur fractures, distal forearm fractures, and supracondylar fractures [48, 56]. This change resulted in an average reduction in patient clinic wait time by 23 min [48]. However, the authors also reported increased skin radiation exposure to patients, which may be attributed to the closer proximity of the extremity to the radiation source [48].

Improved clinic efficiency, productivity, and value have also been observed with the incorporation of the mini-C-arm into adult clinic visits. Using the mini-C-arm for postoperative adult hand radiographs reduced the length of clinic visits [49, 50] and saved an estimated $734 per appointment [49]. Additionally, the mini-C-arm has been safely used to assist with injections in adult clinics [51].

Limitations

(a) *Concern for Sterility*

One advantage of the mini-C-arm is its portability; however, in the operating room, portability can pose challenges regarding sterility. In one study, the mini-C-arm was contaminated in up to 70% of foot and ankle surgical cases [52]. In hand surgeries, the contamination rate was below 50% [53]. While contamination is also common with full-size C-arm use [54], no studies to date have directly compared contamination rates between full-size and mini-C-arm cases.

(b) *Pelvis and Spine Surgery*

The field view of a mini-C-arm is approximately three-quarters that of a full-size C-arm [1]. This reduced field of view, the limited arc of motion, and decreased soft tissue penetration may render the mini-C-arm unsuitable for certain surgical procedures. There is limited evidence supporting the mini-C-arm's use in cervical spine surgery [55]; additional research and clinical experience are necessary before recommending its use in pelvic or thoracolumbar procedures.

Outcome

Appropriate utilization of the mini-C-arm may lead to decreased radiation exposure for patients, surgeons, and the surgical team. Patient outcomes associated with mini-C-arm imaging are comparable to those achieved with traditional full-size C-arm or flat-panel imaging. Additionally, the mini-C-arm offers the potential for cost reduction by enhancing visit efficiency in both the emergency department and clinic settings, as well as by eliminating the reliance on radiographic technicians. The combination of reduced radiation exposure, preserved clinical outcomes, and lower costs supports the mini-C-arm as a high-value tool in pediatric orthopedic surgery.

Case Example

A 14-year-old boy presented to the ED after falling from his bicycle onto an outstretched arm. On examination, he was neurovascularly and sensorimotor intact, with swelling and tenderness over the dorsal wrist. Radiographs revealed a Salter-Harris II distal radius fracture (Fig. 29.3) that underwent reduction and casting. The mini-C-arm was utilized during the reduction, positioned vertically (Fig. 29.4a) to minimize radiation exposure to both the patient and physician. Following manipulation, a short arm cast was applied, and postreduction images were obtained using the mini-C-arm rather than a formal repeat flat-panel radiographs (Fig. 29.5). A total of six mini-C-arm images were obtained, including those taken during the fracture reduction. Both the patient and the physician wore lead aprons throughout the imaging process. The patient was discharged home after recovering from sedation and subsequently followed up in the pediatric orthopedic clinic in 1 week, with an uneventful recovery.

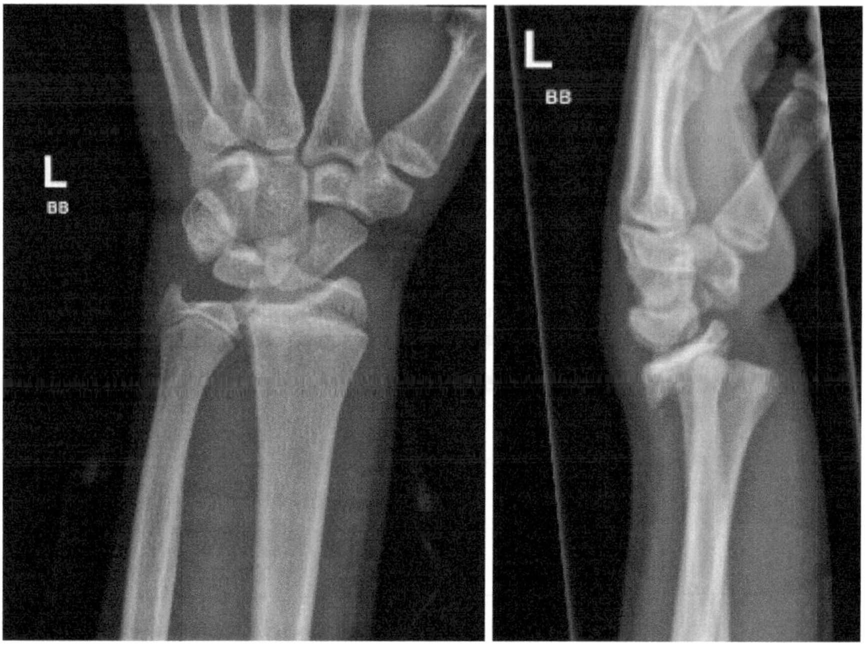

Fig. 29.3 Injury films of a displaced Salter-Harris II fracture of the distal radius

Summary

This chapter reviews the indications for mini-C-arm use and summarizes the evidence supporting its ability to reduce radiation exposure to patients, surgeons, and the surgical team. In addition, the mini-C-arm enhances value by using less hospital resources and reducing costs in the ED, in the operating room, and in the outpatient clinic.

Author Pearls

- All staff should use personal protective equipment, including lead aprons, lead eye protection, and hand protection when appropriate.
- Ensure that each image serves a specific clinical purpose and is properly positioned and optimized before acquisition.
- Whenever possible, surgeons should keep their hands away from the X-ray beam.
- Position yourself on the image receptor side (not the X-ray tube side) to reduce scatter.
- Use collimation and pulse fluoroscopy when available.
- Familiarize residents early with mini-C-arm controls to reduce the learning curve and unnecessary exposures.

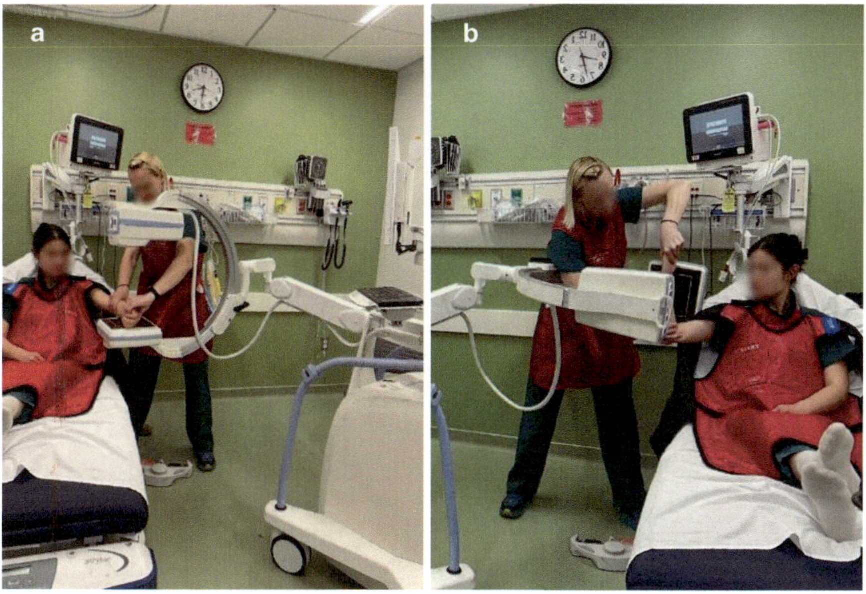

Fig. 29.4 (**a**) Vertical orientation of the mini-C-arm, which is preferred to avoid aiming the beam directly at the patient or surgeon. (**b**) Horizontal orientation of the mini-C-arm (not recommended)

Comments by Editors

WLH

This chapter provides an outstanding overview of the role of the mini-C-arm in pediatric orthopedics, highlighting its contributions to safety, efficiency, and cost savings across clinical settings. The authors have clearly demonstrated how mini-C-arm fluoroscopy aligns with the goals of value-based care—reducing radiation exposure, saving time, optimizing hospital resources, and preserving clinical outcomes. Their comprehensive review offers both evidence-based support and practical guidance for implementation. As mini-C-arm technology becomes increasingly integrated into pediatric orthopedic practice, this chapter will serve as a valuable reference for clinicians, educators, and hospital administrators alike.

RMS

The advantages of mini-C-arm use in pediatric orthopedics are numerous and well-illustrated in this chapter. To contextualize, the radiation exposure from a typical mini-C-arm-assisted upper extremity fracture reduction is equivalent to only a few hours to 2 days of natural background radiation at sea level. In addition to reducing

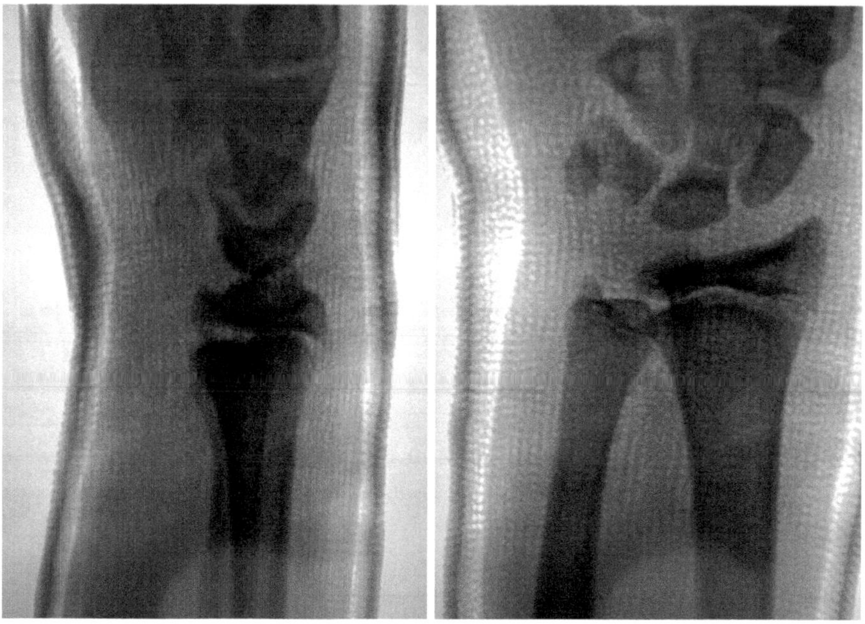

Fig. 29.5 Postreduction and casting mini-C-arm images

radiation, mini-C-arms do not require dedicated architectural shielding, yielding construction cost savings for outpatient clinics or procedure rooms. Importantly, when the operating surgeon interprets and separately documents the fluoroscopic images, such as in the clinic or ED, they may bill for the professional component using CPT code **76000**, enhancing both workflow efficiency and revenue capture. However, the mini-C-arm is not suitable for all patients—its limited penetration and field of view may be inadequate for larger patients or deeper anatomy, such as in the evaluation and treatment of slipped capital femoral epiphysis in obese adolescents.

References

1. Greffier J, Etard C, Mares O, Pereira F, Defez D, Duverger C, Branchereau P, Beregi JP, Coulomb R, Larbi A. Patient dose reference levels in surgery: a multicenter study. Eur Radiol. 2019;29:674–81.
2. Giordano BD, Baumhauer JF, Morgan TL, Ii GRR. Patient and surgeon radiation exposure: comparison of standard and mini-C-arm fluoroscopy. J Bone Joint Surg. 2009;91:297–304.
3. Athwal GS, Bueno RA, Wolfe SW. Radiation exposure in hand surgery: mini versus standard C-arm. J Hand Surg Am. 2005;30:1310–6.
4. Pearce MS, Salotti JA, Little MP, McHugh K, Lee C, Kim KP, Howe NL, Ronckers CM, Rajaraman P, Craft AW, et al. Radiation exposure from CT scans in childhood and subsequent risk of leukaemia and brain tumours: a retrospective cohort study. Lancet. 2012;380:499.
5. Smith-Bindman R, Chu PW, Firdaus HA, Stewart C, Malekhedayat M, Alber S, Bolch WE, Mahendra M, de González AB, Miglioretti DL. Projected lifetime cancer risks from cur-

rent computed tomography imaging. JAMA Intern Med. 2025. https://doi.org/10.1001/JAMAINTERNMED.2025.0505.
6. Madhvani KR, Clark MJR, Kocheta AAJ. Diagnostic reference levels for common orthopedic hand and wrist procedures using intraoperative mini-C-arm fluoroscopy. Hand. 2023;18:153–7.
7. Kropelnicki A, Eaton R, Adamczyk A, Waterman J, Mohaghegh P. Establishing local diagnostic reference levels for common orthopaedic procedures using the mini-C-arm fluoroscope. Br J Radiol. 2020;94:20190878.
8. Gangopadhyay S, Scammell BE. Optimising use of the mini-C-arm in foot and ankle surgery. Foot Ankle Surg. 2009;15:139–43.
9. Duguay T, Housset V, Bouché PA, Hardy A, Bauer T. Prospective observational analysis of intraoperative radiation exposure with a mini-C-arm intensifier in percutaneous forefoot surgery. Orthop Traumatol Surg Res. 2023;109:103705.
10. Li ZX, Wong KPL, Wong JLY, Lim KBL, Mahadev A. The utility of mini-C-arm in the fixation of unstable paediatric supracondylar humeral fractures. Injury. 2019;50:1992–6.
11. Mastrangelo G, Fedeli U, Fadda E, Giovanazzi A, Scoizzato L, Saia B. Increased cancer risk among surgeons in an orthopaedic hospital. Occup Med (Chic Ill). 2005;55:498–500.
12. Chou LB, Johnson B, Shapiro LM, Pun S, Cannada LK, Chen AF, Valone LC, Van Nortwick SS, Ladd AL, Finlay AK. Increased prevalence of breast and all-cause cancer in female orthopaedic surgeons. JAAOS: Glob Res Rev. 2022;6:e22.00031.
13. ALARA | NRC.gov. at https://www.nrc.gov/reading-rm/basic-ref/glossary/alara.html.
14. Guidelines for ALARA – as low as reasonably achievable | Radiation and your health | CDC. at https://www.cdc.gov/radiation-health/safety/alara.html.
15. Patel AA, Patel AA, Kaplan FTD. Radiation exposure safety patterns with the use of intraoperative fluoroscopy. Bull NYU Hosp Jt Dis. 2018;76:183–92.
16. van Rappard JRM, de Jong T, Hummel WA, Ritt MJPF, Mouës CM. Radiation exposure to surgeon and assistant during flat panel mini-C-arm fluoroscopy in hand and wrist surgical procedures. J Hand Surg Am. 2019;44:68.e1–5.
17. Giordano BD, Ryder S, Baumhauer JF, DiGiovanni BF. Exposure to direct and scatter radiation with use of mini-C-arm fluoroscopy. J Bone Joint Surg. 2007;89:948–52.
18. Gausden EB, Christ AB, Zeldin R, Lane JM, McCarthy MM. Tracking cumulative radiation exposure in orthopaedic surgeons and residents. J Bone Joint Surg Am. 2017;99:1324–9.
19. Shoaib A, Rethnam U, Bansal R, De A, Makwana N. A comparison of radiation exposure with the conventional versus mini-C-arm in orthopedic extremity surgery. Foot Ankle Int. 2008;29:58–61.
20. Vosbikian MM, Ilyas AM, Watson DD, Leinberry CF. Radiation exposure to hand surgeons' hands: a practical comparison of large and mini-C-arm fluoroscopy. J Hand Surg Am. 2014;39:1805–9.
21. Singer G. Radiation exposure to the hands from mini-C-arm fluoroscopy. J Hand Surg Am. 2005;30:795–7.
22. Hohendorff B, Sauer H, Biber F, Franke J, Müller LP, Ries C. Radiation exposure caused by the orthoScan mini-C-arm in hand surgery: a one-year case series. Handchir Mikrochir Plast Chir. 2019;51:177–84.
23. Edward Hoffler C, Ilyas AM. Fluoroscopic radiation exposure are we protecting ourselves adequately? J Bone Joint Surg Am. 2015;97:721–5.
24. Wang ML, Hoffler CE, Ilyas A, Beredjiklian P, Leinberry C. Fluoroscopic exposure with use of mini-C-arm during routine hand surgery: a prospective comparison of hand versus eye radiation dosage. J Surg Orthop Adv. 2018;26(2):102–5.
25. Fuller CB, Wongworawat MD, Riedel BB. Radiation exposure and hand dominance using mini-C-arm fluoroscopy in hand surgery. Hand (N Y). 2016;11:188.
26. Cantlon MB, Ilyas AM. Assessment of radiation protection in hand-shielding products with mini-C-arm fluoroscopy. Hand. 2021;16:505–10.
27. Groover MT, Hinkley JR, Gerow DE, Bamberger HB, Evans J, Gazaille RE. The effect of metal instrumentation on patient and surgical team scatter radiation exposure using mini-C-arm in a simulated forearm fracture fixation model. JAAOS: Glob Res Rev. 2019;3:e18.

28. Gendelberg D, Hennrikus W, Slough J, Armstrong D, King S. A radiation safety training program results in reduced radiation exposure for orthopaedic residents using the mini-C-arm. Clin Orthop Relat Res. 2015;474:580.
29. Gendelberg D, Hennrikus WL, Sawyer C, Armstrong D, King S. Decreased radiation exposure among orthopedic residents is maintained when using the mini-C-arm after undergoing radiation safety training. Orthopedics. 2017;40:e788–92.
30. Sumko MJ, Hennrikus W, Slough J, Jensen K, Armstrong D, King S, Urish K. Measurement of radiation exposure when using the mini-C-arm to reduce pediatric upper extremity fractures. J Pediatr Orthop. 2016;36:122–5.
31. Chapman T, Martin DP, Williamson C, Tinsley B, Wang ML, Ilyas AM. Mini-C-arm fluoroscopy: does its configuration matter for radiation exposure to the surgeon? Hand. 2018;13:552–7.
32. Martin DP, Chapman T, Williamson C, Tinsley B, Ilyas AM, Wang ML. Elevated radiation exposure associated with above surface flat detector mini-C-arm use. Hand (NY). 2017;14:565.
33. Hong T, Hones KM, Ballard B, Dell PC, Wright TW, Matthias RC. Role of laser pointer in budgeting fluoroscopy-time and radiation exposure. Hand (NY). 2022;19:316.
34. Guyonnet C, Mulliez A, Fessy MH, Besse JL. Prospective analysis of intraoperative radiation dose in foot and ankle surgery using mini-C-arm fluoroscopy. Continuous series of 1064 procedures. Orthop Traumatol Surg Res. 2021;107:102994.
35. Mesbahi A, Rouhani A. A study on the radiation dose of the orthopaedic surgeon and staff from a mini-C-arm fluoroscopy unit. Radiat Prot Dosim. 2008;132:98–101.
36. Wilson CR. Potential radiation hazard associated with the unprotective use of mini-C-arm fluoroscopy systems. Med Phys. 1997;24:1331.
37. College of Physicians and Surgeons of British Columbia: Non-Hospital Medical and Surgical Facilities Accreditation Program accreditation standards X-ray and Radiation Safety. 2024.
38. Naidu J, Botchu R, Iyengar KP. Safe usage of mini 'C'-arm in operating room environment: implications for clinical practice. J Perioper Pract. 2024. https://doi.org/10.1177/17504589241228138/ASSET/7CA094F4-8A99-4BD6-8069-BD16E1396FA2/ASSETS/IMAGES/LARGE/10.1177_17504589241228138-FIG2.JPG.
39. Lee MC, Stone NE, Ritting AW, Silverstein EA, Pierz KA, Johnson DA, Naujoks R, Smith BG, Thomson JD. Mini-C-arm fluoroscopy for emergency-department reduction of pediatric forearm fractures. J Bone Joint Surg. 2011;93:1442–7.
40. Goodman AD, Walsh DF, Zonfrillo MR, Eberson CP, Cruz AI. Fluoroscopy as definitive Postreduction imaging of pediatric wrist and forearm fractures is safe and saves time. J Pediatr Orthop. 2020;40:E14–8.
41. Sharieff GQ, Kanegaye J, Wallace DC, McCaslin IR, Harley JR. Pediatric emergency care. Pediatr Emerg Care. 1999;15:249–51.
42. Goodman AD, Zonfrillo MR, Chiou D, Eberson CP, Cruz AI. The cost and utility of postreduction radiographs after closed reduction of pediatric wrist and forearm fractures. J Pediatr Orthop. 2019;39:e8–e11.
43. Dailey SK, Miller AR, Kakazu R, Wyrick JD, Stern PJ. The effectiveness of mini–C-arm fluoroscopy for the closed reduction of distal radius fractures in adults: a randomized controlled trial. J Hand Surg Am. 2018;43:927–31.
44. Kazum E, Kadar A, Sharfman ZT, Otremsky H, Gigi R, Rosenblatt Y, Dolkart O, Pritsch T. Adult closed distal radius fracture reduction: does fluoroscopy improve alignment and reduce indications for surgery? Hand. 2017;12:557–60.
45. White SP. Effect of introduction of mini-C-arm image intensifier in orthopaedic theatre. Ann R Coll Surg Engl. 2007;89:268.
46. Dawe EJC, Fawzy E, Kaczynski J, Hassman P, Palmer SH. A comparative study of radiation dose and screening time between mini-C-arm and standard fluoroscopy in elective foot and ankle surgery. Foot Ankle Surg. 2011;17:33–6.
47. Gieroba TJ, Williams N, Antoniou G, Cundy PJ. Mini-C-arm: faster, cheaper, safer? ANZ J Surg. 2017;87:282–6.

48. Fanelli MG, Hennrikus WL, Slough Hill JM, Armstrong DG, King SH. The mini-C-arm adds quality and efficiency to the pediatric orthopedic outpatient clinic. Orthopedics. 2016;39:e1097–9.
49. Kesler K, Buckwalter JA. Efficiency benefits of live fluoroscopy in hand clinics. Iowa Orthop J. 2022;42:118.
50. Swindells MG, O'Brien CM, Armstrong DJ, Arundell MK, Quinton DN, Burke FD. The use of the mini-C-arm in the outpatient setting: evolving practice. J Plast Reconstr Aesthet Surg. 2011;64:688–9.
51. Hasham S, Burke FD, Evans SJ, Arundell MK, Quinton DN. An audit of the safe use of the mini-C-arm image intensifier in the out-patient setting. J Hand Surg Eur. 2007;32:563–8.
52. Momenzadeh K, Williams C, Czerwonka N, Kwon JY, Nazarian A, Miller CP. Contamination of the mini-C-arm during foot and ankle surgery. Foot Ankle Int. 2021;42:994–1001.
53. Hovis JP, Moore-Lotridge SN, Mansour A, Gibson BHY, Weikert DR, Desai MJ, Gebhart SS, Schoenecker JG, Lee DH, Lee H. Sterility of miniature C-arm fluoroscopy in hand and upper extremity surgery. J Hand Microsurg. https://doi.org/10.1055/s-0040-1714434.
54. Magee LC, Piazza B, Harwood K, Lawrence JTR. C-arm contamination of the surgical field: can contamination be reduced with an intervening drape? Injury. 2022;53:1994–8.
55. Giordano BD, Baumhauer JF, Morgan TL, Rechtine GR. Cervical spine imaging using mini--C-arm fluoroscopy: patient and surgeon exposure to direct and scatter radiation. J Spinal Disord Tech. 2009;22:399–403.
56. Flood MG, Bauer MR, Sullivan MP. Radiographic considerations for pediatric supracondylar humerus fractures. J Pediatr Orthop B. 2023;32:110–6.

Improving Value During Overseas Surgical Trips: Keep It Safe and Simple

30

Matthew R. Schmitz

Introduction

Orthopedic surgical mission programs reduce disability and enhance quality of life in underserved nations where access to specialized surgical care is either limited or nonexistent. Orthopedic mission surgery addresses conditions like trauma, deformities, infections, congenital abnormalities, and degenerative diseases. However, the effectiveness and sustainability of short-term orthopedic missions have increasingly come under scrutiny, prompting a reevaluation of strategies to maximize value.

The current chapter reviews strategies to enhance the value of orthopedic surgical mission programs, with a focus on ethics, education, community engagement, capacity building, sustainability, and measuring outcomes. One goal is to transition from episodic interventions to sustainable, ethical, and impactful programs that provide long-term health benefits. A successful orthopedic surgical mission program must strike a balance between maximizing healthcare impact and minimizing costs. The chapter outlines strategies to reduce costs and enhance value through careful planning, efficient resource management, and innovative approaches.

The Role of Orthopedic Surgery in Global Health

Orthopedic conditions are among the leading causes of disability worldwide. The 2017 Global Burden of Disease Study (GBD) reported that musculoskeletal disorders contribute significantly to years lived with disability (YLDs) globally [1]. In LMICs, trauma from road traffic accidents, falls, and violence results in a major

M. R. Schmitz (✉)
Rady Children's Hospital San Diego, Department of Orthopaedics, University of California San Diego, San Diego, CA, USA

W. L. Hennrikus, R. M. Schwend (eds.), *Value in Pediatric Orthopaedics*,
https://doi.org/10.1007/978-3-032-19570-8_30

portion of the orthopedic burden that is further exacerbated by a shortage of trained surgeons and limited surgical infrastructure [2].

Orthopedic surgery such as fracture fixation, limb deformity correction, and joint replacements can restore function and reduce disability. However, in many LMICs, access to orthopedic surgery is limited, resulting in prolonged suffering, deformity, and social isolation. Surgical mission trips aim to address this gap but often face challenges, including episodic care, limited resources, logistical hurdles, and ethical dilemmas. Some of these challenges can be overcome by supporting local communities, emphasizing cultural competence, bidirectional education, and capacity building [3].

Challenges in Orthopedic Surgical Mission Trips

While well-intentioned, many short-term orthopedic missions encounter challenges that jeopardize their long-term impact and ethical integrity. These challenges include the following:

1. *Limited Infrastructure*: Many missions take place in facilities lacking essential resources such as proper sterilization, anesthesia, and postoperative rehabilitation services [4]. Performing complex surgeries in these conditions increases the risk of complications. The principle of "first, do no harm" must always be prioritized.
2. *Short Duration and Lack of Follow-Up*: Episodic missions often fail to provide postoperative care, which can result in complications, poor outcomes, and sometimes the need for reoperations [5]. Follow-up is essential for patient safety and assessing outcomes.
3. *Workforce Limitations*: Volunteer surgeons are often unfamiliar with local protocols. Local capacity may be inadequate to sustain ongoing surgical services [4]. Surgical missions can deplete local resources, disrupt operations, and sometimes reduce income for local surgeons.
4. *Cultural and Language Barriers*: Miscommunication can hinder informed consent, patient understanding, and adherence to postoperative instructions.
5. *Ethical Concerns*: Performing complex surgeries without adequate infrastructure or follow-up can lead to harm, often referred to as "parachute surgery" [5]. In addition, conflicts over resource allocation and concerns about justice and equity may develop.

Value Based Themes

1. Needs Assessment and Community Engagement

Tailoring interventions to local needs ensures relevance and sustainability. This can be achieved by collaborating with local surgeons and community leaders to identify priority conditions or surgical cases that local surgeons desire assistance. Epidemiological surveys can help pinpoint the most prevalent and critical orthopedic issues. Community involvement enhances the acceptability and sustainability of global health missions [6]. A needs assessment ensures that resources are allocated to address actual burdens, rather than perceived needs. During the needs assessment, it is crucial to engage local surgeons and healthcare leaders. Targeted interventions help prevent unneeded procedures and, instead, focus on high-impact treatments. In addition, understanding local cultural perceptions of disability and treatment preferences is important because local perceptions may differ from those in the surgeon's home country. A mission team should establish specific, measurable goals that align with the community's needs. Clear objectives help prioritize cases, optimize resource allocation, and assess outcomes.

2. Capacity Building and Sustainability

While short-term surgical missions can be beneficial, they can fail to produce lasting health improvements unless paired with local education. Therefore, providing hands-on training for local surgeons, nurses, and rehabilitation staff in fracture fixation, deformity correction, and postoperative care is essential. Establishing ongoing mentorship through email, telemedicine, and periodic visits strengthens the relationship between host and visiting surgeons. The ultimate goal is for the surgical mission trip to become unnecessary, as local surgeons, nurses, rehab specialists, and orthotics/prosthetics professionals acquire the skills and resources needed to provide care independently. Training local staff fosters sustained improvements in surgical capacity [7].

Investing in surgical instruments, sterilization tools, and rehabilitation equipment is a wise strategy if the team plans to return to the same location regularly. Furthermore, providing infrastructure support helps to reduce dependency on visiting mission teams. The added infrastructure will help the local community become self-sufficient between visits and improve efficiency at the start of each mission trip, as these resources will have been in continuous use throughout the year.

3. Resource Utilization

Maximizing resources and minimizing waste are crucial for enhancing value. One effective approach is to partner with local hospitals and clinics. This collaboration saves costs by reducing the need to establish temporary clinics and integrating services into the existing healthcare system. Training local surgeons, nurses, and technicians during mission visits helps build local capacity and reduces future dependency on external mission teams.

The mission surgical team must also optimize equipment and supplies. Using portable surgical kits and reusable instruments helps reduce disposable costs and logistical burdens. Sourcing supplies through donations or bulk procurement lowers costs. The team should maintain a well-managed inventory to avoid overstocking or shortages, minimizing both waste and expenses. Tracking equipment and supply levels between trips is crucial if multiple teams are using the same resources at a single location. Securing a local storage space and monitoring supply levels and expiration dates improved efficiency. Using materials before expiration and only restocking items that are running low reduce shipping and travel costs. Clear communication between teams is necessary if multiple mission teams are visiting the same site during the year.

Another way to save cost is through efficient travel and accommodation planning. Coordinating travel and lodging can minimize expenses while fostering teamwork and a sense of community among the mission team. Sharing accommodations reduces lodging costs and potentially strengthens camaraderie. When safety permits, using local transportation instead of renting or chartering vehicles can also reduce costs. Simple measures, like using airline miles or securing baggage discounts, can also significantly cut travel expenses. Team members should commit well in advance to ensure access to reasonably priced airfares. To minimize last-minute team member cancellations, it may be potentially beneficial to require mission members to donate a predetermined amount to the mission trip when they sign up.

4. Funding and Partnership Strategies

Funding is crucial for a successful mission program, and multiple strategies can be employed to offset costs. Grants, corporate sponsorships, foundation sponsorships, and community donations can be used for patient care. Cost-sharing from volunteers for travel or lodging can be utilized. Medical device companies can assist by donating equipment and supplies. Collaborating with academic institutions or nongovernmental organizations (NGOs) can help provide in-kind donations, and shared resources, and, in some cases, travel funding. Maintaining a database of patients in need of surgery and scheduling procedures months in advance allows for the targeted request of foundations funding for specific cases. Moreover, fundraising campaigns led by mission team members using social media and often collaborating with local service organizations such as Rotary, Kiwanis, and Lions club can be effective.

5. Ethical and Cultural Competence

Respecting local customs, obtaining informed consent, and providing culturally sensitive care are essential for building trust and improving outcomes in LMICs. Volunteers should be trained in cultural competence before traveling. An informational document should be shared in advance, allowing new mission team members to review the material and ask questions about past experiences and shared knowledge from previous mission teams.

Aligning with cultural norms and local practices enhances both the acceptance and effectiveness of surgical procedures. For instance, in some LMICs, performing an amputation may place an additional burden on the patient and family due to the lack of access to ongoing prosthetic care. Additionally, cultural considerations in certain regions may make amputation unacceptable. Understanding these factors helps in selecting a treatment plan that improves patient outcomes.

To ease patient and family concerns, utilize interpreters and culturally adapted educational materials. Align informed consent with local norms and language. Culturally sensitive care reduces patient anxiety and improves compliance [8]. Adhering to ethical principles and practices is crucial to prevent harm and uphold global health standards.

Perform evidence-based procedures. Avoid unneeded surgery. Use proven, safe, and resource-appropriate techniques to maximize benefits, minimizing risks and costs. The World Health Organization (WHO) has published guidelines that advocate for contextually appropriate surgical techniques to optimize outcomes in resource-limited settings [9]. These guidelines are particularly relevant in trauma and deformity management, where treatment is often adapted to available resources. WHO's recommendations favor external fixation for fracture stabilization or limb lengthening when internal fixation is unavailable and advise against high-cost, complex procedures when postoperative follow-up and rehabilitation are not available. Performing complex surgeries without adequate infrastructure or follow-up violates ethical principles, risks harm, and can foster dependency.

6. Continuity of Care and Follow-Up

In addition to the surgical procedure, postoperative care, rehabilitation, and follow-up are crucial for success and optimal outcomes. Kruk et al. demonstrated that programs focusing on continuity of care improve functional outcomes and reduce the need for reoperations [10]. Continuity of care also helps build long-term relationships with local surgeons, fostering trust and collaboration and a shared commitment to good outcomes. Pre-trip discussions about cases that local surgeons desire assistance help in surgical planning. It is also important to coordinate with local surgeons about the postoperative visits. Providing detailed postoperative plans to the local surgeons, patient, and family ensures smoother recovery and continuity of care. Telemedicine consultations can facilitate remote monitoring and collaboration with local physicians for postoperative follow-up and for preoperative planning ahead of the next mission trip. In addition, telehealth or email can be used for patient education, follow-up reminders, and data collection, all of which have been shown to improve compliance with postoperative instructions [11].

7. Partnerships and Collaboration

Collaborating with local health leaders, NGOs, medical schools, and private practices helps to align the mission program with national health priorities. These partnerships build long-term relationships and foster continued improvement. Sharing data and outcomes can help better understand the scope of health challenges faced by the community. Hoffman et al. found that collaborative programs promote sustainability and local ownership, resulting in improved health outcomes [12]. By working alongside local surgeons and integrating with the local medical system, these collaborations potentially improve the care of future patients.

8. Monitoring, Evaluation, and Data-Driven Improvement

Data collection enables impact assessment, identification of gaps, and measurable continuous improvement. Prospective data can help refine processes, eliminate inefficiencies, and enhance future operations. The mission team should establish standardized metrics including complication rates, functional scores, and patient-reported outcomes. Baseline clinical data should be gathered prior to surgery, and results should be shared with mission team members to foster transparency and learning and improve program efficacy [13]. Patient outcomes, complication rates, and patient/parent satisfaction should be tracked to evaluate the effectiveness of interventions.

9. Empowerment Through Education

Improving the quality of care provided by local surgeons should be one primary outcome of a surgical mission. Workshops and training sessions for local surgeons should focus on low-cost, high-impact techniques including screening and prevention. Fundamental concepts for treating common conditions such as infections, trauma, developmental hip dysplasia, and clubfoot should be emphasized. Providing educational materials and resources for continuous learning can potentially help reduce the need for surgical interventions over time. For example, developing a screening and bracing program for developmental hip dysplasia or an early casting program for clubfoot can prevent complex deformities that might require surgery and reduce costs. In addition, giving lectures to local medical students and residents can improve knowledge and stimulate interest in identifying and managing musculoskeletal pathologies early on, leading to improved detection, treatment, and outcomes.

Hands-on surgical training of local surgeons during surgical mission trips provides invaluable learning opportunities for host surgeons. The primary focus of an orthopedic surgical mission trip is to train local surgeons. The purpose of surgical mission trips is not to train inexperienced surgeons from the USA on complex procedures they haven't mastered at home. A senior lead US surgeon should prioritize mentorship and skill development for the local doctors. Mentorship can be further strengthened by offering scholarship programs that bring local surgeons from LMICs to the USA for training. Although training in the USA for LMIC surgeons may involve initial upfront costs, the improved surgical skills that they gain may eventually make mission trips to that LMIC site unnecessary, thereby saving costs and enhancing value.

Case Example

During an orthopedic surgical mission trip to Ecuador, a 12-month-old girl is brought in by her family with a left hip dislocation (DDH). The parents express concern that without surgery from the visiting US physicians, their daughter may face a life of disability (Fig. 30.1). The surgical team determines that surgery is necessary. However, due to time constraints in the operating room and more urgent cases requiring attention during that week, they decide to delay the procedure until a future trip.

Developmental hip dysplasia (DDH) can often be successfully treated with open reduction and pelvic/femoral osteotomies at this age or older. The surgical team, with a Spanish interpreter, explains the plan. The mission team keeps detailed notes and contact information for the family and schedules a follow-up appointment with a visiting mission team in 6 months. Her case is prioritized on the surgical list. In the meantime, the mission team reaches out to a nonprofit organization to secure a grant, which will help offset the costs associated with the procedure during the next surgical trip.

Six months later, surgery is performed, including an open reduction of the hip, femoral shortening and derotational osteotomy, capsulorrhaphy, and acetabuloplasty. The surgery is done in collaboration with local surgeons (Fig. 30.2). Postoperatively, she is placed in a hip spica cast with instructions for the local surgeons to remove the cast in 6 weeks and obtain follow-up X-rays. Approximately 3 months after surgery, a video conference is held between the visiting US and local Ecuadorian surgeons to discuss the patient's progress and additional plans. The patient returns for a follow-up with the visiting mission surgical team the following year, and X-rays show good hip reduction. At that time, she is scheduled for removal of the femoral plate (Fig. 30.3).

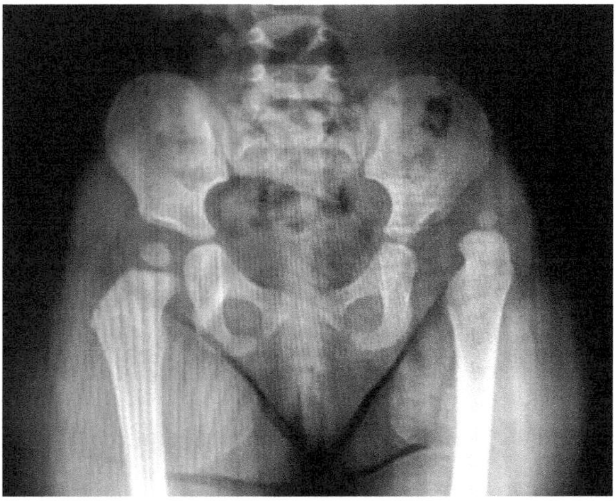

Fig. 30.1 Preoperative AP pelvic radiograph showing a dislocated left hip in a 12-month-old girl with DDH

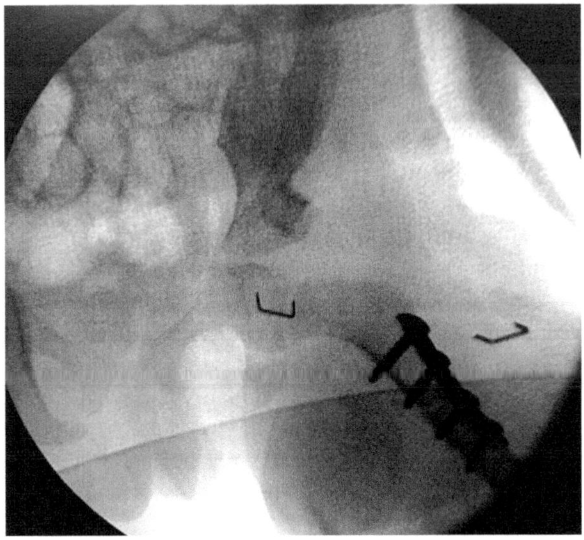

Fig. 30.2 Intraoperative fluoroscopy showing reduction of the left hip, femoral shortening osteotomy, and correction of the acetabular dysplasia

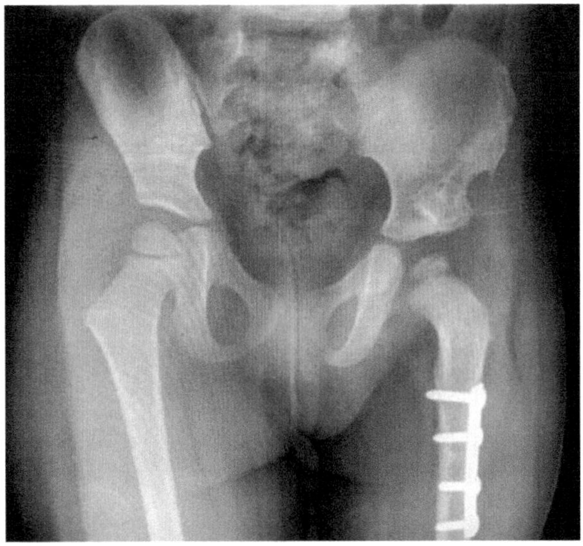

Fig. 30.3 Follow-up imaging 1 year post-op showing good overall correction, reduced left hip, and acetabular remodeling

Summary

Maximizing outcomes while minimizing costs in orthopedic surgical mission trips requires strategic planning, local collaboration, resource optimization, and innovation. By training local staff, utilizing existing infrastructure, using cost-effective techniques, and incorporating telemedicine, mission trips can provide high-impact orthopedic care that benefits LMIC communities in the long term. Value is enhanced by creating a model where orthopedic care is accessible, affordable, efficient, and sustainable and outcomes are excellent.

Recommendations and Author Pearls for Increasing Value

1. Conduct a needs assessments in collaboration with the local doctors to ensure interventions address local healthcare burdens.
2. Train local surgeons, nurses, and rehabilitation staff.
3. Align surgery with available resources and local cultural norms, prioritizing simple, effective, and sustainable procedures.
4. Establish systems for follow-up and continuity of care, utilizing local doctors and telemedicine.
5. Develop partnerships with local doctors, NGOs, and healthcare teams.
6. Support local infrastructure improvements including sterile processing, orthotics and prosthetics, blood banking, infection control, and other programs that enhance local capacity and safety.
7. Educate local surgeons, residents, and medical students to empower them to manage the pathologies encountered, with the goal of making surgical mission trips unnecessary in the future.

Useful Websites

1. https://global-help.org/—free medical/healthcare information with a primary focus on children's musculoskeletalhealth
2. https://www.miraclefeet.org/—NGO focused on the treatment of clubfoot
3. https://hipdysplasia.org/—NGO for the diagnosis, treatment, and prevention of hip dysplasia
4. https://hopewalks.org/ NGO focused on the treatment of clubfoot

Editor Comments

WLH

Short-term orthopedic surgical mission trips offer an opportunity to positively impact the lives of those in need. However, these trips come with risks and costs for the volunteers. Once you have chosen your LMIC destination, register with *Smart Traveler*, a free service that allows US citizens traveling abroad to enroll with the nearest US embassy. At least 8 weeks before departure, check the CDC's travel health page to determine which immunizations you may need. Ensure your US passport is up to date (with an expiration date at least 6 months after your planned return), and apply for any required visas. It's also wise to bring at least one extra color copy of your passport's photo page. Consider obtaining travel insurance, international health insurance, and medical evacuation coverage. Pack your personal medications, along with antibiotics for diarrhea, Tylenol, Motrin, Benadryl, electrolyte replacement tablets, and water purification tablets. Bring quick-dry clothing and a small amount of cash, and make sure your cell phone and credit card are updated for international use. Above all, have fun, travel, and learn from other cultures, as you help children with orthopedic deformities and conditions.

RMS

Parents around the world love their children. When a child faces a condition that limits his or her function or leads to social isolation, parents may feel an urgent need for immediate surgery, hoping it will offer a better future. However, not all surgeries are beneficial and some procedures may result in unforeseen harm. Culturally sensitive shared decision-making and informed consent are very important. In some cases, rather than performing elective surgery during a child's first visit, scheduling the surgery for the next surgical mission gives families time to reflect, consult with grandparents, and speak to others who have undergone similar procedures. To prevent staff moral distress, if any team member feels a surgery cannot be safely performed, pause and do not perform that procedure during that trip. When parents are engaged in shared decision making, it is not uncommon for some parents to choose to postpone surgery. Senior orthopedic surgeons can mentor and guide younger surgeons on mission trips.

References

1. Demyttenaere K, et al. The global burden of musculoskeletal disorders and the role of orthopaedic surgery. Lancet Glob Health. 2018;6(11):e1224–5. https://doi.org/10.1016/S2214-109X(18)30354-9.
2. Mock C, et al. The global burden of injuries: challenges and opportunities. Lancet. 2004;363(9421):2133–40. https://doi.org/10.1016/S0140-6736(04)16569-3.
3. Fornari E, et al. Development of a global pediatric orthopeadic outreach program in Ecuador through project perfect world: past, present, and future directions. Orthop Clin N Am. 2020;51:219–25.
4. Khan MJ, et al. Challenges and opportunities in global orthopaedic surgery. J Orthop Surg Res. 2019;14:297.
5. Ntakiyica R, et al. Postoperative follow-up in global orthopaedic surgery: challenges and solutions. World J Orthop. 2019;10(6):210–9.
6. Crowe S, et al. Developing a framework for community engagement in health research. BMC Med Ethics. 2013;14:4.
7. Kagan JM, et al. Building local capacity in resource-limited settings: a review. Glob Health Sci Pract. 2018;6(2):245–55.
8. Boulware LE, et al. Ethical dilemmas in international health volunteer work. Glob Health Sci Pract. 2014;2(2):251–9.
9. WHO. Musculoskeletal conditions. 2019. Retrieved from https://www.who.int/news-room/fact-sheets/detail/musculoskeletal-conditions.
10. Hoffman S, et al. Collaborations for health: the role of partnerships in global health initiatives. Int J Health Policy Manag. 2017;6(9):511–4.
11. Tomlinson M, et al. mHealth for maternal health in developing countries: context matters. JMIR Mhealth Uhealth. 2013;1(1):e7.
12. Kruk ME, et al. The future of health systems strengthening: a focus on sustainability and resilience. Lancet. 2018;392(10146):1150–61.
13. Garg A, et al. Standardized metrics for evaluating global health programs. Glob Health. 2016;12:31.

Methods to Improve Value in Using Cost-Effective K-Wires Over Expensive Implants in Pediatric Orthopedic Surgery

31

K. Aaron Shaw and Brian A. Shaw

Introduction

The annual cost of inpatient medical and surgical services has increased by over 2.5% per year [1]. This cost trend is especially pronounced in pediatric healthcare, in which the median unadjusted cost of care at US pediatric hospitals is nearly double that of non-pediatric hospitals [2]. Facility costs account for up to 92% of total 90-day expenses for inpatient orthopedic procedures, such as posterior spinal fusion (PSF) for adolescent idiopathic scoliosis (AIS) [3]. In response, there is a growing trend toward shifting orthopedic procedures to outpatient surgical centers, where comparable outcomes can be achieved at approximately half the total cost [4–6].

Beyond facility costs, implant costs represent a large portion of surgical expenses. For example, implant costs account for up to 48% of total surgical costs in various orthopedic procedures [7–11]. While using fewer implants often produces comparable outcomes [12], the use of more implants results in higher hospital charges [13]. One study estimates that reducing the number of orthopedic implants could result in potential annual cost savings of $11–20 million [14].

The use of K-wires offers one practical opportunity for cost reduction in the treatment of pediatric orthopedic surgical patients. At about $24 per wire, the cost of a single K-wire is a fraction of the cost of other implants. In addition, in many surgical cases, K-wires provide comparable fixation strength to more expensive options [15, 16]. Lastly, for many orthopedic trauma cases, K-wires can be removed

K. A. Shaw (✉)
University of Missouri Kansas City Medical School, Children's Mercy Hospital, Kansas City, MO, USA

B. A. Shaw
University of Colorado Medical School, Children's Hospital of Colorado-Colorado Springs, Colorado Springs, CO, USA

W. L. Hennrikus, R. M. Schwend (eds.), *Value in Pediatric Orthopaedics*, https://doi.org/10.1007/978-3-032-19570-8_31

in the clinic, eliminating the need for secondary anesthetic and surgery and further reducing costs and enhancing value [17].

Value-Based Themes

K-Wire Fixation Technical Considerations

K-wires come in a variety of sizes determined by the pin diameter. K-wires also differ from Steinmann pins by the implant diameter. For example, K-wires are defined as having a diameter of 0.062 in (1.5 mm) or smaller, while Steinmann pins have a diameter greater than 0.062 in (1.5 mm), ranging up to 0.25 in (6.5 mm) [18]. The strength of torsional fixation is directly related to the fourth power of the radius. As such, larger-diameter K-wires provide greater strength and stiffness [19]. Additionally, both wires and pins come in smooth and threaded options. Threaded pin/wires demonstrate enhanced fixation pullout strength compared to the same-sized smooth pin/wire [20]. However, threaded pin/wires are more difficult, if not impossible, to remove in a clinic. As a result, threaded pin/wires are often used as buried implants in cases where longer fixation time is required. The threaded pin/wire can be surgically removed later, such as in the case of a Salter innominate osteotomy.

K-Wire Fixation of Forearm Fractures

Internal fixation is common practice in the treatment of displaced pediatric forearm fractures that cannot be successfully aligned and stabilized with reduction and casting. In such cases, fixation can be achieved with both open reduction and internal plate fixation (ORIF) or intramedullary (IM) wire or nail fixation. A 2024 systematic review and meta-analysis reported that ORIF and IM fixation both achieve similar functional outcomes in the treatment of skeletally immature patients [21].

Elastic stable intramedullary nailing (ESIN) is a common procedure used for the treatment of pediatric diaphyseal forearm fractures. IM fixation with ESIN provides comparable outcomes to K-wire IM fixation [15, 22]. Heare et al. compared 100 pediatric patients treated with either titanium ESIN, stainless steel ESIN, or K-wire IM fixation [15]. The time to union and complication rates were similar between the three fixation methods. However, the implant cost for the K-wires was 26 times less than the titanium ESINs and 7 times less than the stainless steel ESINs. K-wires added value.

K-wire IM fixation enables surgeons to perform a standard ESIN mini open approach and bury the K-wire for later surgical removal. Alternatively, in select cases, K-wire IM fixation allows for a percutaneous technique, where the K-wire is bent and cut outside the skin to permit later in-clinic removal (Fig. 31.1).

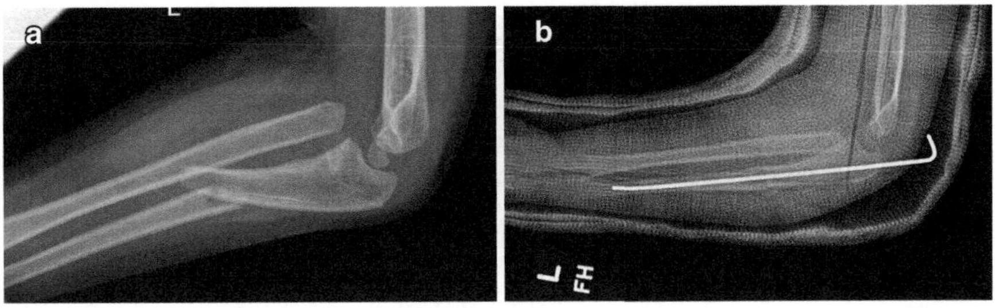

Fig. 31.1 Lateral radiographs of a 5-year-old boy with a left Monteggia variant fracture, including an ulnar shaft fracture and a radial neck fracture (**a**). He underwent closed reduction and K-wire intramedullary fixation of the ulna (**b**). Four weeks later, the K-wire was removed in the clinic, and the limb healed uneventfully

K-Wires for Medial Epicondyle Fractures

The treatment of pediatric medial epicondyle fractures remains controversial, with acceptable displacement reported to range from 5 to 15 mm [23, 24]. Absolute indications for surgery include incarcerated fragment(s) in the setting of an elbow dislocation and an open fracture. A common challenge in these injuries is the small medial epicondyle fragment size and the risk of comminution with screw fixation. K-wire fixation offers a way to mitigate this risk and is also well suited for open fractures, as it minimizes infection risk associated with larger permanent implants (Fig. 31.2).

Rickert et al. reported a clinical and biomechanical analysis of medial epicondyle fractures managed with either cannulated screw fixation, suture anchor, or buried K-wire fixation [16] (Fig. 31.3). The biomechanical analysis demonstrated that all three constructs withstood forces exceeding those observed in the intact medial epicondyle. All fractures showed radiographic healing. Due to the buried position of the K-wires, the rate of metal removal was comparable between the screw and K-wire groups. Not burying the K-wires would allow removal later in clinic and add value.

K-Wires for Lateral Condyle Fractures

Pediatric lateral condyle fractures are a common fracture, with an estimated incidence of 14 per 100,000. Traditional management consists of obtaining an anatomic reduction by closed or open methods followed by fixation with divergent K-wires. Recently, screw fixation has been advocated for these injuries. Biomechanically, bi-cortical fixation with a 4.0 mm lag screw is superior to two divergent 0.062-inch K-wires [25]. Therefore, some surgeons will use three divergent K-wires [26].

Cummings et al. reported a multicenter analysis of 762 lateral condyle fractures, with 72% managed using K-wire fixation [27]. At a minimum of 1-year follow-up, K-wire and screw fixation resulted in similar union rates and no difference in

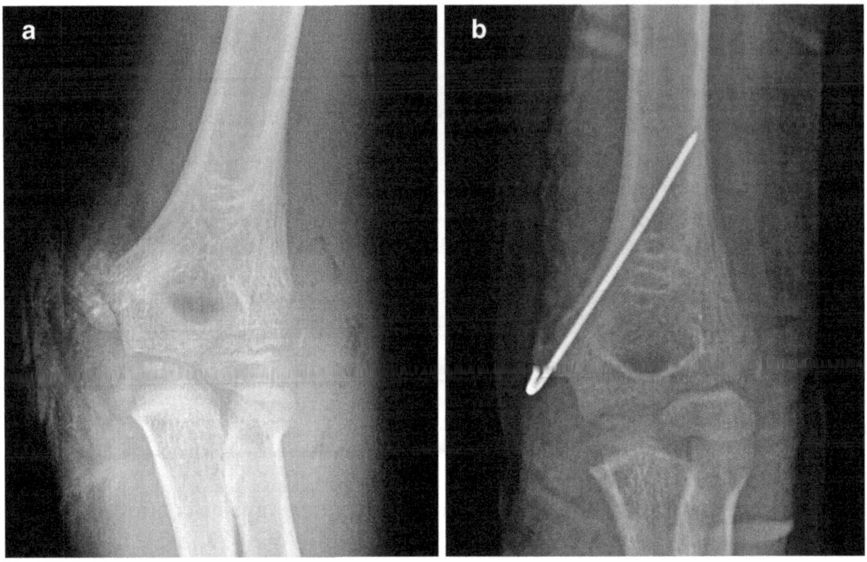

Fig. 31.2 An 8-year-old female with an open left medial epicondyle fracture (**a**) sustained in an all-terrain vehicle rollover accident. The displaced fracture was associated with an elbow dislocation. She underwent operative debridement and fixation of the medial epicondyle using a buried K-wire (**b**)

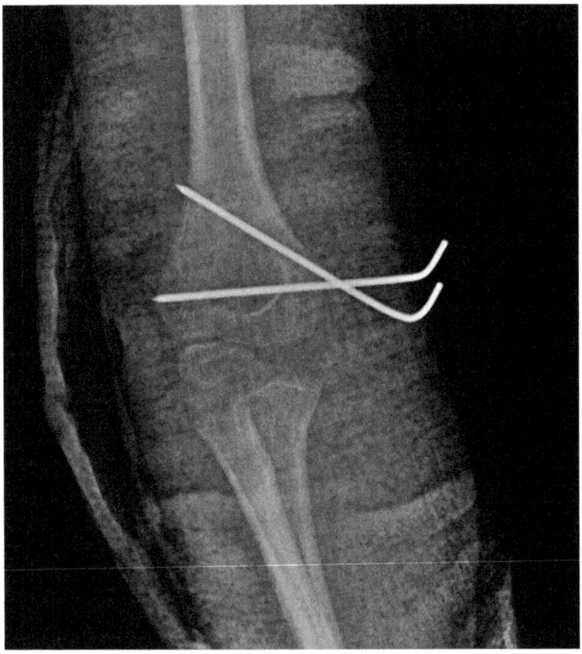

Fig. 31.3 AP radiograph demonstrating unburied K-wire fixation for a displaced medial epicondyle fracture

nonunion rates. The K-wire cohort had a higher rate of residual stiffness and subsequent physical therapy utilization (21% vs. 14%). Stiffness can also be associated with a medial epicondyle fracture and a concomitant elbow dislocation [28]. In addition, an increased risk of superficial infection has been reported with percutaneous K-wire fixation of medical epicondyle fractures but has not resulted in a negative impact on outcomes [27–30].

K-Wires for Distal Radius Fractures

Distal radius fractures are common in pediatric and adolescent patients. While the vast majority can be successful with closed reduction and casting, some cases require operative intervention. In skeletally mature or near-mature adolescents, there is often a dilemma regarding the appropriate rigidity of fixation. Although K-wire fixation is commonly used in younger patients, a more rigid plate-and-screw construct is often employed in patients with closed growth plates.

A review literature focused on patients at or near skeletal maturity can provide insight to guide treatment decisions. Chaudhry et al. performed a meta-analysis comparing clinical outcomes in skeletally mature patients treated with either volar locking plate or K-wire fixation [31]. Early functional outcomes, assessed using both patient-reported outcome measures and range of motion, were slightly better with volar locking plates. However, results were comparable between the two groups at 1-year follow-up. Nandyala et al. reviewed clinical and financial outcomes in 40 skeletally mature patients randomized to volar locking plate versus K-wire fixation [32]. Nandyala noted significantly higher direct treatment costs associated with volar plating, with cost ratios of 2.03:1 at 90 days and 1.6:1 at 1 year. Due to the excellent stability and lower cost of K-wires, most authors recommend primary fixation with K-wires (Fig. 31.4), reserving more rigid fixation methods for cases in which satisfactory stability cannot be achieved with K-wire fixation alone.

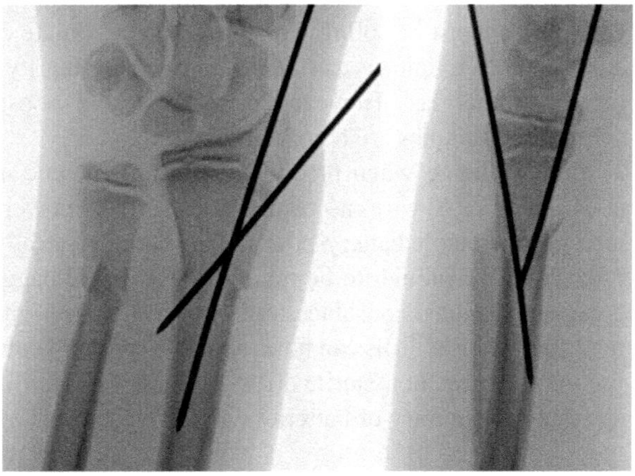

Fig. 31.4 A 12-year-old boy sustained an unstable distal radius and ulna fracture treated with closed reduction, unburied K-wire fixation, and casting. The K-wires were removed in clinic 4 weeks after placement

K-Wires and Steinmann Pins for Pelvic Osteotomy

Pelvic osteotomies are an important technique in the treatment of hip dysplasia. K-wires are commonly used to fix innominate osteotomies [33, 34]. Periacetabular osteotomies (PAOs) have emerged as a powerful technique for the treatment of residual or late-diagnosed acetabular dysplasia in adolescents and young adults. These osteotomies can be fixed with screws or Steinmann pins [35]. Leopold et al. reviewed 191 consecutive patients who underwent periacetabular osteotomy (PAO) for acetabular dysplasia, comparing fixation with unthreaded 2.5 mm Steinmann pins ($n = 99$) versus 4.5 mm screws ($n = 92$) [36]. Leopold reported that Steinmann pins provided stable fixation, with no differences in implant migration or loss of correction compared to screws. However, patients in the Steinmann pin group reported greater soft tissue irritation at 3 months postoperatively. In a subsequent study, the same authors evaluated 120 patients (Steinmann pin: 63; screws: 57) at a mean follow-up of 63 months [37]. This study reported similar patient satisfaction scores between groups, supporting unthreaded 2.5 mm Steinmann pins as a fixation option in these cases.

K-Wires for Surgery in Developing Nations

Many North American surgeons seek opportunities to serve under-resourced communities or patients in developing nations. These settings present unique challenges that must be carefully considered before proceeding with surgical treatment. In pediatric patients, the enhanced healing and remodeling potential can support the use of more limited and less expensive fixation methods, such as K-wires. In addition, due to the limited resources in many of these settings, it is important to use implants that can be easily removed without specialized equipment, such as K-wires.

K-wire fixation is a widely used and versatile technique with broad applications. K-wires can be employed for fracture stabilization (Fig. 31.5), as a substitute for staple fixation (Fig. 31.6), or for fixation following corrective osteotomy (Fig. 31.7). In cases involving limited K-wire fixation, augmenting the construct stability with a well-molded cast or splint is recommended. Climate conditions should be considered, as high humidity can compromise the integrity of plaster casts and splints more than fiberglass. However, in settings where cast saws are not available, plaster splinting techniques are recommended.

One challenge when practicing in a low-income nation is limited access to a power drill for K-wire insertion. When surgical power drills are unavailable, commercially available battery-powered drills can serve as effective alternatives and are often portable enough to be transported in travel baggage. Several medical device companies offer disposable sterile covers for use with non-sterile drills; alternatively, non-sterile drills can be wrapped in sterile towels or sterile drapes for clinical use. Importantly, non-sterile drills should not be sterilized, as the process can damage internal circuitry or batteries.

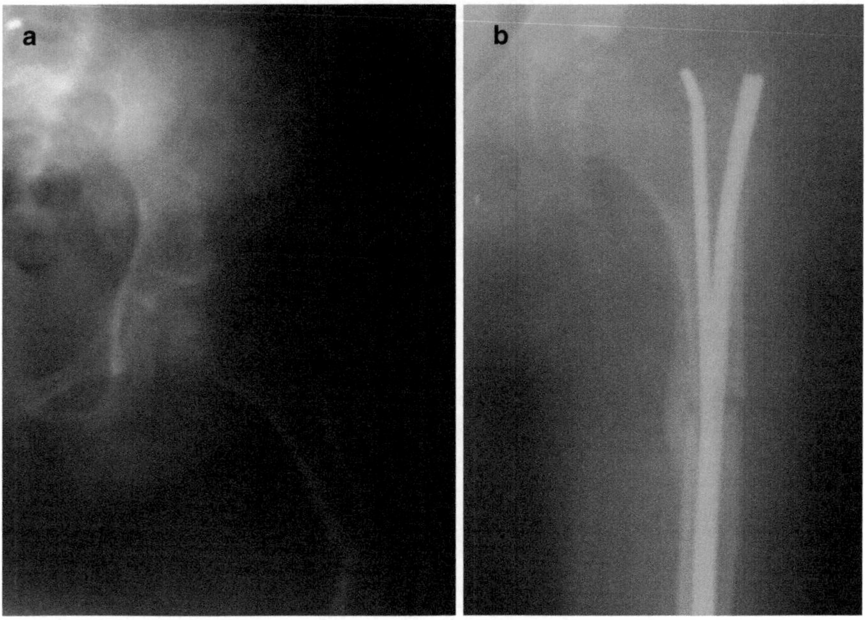

Fig. 31.5 AP radiographs of a young girl who sustained a proximal femoral shaft fracture at the site of a previous femoral shortening osteotomy. The osteotomy had been fixed with a four-hole plate and screws for hip dysplasia and later removed (**a**). She was treated with intramedullary Steinmann pin fixation to stabilize the fracture (**b**)

Summary

K-wires are versatile and stable implants used in the treatment of a wide range of orthopedic conditions. When appropriately indicated, the use of K-wires can enhance the value of pediatric orthopedic surgical care by reducing costs while achieving comparable clinical outcomes. This chapter highlights the utility of K-wire fixation through a series of illustrative cases.

Author Pearls

- For IM fixation of forearm fractures, consider trimming the tip of the K-wire to reduce the risk of iatrogenic cortical penetration during insertion.
- To enhance safety, avoid using double-ended K-wires, which pose a risk of accidental injury to the surgical team during placement.
- When performing retrograde intramedullary nailing for displaced both-bone forearm fractures, a radial entry point is preferred to minimize the risk of extensor pollicis longus injury associated with a dorsal approach.
- Consider augmenting limited K-wire fixation with a well-molded cast or splint to help maintain alignment and correction.

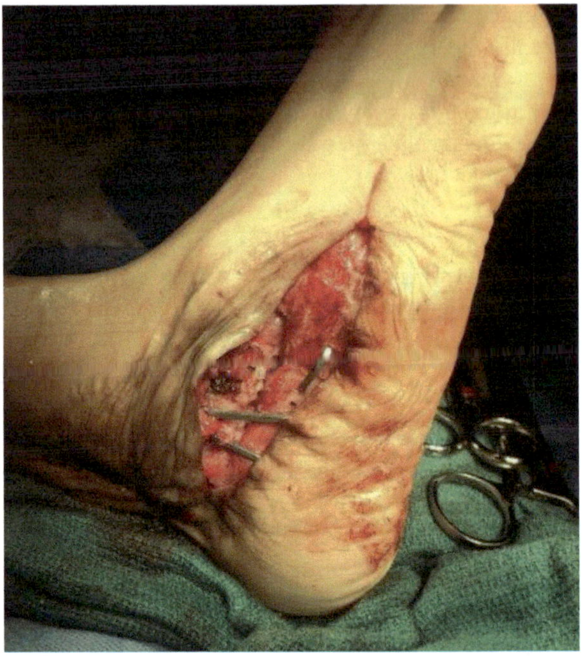

Fig. 31.6 Clinical image of a clubfoot showing K-wires that has been bent and used as staples for fixation during a triple arthrodesis

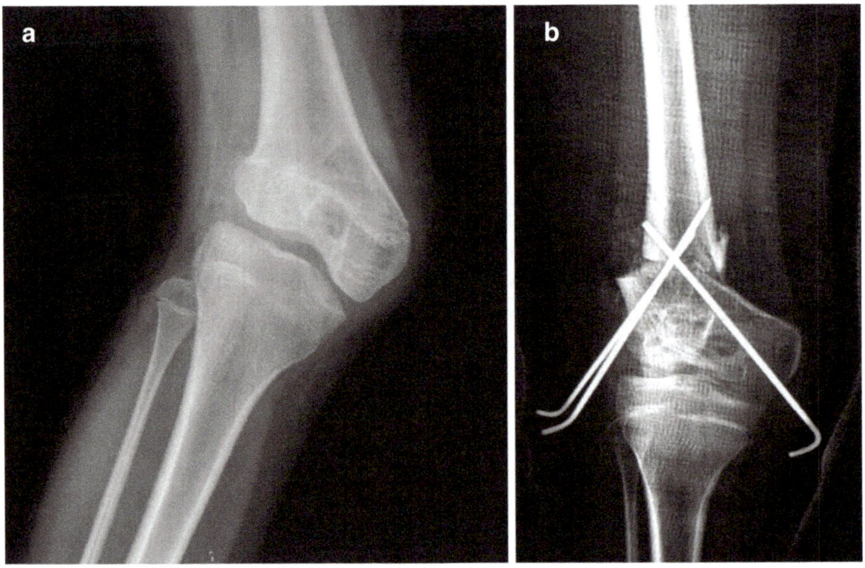

Fig. 31.7 AP radiograph of a 14-year-old girl with genu valgum secondary to a lateral distal femoral growth arrest following a bus-related injury in early childhood (**a**). She was treated with a corrective osteotomy stabilized with K-wire fixation and cast immobilization (**b**)

- In pediatric patients, it is generally safe to remove K-wire implants after 4 weeks, followed by continued immobilization with a cast or splint.
- In resource-limited settings, commercially available, non-sterile, battery-powered drills can serve as an alternative for K-wire placement.
- Several medical device companies offer disposable sterile drill covers, or the drill can be wrapped in sterile towels or drapes for clinical use.
- Do not sterilize non-sterile drills, as the process may damage internal circuitry or batteries, rendering the drill unusable.

Editor Comments

WLH

We congratulate Drs. Shaw and Shaw for an entertaining and practical chapter that could be entitled, “K-wires gone wild with value!” K-wires are undoubtedly the most widely used implant in pediatric orthopedic surgery. They are inexpensive and readily available even in low-income nations. K-wires are remarkably versatile and can be used to treat a wide variety of fracture types across multiple anatomic locations. Their placement typically results in minimal soft tissue disruption, reduced blood loss, and a lower risk of infection. Once healing is complete, K-wires can often be removed in the clinic without the need for general anesthesia or specialized equipment.

RMS

Larger-diameter K-wires tend to provide better stability, especially in active children who may place greater stress on the fracture site despite immobilization. Most metaphyseal and physeal injuries heal rapidly, allowing for wire removal as early as 4 weeks. In contrast, diaphyseal fractures require a longer healing period, necessitating longer retention of intramedullary K-wires. A practical tip for pin site care: the sterile scratch pad included with Bovie electrocautery units works well to protect the skin from pin irritation. Placing the adhesive side against the skin and allowing the pins to pass through the foam with the rough side facing the bent pin can help prevent pin migration into the skin. For safety, avoid using K-wires with sharp tips on both ends, as they pose a risk of impalement to scrub staff or the surgeon. Safety should always come first.

References

1. Russell H, Hall M, Morse RB, et al. Longitudinal trends in costs for hospitalizations at children’s hospitals. Hosp Pediatr. 2020;10(9):797–801. (In eng). https://doi.org/10.1542/hpeds.2020-0009.

2. Merenstein D, Egleston B, Diener-West M. Lengths of stay and costs associated with children's hospitals. Pediatrics. 2005;115(4):839–44. (In eng). https://doi.org/10.1542/peds.2004-1622.
3. Malik AT, Yu E, Kim J, Khan SN. Understanding costs in a 90-day episode of care following posterior spinal fusions for adolescent idiopathic scoliosis. World Neurosurg. 2019;130:e535–41. (In eng). https://doi.org/10.1016/j.wneu.2019.06.149.
4. Modest JM, Brodeur PG, Lemme NJ, Testa EJ, Gil JA, Cruz AI Jr. Outpatient operative Management of Pediatric Supracondylar Humerus Fractures: an analysis of frequency, complications, and cost from 2009 to 2018. J Pediatr Orthop. 2022;42(1):4–9. (In eng). https://doi.org/10.1097/bpo.0000000000001999.
5. Makarewich CA, Stotts AK, Yoo M, Nelson RE, Rothberg DL. Inpatient versus outpatient treatment of Gartland type II supracondylar Humerus fractures: a cost and safety comparison. J Pediatr Orthop. 2020;40(5):211–7. (In eng). https://doi.org/10.1097/bpo.0000000000001442.
6. Beagles CB, Watkins IT, Lechtig A, Blazar P, Chen NC, Lans J. Trends in inpatient versus outpatient upper extremity fracture surgery from 2008 to 2021 and their implications for equitable access: a retrospective cohort study. Eur J Orthop Surg Traumatol. 2024;34(8):4049–56. (In eng). https://doi.org/10.1007/s00590-024-04106-2.
7. Zeidan M, Stephens AR, Zhang C, Presson AP, Tyser AR, Kazmers NH. Evaluation of factors driving cost variation for distal humerus open reduction internal fixation. JSES Int. 2021;5(1):18–23. (In eng). https://doi.org/10.1016/j.jseint.2020.09.009.
8. Feller R, Illing D, Allen C, Presson A, Tyser A, Kazmers N. Evaluation of factors influencing surgical treatment costs for distal biceps rupture. J Shoulder Elb Surg. 2020;29(6):e229–37. (In eng). https://doi.org/10.1016/j.jse.2020.01.082.
9. Okelana AB, McMillan LJ, Kibble K, et al. Variation in implant selection for ankle fractures: identifying cost drivers. J Orthop Trauma. 2019;33(Suppl 7):S26–s31. (In eng). https://doi.org/10.1097/bot.0000000000001623.
10. Kazmers NH, Judson CH, Presson AP, Xu Y, Tyser AR. Evaluation of factors driving cost variation for distal radius fracture open reduction internal fixation. J Hand Surg Am. 2018;43(7):606–614.e1. (In eng). https://doi.org/10.1016/j.jhsa.2018.04.015.
11. Kamerlink JR, Quirno M, Auerbach JD, et al. Hospital cost analysis of adolescent idiopathic scoliosis correction surgery in 125 consecutive cases. J Bone Joint Surg Am. 2010;92(5):1097–104. (In eng). https://doi.org/10.2106/jbjs.I.00879.
12. Larson AN, Polly DW Jr, Diamond B, et al. Does higher anchor density result in increased curve correction and improved clinical outcomes in adolescent idiopathic scoliosis? Spine (Phila Pa 1976). 2014;39(7):571–8. (In eng). https://doi.org/10.1097/brs.0000000000000204.
13. Baky FJ, Echternacht SR, Milbrandt TA, et al. Predictors of cost for posterior spinal fusion in adolescent idiopathic scoliosis. Spine Deform. 2020;8(3):421–6. (In eng). https://doi.org/10.1007/s43390-020-00053-0.
14. Larson AN, Polly DW Jr, Ackerman SJ, et al. What would be the annual cost savings if fewer screws were used in adolescent idiopathic scoliosis treatment in the US? J Neurosurg Spine. 2016;24(1):116–23. (In eng). https://doi.org/10.3171/2015.4.Spine131119.
15. Heare A, Goral D, Belton M, Beebe C, Trizno A, Stoneback J. Intramedullary implant choice and cost in the treatment of pediatric Diaphyseal forearm fractures. J Orthop Trauma. 2017;31(10):e334–8. (In eng). https://doi.org/10.1097/bot.0000000000000925.
16. Rickert KD, Sarrel KL, Sanders JS, et al. Medial epicondyle fractures: biomechanical evaluation and clinical comparison of 3 fixation methods used in pediatric patients. J Pediatr Orthop. 2020;40(9):474–80. (In eng). https://doi.org/10.1097/bpo.0000000000001601.
17. Boulos A, DeFroda SF, Kleiner JE, Thomas N, Gil JA, Cruz AI Jr. Inpatient orthopaedic hardware removal in children: a cross-sectional study. J Clin Orthop Trauma. 2017;8(3):270–5. (In eng). https://doi.org/10.1016/j.jcot.2017.06.020.
18. Harasen G. Orthopedic hardware and equipment for the beginner: part 1: pins and wires. Can Vet J. 2011;52(9):1025–6. (In eng).
19. Pradhan A, Hennrikus W, Pace G, et al. Increased pin diameter improves torsional stability in supracondlar humerus fractures. J Child Orthop. 2016;10:163–7.

20. Stamatis ED, Navid DO, Parks BG, Myerson MS. Strength of fixation of Ludloff metatarsal osteotomy utilizing three different types of Kirschner wires: a biomechanical study. Foot Ankle Int. 2003;24(10):805–11. (In eng). https://doi.org/10.1177/107110070302401014.
21. Ahmed AM, Said E, Addosooki A, et al. Intramedullary versus plate fixation of both bone forearm fractures in skeletally immature patients: a systematic review and meta-analysis. Eur J Orthop Surg Traumatol. 2024;34(5):2263–78. (In eng). https://doi.org/10.1007/s00590-024-03925-7.
22. Calder PR, Achan P, Barry M. Diaphyseal forearm fractures in children treated with intramedullary fixation: outcome of K-wire versus elastic stable intramedullary nail. Injury. 2003;34(4):278–82. (In eng). https://doi.org/10.1016/s0020-1383(02)00310-8.
23. Shaw KA, Murphy JS. Methods to facilitate reduction of medial epicondyle fractures in the supine position. J Pediatric Orthop Soci North America. 2022;4(3):495. https://doi.org/10.55275/JPOSNA-2022-0081.
24. Dias JJ, Johnson GV, Hoskinson J, Sulaiman K. Management of severely displaced medial epicondyle fractures. J Orthop Trauma. 1987;1(1):59–62. (In eng). https://doi.org/10.1097/00005131-198701010-00009.
25. Schlitz RS, Schwertz JM, Eberhardt AW, Gilbert SR. Biomechanical analysis of screws versus K-wires for lateral humeral condyle fractures. J Pediatr Orthop. 2015;35(8):e93–7. (In eng). https://doi.org/10.1097/bpo.0000000000000450.
26. Jeon S, Ahn W, Oh J, Chung J, Choi J, Lee S. Finite element analyses of lateral condyle fracture fixation in paediatrics regarding configuration of Kirschner-wire. BMC Musculoskelet Disord. 2022;23(1):940. (In eng). https://doi.org/10.1186/s12891-022-05897-3.
27. Cummings JL, Schwabe MT, Rivera AE, et al. K-wire versus screw fixation in displaced lateral condyle fractures of the Humerus in children: a multicenter study of 762 fractures. J Pediatr Orthop. 2023;43(4):e284–9. (In eng). https://doi.org/10.1097/bpo.0000000000002348.
28. Masquijo JJ, Sanchez Ortiz M, Ponzone A, Fernández Korosec L, Arkader A. Management of Lateral Condyle Humeral Fracture Associated with Elbow Dislocation in children. A retrospective international multicenter cohort study. J Pediatr Orthop. 2024;44(2):82–8. (In eng). https://doi.org/10.1097/bpo.0000000000002574.
29. Li WC, Xu RJ. Comparison of Kirschner wires and AO cannulated screw internal fixation for displaced lateral humeral condyle fracture in children. Int Orthop. 2012;36(6):1261–6. (In eng). https://doi.org/10.1007/s00264-011-1452-y.
30. Cho YJ, Kang SH, Kang MH. K-wire versus screws in the fixation of lateral condyle fracture of humerus in pediatrics: a systematic review and meta-analysis. BMC Musculoskelet Disord. 2023;24(1):649. (In eng). https://doi.org/10.1186/s12891-023-06780-5.
31. Chaudhry H, Kleinlugtenbelt YV, Mundi R, Ristevski B, Goslings JC, Bhandari M. Are volar locking plates superior to percutaneous K-wires for distal radius fractures? A meta-analysis. Clin Orthop Relat Res. 2015;473(9):3017–27. (In eng). https://doi.org/10.1007/s11999-015-4347-1.
32. Nandyala SV, Giladi AM, Parker AM, Rozental TD. Comparison of direct perioperative costs in treatment of unstable distal radial fractures: open reduction and internal fixation versus closed reduction and percutaneous pinning. J Bone Joint Surg Am. 2018;100(9):786–92. (In eng). https://doi.org/10.2106/jbjs.17.00688.
33. Salter RB. Role of innominate osteotomy in the treatment of congenital dislocation and subluxation of the hip in the older child. J Bone Joint Surg Am. 1966;48(7):1413–39. (In eng).
34. Sucato DJ, Brabham CE, De La Rocha A, Podeszwa DA, Karol LA. Radiographic outcome following treatment of residual hip dysplasia with pemberton versus salter osteotomy: comparison of results in patients followed to skeletal maturity. J Bone Joint Surg Am. 2024. (In eng). https://doi.org/10.2106/jbjs.23.01346.
35. Leunig M, Ganz R. The Bernese method of periacetabular osteotomy. Orthopade. 1998;27(11):743–50. (In ger). https://doi.org/10.1007/pl00003460.
36. Leopold VJ, Conrad J, Zahn RK, Hipfl C, Perka C, Hardt S. Fixation stability and implant-associated complications in periacetabular osteotomy: a comparison of screw and K-wire

fixation. Arch Orthop Trauma Surg. 2023;143(2):691–7. (In eng). https://doi.org/10.1007/s00402-021-04112-7.
37. Leopold VJ, Hipfl C, Zahn RK, Pumberger M, Perka C, Hardt S. Periacetabular osteotomy with a modified fixation technique using K-wires shows clinical results comparable to screw fixation at mid-term follow-up. J Clin Med. 2023;12(19). (In eng). https://doi.org/10.3390/jcm12196204.

Part V

Spine

Methods to Improve Value: Scoliosis Screening

32

Joseph L. Petfield

Introduction

AIS has an estimated prevalence of 0.5–4% [1]. Most cases are mild, occur during adolescence, and do not require treatment. However, larger curves can lead to pain, pulmonary issues, cosmetic concerns, and negative body image [2, 3]. High-magnitude curves exceeding 50° are often treated with surgery due to these complications. Scoliosis tends to worsen with growth [4, 5], making younger children with larger deformities susceptible to curve progression that may reach a surgical threshold. When diagnosed early, bracing can effectively manage AIS [6], potentially preventing the need for surgery and the challenges associated with nonoperative treatment of curves greater than 50°.

The role of universal scoliosis screening remains controversial due to the variable effectiveness of screening tools and the high costs associated with identifying patients who may require treatment. Furthermore, confirmatory diagnostic testing involves X-rays, which carries the risk of radiation exposure. As a result, the optimal approach to scoliosis screening is a subject of ongoing global debate.

Value-Based Themes

History and Physical Examination Should Be the Workhorse of Screening

A skilled and detailed examiner can enhance the sensitivity and specificity of any screening test. For AIS screening, the examiner should be familiar with the demographics of scoliosis, noting that AIS occurs in females at a 5:1 ratio compared to

J. L. Petfield (✉)
Penn State College of Medicine, Hershey, PA, USA

W. L. Hennrikus, R. M. Schwend (eds.), *Value in Pediatric Orthopaedics*,
https://doi.org/10.1007/978-3-032-19570-8_32

males [1]. Additionally, the examiner should inquire about a family history of scoliosis, Marfan syndrome, neurofibromatosis, and whether any relatives have required bracing or surgery for scoliosis. It's also important to ask the patient and parents if they notice any asymmetry in the patient's shoulders, breasts, or flank contours.

The forward bending test is the most commonly used physical examination method for assessing scoliosis [7]. During the test, the child faces away from the examiner and bends forward until their spine is parallel to the ground [8]. The examiner then evaluates asymmetry in the posterior ribs, paraspinal muscles, and scapulae. In addition, the examiner should assess asymmetry in the ribs, scapulae, flanks, and shoulders while the child is standing upright. Palpation of the posterior superior iliac spines (PSIS) or iliac crests is helpful to evaluate pelvic obliquity. Pelvic tilt in the coronal plane may indicate a limb length discrepancy, which could potentially mimic scoliosis during the forward bend test. The forward bend test has demonstrated a sensitivity of 85% and specificity of 93% [9].

A scoliometer can improve the diagnostic accuracy of the forward bend examination [10]. The scoliometer measures the degree of spinal and rib rotation in the transverse plane. It is placed on the back at the point of maximal asymmetry while the child bends forward [11]. A reading of 5–7° is considered a positive test, indicating the need for further evaluation (Fig. 32.1). The scoliometer has demonstrated a sensitivity of up to 90%. A digital version of the scoliometer, which has been clinically validated, is also available for download on smartphones [12, 13].

Other advanced tools for scoliosis assessment have been developed but are not widely adopted. For example, Moiré topography projects lines onto the back, which are then analyzed with photography. However, the false positive rate for this method can range from 12% to 67% [14, 15]. Additionally, other experimental surface topography systems have been developed [13, 14].

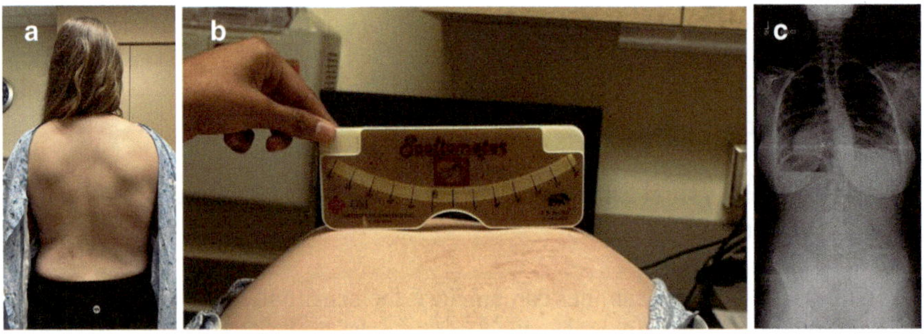

Fig. 32.1 Scoliosis screening exam with radiology correlation. This 12-year-old female was diagnosed following a screening examination by her pediatrician. On standing observation (**a**), scapular and flank asymmetry are noted. Upon forward bending (**b**), a right thoracic prominence is observed, with a scoliometer measurement of 5°. A PA radiograph obtained at the time of examination (**c**) shows a 30° right thoracic curve, measured from T6 to T12. Note that the hips and one proximal humerus are included in the image, and no shielding was used. Slot scanning radiography would have provided lower radiation exposure and would have also included a lateral view

Screening Programs for Scoliosis Are Heterogeneous and Can Be Costly

Scoliosis screening programs were widely implemented in many countries and hospitals from the 1960s to the 1990s. However, several nations and states that previously mandated screening have since abandoned screening due to concerns about radiation exposure, the variability of referral guidelines, and uncertain cost-effectiveness [7]. A cost analysis conducted by Yawn and colleagues in 2000 revealed that in Rochester, Minnesota, the screening program costs about $25 per child screened and over $10,000 to identify a single child requiring treatment [16]. Although the cost of scoliosis surgery exceeds $150,000 per patient, there is no published study on the cost-effectiveness of screening relative to the expense of surgical treatment.

Orthopedic Surgeons and Pediatricians Should Be Aware of Established Guidelines

In the USA, orthopedic surgeons, pediatricians, and primary care clinicians should be aware that the US Preventive Services Task Force (USPSTF) assigns a grade of "I" to scoliosis screening. The "I" designation indicates insufficient evidence to determine whether the benefits of screening outweigh the potential harms [17]. Notably, the USPSTF initially issued an "I" rating in 1994, which was changed to a "D" (recommending against screening) in 2004. However, after the publication of the BRAIST study by Weinstein and colleagues, which demonstrated the effectiveness of bracing in halting curve progression and preventing the need for surgery [6], the rating was reverted to "I."

Clinicians should also be familiar with the 2008 and 2015 position statements from the American Academy of Pediatrics, American Academy of Orthopaedic Surgery, Scoliosis Research Society, and Pediatric Orthopaedic Society of North America [18, 19]. These statements recommend that if scoliosis screening is performed, screening should include both the forward bending test and the use of a scoliometer. Screenings should be conducted at age 10 and 12 years for females and at age 13 or 14 years for males.

Lastly, the International Society on Scoliosis Orthopaedic and Rehabilitation Treatment (SOSORT) recommends school-based scoliosis screening for females only and with the patient in a seated position to minimize the effects of pelvic obliquity. Additionally, SOSORT recommends screening at a later age for patients in northern latitudes, due to the later onset of menarche in these regions [20]. In contrast, the American Academy of Pediatrics (AAP) specifically does not endorse school-based screening.

Optimize Your Gold Standard Imaging

Radiographs with the measurement of the Cobb angle for the major curve remain the generally preferred method for diagnosing scoliosis [21]. While this is not a practical screening test, it is the next logical step for patients who test positive with the scoliometer. Developing an optimal imaging protocol for AIS can help streamline workflow, minimize radiation exposure, and enhance value.

If available, clinicians should perform imaging with a biplanar slot scanning device, as this device has been shown to reduce radiation exposure to the patient [22]. A modified biplanar slot scanning technique also allows for the simultaneous assessment of hand bone age and Sanders classification on the PA image, further minimizing both radiation exposure and time in the radiology suite [23]. If slot scanning technology is unavailable, clinics can adopt other strategies to reduce radiation exposure using conventional radiographs, including modifying imaging techniques and avoiding shielding [24].

Major Changes May Be Around the Corner: Stay Tuned

The rise of genomic analysis, high-volume data processing, widespread smartphone use, and artificial intelligence (AI) is poised to bring major changes to scoliosis screening. Early reports on several promising technologies have recently been published.

For example, a new smartphone-based scoliosis assessment app, the Scoliosis Assessment App (NSite Medical, Inc., Menlo Park, California, USA), received FDA clearance in 2023 [25]. This technology utilizes the optical sensors of a smartphone to diagnose scoliosis through a 3D scan of the back. The app can estimate the likelihood of clinically significant scoliosis, aiding both diagnosis and monitoring. In a validation study, Rohde and colleagues evaluated 55 adolescent patients using the Scoliosis Assessment App, a scoliometer, and radiographs [26]. The app generated an asymmetry index, which was analyzed to estimate the probability of scoliosis based on previously collected data. When identifying a curve magnitude greater than 20°, the app demonstrated 96% sensitivity and 85% specificity, while scoliometer assessment showed 50% sensitivity and 89% specificity. The app had four false negatives and one false positive result, with all false cases having spinal curves with radiographic coronal scoliosis angles between 9 and 21 degrees. While not yet widely available, apps linked to smartphone technology hold promise for improving scoliosis diagnosis in the future.

Another emerging diagnostic test of note is Collagen X Biomarker (CXM). CXM is a stable breakdown product of Collagen type X that can be detected using an immunoassay [27]. Welborn and colleagues have shown that CXM closely correlates with growth velocity and the cessation of growth [28]. If further developed, this test could enhance value by more accurately identifying which patients with scoliosis are at the highest risk for curve progression.

Conclusions

Clinicians should be aware of the relevant scoliosis screening guidelines specific to their state and practice locality. An examiner who takes a detailed history and performs a reproducible examination can increase the efficiency of scoliosis screening. Adding a scoliometer to the physical examination can improves diagnostic accuracy. While universal screening of adolescents for AIS remains controversial, future technologies hold promise for enhancing value in the diagnosis of scoliosis.

Author Pearls

- Our standard protocol for new scoliosis patients is to have them change into disposable exam shorts, a gown that opens in the back, and another gown that opens in the front.
- Outside radiographs should be uploaded in advance, when possible. I typically analyze the radiographs at the workstation in the patient's room, allowing the parent and child to observe the process directly.
- Educating community partners, such as school nurses, family medicine doctors, and pediatricians, about screening best practices is a valuable exercise. Providing education helps strengthen relationships and improve orthopedic referrals, ultimately making care more efficient and effective.

Comments by the Editors

WLH

In the USA, less than 50% of states mandate school-based scoliosis screenings. However, the implementation of these screenings varies from state to state, including the specific grades targeted and the details of the screening process. The effectiveness of screening programs for AIS has been a subject of ongoing debate and research. For example, the US Preventive Services Task Force (USPSTF) has reviewed the evidence and found no conclusive evidence to support or refute school screening for scoliosis, citing a lack of randomized controlled trials and observational studies on the outcomes of these programs. In addition, the American Academy of Pediatrics (AAP) recommends against school-based screening for AIS, expressing concern over low predictive value, potential overdiagnosis, unnecessary referrals, and unclear long-term outcomes. Physicians are encouraged to research this topic in more detail for themselves when developing or evaluating school screening policies in their state or city.

RMS

As imaging practices have advanced, so too have recommendations for radiation protection during scoliosis radiography. Historically, gonadal and breast shielding was standard practice in pediatric imaging to protect radiosensitive tissues from potential long-term radiation effects. However, recent guidance from the FDA and the American Association of Physicists in Medicine now recommends against routine shielding. This shift reflects the use of modern imaging systems that operate at much lower radiation doses and concerns that shielding may interfere with automatic exposure control, obscure critical anatomy, or lead to repeat exposures. The focus has now shifted toward techniques that reduce radiation dose, such as posteroanterior (PA) imaging, collimation, and proper patient positioning.

References

1. Konieczny MR, Senyurt H, Krauspe R. Epidemiology of adolescent idiopathic scoliosis. J Child Orthop. 2013;7(1):3–9.
2. Weinstein SL. The natural history of adolescent idiopathic scoliosis. J Pediatr Orthop. 2019;39(Issue 6, Supplement 1 Suppl 1):S44–6.
3. Agabegi SS, Kazemi N, Sturm PF, Mehlman CT. Natural history of adolescent idiopathic scoliosis in skeletally mature patients: a critical review. J Am Acad Orthop Surg. 2015;23(12):714–23.
4. Sanders JO, Khoury JG, Kishan S, Browne RH, Mooney JF, Arnold KD, et al. Predicting scoliosis progression from skeletal maturity: a simplified classification during adolescence. J Bone Joint Surg Am. 2008;90(3):540–53.
5. Charles YP, Daures JP, de Rosa V, Diméglio A. Progression risk of idiopathic juvenile scoliosis during pubertal growth. Spine. 2006;31(17):1933–42.
6. Weinstein SL, Dolan LA, Wright JG, Dobbs MB. Effects of bracing in adolescents with idiopathic scoliosis. N Engl J Med. 2013;369(16):1512–21.
7. Oetgen ME, Heyer JH, Kelly SM. Scoliosis screening. J Am Acad Orthop Surg. 2021;29(9):370–9.
8. SRS Educational Video: Scoliosis Screening Exam [Internet]. 2015 [cited 2025 May 18]. Available from: https://www.youtube.com/watch?v=7bfp0fcfH7E
9. Karachalios T, Sofianos J, Roidis N, Sapkas G, Korres D, Nikolopoulos K. Ten-year follow-up evaluation of a school screening program for scoliosis. Is the forward-bending test an accurate diagnostic criterion for the screening of scoliosis? Spine. 1999;24(22):2318–24.
10. Fong DYT, Lee CF, Cheung KMC, Cheng JCY, Ng BKW, Lam TP, et al. A meta-analysis of the clinical effectiveness of school scoliosis screening. Spine. 2010;35(10):1061–71.
11. SRS Educational Video: Use of Scoliometer [Internet]. 2015 [cited 2025 May 18]. Available from: https://www.youtube.com/watch?v=YIthaksm9mY
12. Balg F, Juteau M, Theoret C, Svotelis A, Grenier G. Validity and reliability of the iPhone to measure rib hump in scoliosis. J Pediatr Orthop. 2014;34(8):774–9.
13. Franko OI, Bray C, Newton PO. Validation of a scoliometer smartphone app to assess scoliosis. J Pediatr Orthop. 2012;32(8):e72–5.
14. Yamamoto S, Shigematsu H, Kadono F, Tanaka Y, Tatematsu M, Okuda A, et al. Adolescent scoliosis screening in Nara City schools: a 23-year retrospective cross-sectional study. Asian Spine J. 2015;9(3):407–15.
15. Daruwalla JS, Balasubramaniam P. Moiré topography in scoliosis. Its accuracy in detecting the site and size of the curve. J Bone Joint Surg Br. 1985;67(2):211–3.

16. Yawn BP, Yawn RA. The estimated cost of school scoliosis screening. Spine. 2000;25(18):2387–91.
17. US Preventive Services Task Force, Grossman DC, Curry SJ, Owens DK, Barry MJ, Davidson KW, et al. Screening for adolescent idiopathic scoliosis: US preventive services task force recommendation statement. JAMA. 2018;319(2):165–72.
18. Hresko MT, Talwalkar V, Schwend R, AAOS, SRS, POSNA. Early detection of idiopathic scoliosis in adolescents. J Bone Joint Surg Am. 2016;98(16):e67.
19. Richards BS, Vitale MG. Screening for idiopathic scoliosis in adolescents. An information statement. J Bone Joint Surg Am. 2008 Jan;90(1):195–8.
20. Grivas TB, Hresko MT, Labelle H, Price N, Kotwicki T, Maruyama T. The pendulum swings back to scoliosis screening: screening policies for early detection and treatment of idiopathic scoliosis – current concepts and recommendations. Scoliosis. 2013;8(1):16.
21. Malfair D, Flemming AK, Dvorak MF, Munk PL, Vertinsky AT, Heran MK, et al. Radiographic evaluation of scoliosis: review. AJR Am J Roentgenol. 2010;194(3 Suppl):S8–22.
22. Rose LD, Williams R, Ajayi B, Abdalla M, Bernard J, Bishop T, et al. Reducing radiation exposure and cancer risk for children with scoliosis: EOS the new gold standard. Spine Deform. 2023;11(4):847–51.
23. Jackson TJ, Miller D, Nelson S, Cahill PJ, Flynn JM. Two for one: a change in hand positioning during low-dose spinal Stereoradiography allows for concurrent, reliable Sanders skeletal maturity staging. Spine Deform. 2018;6(4):391–6.
24. Health C for D and R. Reducing Patient Exposure During Scoliosis Radiogr aphy. FDA [Internet]. 2019 Feb. 9 [cited 2025 May 18]. Available from: https://www.fda.gov/radiation-emitting-products/resources-you-radiation-emitting-products/reducing-patient-exposure-during-scoliosis-radiography
25. Tileston K. Prospective Validation of 3D Body Surface Modeling for Patient Monitoring in Adolescent Idiopathic Scoliosis [Internet]. clinicaltrials.gov; 2025 Apr [cited 2025 May 18]. Report No.: NCT05697939. Available from: https://clinicaltrials.gov/study/NCT05697939
26. Rohde MS, Albarran M, Catanzano AA, Sachs EJ, Naz H, Jobanputra A, et al. Smartphone-based surface topography app accurately detects clinically significant scoliosis. Spine Deform. 2025;
27. Coghlan RF, Oberdorf JA, Sienko S, Aiona MD, Boston BA, Connelly KJ, et al. A degradation fragment of type X collagen is a real-time marker for bone growth velocity. Sci Transl Med. 2017;9(419):eaan4669.
28. Welborn MC, Coghlan R, Sienko S, Horton W. Correlation of collagen X biomarker (CXM) with peak height velocity and radiographic measures of growth in idiopathic scoliosis. Spine Deform. 2021;9(3):645–53.

Methods to Improve Value When Treating Children with Adolescent Idiopathic Scoliosis

33

John T. Anderson

Abbreviations

AIS	Adolescent idiopathic scoliosis
EBL	Estimated blood loss
ERAS	Enhanced recovery after surgery
HRQOL	Health-related quality of life
LOS	Length of stay
MRSA	Methicillin-resistant *S. aureus*
POD	Postoperative day
SRS	Scoliosis Research Society
SSI	Surgical site infection
TXA	Tranexamic acid
UBS	Ultrasound bone scalpel

Introduction

With rising healthcare costs, there has been increasing emphasis on improving the value of services provided. From 1997 to 2012, despite decreasing length of hospital stays (LOS) for AIS, hospital charges tripled [1]. The major contributors to the cost of AIS surgical treatment include implants, ICU utilization, LOS, operating room and postanesthesia care unit time, and bone grafts [2]. Lonner et al. analyzed a multicenter, prospective database and found significant variations in factors such

J. T. Anderson (✉)
Children Mercy Hospital, Kansas City, MO, USA
e-mail: jtanderson@cmh.edu

W. L. Hennrikus, R. M. Schwend (eds.), *Value in Pediatric Orthopaedics*,
https://doi.org/10.1007/978-3-032-19570-8_33

as the percentage of posterior approaches, operative time, LOS, estimated blood loss (EBL), use of cell saver, rod material, screw density, number of screws, use of antifibrinolytics, and use of intravenous analgesics. Despite these differences, Lonner reported no variations in curve correction, levels fused, or the need for allogenic blood transfusions [3]. A separate study of 1819 AIS cases over 20 years showed that anterior surgery had largely been abandoned, pedicle screw use had increased, EBL had decreased, operative time and LOS were shorter, antifibrinolytic use had risen, complications had reduced, and SRS scores had improved [4]. Given the variability in the surgical care of AIS, there are many potential areas for improving value.

Value Based Themes

Nonoperative Care Is an Option

Nonsurgical management is a reasonable option for some patients. AIS is not a life-threatening condition, and surgical intervention is elective [5]. This shared decision-making approach with the surgeon, the parents, and the patient requires a thoughtful discussion about the natural history of untreated AIS. For example, according to the landmark study by Weinstein et al., which followed untreated AIS patients for 50 years, these individuals live productive and functional lives. Patients opting for nonoperative treatment should be informed that they may experience more back pain (61%) compared to age-matched controls (35%) and may have cosmetic concerns related to their back. However, the majority (68%) report experiencing only little to moderate back pain [6].

Erwin et al. found that untreated AIS patients had lower SRS-22r scores compared to age- and sex-matched controls. Erwin analyzed a cohort of 275 subjects, divided into three age groups: 20–30 years, 40–59 years, and 60+ years. Females generally scored worse in all domains, except for function in the 20–39 age group. Males, on the other hand, showed no difference in function across all age groups. There were also no differences in the mental health or total score domains for the 40–59 age group. Additionally, Oswestry Disability Index (ODI) scores were positively correlated with age, BMI, and curve size. Subjects with thoracolumbar curves had lower ODI scores than those with thoracic curves [7].

The results comparing surgical and nonsurgical care for AIS show conflicting outcomes. Mayo et al. found that while the coronal Cobb angle did not directly correlate with the frequency of back pain, the deformity itself could serve as a pain generator. Mayo concluded that surgical treatment did not create additional pain beyond what was caused by the deformity itself. The ODI scores indicated that both untreated patients with severe curves and those treated surgically experienced limitations in pain management, lifting, and social activities [8].

Dickson et al. compared symptomatic untreated adults with AIS who were offered surgery, those who had surgery, and a non-scoliotic control group. At a 5-year follow-up, Dickson found that 35% of the surgical group reported substantial or severe pain, compared to 70% of those who did not undergo surgery and 7% of the non-scoliotic control group [9].

Diarbakerli et al. compared surgically treated adults with AIS to those who had been braced or had no treatment. The braced and surgical groups were treated before skeletal maturity. This study included 1187 adults with an average age of 39 years. Diarbakerli found that untreated subjects had similar health-related quality of life (HRQL) scores, based on SRS 22r and EQ-5D, when compared to those who had been braced. Interestingly, both the braced and untreated groups had slightly higher HRQL scores than the surgically treated group [10].

More recently, Ahonen et al. reported a 10-year follow-up study of patients who underwent segmental pedicle screw instrumentation for AIS. This cohort of 53 patients was compared to age- and sex-matched controls with untreated AIS and healthy individuals without scoliosis. Ahonen found that surgically treated AIS patients had better SRS-24 scores than the nonsurgical group, except for the function domain. However, surgically treated patients had significantly lower total scores compared to the healthy control group [11]. This information should be shared with patients and parents considering surgical treatment, as it allows them to make a more informed decision about their care.

Infection Prevention

One of the most concerning complications of any surgery is infection, a risk that is heightened in spinal procedures and other orthopedic surgeries involving implants. To reduce the risk of infection, many hospitals have developed standardized protocols (or "bundles") aimed at minimizing the risk of infection.

Marks et al. reported that the incidence of surgical site infection (SSI) among 1757 patients with AIS was 1.6% [12]. A common theme in many SSI prevention bundles includes nasal decontamination, use of chlorhexidine wipes on the planned surgical site, standardization of timing and dosing for antibiotic prophylaxis, limiting operating room traffic, povidone-iodine irrigation with intrawound vancomycin powder, and consistent dressing care protocols.

Mallet et al. reported that in patients who tested positive for *Staphylococcus aureus* (*S. aureus*), nasal decontamination with mupirocin for 5 days prior to surgery reduced the SSI rate from 5.1% to 1.3%. For patients testing positive for methicillin-resistant *S. aureus* (MRSA), vancomycin was used for antibiotic prophylaxis. All patients showered with Hibiscrub 4% for 5 days before surgery. No patient who underwent mupirocin nasal decontamination developed an SSI [13]. In second study by Mallet et al., the incidence of SSI was 1.1% in patients who received povidone-iodine irrigation and intrawound vancomycin powder, compared to 5.4% in those who did not receive these interventions [14]. In a separate study of 804 pediatric patients undergoing posterior spinal fusion and instrumentation for AIS, the incidence of SSI was 7.2% before implementing an SSI prevention bundle compared to 2.5% after the bundle was introduced [15].

Another controversial theme in spine surgery concerns the duration of post-op antibiotic administration. Abola et al. evaluated 4454 patients who underwent spinal surgery, with 2672 receiving 24 hours of postoperative antibiotics and 1782 receiving no postoperative antibiotics. The study found no significant difference in infection rates (1.8% vs. 1.5%) [16].

The use of post-op drains is also frequently questioned. Diab et al. found that patients with drains did not have a lower incidence of complications, including SSI or neural injury. However, patients with drains did experience a higher rate of postoperative transfusions [17]. Similarly, Helenius et al. conducted a randomized, multicenter study and found no difference in SSI rates between patients with and without a subfascial drain. Interestingly, they noted that patients without a drain required significantly more opioids in the first 48 hours postoperatively [18].

Reducing Blood Loss

Blood loss is a concern shared by all surgeons. Allogeneic blood transfusions carry known risks, including hemolytic and anaphylactic reactions, long-term immunosuppression, and an increased likelihood of SSIs [19–22]. In spine surgery, hypotensive anesthesia is commonly used to reduce bleeding during surgical exposure. However, hypotension during deformity correction adds neurologic risks. Therefore, to mitigate blood loss and the need for allogeneic transfusions, other measures have been implemented. Tranexamic acid (TXA) has become a routine antifibrinolytic agent used in AIS surgery. Tumber et al. reported that high-dose TXA (defined as a > 30 mg/kg loading dose followed by a 10 mg/kg/hour infusion) was safe to administer and effectively reduced estimated blood loss (EBL) and transfusion rates compared to lower doses [23]. On the other hand, in a prospective randomized double-blinded study, Hasan et al. found no significant difference in EBL or transfusion rates between high- and low-dose TXA groups [24]. The high-dose group received a 30 mg/kg loading dose and 10 mg/kg/hour infusion compared to 10 mg/kg loading dose and 1 mg/kg/hour infusion in the low-dose group [24].

Another strategy used in AIS surgery to reduce blood loss is the utilization of intraoperative cell salvage systems. These systems aim to recover the patient's blood during surgery and reinfuse it, potentially reducing the need for allogeneic transfusions. The literature supports blood salvage use under specific circumstances. For example, Bowen et al. found that cell salvage reduced allogeneic transfusion requirements in cases with surgical times exceeding 6 hours and estimated blood loss (EBL) greater than 30% of total body volume [25].

Wahl and Luhmann reported that only 6.5% of their patients received ≥250 cc of salvaged blood, and 59% did not receive any. They concluded that cell salvage should be used in cases involving fusion of 12 or more levels, major Cobb angles ≥55°, anesthesia exposure ≥6 hours, and the use of posterior column osteotomies [26].

On the other hand, Weiss et al. reported that cell salvage did not reduce the need for allogeneic transfusion. In Weiss' study, no patients with EBL <500 cc received salvaged blood. This study included both idiopathic and neuromuscular patients [27]. Following the results of Weiss et al., Chi et al. analyzed cell salvage in 402 AIS patients with an EBL ≥500 cc. They found that patients with EBL ≥1000 cc had fewer allogeneic transfusions when cell salvage was used, but it was not cost-effective until the EBL reached ≥1500 cc [28].

The use of an ultrasonic bone scalpel (UBS) for tasks such as facetectomies and osteotomies is another potentially effective method to reduce blood loss in AIS surgery. The UBS employs an oscillating blade that efficiently cuts the bone while preserving soft tissue structures. The blade is cooled by an irrigation system. Friction between the bone and the blade facilitates coagulation of the cut surfaces. Studies have shown that the UBS can reduce EBL by 30–40% and decrease the amount of salvaged blood transfused and EBL per level fused [29].

A related debate concerns the need for postoperative hemoglobin and hematocrit labs on postoperative day 1 (POD1). Drawing blood the morning after major surgery can cause anxiety and discomfort for the child and additional stress for the parents. Liu et al. suggest that these labs should be drawn if the last intraoperative hematocrit is <26%, if the operative time per level fused exceeds 35 minutes, or if the amount of cell salvage is >241 cc. For asymptomatic patients who do not meet these criteria, morning labs are not necessary [30].

Use Fewer Pedicle Screws

The use of thoracic pedicle screws has become common practice in AIS surgery. Compared to hybrid constructs, pedicle screw constructs offer better correction and fewer revision procedures [31–34]. In addition, the increasing use of posterior pedicle screws has led to a decline in the number of anterior procedures performed [1, 35]. However, screws are expensive, and the question of how many screws are necessary remains debated. The cost of implants, especially pedicle screws, contributes to rising hospital charges for AIS surgery [36].

The debate over whether higher density pedicle screw constructs offer any advantage over lower density constructs continues [4, 37–40]. A recent multicenter, randomized study found that low-density constructs (≤1.4 screws per spinal level) were comparable to high-density constructs (≥1.8 screws per spinal level) in curves ranging from 45° to 65°. Additional controversy remains over whether or not the greater curve correction achieved with pedicle screw constructs leads to improved clinical outcomes justifying the added expense of the screws [4, 34, 38, 40, 41].

Spine Surgical Teams Improve Efficiency

Having a dedicated team of operating room (OR) staff decreases surgical time, total OR time, EBL, LOS, transfusion rates, and overall costs [42–44]. Sarhwahi et al. reported that the presence of a dedicated "scoliosis team" reduced costs by 19%, with results that were transferable across institutions [42].

Enhanced Recovery After Surgery Pathway

Enhanced recovery after surgery (ERAS) pathways have been implemented in many hospitals to reduce LOS, lower costs, and potentially decrease complications [45–48]. ERAS pathways are a multimodal, multidisciplinary approach that standardizes perioperative care through evidence-based interventions. Boylan et al. demonstrated that longer LOS increased costs and was associated with a higher risk of 90-day readmissions and return-to-operating-room procedures [49]. In a meta-analysis and systematic review, Gadiya et al. found that ERAS pathways in AIS surgery reduced LOS without increasing complications or readmission rates [50]. A prospective dual-center study by Fletcher et al. revealed a 55% reduction in LOS with the use of an ERAS pathway. The study also showed that surgery time and EBL were lower in the ERAS group. However, these differences may have been influenced by larger curves, greater use of osteotomies, and more levels fused in the traditional pathway group. Visual analog scores at discharge and quality of recovery (assessed by the QOR9 instrument) were similar between the two groups at 4 weeks [51].

Consider Using Two Attending Surgeons

While this may not be feasible at every hospital or practice, the use of two attending surgeons or AIS cases has been shown to reduce surgical time, total OR time, complications, EBL, allogeneic transfusions, and narcotic use [52–54]. Shorter surgical times have also been linked to reductions in EBL, allogeneic transfusions, LOS, and intraoperative neuromonitoring alerts [55].

Skip the Intensive Care Unit for Some Cases

In many hospitals, AIS patients are receiving postoperative care on the surgical floor rather than in the intensive care unit. Surprisingly, there is limited data on this practice. In one study on this theme, Haber et al. compared a group of patients who maintained mean arterial pressures (MAPs) ≥60 mmHg to another group with multiple episodes of MAPs <60 mmHg. The latter group comprised 31.3% of their subjects. They found that patients who maintained MAPs ≥60 mmHg during the first 4 hours post-surgery did not experience hypotensive events during the subsequent 24 hours. In contrast, those with multiple episodes of MAPs <60 mmHg continued to experience hypotension within the first 24 hours. Therefore, Haber recommended that patients be monitored in a pediatric intensive care unit (ICU) or postanesthesia recovery area for at least 4 hours after surgery. For patients who did not experience hypotensive events during this 4-hour time period, consideration could be given to moving the patient to a less intensive monitoring environment on the surgical ward [56].

Case Example

The patient was a 15-year-and-8-month-old healthy boy with a history of AIS. He failed bracing. He was only wearing the brace for about 8 hours per day. He had a Lenke 6C curve, with a 54° lumbar curve and a 49° main thoracic curve. He was Risser 4. His thoracic kyphosis measured 0° from T4 to T12, and his lumbar lordosis was 44° from L1 to S1. Both curves measured 20° on side-bending supine AP views. His perioperative course followed our hospital's ERAS pathway for AIS (Figs. 33.4, 33.5, and 33.6).

A T4-L3 posterior spinal fusion with instrumentation was performed. Intraoperatively, the patient was given tranexamic acid (TXA) with a loading dose of 30 mg/kg, followed by a 10 mg/kg/hour infusion. An ultrasonic bone scalpel (UBS) was used during the procedure. He also received 30 mg/kg of cefazolin, re-dosed every 3 hours, for 24 hours postoperatively. A dedicated OR team was utilized, and the surgery was performed by two attending surgeons. A pedicle screw construct with a density of 1.75 anchors per level was used (Figs. 33.1, 33.2, and 33.3). Pedicle screws were placed freehand. There were no intraoperative neuromonitoring alerts or concerns. Diluted povidone-iodine irrigation was used, and 1 gram of powdered vancomycin was placed in the allograft-autograft bone. A 15 Fr Blake drain was placed subfascially and removed on postoperative day 2. Liposomal bupivacaine was injected into the peri-wound tissues prior to closure. The total surgical time was 3.5 hours, and the estimated blood loss (EBL) was 360 cc. He received no allogeneic transfusions during his hospitalization and was given 135 cc of salvaged autologous blood intraoperatively (Figs. 33.4, 33.5, and 33.6).

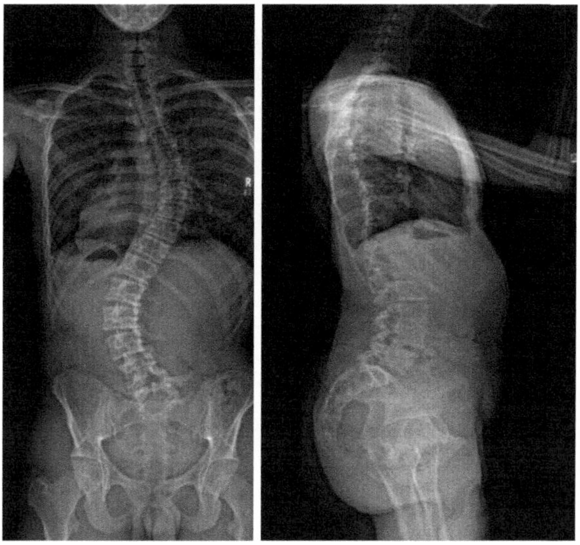

Fig. 33.1 Preoperative PA and lateral standing radiographs

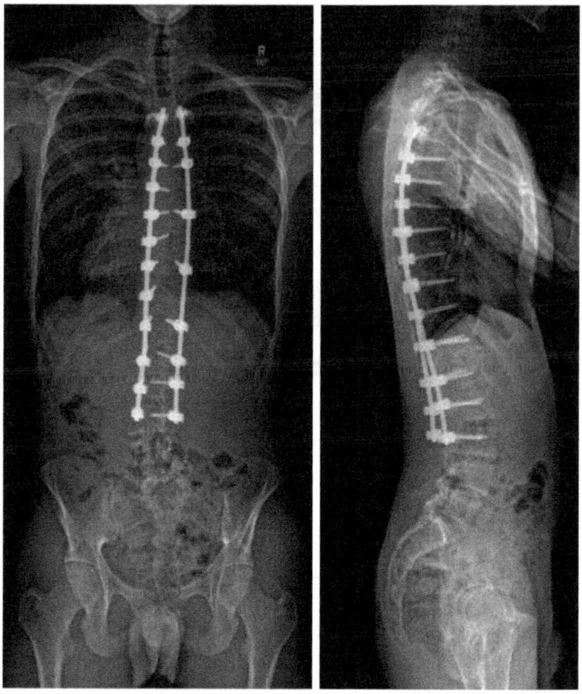

Fig. 33.2 Postoperative PA and lateral standing radiographs

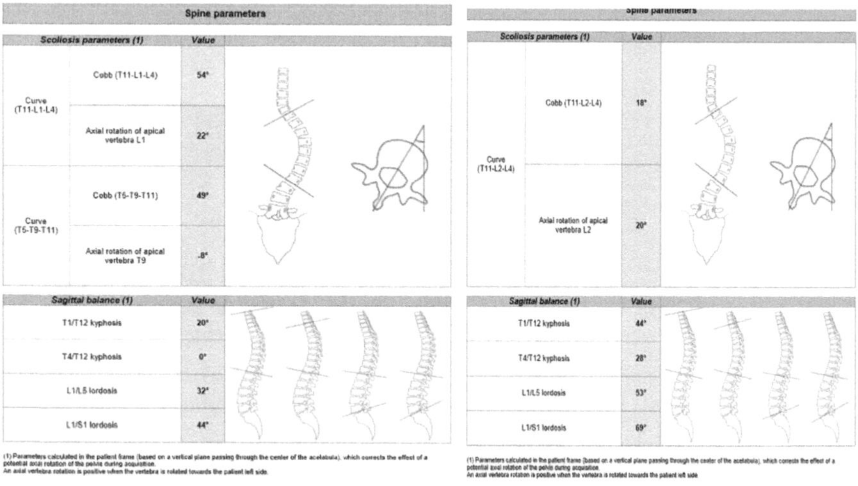

Fig. 33.3 Preoperative (left) and postoperative (right) sterEOS data

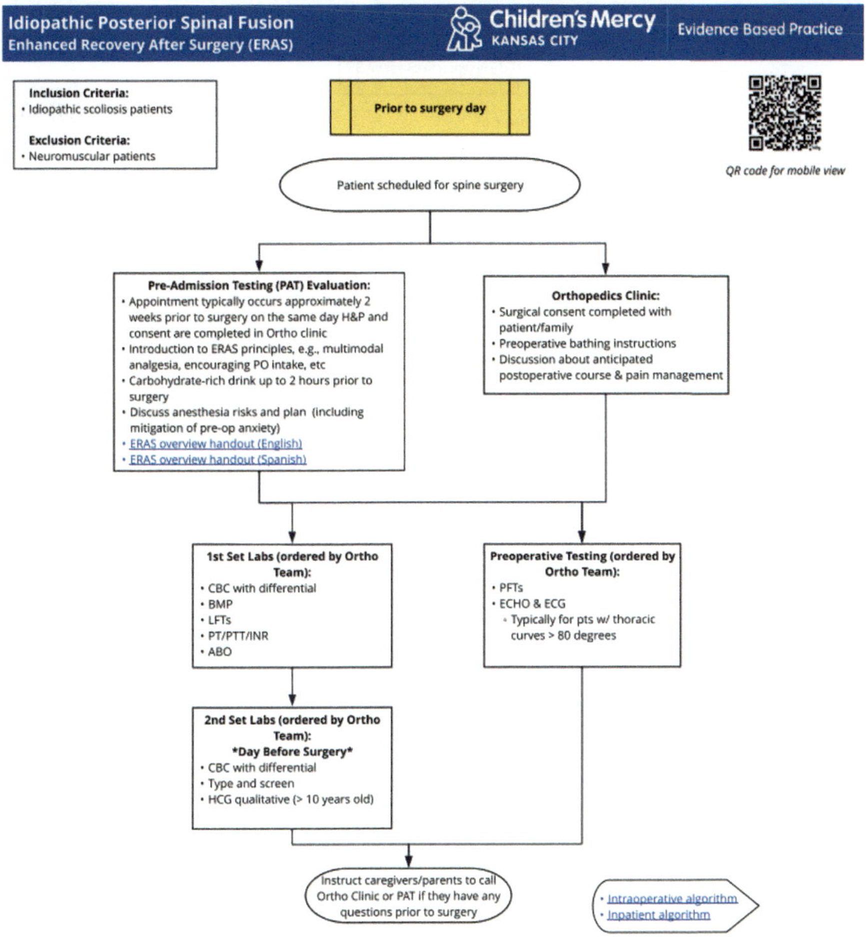

Fig. 33.4 Day before surgery ERAS pathway

After a brief stay in the postanesthesia care unit, he was admitted to the orthopedic surgical floor. Patient-controlled anesthesia was not used. Instead, he was managed with oxycodone, ketorolac, and diazepam, with morphine sulfate provided for breakthrough pain. Postoperative labs were not obtained. He was mobilized by a physical therapist on the day of surgery. The patient was discharged home on postoperative day 2.

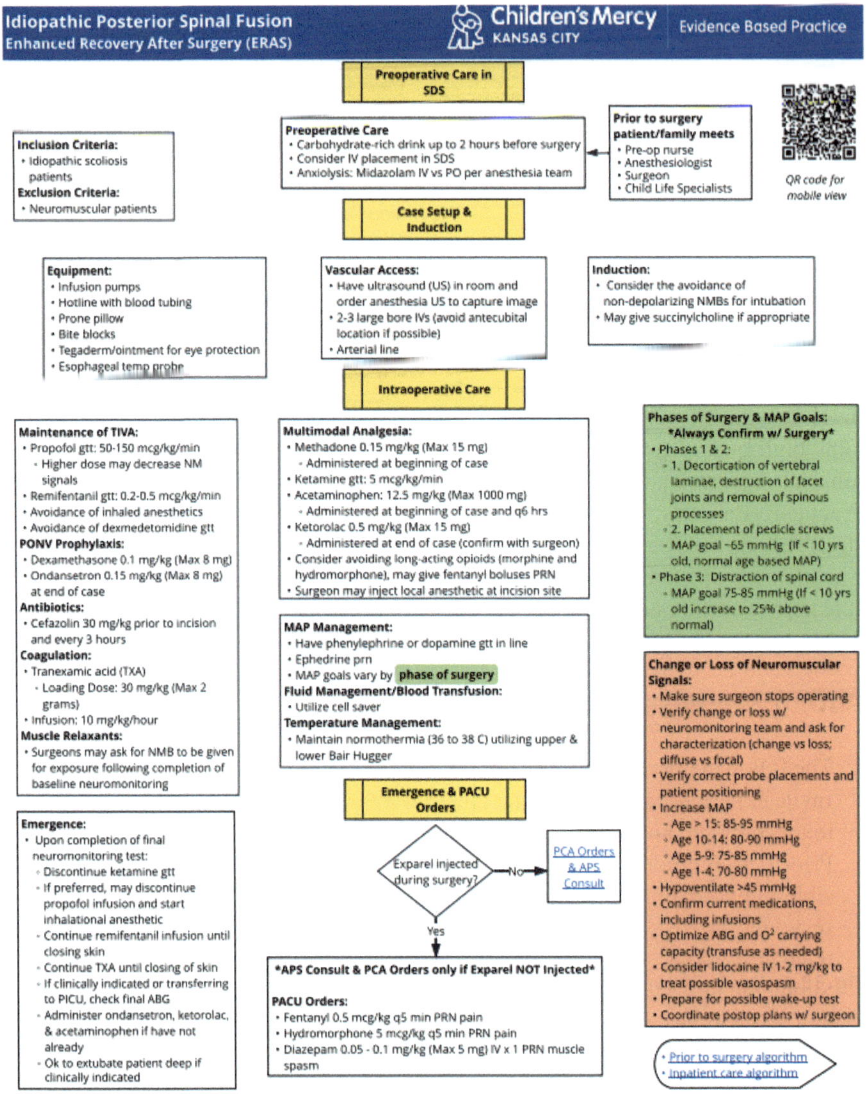

Fig. 33.5 Day of surgery and intraoperative ERAS pathway

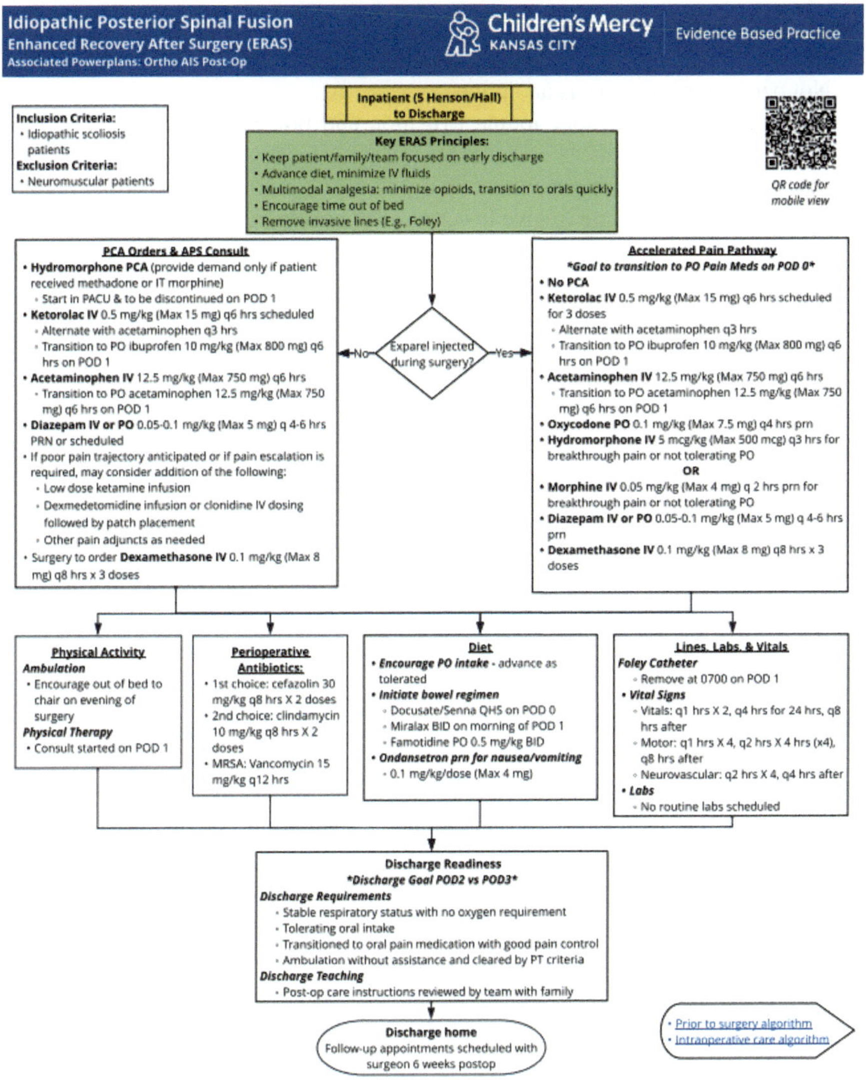

Fig. 33.6 Postoperative ERAS pathway

Conclusions

The current chapter has reviewed eight key evidence-based strategies to enhance the value of surgical care for AIS patients.

Author Pearls

- Not performing surgery is an option.
- Consider adding povidone-iodine irrigation and powered vancomycin to your intraoperative routine.
- Consider giving fewer postoperative doses of antibiotics if you are exceeding 24 hours. It may be safe to give fewer or none postoperative.
- Reduce EBL by using TXA and UBS.
- Use cell salvage in selected cases with anticipated high EBL.
- Consider omitting routine morning labs in certain cases.
- Consider using fewer pedicle screws in certain cases, i.e., flexible curves with less rotation, patients with smaller rib and flank prominences.
- Establish a scoliosis team to improve efficiency and safety.
- Create an ERAS pathway to standardize care with evidence-based measures, shorten LOS, decrease complications, and save money.
- Use two attending surgeons if possible, for certain cases.Consider admitting to the surgical floor rather than the intensive care unit postoperatively for certain cases.

Editor Comments

WLH

This comprehensive and detailed chapter outlines several methods to enhance value in the treatment of AIS. One important suggestion is the use of a dedicated orthopedic spine team. I would extend this recommendation to include the anesthesia team as well. Having a core group of skilled and motivated anesthesia doctors who are experienced in managing complex AIS surgical patients is essential. Additionally, while the current chapter briefly mentions bone grafting, it does not delve into the topic in detail. The choice of bone graft type and methods for achieving fusion can impact the cost, outcomes, and value of care.

RMS

Not all pediatric orthopedic surgeons perform spine surgery; however, most pediatric orthopedic surgeons share the goal of improving the value. At our hospital, the spine team (including our chief, the author of the current chapter) identified practical ways to reduce costs while maintaining excellent outcomes. By collaborating with vendors and hospital supply chain administrators, the spine team standardized implants, simplified contracts, and saved $two million annually. Simultaneously, our spine team and operating room nursing staff applied "Lean" principles to streamline instrument use and reduce instrument and implant trays from 22 to 6 per case. We also began preselecting screw implants the day before surgery. These changes improved efficiency in the OR, reduced contamination risks, and saved about $2400 per case. This effort was truly multidisciplinary, driven by a shared commitment to high-quality, efficient care. This is an example of what can be achieved when a team takes ownership of value improvement.

References

1. Vigneswaran HT, Grabel Z, Eberson CP, et al. Surgical treatment of adolescent idiopathic scoliosis in the United States from 1997 to 2012: an analysis of 20, 346 patients. J Neurosurg Pediatr. 2015;16:322–8.
2. Kamerlink JR, Quirno M, Auerbach JD, et al. Hospital cost analysis of adolescent idiopathic scoliosis correction surgery in 125 consecutive cases. J Bone Joint Surg Am Vol. 2010;92:1097–104.
3. Lonner BS, Toombs CS, Paul JC, Shah SA, Shufflebarger HL, Flynn JM, Newton PO. Resource utilization in adolescent idiopathic scoliosis surgery: is there opportunity for standardization? Spine Deformity. 2017;5:166–71.
4. Lonner BS, Ren Y, Yaszay B, Cahill PJ, Shah SA, Betz RR, Samdani AF, Shufflebarger HL, Newton PO. Evolution of surgery for adolescent idiopathic scoliosis over 20 years: have outcomes improved? Spine. 2018;43(6):402–10.
5. Pehrsson K, Larsson S, Oden A, Nachemson A. Long-term follow-up of patients with untreated scoliosis. A study of mortality, causes of death, and symptoms. Spine. 1992;17:1091–6.
6. Weinstein SL, Dolan LA, Spratt KF, Peterson KK, Spoonamore MJ, Ponseti IV. Health and function of patients with untreated idiopathic scoliosis: a 50-year natural history study. JAMA. 2003;289(5):559–67.
7. Erwin J, Carlson BB, Bunch J, Jackson RS, Burton D. Impact of unoperated adolescent idiopathic scoliosis in adulthood: a 10-year analysis. Spine Deformity. 2020;8:1009–16.
8. Mayo NE, Goldber MS, Poitras B, Scott S, Hanley J. The Ste-Justine adolescent idiopathic scoliosis cohort study. Part III: back pain. Spine. 1994;19:1573–81.
9. Dickson JH, Mirkovic S, Noble PC, Nalty T, Erwin WD. Results of operative treatment of idiopathic scoliosis in adults. J Bone Joint Surg. 1995;77-A:513–23.
10. Diarbakerli E, Grauers A, Danielsson A, Gerdhem P. Health-related quality of life in adulthood in untreated individuals with adolescent or juvenile idiopathic scoliosis. J Bone Joint Surg. 2018;100(10):811–7.
11. Ahonen M, Syvanen J, Helenius L, Mattila M, Perokorpi T, Diarbakerli E, Gerdhem P, Helenius I. Back pain and quality of life 10 years after segmental pedicle screw instrumentation for adolescent idiopathic scoliosis. Spine. 2023;48(10):665–71.
12. Marks MC, Newton PO, Bastrom TP, Betz RR, Sponseller PD, Lonner B, Shah SA, Samdani A, Petcharaporn M, Shufflebarger H, Asghar J. Surgical site infection in adolescent idiopathic scoliosis surgery. Spine Deformity. 2013;1:352–8.
13. Mallet C, Caseris M, Doit C, Simon AL, Michelet D, Madre C, Mazda K, Bonacorsi S, Ilharreborde B. Does Staphylococcus aureus nasal decontamination affect the rate of early surgical site infection in adolescent idiopathic scoliosis surgery? Eur Spine J. 2018;27:2543–9.
14. Mallet C, Meissburger V, Caseris M, Happiette A, Chinnappa J, Bonacorsi S, Simon AL, Ilharreborde B. Does the use of intrawound povidone-iodine irrigation and local vancomycin powder impact surgical site infection rate in adolescent idiopathic scoliosis surgery? Eur Spine J. 2022;31:3020–8.
15. Poe-Kochert C, Shimberg JL, Thompson GH, Song-Hing JP, Hardesty CK, Mistovich RJ. Surgical site infection prevention protocol for pediatric spinal deformity surgery: does it make a difference? Spine Deformity. 2020;8:931–8.

16. Abola MV, Lin CC, Jin LJ, Schreiber-Stainthorp W, Frempong-Boadu A, Buckland AJ, Protopsaltis TS. Postoperative prophylactic antibiotics in spine surgery: a propensity-matched analysis. J Bone Joint Surg Am. 2021;103(3):219–26.
17. Diab M, Smucny M, Dormans JP, Erickson MA, Ibrahim K, Lenke L, Sucato DJ, Sanders JO. Use and outcomes of wound drain in spinal fusion for adolescent idiopathic scoliosis. Spine. 2012;37(11):966–73.
18. Helenius L, Gerdhem P, Ahonen M, Syvanen J, Jalkanen J, Nietosvaara Y, Helenius I. The impact of closed suction wound drainage on chronic pain and health-related quality of life after posterior spinal fusion in patients with adolescent idiopathic scoliosis. Bone Joint J. 2024;106B(10):1176–81.
19. Suddock J, Crookston K. Transfusion reactions. In: Stat-pearls [internet]. StatPearls Publishing; 2020.
20. Youseff LA, Spitalnik SL. Transfusion-related immunomodulation: a reappraisal. Curr Opin Hematol. 2017;24:551–7
21. Fisahn C, Jeyamohan S, Norvell DC, Tubbs RS, Moisi M, Chapman JR, Page J, Oskouian RJ. Association between allogeneic blood transfusion and postoperative infection in major spine surgery. Clin Spine Surg. 2017;30(7):E988–92.
22. Everhart JS, Sojka JH, Mayerson JL, Glassman AH, Scharschmidt TJ. Perioperative allogeneic red blood-cell transfusion associated with surgical site infection after total hip and knee arthroplasty. J Bone Joint Surg Am. 2018;100(4):288–94.
23. Tumber S, Bacon A, Stondell C, Tafoya S, Taylor SL, Javidan Y, Klineberg E, Roberto R. High- versus low-dose tranexamic acid as part of a patient blood management strategy for reducing blood loss in patients undergoing surgery for adolescent idiopathic scoliosis. Spine Deformity. 2022;10:107–13.
24. Hasan MS, Yunus SN, Ng CC, Chan CYW, Chiu CK, Kwan MK. Tranexamic acid in pediatric scoliosis surgery: a prospective randomized trial comparing high-dose and low-dose tranexamic acid in adolescent idiopathic scoliosis undergoing posterior spinal fusion surgery. Spine. 2021;46(22):E1170–7.
25. Bowen RE, Gardner S, Scaduto AA, Egan M, Beckstead J. Efficacy of intraoperative cell salvage systems in pediatric idiopathic scoliosis patients undergoing posterior spinal fusion with segmental spinal instrumentation. Spine. 2010;35(2):246–51.
26. Wahl GE, Luhmann SL. Intraoperative red blood cell salvage in posterior spinal fusions for idiopathic scoliosis: identifying potential criteria for selective use. Spine Deformity. 2021;9(2):355–63.
27. Weiss JM, Skaggs D, Tanner J, Tolo V. Cell saver: is it beneficial in scoliosis surgery? J Child Orthop. 2007;1:221–7.
28. Chi W, Zhenguo L, Zanquing W, Hao J. A cost-effectiveness analysis of intraoperative autologous transfusion in adolescent idiopathic scoliosis surgery: a single-centre retrospective study. BMC Anesthesiol. 2023;23:211.
29. Bartley CE, Bastrom TP, Newton PO. Blood loss reduction during surgical correction of adolescent idiopathic scoliosis utilizing an ultrasonic bone scalpel. Spine Deformity. 2014;2:285–90.
30. Liu DS, Farid AR, Linden GS, Cook D, Birch CM, Hresko MT, Hedequist DJ, Hogue GD. Utility of postoperative laboratory testing after posterior spinal fusion for adolescent idiopathic scoliosis. Spine Deformity. 2024;12(2):375–81.
31. Kim YJ, Lenke LG, Kim J, et al. Comparative analysis of pedicle screw versus hybrid instrumentation in posterior spinal fusion of adolescent idiopathic scoliosis. Spine. 2006;31:291–8.
32. Dobbs MB, Lenke LG, Kim J, et al. Selective posterior thoracic fusions for adolescent idiopathic scoliosis: comparison of hooks versus pedicle screws. Spine. 2006;31:2400–4.
33. Liljenqvist U, Lepsien U, Hackenberg L, et al. Comparative analysis of pedicle screw and hook instrumentation in posterior correction and fusion of idiopathic thoracic scoliosis. Eur Spine J. 2002;11:336–43.

34. Kuklo TR, Potter BK, Lenke LG, et al. Surgical revision rates of hooks versus hybrid versus screws versus combined anteroposterior spinal fusion for adolescent idiopathic scoliosis. Spine. 2007;32:2258–64.
35. Luhmann SJ, Lenke LG, Kim YJ, Bridwell KH, Schootman M. Thoracic adolescent idiopathic scoliosis between 70 degrees and 100 degrees: is anterior release necessary? Spine. 2005;30(18):2061–7.
36. Martin CT, Pugely AJ, Gao Y, Mendoza-Lattes SA, Ilgenfritz RM, Callaghan JJ, Weinstein SL. Increasing hospital charges for adolescent idiopathic scoliosis in the United States. Spine. 2014;39(20):1676–82.
37. Larson AN, Polly DW, Sponseller PD, et al. The effect of implant density on adolescent idiopathic scoliosis fusion. J Bone Joint Surg Am. 2024;106:180–9.
38. Cheng I, Kim Y, Gupta MC, et al. Apical sublaminar wires versus pedicle screws—which provides better results for surgical correction of adolescent idiopathic scoliosis? Spine. 2005;30:2104–12.
39. Larson AN, Aubin CE, Polly DW, et al. Are more screws better? A systematic review of anchor density and curve correction in adolescent idiopathic scoliosis. Spine Deform. 2013;1:237–47.
40. Larson AN, Polly DW, Diamond B, Ledonio C, Richards BS, Emans JB, Sucato DJ, Johnston CE. Does higher anchor density result in increased curve correction and improved clinical outcomes in adolescent idiopathic scoliosis? Spine. 2014;39(7):571–8.
41. Storer SK, Vitale MG, Hyman JE, et al. Correction of adolescent idiopathic scoliosis using thoracic pedicle screw fixation versus hook constructs. J Pediatr Orthop. 2005;25:415–9.
42. Sarwahi V, Hasan S, Rao H, Visahan K, et al. Does a dedicated "scoliosis team" and surgical standardization improve outcomes in adolescent idiopathic scoliosis surgery and is it reproducible? Spine Deformity. 2023;11:1409–18.
43. Murgai RR, Andras LM, Neilsen E, Scott G, Gould H, Skaggs DL. Dedicated spine nurses and scrub technicians improve intraoperative efficiency of surgery for adolescent idiopathic scoliosis. Spine Deformity. 2020;8:171–6.
44. Martin BD, Gordish-Dressman H, Mirzada A, Kelly SM, Pestieau SR, Cronin J, Oetgen ME. A dedicated surgical team for posterior spinal fusion in patients with adolescent idiopathic scoliosis improves OR efficiency. Spine Deformity. 2023;11:643–9.
45. Fletcher ND, Andras LM, Lazarus DE, et al. Use of a novel pathway for early discharge was associated with a 48% shorter length of stay after posterior spinal fusion for adolescent idiopathic scoliosis. J Pediatr Orthop. 2017;37(2):92–7.
46. Gornitzky AL, Flynn JM, Muhly WT, Sankar WN. A rapid recovery pathway for adolescent idiopathic scoliosis that improves pain control and reduces time to inpatient recovery after posterior spinal fusion. Spine Deformity. 2016;4(4):288–95.
47. Muhly WT, Sankar WN, Ryan K, et al. Rapid recovery pathway after spinal fusion for adolescent idiopathic scoliosis. Pediatrics. 2016;137(4):e20151568.
48. Sanders A, Andras L, Sousa T, Kissinger C, Cucchiaro G, Skaggs DL. Accelerated discharge protocol for posterior spinal fusion patients with adolescent idiopathic scoliosis decreases hospital post-operative charges 22. Spine. 2017;42(2):92–7.
49. Boylan MR, Riesgo AM, Chu A, Paulino CB, Feldman DS. Costs and complications of increased length of stay following adolescent idiopathic scoliosis surgery. J Pediatr Orthop B. 2019;28(1):27–31.
50. Gadiya AD, Koch JEJ, Patel MS, Shafafy M, Grevitt MP, Quraishi NA. Enhanced recovery after surgery (ERAS) in adolescent idiopathic scoliosis (AIS): a meta-analysis and systematic review. Spine Deformity. 2021;9:893–904.
51. Fletcher ND, Murphy JS, Austin TM, et al. Short term outcomes of an enhanced recovery after surgery (ERAS) pathway versus a traditional discharge pathway after posterior spinal fusion for adolescent idiopathic scoliosis. Spine Deformity. 2021;9:1013–9.
52. Kwan MK, Chan CYW. Does a dual attending surgeon strategy confer additional benefit for posterior selective thoracic fusion in Lenke 1 and 2 adolescent idiopathic scoliosis (AIS)? A prospective propensity matching score analysis. Spine J. 17:224–9.

53. Kwan MK, Chiu CK, Chan CYW. Single vs two attending senior surgeons: assessment of intraoperative blood loss at different surgical stages of posterior spinal fusion sugery in Lenke 1 and 2 adolescent idiopathic scoliosis. Eur Spine J. 2017;26:155–61.
54. Warren JR, Link RC, Bonanni S, McKenna NC, Anderson JT, Schwend RM. Two AIS cases, 2 surgeons, 1 operating room, 1 day: faster and safer than 1 case in a day. J Pediatr Orthop. 2024;44(8):502–7.
55. McKenna NC, Hagaman D, Sipp B, Qureshi F, Warren JR, Kaji E, Sherman A, Schwend RM. The effect of surgical time on perioperative complications in adolescent idiopathic scoliosis cases. A propensity score analysis. Spine Deformity. 2024;12(4):1053–60.
56. Haber LL, Womack ED, Sathyamoorthy M, Moss JA, Shrader MW. Who needs a pediatric intensive care unit after posterior spinal fusion for adolescent idiopathic scoliosis? Spine Deformity. 2018;6:137–40.

Methods to Improve Value When Treating Children with Early-Onset Scoliosis

34

Ellen Tahmasyan, Tyler A. Tetreault, and Michael J. Heffernan

Introduction

Early-onset scoliosis (EOS) encompasses a complex group of conditions, including congenital, syndromic, neuromuscular, and idiopathic scoliosis [1]. The unifying theme of EOS is the age of onset occurring before 10 years of age [2]. The early development of scoliosis presents unique challenges distinct from scoliosis with later onset. In EOS, treatment involves competing priorities. Preserving spinal and thoracic growth is important for achieving appropriate height and adequate thoracic cage volume. Fusion halts growth at the instrumented segment which is an undesirable outcome for younger, smaller patients. This leads to a fundamental conflict in EOS management: the need to control spinal deformity while simultaneously preserving spinal and thoracic growth.

Value Based Themes

Minimize Anesthetic Events in EOS Patients

Historically, casting had a major role in the treatment of scoliosis. At the turn of the twentieth century, corrective casting combined with spinal fusion was the standard surgical management [3, 4]. Over time, casting and fusion was replaced with

E. Tahmasyan
Children's Hospital Los Angeles, Los Angeles, CA, USA
e-mail: etahmasyan@chla.usc.edu

T. A. Tetreault · M. J. Heffernan (✉)
Department of Orthopaedic Surgery, Children's Hospital Los Angeles, Keck School of Medicine at USC, Los Angeles, CA, USA
e-mail: ttetreault@chla.usc.edu; mheffernan@chla.usc.edu

W. L. Hennrikus, R. M. Schwend (eds.), *Value in Pediatric Orthopaedics*,
https://doi.org/10.1007/978-3-032-19570-8_34

instrumented fusion [5]. More recently, Mehta and colleagues helped reestablish casting as a viable treatment for early-onset scoliosis (EOS) [6]. Multiple studies have shown that casting can serve as definitive treatment for EOS patients with curves under 60 degrees when casting is initiated before the age of 2 years old [7, 8]. Others have highlighted the utility of casting as a means to delay the need for growth-friendly instrumentation [9]. Despite these benefits, casting has drawbacks. Casting is typically performed under general anesthesia, and casts are usually changed every 2–4 months, necessitating repeated anesthetics (Fig. 34.1) [10, 11]. In 2016, the Federal Drug Administration raised concerns about potential negative neurodevelopmental effects of anesthesia in children under 3 years of age [12]. This population overlaps significantly with EOS patients undergoing casting. In response, alternative methods of cast application have been developed. For example, in a series of 155 patients, Kawakami et al. reported the application of casting performed in the clinic rather than the operating room (OR) [13]. Clinic-based casting enhances value by reducing exposure of the child to an anesthetic, saving operating room time, and minimizing costs.

Consider Bracing for Delay Technique in Medically Complex Patients

Although casting can resolve scoliosis in select young patients [6], not all patients experience curve resolution [14]. In these cases, particularly in medically complex children, the goal of casting shifts from definitive treatment to delaying the need for growth-friendly instrumentation [9, 14, 15]. Casting in the OR involves significant use of OR time, surgical and anesthesia services, and hospital resources. For medically complex patients, repeated anesthetic exposures carry additional risks [16]. In EOS cases where the intent is to delay surgical intervention rather than achieve definitive fusion, bracing offers an alternative treatment with less burden to the

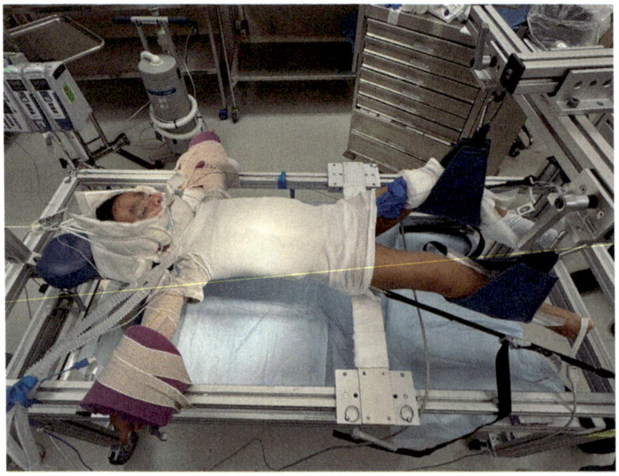

Fig. 34.1 Positioning on the EDF casting table

patient, family, and medical system. Unfortunately, evidence supporting brace effectiveness in one type of EOS, neuromuscular scoliosis, remains limited [17, 18].

Minimize Clinic Visits for Casting Patients

Early-onset scoliosis (EOS) necessitates long-term follow-up until age 18 years old or older. Long-term follow-up places additional burdens on patients and their families [19]. In fact, McFadden et al. reported that parents of children with EOS miss an average of 18 workdays annually, resulting in an associated income loss of $3643, along with a median travel cost of $1656 [20]. For patients undergoing serial casting, reducing unnecessary interim clinic visits can add value. For example, the surgeon can use preoperative and postoperative recovery room discussions at the time of casting to convey key clinical information that would otherwise be discussed during a separate clinic follow-up visit (Fig. 34.2).

Minimize Imaging Studies

Children are especially vulnerable to the harmful effects of ionizing radiation due to their rapidly dividing cells and longer life expectancy [21, 22]. In scoliosis patients, repeated imaging has been linked to later development of breast cancer [23].

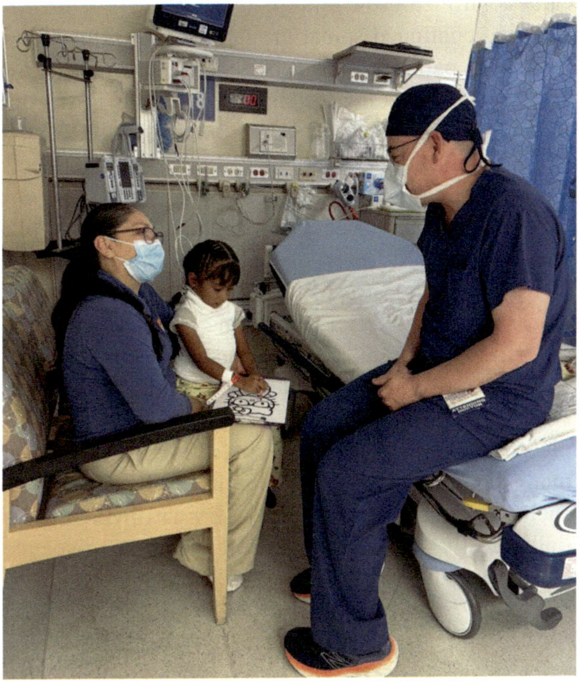

Fig. 34.2 Having a "clinic visit" at the time of casting in the recovery room

Minimizing radiation exposure to children must remain a high priority. The ALARA principle for radiation exposure in children, "as low as reasonably achievable," was established to balance diagnostic utility with patient safety. In pediatric patients, radiation exposure during spine surgery can exceed 30 mSv [24]. Mundis et al. reported that EOS patients treated with growing rods received 3.4 times the annual background radiation dose [25]. Biplanar slot-scan radiography systems have been developed and provide lower radiation dose compared to conventional X-rays [26]. When used in conjunction with thoughtful imaging intervals, biplanar slot-scan technology can substantially decrease the cumulative radiation dose to children with EOS. Further strategies to reduce radiation include the use of ultrasound in place of radiographs to monitor lengthening of magnetically controlled growth rods (MCGR) [27, 28]. Conversely, spinal navigation systems that rely on CT imaging contribute to increased radiation doses [29]. A critical and selective approach to the use of CT-based technologies in EOS care is needed.

Delay the Use of Growth-Friendly Instrumentation

Timing of surgery for EOS presents a challenge due to competing clinical priorities. Growth is critical for achieving sufficient thoracic volume to support long-term cardiac and pulmonary function [30]. At the same time, growth accelerates spinal curve progression. Ideally, growth-friendly instrumentation such as vertical expandable prosthetic titanium ribs (VEPTR), traditional growing rods (TGR), and magnetically controlled growing rods (MCGR) can be used to control the scoliosis while allowing continued spinal growth [31, 32]. However, this goal is not always realized. EOS patients often experience reduced growth over time and are at risk for complications leading to unplanned returns to the operating room (UPROR) [33, 34]. Once growth-friendly instrumentation (GFI) is placed, a finite "treatment clock" begins. For example, Sankar et al. introduced the concept of the "law of diminishing returns," wherein patients experience progressively less spinal lengthening with each subsequent procedure [35]. This likely occurs due to increasing spinal stiffness, or "auto-fusion," that develops over time following GFI placement and lengthening [36]. Most patients experience spinal growth for approximately 5 years after GFI [37]. For example, a patient undergoing GFI at age 2 may demonstrate auto-fusion and diminished growth by age 7. In addition, McIntosh et al. reported a 40% UPROR rate due to complications in patients with MCGR, while Anari et al. found a 23% UPROR rate within the first 2 years after growing rod placement [33, 38]. Due to the reduction in growth over time and expected UPROR, many surgeons delay the initiation of GFI through the use of stalling techniques such as casting and bracing [39]. By narrowing the exposure window to the potentially costly and high-risk complications associated with GFI, this strategy enhances value.

The Cost of Instrumentation for Early-Onset Scoliosis

Advancements in both instrumentation types and treatment strategies for EOS have occurred. Karol et al. reported that instrumented fusion is suboptimal for young patients with significant remaining growth [30]. In response, a variety of distraction-based, growth-friendly techniques have been developed including VEPTR, TGR, and MCGR [40, 41]. The advantage of MCGR lies in its ability to avoid the repeated surgical procedures in the OR required for lengthening with VEPTR and TGR. In contrast, MCGR can be lengthened noninvasively in clinic [42–44]. Multiple studies have compared the costs of TGR versus MCGR [45–48]. Cheung et al. reported that MCGR has a higher initial cost; however, cost neutrality is reached in about 2–3 years postimplantation [46]. Similarly, Charroin et al. reported that over a 4-year time period, MCGR had lower costs [47]. Interestingly, Oetgen noted that the initial costs of MCGR, related primarily to implant pricing, are borne by the hospital, while the long-term cost savings benefit the insurance company rather than the hospital or the patient [48].

One alternative to distraction-based techniques is the Shilla growth technique, which involves selective fusion at the apex of the curve while allowing growth at the proximal and distal ends of the construct [49]. The Shilla method eliminates the need for repeated lengthening. In a cost analysis of Shilla, TGR, and MCGR, Luhmann et al. reported that Shilla resulted in lower costs when evaluated over a 6-year time period [50]. Further research is needed to refine indications for each implant type for EOS. For now, tailoring the instrumentation to the individual patient's needs offers the greatest potential to optimize value.

Lengthen Every 3 Months, Not Every 6 Weeks for MCGR

For patients treated with MCGR, it is important to consider the impact of lengthening frequency on the patient and their family. While the typical interval for MCGR lengthening is every 3 months, some have proposed more frequent lengthening of every 6 weeks [51]. This contrasts with the TGR lengthening schedule, which typically occurs every 6 months and may be extended to every 9–12 months in select cases [52]. However, MCGR replaces repeated surgical lengthening procedures in the OR with noninvasive, office-based lengthening (Fig. 34.3) [53]. Despite the theoretical benefit of less trips to the OR, MCGR has not been shown to improve mental health outcomes [54]. Possibly, the increased frequency of clinic visits required for MCGR lengthening introduces additional stress for EOS patients and families. As such, optimizing lengthening intervals is an important consideration in balancing clinical outcomes with patient mental health outcomes.

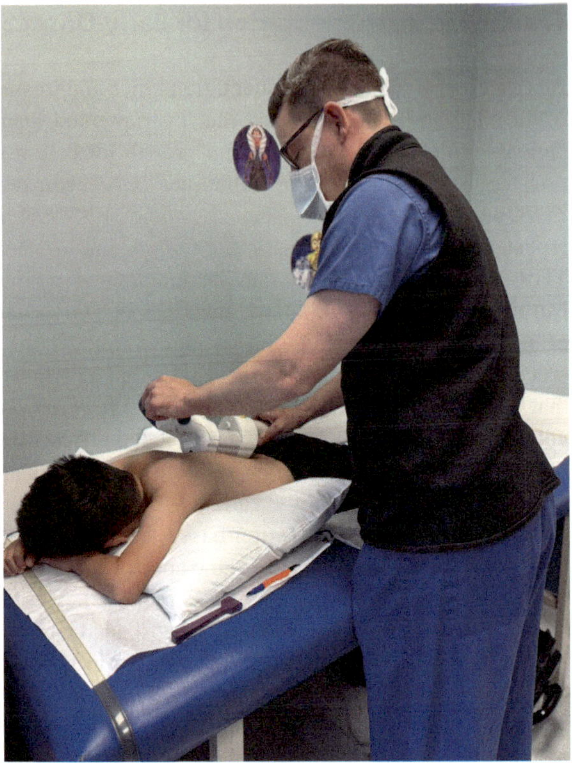

Fig. 34.3 Lengthening MCGR in clinic

Don't Use GFI for Most Tweeners: Wait for a Definitive Fusion

A recent consensus paper defined "tweeners" as females aged 8–10 years and males aged 9–11 years [55]. Although initial enthusiasm surrounded the use of growth-friendly techniques such as MCGR in this age group, recent evidence has prompted a shift toward fusion [56]. Keil et al. found that MCGR resulted in about 2 cm of additional height compared to PSF, but this height benefit came at the cost of increased complications and higher revision surgery rates [57]. In older EOS patients, Mackey et al. demonstrated that both vertebral body tethering and PSF were associated with lower rates of unplanned revision surgery compared to MCGR [58]. Yoshida et al. reported that MCGR patients were more likely to have a caudal lowest instrumented vertebra (LIV) compared to those treated with PSF. This finding may result in later adjacent segment disc degeneration [59]. In the largest single-center study of EOS tweener patients, Xu et al. concluded that PSF was the preferable approach for most patients aged 9–11 years with congenital scoliosis, citing superior deformity correction and fewer complications [60]. Overall, for tweener patients, definitive PSF offers the advantages of fewer surgeries, reduced complication rates, lower overall cost, and improved value.

Outcome

Due to the spectrum of diagnoses and curve patterns included within EOS, treatment outcomes are understandably variable. The treatment of EOS ends in many patients with a definitive PSF; however, select patients undergo continuing observation. Nonetheless, studies consistently show that active management of EOS results in better outcomes compared to the natural history of the untreated disease [61].

Case Example

A 7-month-old boy presented for evaluation of a subtle spinal prominence. His medical history was notable for Larsen syndrome, autism, obstructive sleep apnea, pulmonary hypoplasia, gastrostomy tube dependence, and clubfoot. Initial X-rays revealed a 21-degree scoliosis with a rib-vertebral angle difference (RVAD) of less than 20 degrees. Observation was recommended (Fig. 34.4).

At 33 months of age, the scoliosis had progressed to 36 degrees. MRI revealed a low-lying conus (Fig. 34.5), prompting referral to neurosurgery to evaluate for tethered cord syndrome. The neurosurgical team determined that no intervention was required at that time. Observation continued. At 3.5 years of age, the scoliosis had progressed to 62 degrees and was associated with a significant kyphosis (Fig. 34.6). Casting was initiated at an outside hospital, where the patient received four casts prior to transferring care to our center. We subsequently placed three more elongation-derotation-flexion (EDF) casts in an effort to further delay the placement of GFI (Fig. 34.7).

By age 6, the curve was no longer controlled with casting and MCGR were implanted (Fig. 34.8). Initially, as part of a research protocol, MCGR lengthening were performed every 6 weeks in clinic; however, due to the emotional and

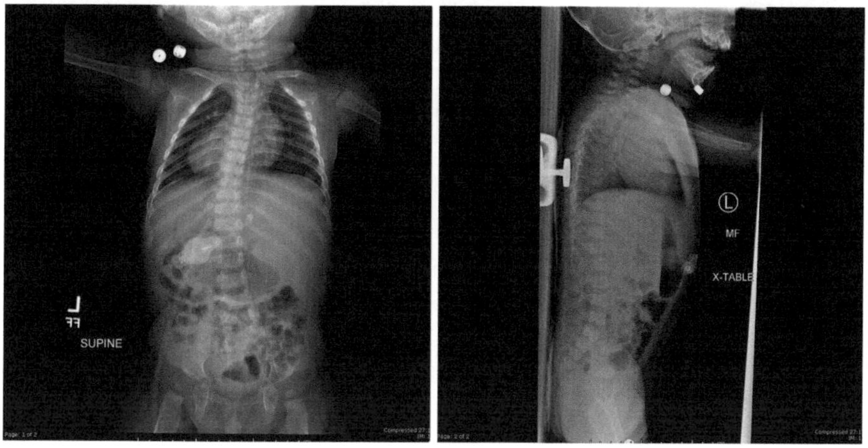

Fig. 34.4 PA and lateral radiographs at 7 months' old

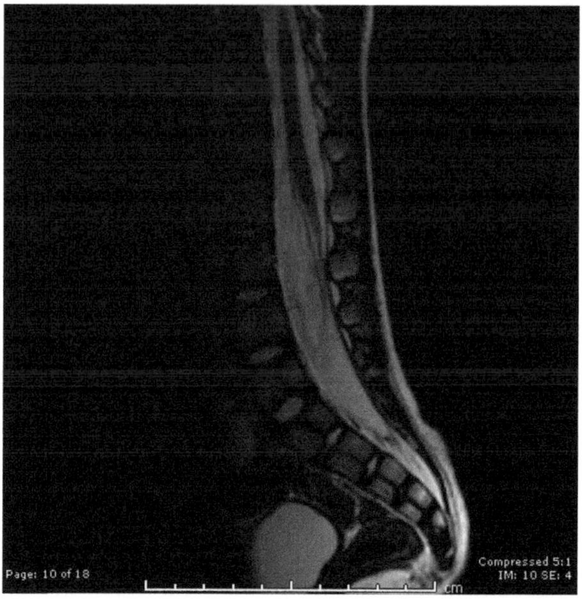

Fig. 34.5 MRI showing low-lying conus

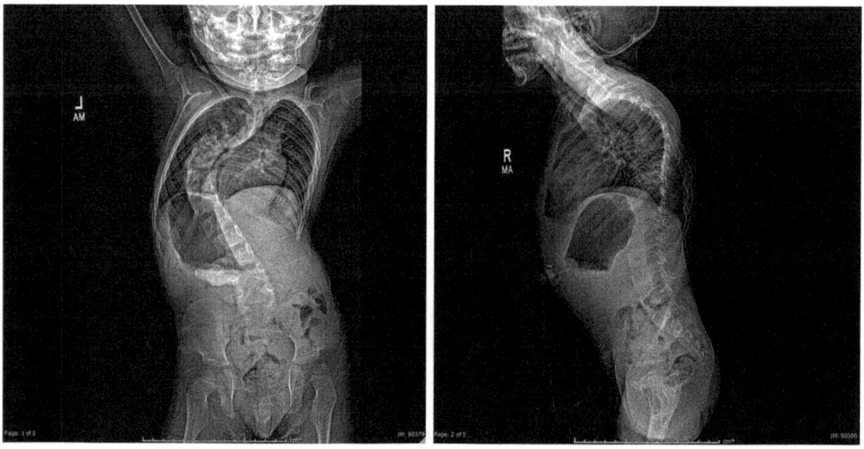

Fig. 34.6 Curve progression at age 3.5 years with new recommendation for casting

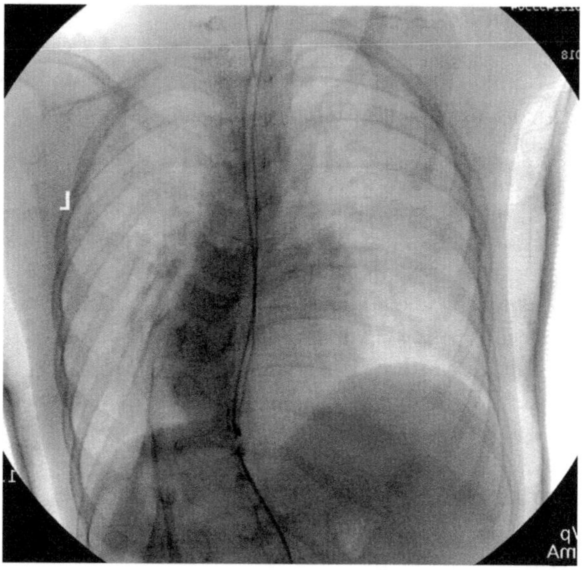

Fig. 34.7 Intraoperative radiograph of in-cast curve correction

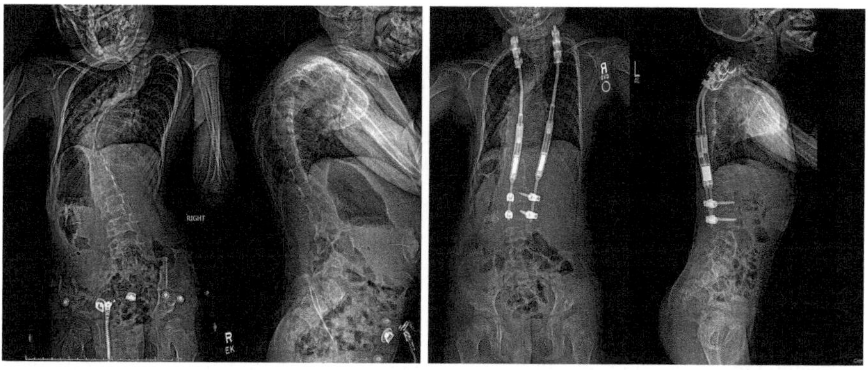

Fig. 34.8 PA and lateral radiographs prior to MCGR and at 1-year follow-up

logistical stress on the family, the interval was adjusted to every 3 months at the parent's request. To date, the patient remains stable and has not experienced any complications such as unplanned return to the operating room.

Summary

Multiple strategies can be employed to enhance value in the care of patients with EOS. The current chapter outlines eight practical recommendations that improve value by reducing costs and decreasing stress on patients and families while maintaining excellent outcomes.

Author Pearls

- Minimize the number of anesthetic exposure in EOS patients.
- Consider bracing for medically complex children when the primary goal is to delay the initiation of GFI.
- Use casting appointments as opportunities for clinical evaluation and family discussion to reduce the need for separate clinic visits and reduce travel burden.
- Follow the ALARA principles as much as possible to reduce radiation exposure.
- Delay the insertion of GFI when possible.
- Tailor the choice of GFI to the individual patient, taking into account clinical needs, expected benefits, and cost implications.
- Schedule MCGR lengthening every 3 months.
- Perform definitive PSF in "tweener" patients when appropriate.

Editor Comments

WLH

EOS is a bear. Treatment continues to evolve and is guided by the severity and progression of the scoliosis. Depending on individual patient factors, management may involve observation, casting, bracing, and/or surgery. The goal is to control scoliosis progression while allowing normal spine and lung development. This comprehensive, evidence-based chapter outlines eight practical, high-value strategies to optimize care for children with EOS.

RMS

One key contributor to value in EOS care is the interdisciplinary care model. Coordinated efforts among orthopedic surgeons, pulmonologists, anesthesiologists, neurologists, hospitalists, and primary care providers improve clinical decision-making, reduce redundant testing, minimize complications, and enhance the family experience particularly for medically complex patients. These collaborative approaches are linked to better outcomes and lower costs in pediatric complex care. Moving forward, value-driven strategies in EOS should continue to formalize and strengthen interdisciplinary collaboration.

References

1. Fletcher ND, Bruce RW. Early onset scoliosis: current concepts and controversies. Curr Rev Musculoskelet Med. 2012;5(2):102–10.
2. Hughes MS, Swarup I, Makarewich CA, Williams BA, Talwar D, Cahill PJ, et al. Expert consensus for early onset scoliosis surgery. J Pediatr Orthop. 2020;40(7):e621–e8.

3. Risser JC. The application of body casts for the correction of scoliosis. Instr Course Lect. 1955;12:255–9.
4. Khan MJ, Srinivasan VM, Jea AH. The history of bracing for scoliosis. Clin Pediatr (Phila). 2016;55(4):320–5.
5. Harrington PR. Treatment of scoliosis. Correction and internal fixation by spine instrumentation. J Bone Joint Surg Am. 1962;44-A:591–610.
6. Mehta MH. Growth as a corrective force in the early treatment of progressive infantile scoliosis. J Bone Joint Surg Br. 2005;87(9):1237–47.
7. Sanders JO, D'Astous J, Fitzgerald M, Khoury JG, Kishan S, Sturm PF. Derotational casting for progressive infantile scoliosis. J Pediatr Orthop. 2009;29(6):581–7.
8. Welborn MC, D'Astous J, Bratton S, Heflin J. Infantile idiopathic scoliosis: factors affecting EDF casting success. Spine Deform. 2018;6(5):614–20.
9. Fletcher ND, McClung A, Rathjen KE, Denning JR, Browne R, Johnston CE 3rd. Serial casting as a delay tactic in the treatment of moderate-to-severe early-onset scoliosis. J Pediatr Orthop. 2012;32(7):664–71.
10. Dede O, Sturm PF. A brief history and review of modern casting techniques in early onset scoliosis. J Child Orthop. 2016;10(5):405–11.
11. Bonsignore-Opp L, Malka MS, Ball J, Simhon ME, Matsumoto H, Sturm P, et al. Institutional variability in anesthesia time for Mehta casting in early-onset scoliosis (EOS). J Pediatr Orthop. 2024;44(5):297–302.
12. Administration USFaD. FDA Drug Safety Communication: FDA review results in new warnings about using general anesthetics and sedation drugs in young children and pregnant women 2016. Available from: https://www.fda.gov/drugs/drug-safety-and-availability/fda-drug-safety-communication-fda-review-results-new-warnings-about-using-general-anesthetics-and
13. Kawakami K, Saito T, Tauchi R, Ohara T, Kawakami N. Nonanesthetized alternatively repetitive cast and brace treatment for early-onset scoliosis. J Pediatr Orthop. 2020;40(8):e720–e7.
14. Waldron SR, Poe-Kochert C, Son-Hing JP, Thompson GH. Early onset scoliosis: the value of serial risser casts. J Pediatr Orthop. 2013;33(8):775–80.
15. LaValva S, Adams A, MacAlpine E, Gupta P, Hammerberg K, Thompson GH, et al. Serial casting in neuromuscular and syndromic early-onset scoliosis (EOS) can delay surgery over 2 years. J Pediatr Orthop. 2020;40(8):e772–e9.
16. Baky FJ, Milbrandt TA, Flick R, Larson AN. Cumulative anesthesia exposure in patients treated for early-onset scoliosis. Spine Deform. 2018;6(6):781–6.
17. Bellamy M, Tung WS, Jayasuriya R, Hind D, Swaby L, Totton N, et al. Bracing effectiveness in idiopathic early onset scoliosis followed to skeletal maturity: a systematic review and meta-analysis. Spine Deform. 2025;13(3):939–50.
18. Li Y, Swallow J, Gagnier J, Thompson GH, Sturm PF, Emans JB, et al. A report of two conservative approaches to early onset scoliosis: serial casting and bracing. Spine Deform. 2021;9(2):595–602.
19. Campbell M, Matsumoto H, St Hilaire T, Roye BD, Roye DP, Vitale MG. Burden of care in families of patients with early onset scoliosis. J Pediatr Orthop B. 2020;29(6):567–71.
20. McFadden RJ, Hauth L, Gregoski M, Anari JB, Brooks JT, Sawyer JR, et al. A multicenter evaluation of the time and travel burden on families with children treated for early-onset scoliosis. Spine Deform. 2024;12(5):1453–8.
21. Law M, Ma WK, Lau D, Chan E, Yip L, Lam W. Cumulative radiation exposure and associated cancer risk estimates for scoliosis patients: impact of repetitive full spine radiography. Eur J Radiol. 2016;85(3):625–8.
22. Luan FJ, Wan Y, Mak KC, Ma CJ, Wang HQ. Cancer and mortality risks of patients with scoliosis from radiation exposure: a systematic review and meta-analysis. Eur Spine J. 2020;29(12):3123–34.
23. Doody MM, Lonstein JE, Stovall M, Hacker DG, Luckyanov N, Land CE. Breast cancer mortality after diagnostic radiography: findings from the U.S. Scoliosis Cohort Study. Spine (Phila Pa 1976). 2000;25(16):2052–63.

24. Sugawara R, Watanabe H, Taki N, Onuma S, Kikkawa I, Takeshita K. Radiation exposure in pediatric patients with early onset scoliosis: a longitudinal single-center study. J Orthop Sci. 2024;29(4):1103–7.
25. Mundis GM Jr, Pawelek JB, Nomoto EK, Hennessy MW, Yaszay B, Akbarnia BA. Longitudinal pilot analysis of radiation exposure during the course of growing rod treatment for early-onset scoliosis. Spine Deform. 2016;4(1):55–8.
26. Deschenes S, Charron G, Beaudoin G, Labelle H, Dubois J, Miron MC, et al. Diagnostic imaging of spinal deformities: reducing patients radiation dose with a new slot-scanning X-ray imager. Spine (Phila Pa 1976). 2010;35(9):989–94.
27. Stokes OM, O'Donovan EJ, Samartzis D, Bow CH, Luk KD, Cheung KM. Reducing radiation exposure in early-onset scoliosis surgery patients: novel use of ultrasonography to measure lengthening in magnetically-controlled growing rods. Spine J. 2014;14(10):2397–404.
28. Cheung JP, Bow C, Samartzis D, Ganal-Antonio AK, Cheung KM. Clinical utility of ultrasound to prospectively monitor distraction of magnetically controlled growing rods. Spine J. 2016;16(2):204–9.
29. Mendelsohn D, Strelzow J, Dea N, Ford NL, Batke J, Pennington A, et al. Patient and surgeon radiation exposure during spinal instrumentation using intraoperative computed tomography-based navigation. Spine J. 2016;16(3):343–54.
30. Karol LA. Early definitive spinal fusion in young children: what we have learned. Clin Orthop Relat Res. 2011;469(5):1323–9.
31. Akbarnia BA, Marks DS, Boachie-Adjei O, Thompson AG, Asher MA. Dual growing rod technique for the treatment of progressive early-onset scoliosis: a multicenter study. Spine (Phila Pa 1976). 2005;30(17 Suppl):S46–57.
32. Murphy RF, Barfield WR, Emans JB, Akbarnia B, Thompson G, Sponseller P, et al. Minimum 5-year follow-up on graduates of growing spine surgery for early onset scoliosis. J Pediatr Orthop. 2020;40(10):e942–e6.
33. Anari JB, Flynn JM, Cahill PJ, Vitale MG, Smith JT, Gomez JA, et al. Unplanned return to OR (UPROR) for children with early onset scoliosis (EOS): a comprehensive evaluation of all diagnoses and instrumentation strategies. Spine Deform. 2020;8(2):295–302.
34. Bess S, Akbarnia BA, Thompson GH, Sponseller PD, Shah SA, El Sebaie H, et al. Complications of growing-rod treatment for early-onset scoliosis: analysis of one hundred and forty patients. J Bone Joint Surg Am. 2010;92(15):2533–43.
35. Sankar WN, Skaggs DL, Yazici M, Johnston CE 2nd, Shah SA, Javidan P, et al. Lengthening of dual growing rods and the law of diminishing returns. Spine (Phila Pa 1976). 2011;36(10):806–9.
36. Cahill PJ, Marvil S, Cuddihy L, Schutt C, Idema J, Clements DH, et al. Autofusion in the immature spine treated with growing rods. Spine (Phila Pa 1976). 2010;35(22):E1199–203.
37. Menapace B, Jain V, Sturm P. Autofusion in early-onset scoliosis growing constructs: occurrence, risk factors, and impacts. Spine Deform. 2024;12(4):1155–63.
38. McIntosh AL, Booth A, Oetgen ME. Unplanned return to the operating room (UPROR) occurs in 40% of MCGR patients at an average of 2 years after initial implantation. Spine Deform. 2024;12(6):1823–9.
39. Cetik RM, Yazici M. The hidden cost of growth-friendly treatment for early onset scoliosis. J Pediatr Orthop Soc North Am. 2022;4(4)
40. Maccaferri B, Vommaro F, Cini C, Filardo G, Boriani L, Gasbarrini A. Surgical treatment of early-onset scoliosis: traditional growing rod vs. magnetically controlled growing rod vs. vertical expandable prosthesis titanium ribs. J Clin Med. 2024;14(1)
41. Bachabi M, McClung A, Pawelek JB, El Hawary R, Thompson GH, Smith JT, et al. Idiopathic early-onset scoliosis: growing rods versus vertically expandable prosthetic titanium ribs at 5-year follow-up. J Pediatr Orthop. 2020;40(3):142–8.
42. Peiro-Garcia A, Bourget-Murray J, Suarez-Lorenzo I, Ferri-De-Barros F, Parsons D. Early complications in vertical expandable prosthetic titanium rib and magnetically controlled growing rods to manage early onset scoliosis. Int J Spine Surg. 2021;15(2):368–75.

43. Hickey BA, Towriss C, Baxter G, Yasso S, James S, Jones A, et al. Early experience of MAGEC magnetic growing rods in the treatment of early onset scoliosis. Eur Spine J. 2014;23 Suppl 1(Suppl 1):S61–5.
44. Garg S, Kim E, Gupta P, Pediatric Spine Study G. Optimizing expansion clinic for patients with magnetic controlled growth rods. J Am Acad Orthop Surg. 2022;30(10):437.
45. Polly DW Jr, Ackerman SJ, Schneider K, Pawelek JB, Akbarnia BA. Cost analysis of magnetically controlled growing rods compared with traditional growing rods for early-onset scoliosis in the US: an integrated health care delivery system perspective. Clinicoecon Outcomes Res. 2016;8:457–65.
46. Cheung PWH, Wong CKH, Sadiang-Abay JT, Lau ST, Cheung JPY. Longitudinal comparison of direct medical cost, radiological and health-related quality of life treatment outcomes between traditional growing rods and magnetically controlled growing rods from preoperative to maturity. BMC Musculoskelet Disord. 2022;23(1):791.
47. Charroin C, Abelin-Genevois K, Cunin V, Berthiller J, Constant H, Kohler R, et al. Direct costs associated with the management of progressive early onset scoliosis: estimations based on gold standard technique or with magnetically controlled growing rods. Orthop Traumatol Surg Res. 2014;100(5):469–74.
48. Oetgen ME, McNulty EM, Matthews AL. Cost-effectiveness of magnetically controlled growing rods: who really benefits? Spine Deform. 2019;7(3):501–4.
49. McCarthy RE, McCullough FL. Shilla growth guidance for early-onset scoliosis: results after a minimum of five years of follow-up. J Bone Joint Surg Am. 2015;97(19):1578–84.
50. Luhmann SJ, McAughey EM, Ackerman SJ, Bumpass DB, McCarthy RE. Cost analysis of a growth guidance system compared with traditional and magnetically controlled growing rods for early-onset scoliosis: a US-based integrated health care delivery system perspective. Clinicoecon Outcomes Res. 2018;10:179–87.
51. Saw SZW, Wei JZ, Cheung JPY, Kwan KYH, Pediatric Spine Study G, Cheung KMC. Increased lengthening frequency does not adversely affect the EOSQ scores in magnetically controlled growing rod surgeries in 133 subjects followed to final fusion. Spine Deform. 2024;12(6):1841–50.
52. Helenius IJ. Standard and magnetically controlled growing rods for the treatment of early onset scoliosis. Ann Transl Med. 2020;8(2):26.
53. Aslan C, Olgun ZD, Ayik G, Karaokur R, Ozusta S, Demirkiran GH, et al. Does decreased surgical stress really improve the psychosocial health of early-onset scoliosis patients?: a comparison of traditional growing rods and magnetically-controlled growing rods patients reveals disappointing results. Spine (Phila Pa 1976). 2019;44(11):E656–E63.
54. Doany ME, Olgun ZD, Kinikli GI, Bekmez S, Kocyigit A, Demirkiran G, et al. Health-related quality of life in early-onset scoliosis patients treated surgically: EOSQ scores in traditional growing rod versus magnetically controlled growing rods. Spine (Phila Pa 1976). 2018;43(2):148–53.
55. Quan T, Matsumoto H, Bonsignore-Opp L, Ramo B, Murphy RF, Brooks JT, et al. Definition of Tweener: consensus among experts in treating early-onset scoliosis. J Pediatr Orthop. 2023;43(3):e215–e22.
56. Li Y, Swallow J, Gagnier J, Cahill PJ, Sponseller PD, Garg S, et al. Growth-friendly surgery results in more growth but a higher complication rate and unplanned returns to the operating room compared to single fusion in neuromuscular early-onset scoliosis: a multicenter retrospective cohort study. Spine Deform. 2021;9(3):851–8.
57. Keil LG, Nash AB, Sturmer T, Golightly YM, Lin FC, Stone JD, et al. When is a growth-friendly strategy warranted? A matched comparison of growing rods versus primary posterior spinal fusion in juveniles with early-onset scoliosis. J Pediatr Orthop. 2021;41(10):e859–e64.
58. Mackey C, Hanstein R, Lo Y, Vaughan M, St Hilaire T, Luhmann SJ, et al. Magnetically Controlled Growing Rods (MCGR) versus Single Posterior Spinal Fusion (PSF) versus Vertebral Body Tether (VBT) in older early onset scoliosis (EOS) patients: how do early outcomes compare? Spine (Phila Pa 1976). 2022;47(4):295–302.

59. Yoshida B, Leonardi C, Valenzuela-Moss J, Andras LM, Tetreault TA, Emans JB, et al. LIV selection in 'tweener' patients treated with magnetically controlled growing rods vs. posterior spinal fusion. Spine Deform. 2025;13(3):765–71.
60. Xu L, Sun X, Du C, Zhou Q, Shi B, Zhu Z, et al. Is growth-friendly surgical treatment superior to one-stage posterior spinal fusion in 9- to 11-year-old children with congenital scoliosis? Clin Orthop Relat Res. 2020;478(10):2375–86.
61. Karol LA. The natural history of early-onset scoliosis. J Pediatr Orthop. 2019;39(Issue 6, Supplement 1 Suppl 1):S38–43.

35 Value-Based Care for Pediatric Patients with Spondylolysis

Kyriakos Chatzis and Douglas Armstrong

Introduction

Back pain is a common reason for visits to pediatric orthopedic practices [1]. For clinicians, the primary challenge is distinguishing between those with spine disorders that need surgical intervention and those that can be treated conservatively.

Spondylolysis is the most common cause of lower back pain in pediatric athletes [2, 3]. Prompt treatment can alleviate pain and facilitate an earlier return to play. In this chapter, we explore the evaluation and management of spondylolysis in children and adolescents through the lens of value-based care. There are opportunities to enhance value-based care in both the evaluation and treatment of spondylolysis.

Spondylolysis is a defect in the vertebral pars interarticularis. Traditionally, it was believed that 90% of lesions occurred at the L5 level [4]. However, with advances in MRI technology, clinicians are increasingly identifying pars abnormalities in the upper lumbar spine, both singly and in combination [5, 6]. For example, Kriz et al., in a study including both stress lesions and pars defects in 902 athletes with an average age of 14.5 (range 8–21) years, reported a prevalence of 60% at L5, 22% at L4, 8% at L3, and 1% at L2 [6]. In addition, 7% of cases involved multilevel involvement.

The prevalence of spondylolysis increases during growth, from 4% at age 6 years to about 6% in young adults [6]. Most children with a pars defect and/or mild spondylolisthesis are asymptomatic [7]. Spondylolysis is present in 11% of pediatric athletes, compared to 3% in nonathletes [4]. A systematic review of MRI studies on spine abnormalities in children found a prevalence of 30% in symptomatic athletes and 6% in asymptomatic athletes [8].

K. Chatzis · D. Armstrong (✉)
Penn State College of Medicine, Hershey, PA, USA
e-mail: kchatzis@pennstatehealth.psu.edu

W. L. Hennrikus, R. M. Schwend (eds.), *Value in Pediatric Orthopaedics*,
https://doi.org/10.1007/978-3-032-19570-8_35

Spondylolysis follows a progressive course. The earliest detectable sign on imaging is bone edema of the pars [4–6], followed by an incomplete fracture and eventually a complete fracture. Fibrous union typically develops next, with progression to bony union depending on the stage of the defect at the time of diagnosis [4]. Early, unilateral, incomplete lesions often heal with bony union [4], while late terminal defects (characterized by rounded edges or sclerosis of the fracture lines) generally do not heal. Between 43% and 74% of patients with chronic bilateral pars defects will progress to a grade 1 or 2 spondylolisthesis (Figs. 35.1 and 35.2).

Spondylolysis should be the primary diagnostic consideration when a pediatric athlete presents with low back pain. On the other hand, the likelihood of low back pain being linked to spondylolysis in a patient who is not involved in sports is relatively low [9]. Typically, symptomatic patients are engaged in sports that involve frequent, repetitive, or extreme loading of the lumbar spine in extension and/or rotation [6]. Sports such as soccer, gymnastics, baseball, basketball, and football (particularly linemen) are associated with spondylolysis [5, 6]. However, spondylolysis is not "sport-specific," and its frequency can vary depending on the local popularity of the sport.

Several additional factors are associated with the development of spondylolysis. Males are at higher risk [5–7, 10]. The condition can be familial [11, 12]. Spina bifida occulta at L5 and/or S1 is present in up to 93% of cases [13]. In

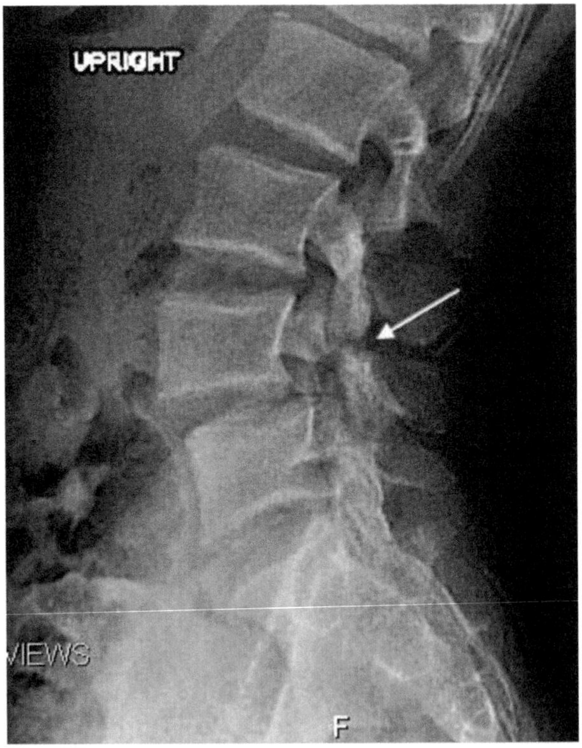

Fig. 35.1 Standing lateral radiograph of the lumbosacral spine of a 14-year-old soccer player showing an L4 pars defect (arrow) and grade 1 L4/L5 spondylolisthesis

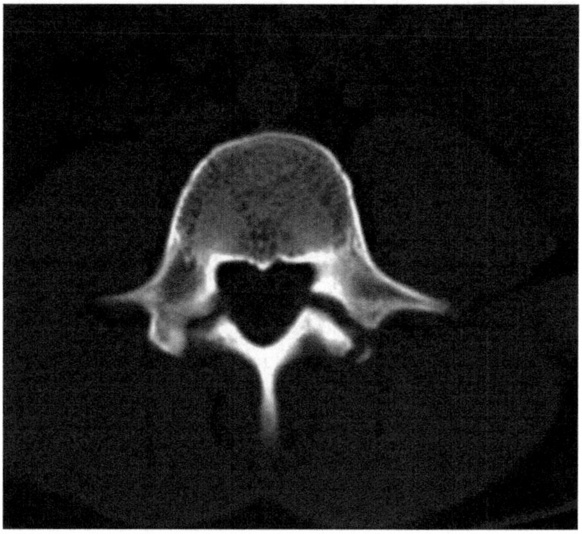

Fig. 35.2 Axial CT of the same patient showing well-defined bilateral L4 pars defects with sclerosis and rounded edges indicating chronic spondylolysis

addition, increased pelvic incidence, horizontal alignment of the L5 pars, and subluxation of the L4/L5 facet joint have been identified in patients with spondylolysis [13, 14].

Value-Based Themes

A Thorough History and Physical Adds Value

The typical patient is a 14-year-old competitive athlete. There frequently is a recent history of increased amount and intensity of training. Offseason strength training or conditioning is another common theme [5, 6]. Low back pain is typically focal, worse with activity and relieved by rest [15]. Referred pain to the posterior hip and thigh is common. The primary site of pain may be localized to the posterior hip or thigh, instead of the low back. Radicular pain or pain radiating below the level of the knee is uncommon.

Carefully examine the gait, spine, and lower limbs. Limitation of active lumbar spine motion (stiffness) is typical. Occasionally, patients may present with painful paraspinal muscle spasms. Have the patient attempt lumbar spine extension in both double-leg and single-leg stances, as well as while prone on the examination table. These maneuvers often reproduce the pain. Tenderness may be noted in the midline or laterally near the lower lumbar spinous processes. Hamstring tightness is common and may limit straight-leg raising or reaching the floor, but without signs of nerve root tension. The neurologic examination is typically normal. Check for tenderness over the SI joints and that the hip joints have full, painless range of motion.

Tiered Diagnostic Imaging

A tiered approach to imaging balances diagnostic accuracy, cost-effectiveness, and radiation safety.

Standing AP and Lateral Radiographs

Standing anteroposterior and lateral radiographs are low cost and offer minimal radiation exposure. Oblique views are not helpful and add radiation exposure [16]. The orientation of the pars defect often does not align with standard radiographic planes [17]. Therefore, the accuracy of radiography in detecting spondylolysis in children is uncertain, with sensitivity reported to be less than 50% [18, 19].

MRI

When radiographs are inconclusive and clinical suspicion remains high, many clinicians prefer MRI as the next step. MRI offers two main advantages: MRI avoids radiation exposure and provides detailed imaging of the neurological system. In addition, MRI can detect the earliest stage of spondylolysis, characterized by bone edema in the affected pars and/or pedicle [5, 6, 18]. MRI techniques, such as T1-weighted Volumetric Interpolated Breath-hold Examination (VIBE) sequences, have shown over 95% accuracy in detecting pars injuries in young adults [6, 20]. However, the reliability of MRI for detecting spondylolysis in children may not be as consistent as the results reported in young adults [21, 22]. Furthermore, depending on the technique and equipment, MRI of the upper lumbar spine may not always provide reliable results [23]. Recently, a new technique, MRI-generated synthetic CT, has been utilized for diagnosing spine pathology in the pediatric population [24].

CT Scan

CT scans are the preferred method for imaging bony anatomy and detecting facet joint fractures [18]. CT may be indicated when MRI results are inconclusive. For various reasons, clinicians and families may opt for a CT scan as a "second-tier" test, with advantages such as lower cost, greater accessibility, shorter wait times, and reliable imaging. Most pediatric centers use low-dose CT protocols to minimize radiation exposure. However, due to the inherent risks of radiation, CT use in children should be approached judiciously, with shared decision-making involving the family. When available, MRI-generated synthetic CT can improve diagnostic accuracy in this patient population with less radiation.

Other Imaging Modalities

Single-photon emission computed tomography (SPECT) and bone scintigraphy are rarely used today and are primarily of historical interest. Both tests have high rates of false positives and false negatives and expose patients to more radiation [18].

A Value-Based Approach to Advanced Imaging for Spondylolysis

Advanced imaging can incur financial costs for families, and delays in insurance approval or long wait times can occur. Unlike radiographs and CT scans, MRI techniques, quality, and interpretation can vary widely between sites and radiologists. This variability can lead to frustration, particularly when a family presents with a nondiagnostic, low-quality MRI for which they have paid out-of-pocket. Therefore, when spondylolysis is strongly suspected clinically but radiographs are inconclusive, it is reasonable and acceptable to proceed with treatment without advanced imaging [5]. In such cases, shared decision-making between the family and physician may lead to initiating treatment with close clinical and radiographic follow-up. If an MRI is requested, clear communication with the radiologist is essential to ensure that the radiologist is aware of the suspected diagnosis and the need for high-quality imaging of the entire lumbar spine. If syringomyelia or other intraspinal anomaly is suspected, an MRI of the entire cervical, thoracic, and lumbosacral spine is ordered.

Treatment

Nonoperative Treatment Is Usually Successful: Patience Is Required

Education and reassurance are key for successful management and patient satisfaction. Misperceptions about spondylolysis exist. Commonly families visit a pediatric orthopedic surgeon after being told their child has a "spine fracture." Although it may take time, counseling the patient and family about the prognosis of spondylolysis is beneficial. The long-term prognosis for spondylolysis is generally good. Bone healing of the pars defect is not required for symptom resolution or a return to previous sports activities. Typically, symptoms resolve regardless of whether there is evidence of bone healing and despite low-grade spondylolisthesis [4, 17, 25]. A meta-analysis found that approximately 84% of children and adolescents treated conservatively for spondylolysis or grade 1 spondylolisthesis returned to pain-free or near pain-free, unrestricted activity after at least 1 year of follow-up [25]. In a study by Sousa et al., with 8 years' follow-up, 90% of spondylolysis patients had returned to playing sports, with 29% playing at a higher level, 40% at the same level, and 31% at a lower level. About 60% reported no pain, and 78% had pain levels of less than 3/10. In adulthood, most patients with spondylolysis experience back pain symptoms no worse than those of the general population [4]. The wise surgeon ensures that both the patient and family have realistic expectations. While most children experience pain relief, the clinical course can be variable. Some athletes return to their sport at a different level, and a few may not be able to return to play at all [26].

Exercise Avoidance

Avoiding the inciting activity is the cornerstone and highest-value treatment for children and adolescents with spondylolysis. While no specific clinical guidelines exist for spondylolysis, the American Medical Society for Sports Medicine recommends a minimum of 3 months of rest from sports [27]. While persuading athletes to adhere to this recommendation may be challenging, those who follow the rest advice are more likely to achieve excellent clinical outcomes compared to those who do not [28]. During this rest from sport period, activities that do not overload the lumbar spine or cause pain, such as walking, cycling, and swimming (avoiding butterfly or breaststroke), are allowed. Once pain resolves and the physical examination normalizes, a gradual return to play program over 3–6 months can begin [29].

Physical Therapy

Along with temporary activity restrictions, physical therapy (PT) is prescribed [4, 25, 29, 30]. Although there is no standard timeline for initiating PT, a period of 4–6 weeks of exercise avoidance before beginning therapy is generally prudent [17, 29, 30]. Patients who begin therapy too soon, without adequate rest, may experience pain exacerbation. PT typically focuses on core strengthening, hamstring stretching, lumbar flexibility, manual therapy, and low-impact aerobic conditioning [30]. While PT has been shown to be effective in alleviating symptoms in adults with spondylolysis, corresponding studies in the children and adolescents are lacking [31]. An experienced therapist will provide a structured treatment plan, as outlined by Selhorst and colleagues [30]. This approach helps motivate the patient and family to take ownership, improve strength, prevent further injury, and avoid deconditioning during the nonparticipation period.

Value-Based Physical Therapy

To reduce costs and enhance value, in-person outpatient PT visits may be minimized. For example, a recent randomized trial in patients with total knee arthroplasty found that virtual PT with telerehabilitation reduced costs by over 50% while maintaining similar effectiveness [32]. Although no studies on telehealth PT for children and adolescents have been published, the age group typically affected by spondylolysis would likely be receptive to this approach. The growing popularity of wearable devices and smartwatches also offers an opportunity to monitor patient compliance with prescribed therapy exercises.

Bracing

Bracing is a commonly prescribed but controversial treatment for spondylolysis. There is variation in recommended types of braces, wear hours, permitted activities, and duration of bracing. Unlike scoliosis, there are no studies on bracing for spondylolysis that include monitoring of compliance. In addition, acceptable clinical outcomes can be achieved without bracing [25, 33]. Formal rigid bracing, obtained from an orthotist, is expensive for families and can reduce value. Adolescent athletes may not share the same enthusiasm for rigid thoraco-lumbosacral orthosis (TLSO). In the senior author's experience, some families, after paying out-of-pocket for a TLSO, are dismayed when their teenager refuses to wear it after just a week. A study comparing rigid bracing to a simple inexpensive elastic support brace found no difference in bony healing rates or health-related quality of life outcomes [34]. Likely, some of the clinical benefits of bracing may be attributable to a placebo effect.

Value-Based Bracing

Rather than following a strict protocol, an individualized treatment approach is the value-based strategy. For most patients, an initial period of rest from sports followed by physical therapy is optimal. Bracing can be considered if there is no improvement upon reevaluation after 2–4 weeks. Patients with severe muscle spasms or sleep disturbances may benefit from bracing, and some may request a brace. In these cases, the surgeon may suggest an affordable, "off-the-shelf" elastic lumbar support, which is less expensive and may be better tolerated than a rigid TLSO.

Other nonoperative treatments for spondylolysis include corticosteroid injections, external bone stimulators, and epidural injections when disc herniation is present [5, 26]. However, the evidence supporting these treatments is based mostly on expert opinion.

Operative Care

Surgery is rarely indicated for spondylolysis. When appropriately selected, surgical patients may often experience long-term pain relief [35], and many, though not all, can return to play. Surgical options include direct pars repair, typically used for L4 defects, and posterolateral fusion for defects at L5 [36]. Several techniques for pars repair have been described [36].

Case Example

A 14-year-old high school football linebacker presented with a monthlong history of low back pain, radiating down the posterior aspect of his left thigh. He also experienced intermittent pain over the past 9 months, particularly after several hard tackles, which had worsened the pain and temporarily prevented him from continuing to play. On physical examination, he appeared to be a robust adolescent with a normal gait. Pain was elicited with active lumbar spine extension, which was limited to about 10 degrees. Forward bending was restricted to 45 degrees, and there was midline tenderness at the lumbosacral junction. Straight-leg raising was 30 degrees bilaterally. A lateral radiograph of the lumbosacral spine is shown (Fig. 35.3). After discussing the case with the family, MRI was obtained (Fig. 35.4), which revealed

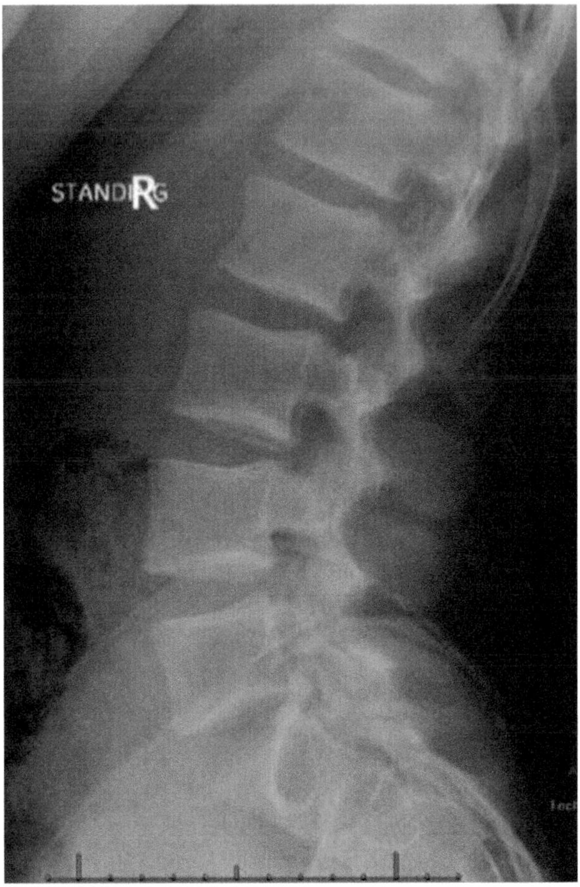

Fig. 35.3 Standing lateral radiograph of the lumbosacral spine of a 14 year-old linebacker. No abnormalities are apparent. (Figure courtesy of Joseph L. Petfield, MD)

bone edema. Subsequent CT imaging provided clearer visualization of the bone pathology (Fig. 35.5).

He was advised to end football, limiting activities to cycling and walking. At the 1-month follow-up, he showed improvement. Physical therapy (PT) was prescribed, and activity restrictions were continued. After 2 months and four PT sessions, he reported continued improvement, though tenderness and limited motion persisted. On the 12-week visit, he reported further improvement, but PT noted steady progress and felt he was not yet ready to return to play. Examination findings were unchanged. During the 4-month visit, he reported feeling well, with no pain during daily activities. On examination, he had full active lumbar extension, could touch his toes with forward bending, and performed a hop test and jogging without pain. Although the football season had ended, baseball practice was starting. He was advised to gradually return to activity over 6 weeks, with the assistance of his high school athletic trainer.

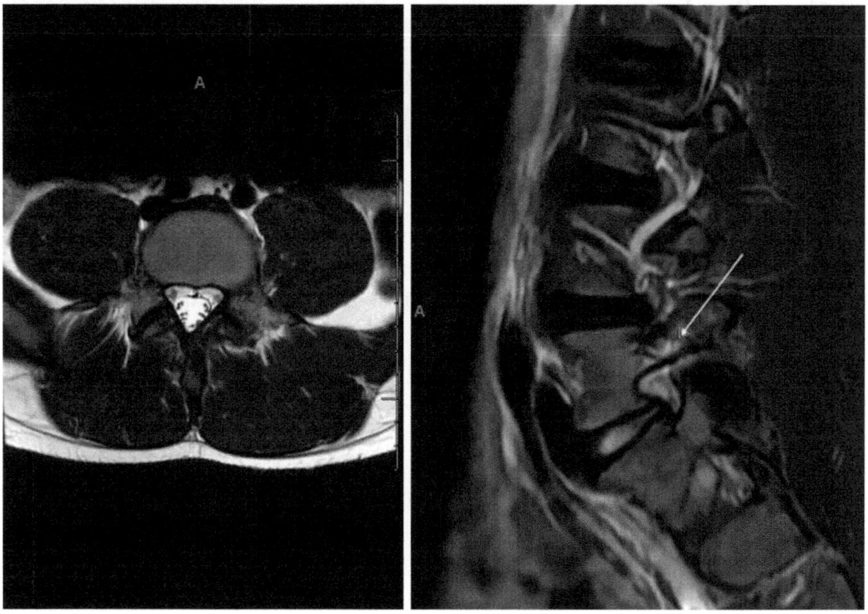

Fig. 35.4 MRI of the lumbar spine showing bone edema within the left pedicle at L5 (thin arrow). (Figure courtesy of Joseph L. Petfield, MD)

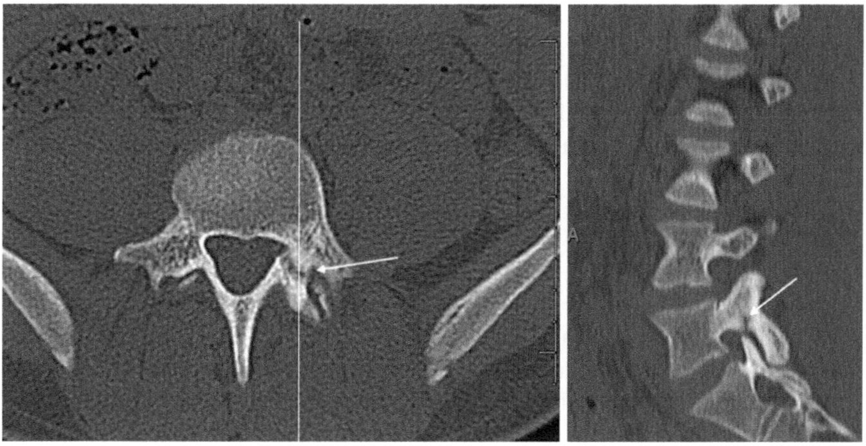

Fig. 35.5 CT showing incomplete unilateral defect of the left pars interarticularis at L5. (Figure courtesy of Joseph L. Petfield, MD)

Authors Pearls

- Start with a thorough history, physical exam, and standing AP and lateral radiographs of the lumbosacral spine.
- If radiographs are normal but clinical suspicion remains high, discuss the pros and cons of advanced imaging with the family. MRI is preferred to minimize radiation and detect early lesions. Inform the radiologist of the suspected diagnosis to guide appropriate sequence selection.
- Patient education and reassurance and a minimum of 3 months of rest from the inciting activity are the most valuable interventions. Set realistic expectations with both the patient and family.
- For patients who may benefit from or request bracing, start with a low-cost "off-the-shelf" elastic brace.
- Introduce physical therapy after a period of rest.

Editor Comments

WLH

For gymnasts, weightlifters, football players, and rowers presenting with low back pain, consider spondylolysis. Repetitive hyperextension stress to the pars interarticularis is the primary cause. As the authors of the current study wisely recommend, conservative treatment remains the cornerstone of care, including rest from sports, NSAIDs (avoiding opioids), simple over-the-counter back supports, and focused physical therapy. Value is enhanced by making the correct diagnosis, utilizing appropriate imaging, opting for low-cost over-the-counter bracing, minimizing in-person PT visits, and reserving surgery as a last resort.

RMS

While spondylolysis is a very common cause of low back pain in adolescent athletes, clinicians must keep a broad differential in mind. Conditions like endplate fractures, lumbar Scheuermann's disease, and even discitis from overtraining can present similarly. My son who was overly competitive in crew was initially diagnosed with L5 spondylolysis, but further evaluation revealed an L5–S1 disc herniation. Young athletes can push their bodies beyond safe limits. As physicians, we must not only guide diagnosis and treatment but also advocate for prevention, recovery, and the long-term health of children and the growing spine.

References

1. Shah SA, Saller J. Evaluation and diagnosis of Back pain in children and adolescents. J Am Acad Orthop Surg. 2016;24(1):37–45.
2. Micheli LJ, Wood R. Back pain in young athletes. Significant differences from adults in causes and patterns. Arch Pediatr Adolesc Med. 1995;149(1):15–8.
3. Wall J, Meehan WP 3rd, Trompeter K, Gissane C, Mockler D, van Dyk N, Wilson F. Incidence, prevalence and risk factors for low back pain in adolescent athletes: a systematic review and meta-analysis. Br J Sports Med. 2022;56(22):1299–306.
4. Crawford CH 3rd, Ledonio CG, Bess RS, Buchowski JM, Burton DC, Hu SS, Lonner BS, Polly DW, Smith JS, Sanders JO. Current evidence regarding the etiology, prevalence, natural history, and prognosis of pediatric lumbar spondylolysis: a report from the Scoliosis Research Society evidence-based medicine committee. Spine Deform. 2015;3(1):12–29.
5. Choi JH, Ochoa JK, Lubinus A, Timon S, Lee YP, Bhatia NN. Management of lumbar spondylolysis in the adolescent athlete: a review of over 200 cases. Spine J. 2022;22(10):1628–33.
6. Kriz PK, Kriz JP, Willwerth SB, Hunt DL, Beasley MA, Stein CJ, Micheli LJ, O'Brien MJ, Hedequist DJ, Meehan WP 3rd. Characteristics of lumbar pars Interarticularis and pedicle stress injuries by sport in 902 pediatric and adolescent athletes: a retrospective study. Am J Sports Med. 2024;52(13):3388–95.
7. Fredrickson BE, Baker D, McHolick WJ, Yuan HA, Lubicky JP. The natural history of spondylolysis and spondylolisthesis. J Bone Joint Surg Am. 1984;66(5):699–707.
8. van den Heuvel MM, Oei EHG, Renkens JJM, Bierma-Zeinstra SMA, van Middelkoop M. Structural spinal abnormalities on MRI and associations with weight status in a general pediatric population. Spine J. 2021;21(3):465–76.
9. Yang S, Werner BC, Singla A, Abel MF. Low back pain in adolescents: a 1-year analysis of eventual diagnoses. J Pediatr Orthop. 2017;37(5):344–7.
10. Lemoine T, Fournier J, Odent T, Sembély-Taveau C, Merenda P, Sirinelli D, Morel B. The prevalence of lumbar spondylolysis in young children: a retrospective analysis using CT. Eur Spine J. 2018;27(5):1067–72.
11. Wynne-Davies R, Scott JH. Inheritance and spondylolisthesis: a radiographic family survey. J Bone Joint Surg Br. 1979;61-B(3):301–5.
12. Albanese M, Pizzutillo PD. Family study of spondylolysis and spondylolisthesis. J Pediatr Orthop. 1982;2(5):496–9.
13. Sakai T, Goda Y, Tezuka F, Takata Y, Higashino K, Sato M, Mase Y, Nagamachi A, Sairyo K. Characteristics of lumbar spondylolysis in elementary school age children. Eur Spine J. 2016;25(2):602–6.
14. Finkel RA, Narendran N, Farivar D, Nilssen P, Metzger MF, Skaggs DL, Illingworth KD. Lumbosacral anatomy is unique in pediatric spondylolysis. Spine Deform. 2025. Epub ahead of print;13:1197.
15. Hensinger RN. Spondylolysis and spondylolisthesis in children and adolescents. J Bone Joint Surg Am. 1989;71(7):1098–107.
16. Beck NA, Miller R, Baldwin K, Zhu X, Spiegel D, Drummond D, Sankar WN, Flynn JM. Do oblique views add value in the diagnosis of spondylolysis in adolescents? J Bone Joint Surg Am. 2013;95(10):e65.
17. Standaert CJ, Herring SA. Spondylolysis: a critical review. Br J Sports Med. 2000;34(6):415–22.
18. Ledonio CG, Burton DC, Crawford CH 3rd, Bess RS, Buchowski JM, Hu SS, Lonner BS, Polly DW Jr, Smith JS, Sanders JO. Current evidence regarding diagnostic imaging methods for pediatric lumbar spondylolysis: a report from the Scoliosis Research Society evidence-based medicine committee. Spine Deform. 2017;5(2):97–101.
19. Kobayashi A, Kobayashi T, Kato K, Higuchi H, Takagishi K. Diagnosis of radiographically occult lumbar spondylolysis in young athletes by magnetic resonance imaging. Am J Sports Med. 2013;41(1):169–76.

20. Ang EC, Robertson AF, Malara FA, O'Shea T, Roebert JK, Schneider ME, Rotstein AH. Diagnostic accuracy of 3-T magnetic resonance imaging with 3D T1 VIBE versus computer tomography in pars stress fracture of the lumbar spine. Skeletal Radiol. 2016;45(11):1533–40.
21. West AM, d'Hemecourt PA, Bono OJ, Micheli LJ, Sugimoto D. Diagnostic accuracy of magnetic resonance imaging and computed tomography scan in young athletes with spondylolysis. Clin Pediatr (Phila). 2019;58(6):671–6.
22. Yamaguchi KT Jr, Skaggs DL, Acevedo DC, Myung KS, Choi P, Andras L. Spondylolysis is frequently missed by MRI in adolescents with back pain. J Child Orthop. 2012;6(3):237–40.
23. Ganiyusufoglu AK, Onat L, Karatoprak O, Enercan M, Hamzaoglu A. Diagnostic accuracy of magnetic resonance imaging versus computed tomography in stress fractures of the lumbar spine. Clin Radiol. 2010;65(11):902–7.
24. Michael GE, Etigunta SK, Liu A, Perales M, Alexander C, Watterson C, Hoghoughi D, Gellada N, Skaggs DL, Illingworth KD. Magnetic resonance imaging-generated synthetic computed tomography in pediatric spine patients. JB JS Open Access. 2025;10(2):e25.00099
25. Klein G, Mehlman CT, McCarty M. Nonoperative treatment of spondylolysis and grade I spondylolisthesis in children and young adults: a meta-analysis of observational studies. J Pediatr Orthop. 2009;29(2):146–56.
26. Sousa T, Skaggs DL, Chan P, Yamaguchi KT Jr, Borgella J, Lee C, Sawyer J, Moisan A, Flynn JM, Gunderson M, Hresko MT, D'Hemecourt P, Andras LM. Benign natural history of spondylolysis in adolescence with midterm follow-up. Spine Deform. 2017;5(2):134–8.
27. DiFiori JP, Benjamin HJ, Brenner J, Gregory A, Jayanthi N, Landry GL, Luke A. Overuse injuries and burnout in youth sports: a position statement from the American Medical Society for Sports Medicine. Clin J Sport Med. 2014;24(1):3–20.
28. El Rassi G, Takemitsu M, Glutting J, Shah SA. Effect of sports modification on clinical outcome in children and adolescent athletes with symptomatic lumbar spondylolysis. Am J Phys Med Rehabil. 2013;92(12):1070–4.
29. Selhorst M, Fischer A, Graft K, Ravindran R, Peters E, Rodenberg R, Welder E, MacDonald J. Timing of physical therapy referral in adolescent athletes with acute spondylolysis: a retrospective chart review. Clin J Sport Med. 2017;27(3):296–301.
30. Selhorst M, Allen M, McHugh R, MacDonald J. Rehabilitation considerations for spondylolysis in the youth athlete. Int J Sports Phys Ther. 2020;15(2):287–300.
31. Lin LH, Lin TY, Chang KV, Wu WT, Özçakar L. Effectiveness of lumbar segmental stabilization exercises in managing disability and pain intensity among patients with lumbar spondylolysis and spondylolisthesis: a systematic review and meta-analysis of randomized controlled trials. Spine (Phila Pa 1976). 2024;49(21):1512–20.
32. Prvu Bettger J, Green CL, Holmes DN, Chokshi A, Mather RC 3rd, Hoch BT, de Leon AJ, Aluisio F, Seyler TM, Del Gaizo DJ, Chiavetta J, Webb L, Miller V, Smith JM, Peterson ED. Effects of virtual exercise rehabilitation in-home therapy compared with traditional care after Total knee arthroplasty: VERITAS, a randomized controlled trial. J Bone Joint Surg Am. 2020;102(2):101–9.
33. Boyd ED, Mundluru SN, Feldman DS. Outcome of Conservative Management in the Treatment of symptomatic spondylolysis and grade I spondylolisthesis. Bull Hosp Jt Dis (2013). 2019;77(3):172–82.
34. Virkki E, Holstila M, Kolari T, Lastikka M, Mattila K, Malmi S, Pajulo O, Helenius I. Rigid thoracolumbar orthosis does not improve outcomes of acute adolescent spondylolysis as compared with placebo. Bony union predicts improved health-related quality of life outcomes at 2-year follow-up. Spine (Phila Pa 1976). 2025;50(7):454–62.
35. Helenius I, Lamberg T, Österman K, Schlenzka D, Yrjönen T, Seitsalo S, et al. The Scoliosis Research Society outcome instrument in the evaluation of long-term surgical results of spondylolysis or low-grade isthmic spondylolisthesis in young patients. Spine. 2005;30(3):336–41.
36. Wu HH, Brown K, Flores M, Cazzulino A, Swarup I. Diagnosis and management of spondylolysis and spondylolisthesis in children. JBJS Rev. 2022;10(3).

Value Based Care in Treating Pediatric Spondylolisthesis

36

Robert D. Garner and Aaron Shaw

Introduction

Spondylolisthesis has an incidence of 3.5% in pediatric patients [1, 2]. Spondylolisthesis is defined as the anterior displacement of a vertebral body in relation to an adjacent vertebral body [3]. The condition typically results from a spectrum of disease beginning with spondylolysis and progressing to spondylolisthesis. About 90% of spondylolysis occurs at the L5 vertebra and can be either unilateral or bilateral [3]. Repetitive hyperextension stress places strain on the pars interarticularis and is a common cause of spondylolysis [3]. Congenital and developmental anatomical abnormalities can contribute to higher degrees of spondylolisthesis [4, 5]. Common sports associated with spondylolysis and spondylolisthesis include football, gymnastics, ballet, figure skating, and weightlifting [2, 3]. Patients often present with low back pain, numbness, tingling, lower extremity weakness, hamstring tightness, and/or exacerbation of pain with lumbar extension [1, 3].

Several classification systems exist to describe the degree of anterior displacement of the vertebral body relative to adjacent vertebrae. The Meyerding classification, introduced in 1941 (Table 36.1), uses the degree of vertebral slip to guide both nonsurgical and surgical management [3]. More recently, the Spinal Deformity Study Group (SDSG) classification has been proposed for spondylolisthesis at the L5-S1 level and has shown utility in guiding surgical treatment [6]. The SDSG classification divides spondylolisthesis into six types, categorizing it as either low grade (Types 1–3) or high grade (Types 4–6). The classification further subdivides these categories based on sagittal spinopelvic alignment and global balance.

R. D. Garner
Kansas City University-HCA at Research Medical Center, Kansas City, MO, USA

A. Shaw (✉)
Children's Mercy Kansas City, University of Missouri-Kansas City, Kansas City, MO, USA

W. L. Hennrikus, R. M. Schwend (eds.), *Value in Pediatric Orthopaedics*,
https://doi.org/10.1007/978-3-032-19570-8_36

Table 36.1 Meyerding classification

Grade	Percentage of slip
I	0–25%
II	26–50%
III	51–75%
IV	75–100%
V	>100% (spondyloptosis)

Treatment for spondylolisthesis is generally categorized based on grade: low vs. high. Low-grade spondylolisthesis is typically managed conservatively with a combination of rest, cessation of sports or aggravating activities, a thoraco-lumbo-sacral orthosis (TLSO), a bone stimulator, and physical therapy. Low-grade spondylolisthesis treated conservatively usually results in good outcomes [1, 3, 7, 8]. High-grade spondylolisthesis is typically managed surgically due to the risk of progression. Surgical options are aimed at restoring spinal alignment and promoting bone fusion. Surgical treatments include both non-instrumented and instrumented fusion, transdiscal screws, posterior lumbar interbody fusion (PLIF), and anterior lumbar interbody fusion (ALIF) [1, 9]. Selecting the most appropriate surgical method can be challenging but is often guided by the specific characteristics of the underlying deformity.

Value Based Themes

Improving value in the care of spondylolisthesis involves achieving the best outcomes at the lowest cost. Treatment for spinal disorders such as spondylolisthesis can be expensive, particularly when surgery is involved, with implants alone making up more than 30% of the total costs [10].

Nonoperative Management of Low-Grade Spondylolisthesis

Nonoperative methods are typically the first line of treatment for low-grade pediatric spondylolisthesis. Nonoperative measures focus on rest and managing underlying back pain. Physical therapy is often included in nonoperative care and has been shown to reduce physical disability in cases of acute, symptomatic spondylolysis and spondylolisthesis [11].

Spinal orthoses are frequently incorporated into nonoperative treatment. A variety of orthotic devices are used, including lumbar corsets, off-the-shelf braces, soft orthoses, and custom-made options. Fujimoto et al. evaluated lumbar motion restriction with different braces and found that custom-made orthoses provided the greatest restriction [12]. However, a 2009 meta-analysis on the effectiveness of nonoperative treatments for lumbar spondylolysis and Grade 1 spondylolisthesis concluded that bracing did not significantly impact outcomes [13]. Given these findings, along with the financial costs of braces and the lack of reliable compliance data, bracing does not add value in most cases of pediatric spondylolisthesis.

Indications to Surgically Treat Low-Grade Spondylolisthesis

Initial treatment for low-grade spondylolisthesis (Grade I/II, Meyerding classification) typically involves conservative management [1, 3, 7]. Pain improvement is reported in up to 90% of patients [1]. In children with spondylolysis and a pars nonunion, there is a 25% risk of developing low-grade spondylolisthesis, with slip progression greater than 10% occurring in 4% of these cases [2]. However, Beutler et al. reported that after a 45-year follow-up, no cases of nonoperatively managed low-grade spondylolisthesis progressed to high-grade spondylolisthesis [14]. Adolescents are at the highest risk for progression, though this risk decreases with age [3]. The risk of progression was not correlated with back pain or lower quality of life measures, suggesting that nonoperative management is a viable treatment option [14].

Indications for surgical management of low-grade spondylolisthesis include active slip progression indicating instability and/or failure of conservative treatment for more than 6 months [1, 15]. Scheepers et al. reported that for athletes in whom conservative measures have failed, surgery is more likely to facilitate a return to sports, reduce pain, and improve overall function [16]. Postoperative timing for recommendations for return to sports vary by surgeon, typically ranging from 6 to 12 months, with a more cautious approach regarding contact sports [8]. Patients who undergo surgery have reported lower rates of low back pain in mid- and long-term follow-up studies compared to those treated conservatively [2]. Long-term clinical and radiographic outcomes following posterolateral fusion for low-grade spondylolisthesis have been satisfactory [17].

To provide the best value in care, the initial treatment for symptomatic low-grade spondylolisthesis is nonsurgical, with surgery reserved for patients who do not respond to conservative treatment.

Indications to Surgically Treat High-Grade Spondylolisthesis

High-grade spondylolisthesis (Meyerding Grade $\geq$ III or SDSG Types 4–6) typically warrants surgical treatment to prevent further progression and improve long-term function and outcomes [2] (Fig. 36.1). Patients with high-grade slips who do not undergo surgery have up to a 50% chance of progressing to spondyloptosis (Meyerding Grade V), often accompanied by severe neurological symptoms [2]. For symptomatic patients, surgical intervention yields long-term outcomes comparable to those of patients with minimal symptoms who are not indicated for surgery. On the other hand, a few patients without neurological symptoms have experienced clinical success with nonoperative treatment. In addition, delayed surgical

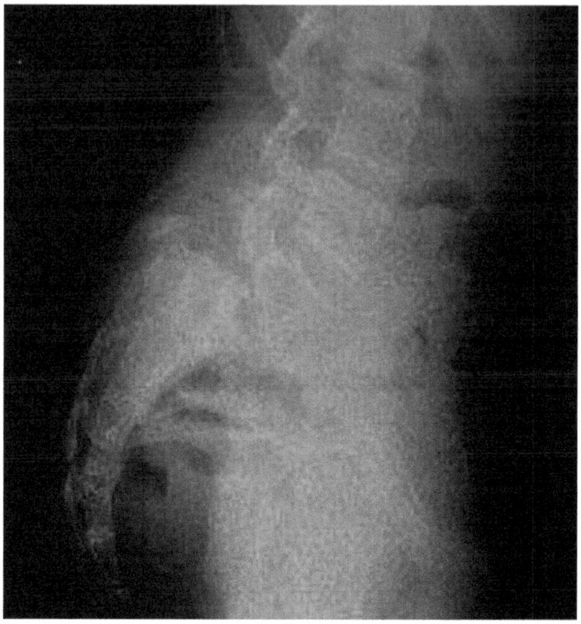

Fig. 36.1 Lateral radiograph of a 16-year-old boy with a high-grade spondylolisthesis (Meyerding Grade IV, SDSG Type 5). Note the anterior-superior defect in the sacrum, trapezoidal shape of L5, marked separation of the pars interarticularis

intervention in these patients has not been shown to result in worse outcomes, supporting the efficacy of an initial trial of nonoperative management [18].

Long-term follow-up surveys show that health-related quality of life (HRQoL) scores improve following surgery for high-grade spondylolisthesis. Patients with lower baseline HRQoL scores tend to benefit more from surgery compared to those with higher baseline scores [19]. A 24-year follow-up study found that 95% of patients treated with a simple in situ posterior fusion experienced minimal or no symptoms [2].

Sagittal Balance Is Key

Sagittal balance correlates with improved outcomes in patients with lumbar spondylolisthesis [20, 21]. A detailed analysis of sagittal spinopelvic alignment and balance is important, as it helps differentiate the various types of high-grade spondylolisthesis in the SDSG classification, as outlined below. An important measure in assessing spinopelvic balance is the L5 incidence (Table 36.2).

Patients with greater local kyphotic deformity preoperatively, indicating spine and pelvic imbalance, generally have a poorer prognosis [18]. Although surgical reduction alone has not been shown to directly improve health-related quality of life (HRQoL) outcomes [22], another study suggests that achieving balanced pelvic alignment after surgery is associated with improved HRQoL and better self-image [22]. Patients who undergo surgical reduction to achieve a low-grade spondylolisthesis, with an L5 incidence of $\leq 60^\circ$, are more likely to experience improved mental

Table 36.2 Differentiation of high-grade L5-S1 spondylolisthesis using the Spinal Deformity Study Group classification system[4]

SDSG classification types	Spinopelvic balance	Global spinal balance	Treatment recommendation
4	Balanced (SS > PT)[%]	–	In situ fusion Unless spine is unbalanced
5	Unbalanced (SS < PT)	Balanced	In situ fusion
6	Unbalanced (SS < PT)	Unbalanced	Reduction and fusion

Global spinal balance is defined using the C7 sagittal vertical axis, determining if this is anterior to the hip axis (unbalanced) or posterior to the hip axis (balanced)
SS sacral slope, *PT* pelvic tilt
% Patients with L5 incidence >60° should be considered as being unbalanced

health and quality of life compared to those who do not achieve a low-grade slip and/or an L5 incidence >60° [22]. These findings underscore the importance of a careful assessment of sagittal alignment preoperatively in decision-making for high-grade spondylolisthesis, with surgical reduction typically reserved for patients with SDSG Types 5 and 6 [16, 20] (Fig. 36.2).

Surgical Techniques

Multiple surgical techniques are available, depending on the neurological status, grade of spondylolisthesis, and the extent of the sagittal deformity. An in situ fusion, with or without instrumentation and nerve root decompression, reduces the risk of postoperative nerve root injury compared to reduction with instrumentation [2]. An in situ fusion is beneficial for patients with good preoperative sagittal spinopelvic alignment, such as those with low-grade and high-grade spondylolisthesis (SDSG Types 4 and 5) (Fig. 36.3). In situ fusion in patients with high-grade slips results in pain and neurological symptom relief in 74% of cases [1]. Patients who undergo in situ fusion with instrumentation demonstrate higher union rates, lower pseudoarthrosis rates, no increased risk of motor deficits, no increased reoperation rates, higher patient satisfaction, and lower pain scores, when compared to un-instrumented in situ lumbar fusions [2, 23].

A circumferential fusion, posteriorly and anteriorly, is biomechanically advantageous in preventing slip progression and further kyphosis. Grade B evidence supports the inclusion of circumferential fusion in patients with high-grade spondylolisthesis, with benefits including a reduced risk of pseudarthrosis [15, 23, 24] (Fig. 36.4). Additionally, health-related quality of life (HRQoL) scores have shown significant improvement following circumferential spinal instrumented fusion in adolescents with spondylolisthesis, offering higher HRQoL scores compared to posterolateral or anterior fusions [2, 25, 26]. An anterior fusion alone, incorporating an anterior lumbar interbody fusion (ALIF), is also a viable option for

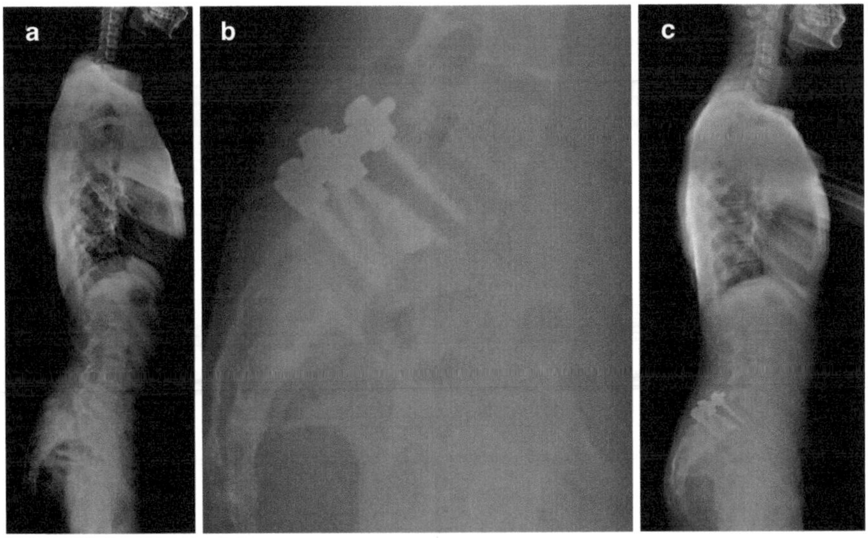

Fig. 36.4 A 16-year-old boy with a grade 3 spondylolisthesis at L5-S1 presented with radicular leg pain and back pain, unresponsive to 6 months of nonoperative treatment (**a**). Based on his deformity parameters including sacral slope 39°, pelvic tilt 25°, L5 incidence 66°, and C7 sagittal vertical axis anterior to the hip axis, he was classified as having a SDSG Type 6 deformity. He was treated with L5-S1 TLIF, decompression, and reduction to a Meyerding grade I spondylolisthesis (**b**). At the 1-year follow-up, he had a solid fusion and returned to playing basketball and baseball without symptoms (**c**)

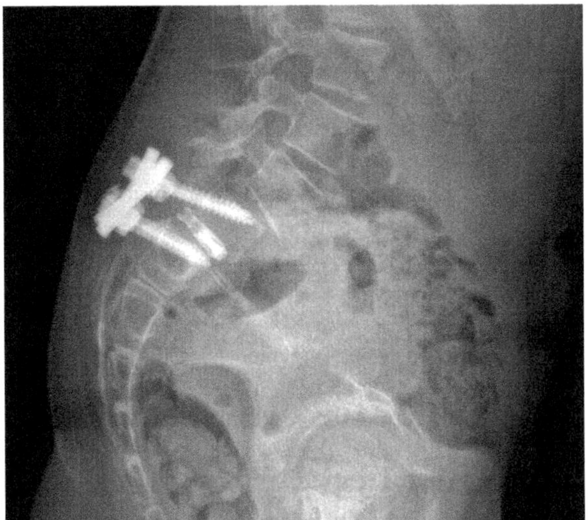

Fig. 36.5 Lateral radiograph of a patient with a symptomatic high-grade L5-S1 spondylolisthesis, SDSG Type 6, with an L5 incidence of 95° that was treated with reduction and circumferential fusion from L5 to S1. However, 6 months postoperatively, this was complicated by adjacent segment antero-listhesis

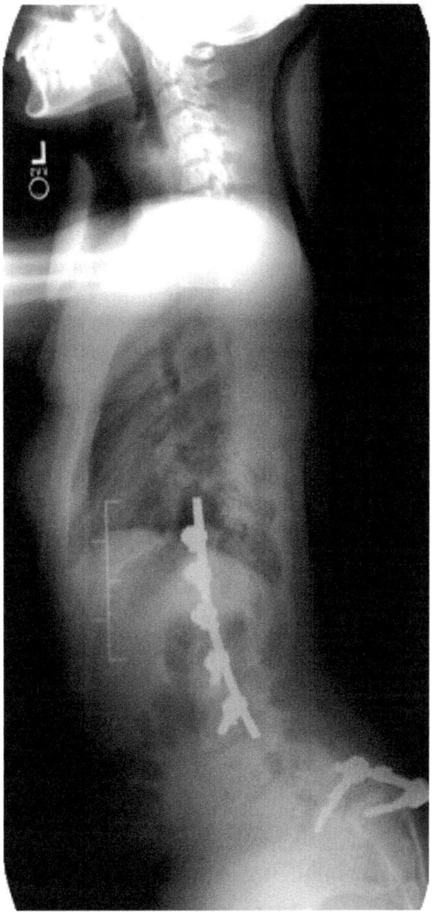

Fig. 36.6 Adolescent female with symptomatic high-grade L5-S1 spondylolisthesis and lumbar scoliosis, initially treated with an anterior spinal fusion. She later underwent an instrumented posterior fusion without reduction or interbody fixation of L5-S1. Due to the lack of reduction and interbody fixation, persistent sagittal spinal malalignment led to nonunion and implant failure

Author Pearls

- Obtain full-length lateral spinal radiographs to assess sagittal spinal alignment.
- Consider reduction when treating Type 5 and 6 deformities.
- When performing a reduction for high-grade spondylolisthesis, be cautious about the extent of the reduction. For example, reducing to a Grade 1 spondylolisthesis is sufficient to minimize nerve root tension.
- Adequate foraminal decompression is necessary during reduction to minimize the risk of postoperative nerve root deficits. In addition, direct nerve root stimulation may be used to assess decompression quality and ensure there is no excessive nerve tension.
- Incorporating an interbody device reduces the risk of nonunion.
- In cases with kyphotic deformity and sagittal imbalance, consider extending the fusion construct to L4.

Editor Comments

WLH

Spondylolisthesis is a serious and potentially complex spine condition in children and adolescents. Value is especially enhanced by minimizing complications and reducing the need for revision surgery. Fortunately, many cases can be managed conservatively. However, when conservative treatment fails, or when significant nerve compression or spinal instability is present, surgery becomes necessary. The authors of this excellent chapter have thoroughly outlined the indications for surgery, surgical techniques, and potential complications in treating spondylolisthesis in children and adolescents. As the authors have emphasized, minimizing complications and the need for revision surgery requires performing the initial surgery with precision and care.

RMS

High-value care in pediatric spondylolisthesis relies on determining who needs surgery and who does not. Similar to spondylolysis, most low-grade slips can be treated without surgery. In high-grade cases, surgery adds value when guided by symptoms, progression, and spinopelvic imbalance. For L5-S1 spondylolisthesis, overcorrection should be avoided, as it increases the risk of L5 and even L4 nerve injury. Full-length lateral radiographs and a careful assessment of sagittal balance are key to guiding surgical decisions. When surgery is indicated, a well done instrumented circumferential fusion, particularly for SDSG Types 5 and 6, can improve outcomes and reduce complications. Precise, patient-specific care results in optimal function while minimizing harm and cost.

References

1. Cha MJ, Sponseller P. Pediatric spondylolisthesis. JBJS Summary.
2. Helenius I, Virkki E, Toomela T, Studer D, Gehrchen M, Ahonen M. Treatment of pediatric spondylolysis and spondylolisthesis. Acta Orthop. 2025;96:80–6. https://doi.org/10.2340/17453674.2024.42450.
3. Ebraheim N, Elgafy H, Gagnet P, Andrews K, Kern K. Spondylolysis and spondylolisthesis: a review of the literature. J Orthop. 2018;15(2). https://doi.org/10.1016/j.jor.2018.03.008.
4. Sponseller PD. Classification and natural history of Spondyloysis and spondylolisthesis. Semin Spine Surg. 1999;11(1):3–10.
5. Wiltse LL, Newman PH, Macnab I. Classification of spondylolisis and spondylolisthesis. Clin Orthop Relat Res. 1976;117:23–9.
6. Mac-Thiong JM, Duong L, Parent S, et al. Reliability of the spinal deformity study group classification of lumbosacral spondylolisthesis. Spine (Phila Pa 1976). 2012;37(2):E95–102. https://doi.org/10.1097/BRS.0b013e3182233969.

7. Choi JH, Ochoa JK, Lubinus A, Timon S, Lee Y-P, Bhatia NN. Management of lumbar spondylolysis in the adolescent athlete: a review of over 200 cases. Spine J. 2022;22(10). https://doi.org/10.1016/j.spinee.2022.04.011.
8. Bouras T, Korovessis P. Management of spondylolysis and low-grade spondylolisthesis in fine athletes. A comprehensive review. Eur J Orthop Surg Traumatol. 2015;25. https://doi.org/10.1007/s00590-014-1560-7.
9. Douleh DG, Albert G, Garg S. Surgical techniques for adolescent lumbar spondylolisthesis. J Pediatr Orthop Soc North Am. 2022;4(4). https://doi.org/10.55275/jposna-2022-545.
10. Kamerlink JR, Quirno M, Auerbach JD, et al. Hospital cost analysis of adolescent idiopathic scoliosis correction surgery in 125 consecutive cases. J Bone Joint Surg Am. 2010;92(5):1097–104. https://doi.org/10.2106/JBJS.I.00879.
11. Lin LH, Lin TY, Chang KV, Wu WT, Özçakar L. Effectiveness of lumbar segmental stabilization exercises in managing disability and pain intensity among patients with lumbar spondylolysis and spondylolisthesis: a systematic review and meta-analysis of randomized controlled trials. Spine (Phila Pa 1976). 2024;49(21):1512–20. https://doi.org/10.1097/BRS.0000000000004989.
12. Fujimoto Y, Sakai T, Sairyo K. What type of orthosis is optimal for conservative treatment of lumbar spondylolysis?: a biomechanical analysis. Spine Surg Relat Res. 2020;4(1):74–80. https://doi.org/10.22603/ssrr.2019-0018.
13. Klein G, Mehlman CT, McCarty M. Nonoperative treatment of spondylolysis and grade I spondylolisthesis in children and young adults: a meta-analysis of observational studies. J Pediatr Orthop. 2009;29(2):146–56. https://doi.org/10.1097/BPO.0b013e3181977fc5.
14. Beutler WJ, Fredrickson BE, Murtland A, Sweeney CA, Grant WD, Baker D. The natural history of spondylolysis and spondylolisthesis: 45-year follow-up evaluation. Spine (Phila Pa 1976). 2003;28(10):1027–35; discussion 1035. https://doi.org/10.1097/01.BRS.0000061992.98108.A0.
15. Wu HH, Brown K, Flores M, Cazzulino A, Swarup I. Diagnosis and management of spondylolysis and spondylolisthesis in children. JBJS Rev. 2022;10(3). https://doi.org/10.2106/JBJS.RVW.21.00176.
16. Scheepers MS, Streak Gomersall J, Munn Z. The effectiveness of surgical versus conservative treatment for symptomatic unilateral spondylolysis of the lumbar spine in athletes: a systematic review. JBI Database System Rev Implement Rep. 2015;13(3). https://doi.org/10.11124/jbisrir-2015-1926.
17. Helenius I, Lamberg T, Österman K, et al. Scoliosis research society outcome instrument in evaluation of long-term surgical results in spondylolysis and low-grade isthmic spondylolisthesis in young patients. Spine (Phila Pa 1976). 2005;30(3). https://doi.org/10.1097/01.brs.0000152375.13316.6a.
18. Lundine KM, Lewis SJ, Al-Aubaidi Z, Alman B, Howard AW. Patient outcomes in the operative and nonoperative management of high-grade spondylolisthesis in children. J Pediatr Orthop. 2014;34(5). https://doi.org/10.1097/BPO.0000000000000133.
19. Bourassa-Moreau É, Mac-Thiong JM, Joncas J, Parent S, Labelle H. Quality of life of patients with high-grade spondylolisthesis: minimum 2-year follow-up after surgical and nonsurgical treatments. Spine J. 2013;13(7). https://doi.org/10.1016/j.spinee.2013.01.048.
20. Gussous Y, Theologis AA, Demb JB, Tangtiphaiboontana J, Berven S. Correlation between Lumbopelvic and sagittal parameters and health-related quality of life in adults with lumbosacral spondylolisthesis. Global Spine J. 2018;8(1):17–24. https://doi.org/10.1177/2192568217696692.
21. Harroud A, Labelle H, Joncas J, Mac-Thiong JM. Global sagittal alignment and health-related quality of life in lumbosacral spondylolisthesis. Eur Spine J. 2013;22(4):849–56. https://doi.org/10.1007/s00586-012-2591-6.
22. Mac-Thiong JM, Hresko MT, Alzakri A, et al. Criteria for surgical reduction in high-grade lumbosacral spondylolisthesis based on quality of life measures. Eur Spine J. 2019;28(9). https://doi.org/10.1007/s00586-019-05954-x.

T